Dynamic Bodyuse
for Effective
Strain-free Massage

Dynamic Bodyuse
for Effective
Strain-free Massage

Darien Pritchard

Lotus Publishing
Chichester, England

North Atlantic Books
Berkeley, California

First published in 2007 by
Lotus Publishing
3. Chapel Street, Chichester, PO19 1BU and
North Atlantic Books
P O Box 12327
Berkeley, California 94712

All Drawings Amanda Williams
Photographs Dave Daggers
Text and Cover Design Wendy Craig
Printed and Bound in the UK by Scotprint

Dedication

To my dad, Hal Pritchard, for encouraging me to think, and for introducing me to my body, to meditative relaxation, and to the Australian bush.

And to my sister Ann Pritchard, who dances.

Disclaimer

This book offers information only. It cannot take the place of personal instruction. If in doubt, consult a doctor, physiotherapist, or other health professional.

Dynamic Bodyuse for Effective Strain-free Massage is sponsored by the Society for the Study of Native Arts and Sciences, a nonprofit educational corporation whose goals are to develop an educational and crosscultural perspective linking various scientific, social, and artistic fields; to nurture a holistic view of arts, sciences, humanities, and healing; and to publish and distribute literature on the relationship of mind, body, and nature.

British Library Cataloguing in Publication Data

A CIP record for this book is available from the British Library
ISBN 978 0 9543188 9 5 (Lotus Publishing)
ISBN 978 1 55643 655 0 (North Atlantic Books)

Library of Congress Cataloguing-in-Publication Data

Pritchard, Darien.
  Dynamic bodyuse for effective strain-free massage / Darien Pritchard.
        p. ; cm.
  Includes bibliographical references and index.
  ISBN 978-1-55643-655-0 (pbk.)
  1. Masseurs--Health and hygiene. 2. Physical therapists--Health and
hygiene. 3. Human mechanics. 4. Overuse injuries--Prevention. I. Title.
II. Title: Dynamic body use for effective strain-free massage.
  [DNLM: 1. Massage--methods. 2. Biomechanics--methods. 3. Cumulative
Trauma Disorders--prevention & control. WB 537 P961d 2007]
  RM722.P75 2007
  615.8'2--dc22

2007026176

Contents

My Personal Journey

In my late teens, without any prior history of back trouble, I 'put my back out'. Over four or five days, I stiffened up with excruciating lower back pain. The family doctor aggravated the pain with his efforts; a chiropractor, consulted in desperation, provided some instant relief and, in subsequent sessions, quietened the condition.

Over the next decade, recurrences of the pain and consequent visits to chiropractors and osteopaths led me to seek alternative ways of looking after my back myself. I attended Yoga classes, studied Tai Chi and creative movement, and trained in massage and the Feldenkrais Method® of movement awareness. In the process, I discovered the wider sense of wellbeing that is possible through physical disciplines.

In addition to inspiring my choice of career, my back has forced me to remain attentive to *how* I work. My original massage trainer spent much of his working life doing fairly routine massages in public baths. He was good with his hands and in communicating his basic routine. However it was exposure to these other body disciplines that reinforced for me the importance to massage of how you use your body and gave me a grounding in this. Focusing on bodyuse has therefore always been an integral part of both my practice and my teaching.

At one stage I pushed my body too hard due to the enthusiasm of youth and my desire to provide the depth of pressure that many of my clients sought. I often felt tired, and occasionally woke at night with painful tingling in my wrists, which is a classic symptom of repetitive strain. This forced me to further fine-tune my bodyuse in order to be able to continue working.

This book summarises three decades of gathering and refining information about this often neglected area of massage. For twenty-five years, I have included good bodyuse as an integral part of training massage students to professional standards. Nearly twenty years ago I started running workshops for practitioners which focused just on this aspect of massage, and, a dozen years ago, I began to expand the workshop notes into book form, little realising the enormous task that I had set myself – turning bodily experience into comprehensible words and pictures. I have been spurred on by the continually emerging stories from massage professionals about strains and injuries that they have developed through their work. It concerns me that so many people do not have the information that will enable them to work effectively and to sustain their careers. I hope that this book will not only benefit individual practitioners but also enrich the profession of massage.

We are often attracted to occupations by learning of their benefits and satisfactions, and only discover the potential problems and pitfalls when they are already affecting us. If you are in this situation, I hope that this book will help you to recover before any difficulties become irreversible.

Hopefully, for the majority of readers, this book will help to steer you away from ways of doing massage that are most likely to lead to problems. My intention is to help you to sustain your working life as a practitioner, rather than have it cut short by not knowing essential information.

I wish you well with it.

Darien Pritchard, Cardiff, South Wales, UK, 2007.

Introduction

An old friend recently reminded me of when she attended a massage class of mine years ago. She was trained in massage and wanted to see if I had any new 'tricks' to offer. After watching her massaging for a couple of minutes, I asked her: "How does your back feel?" She immediately asked the client how his back was feeling. I said to her: "No, it's *your* back I'm asking about. The way that you are working looks awkward; how does *your* back feel?" She was quite bemused by this. Because of the way that she had been trained, it had never occurred to her to consider her own body as she was working.

When she did pay attention, she realised that she was working in a stiff and awkward way that was quite taxing on her body. She was intrigued to discover that she was in fact straining her body, tightening her back and holding her breath much of the time. On reflection she realised that the soreness and tiredness she sometimes felt after doing massages could be directly attributed to this. With my coaching she began to apply some of the principles of movement that she'd been learning in a martial arts class. She immediately felt easier in her body and also discovered that she could be more effective.

What had made me focus on this aspect of massage? It was not part of my own original training, which only covered techniques and was not concerned with *how* the practitioner delivered them. In a way I was 'lucky' – problems that I'd had with my back from my late teens onwards had not only led me in the direction of massage as a career, but also had made it second nature to look after my back.

Teaching experiences such as the one described above made me appreciate that my concern with how I used my body was not just a source of difficulties because I found some strokes awkward and uncomfortable. By forcing me to find alternatives, it had actually helped me to develop useful perceptions that I could offer others in my teaching.

At the beginning of my career, I was lucky enough to discover physically-based disciplines such as yoga and Tai Chi that incorporated elements of bodyuse that I could apply to massage, and that also encouraged self-monitoring to gauge how you were applying them. They also introduced me to the concept of creating an atmosphere through movement that was both relaxed *and* dynamic, and simultaneously powerful and centered – the combination that I was seeking. That started my journey into the area of growing concern to massage practitioners and teachers that is the subject of this book – how to look after your body and use it well when doing massages.

Monitoring Yourself as You Massage

Once you start observing yourself, it becomes obvious that if you are straining your own body as you do a massage, you will not deliver it well. You will not be particularly effective and the client will often feel that you are not very competent.

Observing the client's reactions to how you, the practitioner, use your body becomes clear once your eyes (and sense of touch) are opened. Clients are often not even conscious of their reactions, but there is a 'body-to-body' dialogue going on below the level of words. If you are tensing your body in order to deliver the massage, this tension communicates itself and is likely to invoke an instinctive wariness (often unconscious) in clients who will therefore be less responsive. And, if you are holding your breath, it doesn't encourage clients to breathe in a free, relaxed manner. You cannot *make* someone relax, but if you are relaxed in your own body as you work, clients are more likely to be receptive (even to firm strokes, as long as they are within their range of comfort); they 'go with it' more.

The Cumulative Strains of Massage

How to apply pressure without straining your body or damaging your hands is one of the greatest challenges involved in massage.

One of the major causes of early retirement by established massage practitioners is the *cumulative* strains on the body *developed in the course of doing massages.* The growth of the profession in recent years has been accompanied by an increase in the number of work-induced problems. Ironically these strains are sustained in the course of helping others to look after their bodies. Practitioners too often strain their hands, particularly their thumbs and wrists, and sometimes their fingers, through doing massage. They can also strain their shoulders and backs.

People with the 'classic' massage build – a large, strong body and hands – may never encounter problems in their careers. However, for the majority of us who don't have this build, this book presents ways of doing massage that address these problems. It gives you practical information that will enable you to approach massage with an attitude of self-preservation.

Doing one massage awkwardly is unlikely to produce lasting physical damage. However it is the *cumulative* effect of doing many massages that is of concern. The amount of force that you apply through your body in one massage treatment can be equivalent to what you'd need to push a car for a few minutes. One day of doing massages could therefore be the equivalent of pushing a car for ten to fifteen minutes. Consider the toll on your body if you were to do that awkwardly.

What the Book Covers

The book focuses on two aspects of massage:

1. How you use your working tools (your hands/forearms, etc.) to deliver the massage, and;
2. How you use your body to support these working tools.

It highlights the aspects of massage that are most likely to cause problems and which, over time, could lead to permanent damage. It looks at how to *minimise the strain* on your body in massage sessions, whilst *being most effective*. This includes:

*   *Involving your whole body* to generate the power and movement that supports your working hands;
*   *Conserving your hands* by using them skilfully, and;
*   *Saving them* by using other body areas such as your forearms and elbows whenever possible.

The potential problems of different working situations are covered – at the massage table, with the client seated or lying on a futon on the floor; and also with the practitioner standing, seated or kneeling. The book also covers the role of warm-ups and wind-down exercises. In addition, ways of managing the general demands of working as a massage professional are covered.

This book assumes a familiarity with basic massage strokes. While it focuses on the practitioner, you obviously need to take the client into account as you apply the information presented here. The long-term ideal is for you to develop the ability to pay attention to the client and their responses *and simultaneously* to focus on how you are using your own body to deliver the massage.

This book presents *general information* and offers *guidelines* for you to explore. Try out the suggestions with colleagues who will give you useful feedback. Experiment to find out how the information works best *for you* and how to apply it in massage sessions – observing your habits, experimenting with different ways of working and incorporating those that seem least stressful and most effective. If you experience difficulties in applying the information, find an experienced colleague or teacher who can give you *individual coaching* that is *personally tailored* for you.

Acknowledgements

To Frankie Armstrong, for her love and encouragement, which helped me to find my voice in many ways.

To Ahn Mathews, Tai Chi teacher extraordinaire, and Eric Maddern who introduced me to creative movement. To Frank Wildman and Ruthy Alon, inspiring Feldenkrais trainers. To Jude Gooden and Jane Crabtree for belief and support.

To Alex for my first formal massage, and to Billy Barber for my first formal training, and to all the massage teachers that I've learnt from since then.

To colleagues who have inspired and challenged me: Sue Fraser and Leanne Steer, Maureen Moss and Mario Monteleone, Zoe Balfour and John Morgan, Andy Fagg, Su Fox, Vicky Gaughan, Richard Leadbeater, Sally Morris, Anja Saunders, Sara Thomas, Anne Whall and Chris Way.

To many people for support and sharing ideas, especially Richard (Tig) Bidmead, Bob Evans, Ally Fitzpatrick, Miranda James, Wendy Kavanagh, Viv Lancey, Annie McCloud, Andrew McNicholl, Jacqui Showell, Clive Taylor, Carole Walker, Meg Ward, Jackie Zaslona, and to David Woodhouse, Helen Woodhouse and Kelly Allan at the Massage Table Store.

To all those who I've trained over the years, and to all my clients, whose needs, comments and questions have forced me to extend my understanding and my communication of my knowledge.

To all those who have developed massage over the millenia and to those who have written about it, especially the inspiring writers who have documented significant developments in recent decades: Ben Benjamin, Leslie Bruder, Mel Cash, Mario-Paul Cassar, John H. Clay, George Downing, Barbara Frye, Lauriann Greene, Gordon Inkeles, Clare Maxwell-Hudson, Tom Myers, Gerry Pyves, Art Riggs and Ralph R. Stephens.

Thanks to the models and practitioners who appear in the photographs: Frankie Armstrong, 'Tig' Bidmead, Paul Clarke, Ryan Condon, Bob Evans, Ally Fitzpatrick, Nadine Maddocks, Tom O'Reilly, Leilah Porter, Mary-Anne Roberts, Frank Rozelaar-Green, Hiromi Shirai, Sally Styles, Cynthia Thomas, Dave Tolcher-James at Cardiff Sports Gear, and Jackie Zaslona.

Thanks to Dave Daggers for doing your job so well in the studio which enabled me to get on with mine, for your hospitality and willingness to be flexible and accommodating, and for a good eye and an eclectic taste in music.

Thanks to Wendy Craig for the clean and inspired design (and for burning the midnight oil). And special thanks to my editor Jon Hutchings, for patience, understanding, belief, and support.

How to Use This Book

The central focus of this book is on using your body *most effectively* in massage sessions with the *least discomfort or strain*. The book looks at the best ways to use your hands (or forearm, etc.) to deliver the massage, and how to use the rest of your body to support them. It highlights common ways of working that can lead to problems and how to avoid these.

The book presents principles of good bodyuse that will enable you to work in a way that is both *dynamic* and *relaxed*. These principles are initially presented so that you can focus on one aspect at a time. The long-term goal is for you to learn to monitor and adapt your bodyuse, whilst also focusing on the *client* and maintaining the 'flow' of the massage and the overall sequence of the treatment session. This takes time and practice. Because an integrated approach is being presented, you will find that many details of bodyuse are repeated throughout the book to link them together from a range of perspectives.

A Few Notes of Caution

Adapt the Ideals Presented in the Book
The guidelines offered in this book are those that have worked for a wide range of people. They are not necessarily immediately or completely achievable, but are goals to aim towards. They won't necessarily be ideal for every practitioner. In any case, you will need to adapt them to suit your build, strengths and weaknesses, and to accommodate physical conditions such as injuries or being pregnant (see Chapter 9).

Get Personal Instruction
One of my biggest concerns in writing this book is that readers might mistake or misuse the ideas presented here because of lack of experience and/or personal instruction. It is not always easy to translate ideas from the pages of a book into the three-dimensional, moving world of massage, particularly when you are working in new, unfamiliar ways. Experienced practitioners will no doubt be able to apply numerous of the ideas in this book without problems. However, if you are unsure of what's being suggested or you run into difficulties, *enlist the help of an experienced teacher or colleague* who can provide you with coaching that is *tailored to your individual needs*.

Monitor Your Client's Responses
As you incorporate ideas from this book, you may feel that you are not working 'hard enough' – not giving everything that you could to each treatment. This is because you won't be. The ideal is to work easier (while working stronger) so that you can pace yourself and conserve your energy.

In fact, you are quite likely to find yourself becoming more effective with considerably less effort. So it is important to monitor your clients and to get verbal feedback, as you could easily be applying more pressure than you realise. Be sensitive to their bodily reactions such as grimaces, holding the breath, or micro-flickers of reaction in the muscles that you're working on, and adapt your technique accordingly.

Respect Your Own Limits

And bear in mind that, no matter how well you have learnt to use your body, there are *limits* to what any of us can physically do, both in each individual treatment and in terms of one's overall workload. There may be times when you need to reduce your workload and/or refer clients on to other practitioners.

I therefore present this book with the hope and the plea that you will approach the ideas presented with care and respect for yourself and your clients.

The Contents

You may decide to systematically work your way through this book, or to just focus on some sections in order to improve aspects of your massage. Or you might just use the book as a resource when you are having difficulties. Whichever way you approach it, read the chapters in the first two sections: *General Principles* (see Chapters 1–6) and *Preparations* (see Chapters 7–10) – before moving on to the other sections, as they lay the groundwork for the more detailed information of the later chapters.

There are three sections which look in detail at the best use of each part of your body in massage. Section 3 (see Chapters 11–17) covers ways of reducing the strain on your hands, the traditional 'tools' of Western massage. Section 4 (see Chapters 18–21) looks at 'hands-free' massage – using substitutes such as the forearm, elbow, knees and feet, in order to save your hands. Section 5 (see Chapters 22–28) focuses on how to use the rest of your body to back up and support these working tools most effectively.

Section 6 (see Chapters 29–32) covers integrating these elements into the overall 'dance' of doing massage. Section 7 (see Chapters 33–40) look at good bodyuse practices and potential problems in common massage strokes when you are working at a massage table. Section 8 (see Chapters 41 & 42) looks at working on a seated client, or when the client is on a futon on the floor. Section 9 (see Chapters 43–46) contains important information on self-maintenance for massage practitioners, ways of avoiding 'burn out', and trouble shooting and recommendations if you are already experiencing problems.

Practising

Try out the ideas from this book with a friend/colleague or in a supervision/study group where you can compare experiences, including how it feels on the receiving side. Or you may want to find a skilled teacher for personal tuition.

You will probably find it easiest to start by trying out each bodyuse suggestion separately. And you may find it helpful at first to exaggerate some of the suggestions to clarify for yourself the difference between poor working practices and good ones. You may also find it useful to exaggerate new ways of working until they become familiar.

Find Out What Works FOR YOU

You will probably find that you can incorporate some ideas quite easily into your massage. Others may initially feel awkward and 'artificial' and demand the use of unfamiliar muscles in 'strange' ways. Do not be discouraged by this. Persistent practice outside of massage sessions may be needed to develop the necessary coordination and familiarity for them to start to feel 'natural' enough to use with paying clients.

Through this practice, you will discover what works for you, and how and where to best incorporate these concepts into your work. Then it will take practice to consolidate using them. And, even when you feel that new ways of working have become familiar, keep monitoring your body consistently as you work to make sure that they remain easy and comfortable.

However do not persevere with new practices if they still remain awkward and strainful after a reasonable trial period. Either they don't work for you, or you need more individual instruction from a skilled teacher.

Being Open to Experiment
The attitude with which you try out the ideas presented in this book is crucial. Of course, you will probably be a little stiff and awkward at first, until you get the sense of what is being suggested and find comfortable ways of incorporating the new practices. However, doing them with a grim determination to 'get them right' will imbue them with a rigidity that defeats the purpose. Instead, try to approach this book with an attitude of curiosity and a willingness to experiment. Try out the suggestions presented to find out how to adapt them to suit *your own body*, particularly your build and the size of your hands (see Chapter 9). Take into account also how you need to vary and adapt your approach to suit clients with different builds.

Continuous Self-monitoring
Trying out the ideas in this book will help you to identify unhelpful postural habits that need changing and good practices to develop. Using your body well in massage needs constant attention. Therefore you need to develop the habit of continually *monitoring* your bodyuse (see Chapter 5) until it becomes an automatic part of every massage. This will enable you to notice points of awkwardness in massage sessions and catch yourself in the early stages of stiffening up or straining. You will then be able to make adjustments before these develop into major problems.

Terminology

As many writers have noted, there is no common third person pronoun in English to cover both sexes together, or either sex when it's unknown. In this book, I have mostly used *you/your*. Occasionally I have used *they/their* which can sound a little strange when used for individuals, but it is sometimes used in everyday language ("Will each passenger make sure that *they* have *their* ticket ready for inspection."). I have tried to use *she* and *he* in relation to clients, depending on the sex of client in the accompanying photos.

The People
I refer to the *massage practitioner* or just *practitioner* (even for the student) to avoid the clumsiness of *masseur/masseuse* or *giver of the massage*, etc.

The person receiving the massage is referred to as the *client* or occasionally as the *recipient* or the *receiver*.

Throughout the book, I have used the term *physiotherapist*, which is used in UK and Australasia. This is the same as *physical therapist* (USA).

Equipment

I generally refer to the massage *table*. It is also called a *couch, bench* or *plinth*.

Prone (face down) and *supine* (face up) refer to the position in which the client lies on the table.

In seated massage, I distinguish between having the client seated in:

- An *upright chair* (an ordinary chair – either four-legged or a swivel chair);
- A *portable massage chair* (in which the client sits on a tilted seat with the chest, head, arms and lower legs supported), and;
- A *desktop unit* (the portable equivalent of the upper part of a massage chair, which is placed on a desk so that the client who is seated in an ordinary chair can lean the trunk and head into it).

> **Note:** Much of the book is written in reference to working with the client lying on a massage table. However, most of the information can be applied directly to working with the client seated in a ***portable massage chair***, or can be easily adapted to it. Chapter 41 focuses on the specific issues of working with the client seated on a portable massage chair.

Parts of the Body

In this book, the general term *massage tool* refers to the part of the practitioner's body that is being used to deliver the massage. This is usually the hands (see Chapters 11–16), the forearm (see Chapter 18) or the elbow (see Chapter 19), but can also be the knees or feet (see Chapter 20). In the few instances in the book which refer to the use of *mechanical tools*, this is specifically stated.

People generally use the term *knuckles* to refer to the first joints of the fingers (the proximal interphalangeal joints, the 'IP' joints, see Chapter 15). When people talk about working with the *fist* (see Chapter 16), they are usually referring to the use of the metacarpo-phalangeal joints of the fingers (the 'MP' joints) or the side of the fist. Although the MP joints are sometimes called 'knuckles', I will refer to them as the 'fist' in this book for simplicity, and call them the MP joints whenever there could be any confusion.

When referring to the practitioner's body, I use the term *pelvis* in the anatomical sense for the combination of the innominate bones (the 'hip' bones) and the sacrum. I use the term *hips* in the common language way to refer to the general area and *hip bones* to refer specifically to the innominate bones. The *hip joint* is the junction between the head of the femur and the innominate bone at the acetabulum.

Massage Techniques

Palpation is the process of identifying body structures via touch.

This book mainly refers to massage done with a lubricant. The most commonly used lubricant is *oil* and this term will be used to include other mediums such as massage balm or powder. In the situations where no lubricant is used (*massage without oil, non-oil massage or dry massage* – see Chapter 36), this is clearly stated.

A *massage stroke/technique* refers to an individual massage movement. Most massage students are initially taught separate massage strokes for clarity and ease of learning. In this book, I refer to individual strokes in the application of massage for the same reason.

(However, bear in mind that a massage made up of distinctly separate units is quite disjointed and not very relaxing for the client. So the student also needs to learn how to join the strokes together to deliver a fluid, continuous massage. Experienced practitioners learn to 'improvise' and further extend their massage by adapting strokes and by blending them together in various ways that open up new ideas and ways of working).

There are differences in the names and categories of massage techniques in various professions and in different countries. I am using the following terminology:

- *Effleurage* strokes (see Chapter 33) are used to begin and end the massage, and to join other strokes and other parts of the body – including 'stroking', 'gliding' and 'draining' techniques.
- *Petrissage* strokes (see Chapter 34) are the group of strokes that are used to stretch and move the skin and muscles – kneading, wringing, squeezing and pinching strokes.

> Note: Kneading can range from a stroke that is focused on pushing muscles along (for example, on the inner forearm) to digging deeply down into the muscles (or can combine elements of both). Whether you are pushing along or digging down has different implications for how you use your hands and the potential pressure on them, and how you position your body behind your working hands. Therefore, throughout the book, I will distinguish between these two aspects of kneading.

- *Compression / friction* strokes (see Chapter 35) are used for applying pressure into muscles – 'knuckling', friction/'frictions' and sliding pressure strokes.
- *Percussion / tapotement* (see Chapter 37) covers the group of percussive strokes that can be applied in a range of ways that vary from very lightly (with the fingertips on the face) to quite forcefully for stimulating the skin and the underlying muscles – for example tapping, cupping, hacking, pounding, 'flicking' and 'plucking'.
- *Vibration* strokes (see Chapter 38) include includes shaking and 'tremoring' muscles.

Other commonly used strokes include:

- *'Holds'* (see Chapter 33), in which the practitioner rests his/her hands on the client's body;
- *Stretches* (see Chapter 39), either *passive* in which the practitioner moves parts of the client's body, or *active* in which the practitioner asks the client to move;
- *Rhythmical body movements* (see Chapter 40), which includes rocking the client's body and rhythmically rolling their limbs.

Experiments
The information in this book is presented for you to explore and try out to see how it works for you. Clear contrasts between good and poor practices are described and shown in the photos. At various points in the book, you will find boxes which invite you to do an *experiment / exercise* to help you to clarify these differences and to explore the implications for your way of working.

About the Photographs
Many of the photographs in this book illustrate good working practices or factual information. There are also groups of photographs which are designed to contrast good and poor bodyuse. Those that illustrate *poor* bodyuse practices are marked with an ⊘. Some of the photographs of poor practices show exaggerated versions of common working habits in order to make them clear. In real life, they will not necessarily be as obvious, so monitor yourself for the more subtle, everyday tendencies.

> Note: The cross-referencing in the book refers to the relevant figure, and its associated text (and not to the page number). For example, a reference to Figure 7.3 refers to Figure 3 (*The width of the massage table*) in Chapter 7 (Equipment).

SECTION 1
Dynamic Bodyuse for Massage: an Overview

This book highlights ways of using your body *in massage sessions* that reduce the potential strains while increasing your effectiveness, particularly when you are applying pressure. It focuses on two main aspects:

- *Involving your whole body* to generate the power and movement that supports your working hands, and;
- *Conserving your hands* by using them skilfully and saving them by using other body areas such as your forearms and elbows whenever possible.

This first section covers the main themes of this approach, laying the groundwork for the more detailed information of the rest of the book. It is therefore useful to read this section in its entirety before moving on to the other chapters.

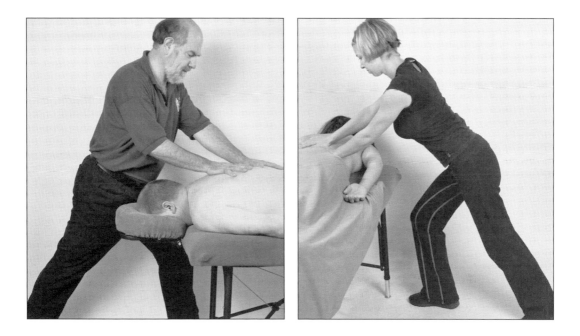

CHAPTER 1

Dynamic Bodyuse for Massage: Main Principles

Massage is one of the easiest professions in which to strain your body and to wear yourself out. It is a physically demanding activity and unfortunately has too often been taught in a way that puts undue strain on the practitioner's body.

How practitioners use their own bodies as they massage has been neglected in much massage teaching until recent years. The focus was primarily on massage techniques, with little or no consideration given to the practitioner's ease and comfort in delivering them. And teachers are often obliged to teach a set routine, with no adaptations to the build and abilities of the individual student.

Many people therefore come out of massage training believing that every massage must follow a set routine, and/or that there are certain strokes that must always be done – *no matter the build or needs of the client, and no matter how much it strains the practitioner's own body*. This attitude is often reinforced by the demands of work situations. For example, practitioners who are employed to do 'on-site' massages in offices are often required to work to a strict routine. In medical insurance cases, practitioners are often expected to work in a set way to deliver the outcomes defined by the insurance company. And many health clinics and spas require practitioners to fit in with the 'house style'.

Practitioners have only recently begun to realise that they can strain and damage their bodies in this field of work. The growing numbers of people working in massage in recent decades has also seen a small but increasing number of massage practitioners who have had to retire early due to work-related strains, particularly in their hands. It is the *cumulative* effect of poor working habits that cause these stresses and strains to the body. So it is important to develop an attitude of working *defensively* – considering the toll on your body of doing particular strokes for an extended time and of regularly working on people with significantly larger builds than yourself.

Practitioners' abilities will also be affected by their build (see Chapter 9). Practitioners with the 'ideal' massage build of a large, strong body and hands may never encounter problems in their careers. A short but robust or wiry build is also likely to sustain a practitioner through years of doing massage without problems. Until recently, most masseurs and masseuses working in public baths and saunas throughout Europe, the Middle East and Asia, were people with these builds and were accustomed to hard physical work. Practitioners with these builds will find the information in this book helpful in maintaining their energy and ease in doing massage.

However practitioners with other builds need to be more careful about how they use their bodies and hands. So do those with old injuries or particular weaknesses. This book is written very much to help these practitioners look after their bodies and maintain their careers – to acquaint them with the potential problems in doing massage and ways of minimising or avoiding these.

When the potential dangers of performing massage are spelled out, as I have done in this book, people can become scared of it. It is not my intention to put people off doing massage. However, I think that it is important to approach it respectfully and defensively, armed with a realistic perspective, good information and the skill of self-monitoring (see Chapter 5). This is similar to learning to drive a car, where it is important to bear in mind that it is a lethal weapon (potentially dangerous to the driver, passengers and bystanders). I do not think that this has stopped anyone from learning to drive, but hopefully it encourages people to do it with care and attention.

The Strains of Massage

Swedish Massage

The *Swedish Movement Cure* was developed by Per Henrik Ling in Stockholm in the early 1800s. It included massage as an adjunct to exercise in the gymnasium. Later in the 19th century his approach to massage was brought to Britain and the United States and later to other parts of the English-speaking world, and is thus known today as *Swedish Massage* in Sweden and throughout the English-speaking world. Similar ways of working are known as *Classical Massage* in other parts of Europe.

Swedish Massage and its derivatives still form the basis of most basic massage training in the English-speaking world. It is important to note that massage was only a small part of Ling's health regime. His synthesis of common massage techniques was planned for use in conjunction with gymnastic coaching. It was not envisaged as a full-time professional activity. Some of the basic techniques of Swedish Massage are not designed for constant, repetitive use. And this style of massage is most suited to a general relaxing 'rub down' and not adequate for the specific, deep massage that many of today's clients expect. Massage practitioners therefore need to take particular care with the techniques that they use and how they apply them.

Applying Pressure

Applying pressure is a significant part of most massage sessions. There is the potential for strain whenever you are applying pressure, whether it is focused on one point or maintained throughout a moving stroke. It puts compressive pressure on all of the joints in your arms and shoulders, and into your back.

Learning how to incorporate pressure without straining your body or doing damage to your hands is one of the greatest challenges in doing massage.

The Common Problems

The most common work-related strains in massage involve the thumbs and wrists. Problems in the thumbs generally arise from overusing them for applying strong and sustained pressure, particularly in kneading and compression strokes and in pressure point techniques. Practitioners can also strain their fingers in similar ways, especially if they have small hands or slender and/or hypermobile fingers.

Wrist strains generally come from consistently having the wrists bent back (hyperextended) when working firmly. Shoulder stiffness and backaches are also common.

Unfortunately, practitioners often try to overcome these strains by tensing up in an attempt to 'muscle through', which is likely to lead into a vicious cycle of stiffening up and further overworking the hands. At the very least, these problems will reduce the practitioner's effectiveness. If they are not addressed, they can become serious enough to stop the practitioner from continuing with their work and may even cause permanent, debilitating damage.

Adapting to Your Abilities

The book covers practices that will get you through a full working day and working week. The overall aim is to help you to establish good habits that will enable you to sustain your career over years. The principles covered are useful to bear in mind when you are doing light massage strokes. They are *crucial* to minimise strain and avoid damage to your hands and body *when you are applying pressure,* as it is the *slowly accumulating effects* of doing many massages, which often go unnoticed, that cause problems.

Bear in mind that the book can only present general guidelines for working. Take time to try them out and find out how they can work best *for you*. Modify or adapt them as you need to, and practice integrating them into your massage work. (And be aware that, no matter how well you use your body, everyone has limits which are determined by your build, natural strength and fitness).

As you incorporate ideas from this book, you may feel that you are not working 'hard enough' – not giving everything that you could to each treatment. This is because you won't be. The ideal is to work easier (while working stronger) so that you can pace yourself and conserve your energy.

Working Defensively

This book emphasises that *the practitioner's ease of working* is *just as important* in massage *as any specific stroke or technique* – the practitioner's comfort should be a significant factor in determining his/her way of working. It takes a long-term perspective on the problems that can arise as the *cumulative effects* of poor working practices take their toll. It describes the common ways that practitioners strain their bodies and offers guidelines for reducing or avoiding these. The aim is to look after your body and simultaneously deliver maximum effect with minimum effort.

Try to develop an attitude of working *defensively* – considering the toll on your own body of doing particular strokes for an extended time, and the general strain of regularly working on people with a significantly larger build than yourself.

So, as you massage, take account of your ease and comfort, so that small awkwardnesses and discomforts do not accumulate into major aches and strains. Monitor and adjust how you are using your body. Pay particular attention to the most commonly strained areas – the thumbs, fingers, wrists, shoulders and back.

Don't Do Strokes That Cause You Strain

It is crucial not to continue doing strokes that strain your hands or your body. Try to find other ways of doing those strokes, or other techniques that can replace them. Discuss this with colleagues who may have helpful ideas. If you can't find satisfactory alternatives, you will need to consider changing the way that you work, and, if necessary, the range and type of clients that you treat. Remember that it is the *cumulative* effect of poor working habits in massage sessions that is of concern – ultimately it may end your career.

The Limits of Good Bodyuse

At the same time, bear in mind that, however effective you are, there are *limits* to everyone's abilities. Your strength, stamina and resilience will be determined by your build and inherited constitution, your age, your level of fitness and medical history, and the pressures that exist in the rest of your life. You *WILL* strain your body if you consistently exceed your comfortable limits.

So try not to push yourself too hard. And take into account how events in your work situation and the rest of your life affect your energy for doing massages. At times, you may need to reduce your workload. Refer clients on to other professionals if you need to, and do things outside your work situation to maintain your energy and zest for life (see Chapter 43).

The Benefits of Good Bodyuse

As well as saving your body and hands, good bodyuse can add depth and effectiveness to the massage that you deliver. Conversely, a massage in which you use your body poorly is less effective for both giver and receiver.

Reducing Strain
The most important reason for learning to use your body well when doing massages is, of course, to reduce the *cumulative strain* on your body. This is particularly crucial for a practitioner with a small build and/or small or slender hands.

Increasing Effectiveness
As you gain experience in using your body well, you can become more efficient and effective in the precision and the power (where appropriate) that you bring to your work. When you are able to apply techniques in an easier way, you will be able to sustain pressure longer, and to pace yourself in order to maintain your energy over the working day/week/year.

Easier to Monitor the Client's Responses
There are other benefits of using your body well. If you do not involve your whole body in the massage, you are likely to be tensing your shoulders and arms unnecessarily to deliver the power. This makes it harder to feel the client's responses, as your brain is preoccupied with how hard you're working. However, the more relaxed that your body and hands are, the easier that you'll find it to *monitor* the responses which happen in the client's tissues under your hands, and to adapt to them. This is especially important when applying pressure – the firmer the pressure that you are using, the more you need to monitor its appropriateness for the client.

The Client Responds Better
And, when *you* use your body well, your *clients* will also have a different experience. If you are tensing your body to deliver the massage, this communicates to the client, who is more likely to react with an instinctive, unconscious wariness than when you use your whole body in a more even, relaxed fashion. If you are using your body well so that your hands are relatively relaxed, your touch will be more acceptable to the client. The client is more likely to relax, which in turn allows you to work more deeply without provoking them into tensing against you. And, if you are in a comfortable position that enables you to stay relaxed when you are applying consistent, continuous pressure, you can wait for the client's tissues to 'melt' and let you through, like butter melting under a hot knife, rather than trying to force your way through.

Good Bodyuse Principles

The main elements of good bodyuse for doing massage are using your hands (or forearms or elbow) effectively without strain, and positioning and using your body to support them.

Look after your working tools by:

- *Conserving your hands* by using them skilfully, and;
- *Saving them* by using other body areas such as your forearms and elbows whenever possible.

Use your body to support your working tools by:

- Getting *your body aligned behind your working hands* (or forearms/elbows, etc.) to use your bodyweight;
- *Leaning and swaying your body to* generate the power and movement for your massage strokes, and;
- Continually *repositioning yourself* around the massage couch for best advantage.

The next chapter covers common problems encountered in doing massage and the following chapter covers good working practices that address these, which the rest of the book looks at in more detail. In this chapter and throughout much of the book, one principle of bodyuse is covered at a time for clarity. Ultimately, these guiding principles need to be blended together into a continuous, moving 'dance' (see Chapter 4), like the 'dance' of a skilled sports player in action.

Looking After Your Hands

If you are positioning and moving your body to provide the power and movement for massage strokes, then your hands can be relatively *relaxed* and you can use them most effectively. This enables you to *monitor* and to *adapt* to the recipient's build, needs and responses.

Conserve Your Thumbs and Fingers

The areas of the hands that are most at risk in massage are the thumbs and the wrists, and, to a lesser extent, the fingers. Practitioners with small hands, or long, slender and/or hypermobile thumbs and fingers need to be especially careful about how they use them. Strains in these areas can lead to permanent, debilitating damage over time if they are not addressed.

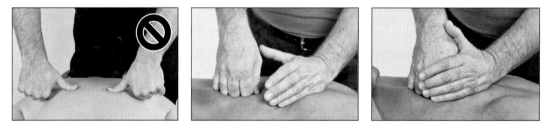

Figure 1.1: Applying pressure; a) with the thumb hyperextended,
b), c) supporting the thumb (fingers behind; wrapping hand around).

Straining the thumbs by overusing them for applying pressure is a common problem in massage. If you need to use your thumb to apply pressure, make sure that it is not bent out to the side (hyperextended). Keep it in line with your hand and forearm and support it with your fingers and the other hand (see figures 13.10–13.15).

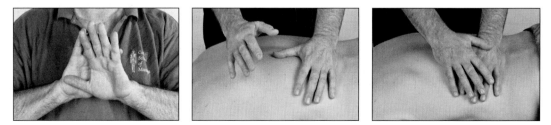

Figure 1.2: The 'reinforced' thumb.

Or learn to use a 'reinforced thumb' (see figure 13.15).

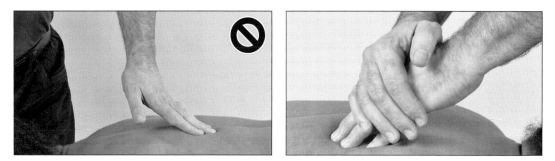

Figure 1.3: Applying pressure through the fingers; a) hyperextended fingers, b) fingers aligned with hand and supported.

Strain can also arise from regularly hyperextending your fingers when applying pressure through them. Keep them in line with your hand and support them.

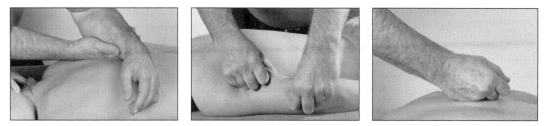

Figure 1.4: Substitutes for the fingers and thumbs; a) the back of the hand, b) the knuckles, c) the fist.

Whenever possible, save your thumb and fingers or thumbs, by using larger 'tools' to deliver the massage. For example, you can use other parts of your hands, such as the back of your hand (see figure 14 13), your knuckles (see Chapter 15) or your fist (see Chapter 16) for applying firm pressure more easily.

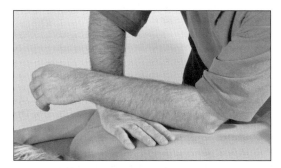

Figure 1.4 (cont.): d) the forearm, e) the elbow.

And find an experienced teacher who can train you in the use of your forearm and elbow to save your hands completely (see Chapters 18 & 19).

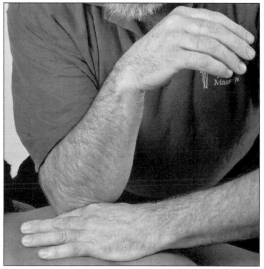

Keep Your Hands Relaxed

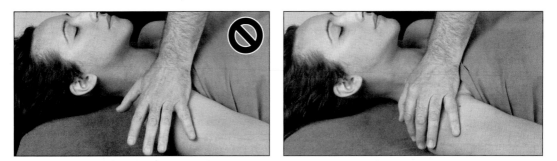

Figure 1.5: The practitioner's hands; a) stiff, b) relaxed.

Massage beginners often use their hands in a stiff, awkward way as they initially struggle to master techniques. With practice, you can learn to gauge the *necessary effort* for each stroke, which conserves energy and makes the delivery of the massage more fluent and effective, and makes it easier to feel the client's responses. Learning to use your bodyweight for the power and movement of massage strokes instead of standing still and relying on upper body effort (below) will also reduce the tendency to stiffen your hands unnecessarily.

Look After Your Wrist

People with small wrists need to be particularly careful of the pressure that they put on them. Learning to use your forearm and elbow also saves your wrists.

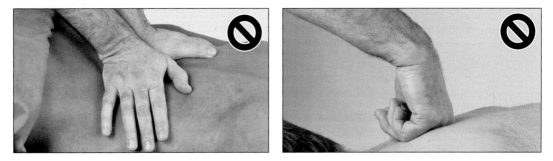

Figure 1.6: Angle of the working wrist; a) overextended, b) overflexed.

Strain in the wrists is generally due to consistently working with them hyperextended when you are applying pressure with your fingers, palm, or knuckles. Less often it can be due to having your wrist overflexed, for example when using your fist.

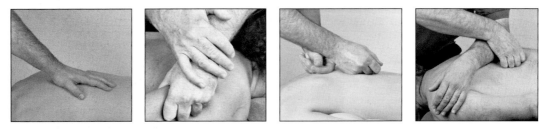

Figure 1.7: Looking after your wrist; a) having a relatively straight wrist, b) holding the wrist, c), d) support under the wrist.

Try to keep your wrist relatively straight (but not *stiff*) whenever possible. And support it with your other hand if you can, either by holding it directly or by supporting it from underneath.

[The only situations in which you can safely have your working wrist *somewhat* bent – to around 30° – is when you are working lightly or when you are applying pressure through the heel of your hand, as *long as the rest of your hand is relaxed* – see figure 17.8].

Using Your Body

Your ability to use your hands in a relaxed, skilful way is dependent on using your body to support them. Do not stand still, but position yourself so that you can sway and lean your body.

Do Not Stand Still

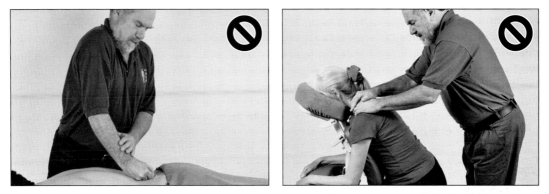

Figure 1.8: Standing still; a) standing still and working awkwardly at the massage table, b) standing stiffly around a massage chair.

One of the biggest problems when doing massage is standing still, which leads the practitioner to rely on 'muscling through'. This makes unnecessary demands of the practitioner's shoulder and arm muscles, and also puts extra pressure on the back and hands. The massage delivery is stilted and less fluid, which is less relaxing for the recipient. It is also less powerful.

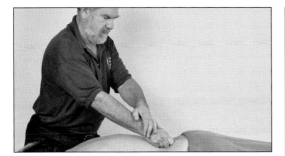

Figure 1.9: Moving into position.

Instead, involve your whole body to reduce the workload on your upper body, and to make the massage easier while delivering greater power and fluidity to your massage strokes.

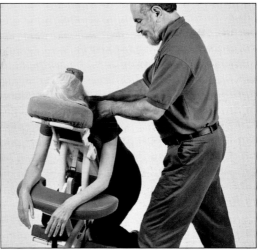

Position Yourself Behind Your Hands

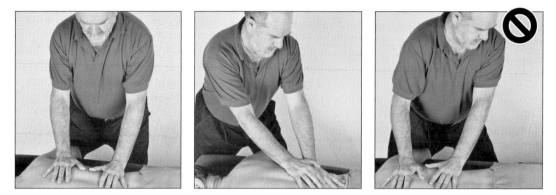

Figure 1.10: Aligning your hips and your working tools; a), b) working tools in front of the hips, c) working tools not in front of the hips.

Position yourself so that your body is behind your hands (or your working forearm/elbow). Otherwise, your trunk will be twisted, which can strain your back and will reduce the effective transmission of force from your body.

Lean Forward for Power

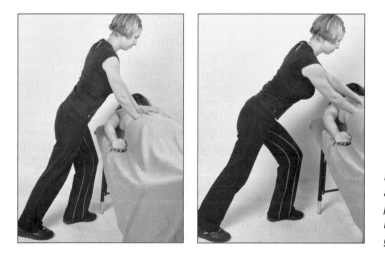

Figure 1.11: Applying pressure; a) leaning forward for light pressure, b) leaning forward more for greater pressure.

Leaning forward enables you to generate power for massage strokes without strain and without stiffening your shoulders or arms. This leaves your hands relatively relaxed for fine-tuning the massage techniques. Lean forward by bending your knees to avoid hunching over (see figure 3.26).

Sway Your Body for Moving Massage Strokes

Initiate pushing or pulling strokes by swaying forward or back. This reduces the strain on your lower back, and the workload on your upper body. It provides fluidity, power and evenness to your massage strokes and enables you to pace yourself throughout a massage session.

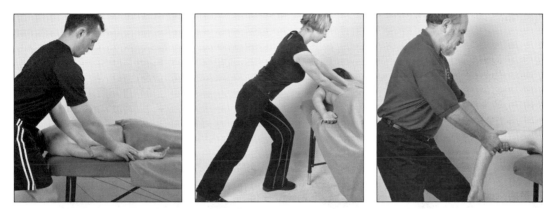

Figure 1.12: Power from the lower body; a), b) swaying forward, c) swaying back for pulling.

When you work in this way, there are two components to balance – the pressure and the movement of the stroke. You can increase the pressure by bringing your weight more directly above your working tools (your hands/forearm, etc.). Lowering your body (by bending your knees) makes it easier to push forward.

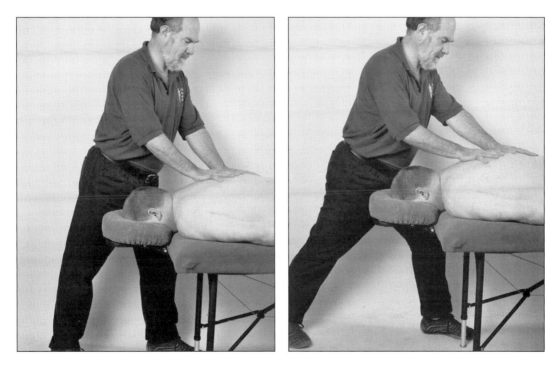

Figure 1.13: Balancing pressure and movement; a) rising up to increase the pressure, b) getting lower behind the hands to push forward.

Blend Effort and Relaxation

The way of working presented in this book encourages you to develop a balance in your body between being *dynamic* and being relatively *relaxed* – not tensing up because you are working too hard or, at the other end of the scale, delivering a listless massage. Using your whole body for the massage, which saves you from tensing and overusing your upper body will help you to achieve this balance. Watch a skilled skater or high diver to see this balance of 'easy power' in action.

The Massage 'Dance'

Just applying these principles in a static way is not enough. Unfortunately, some people take up a single position by the massage table / chair and then work exclusively from there. This limits how far you can comfortably reach and your ability to involve your bodyweight behind your hands.

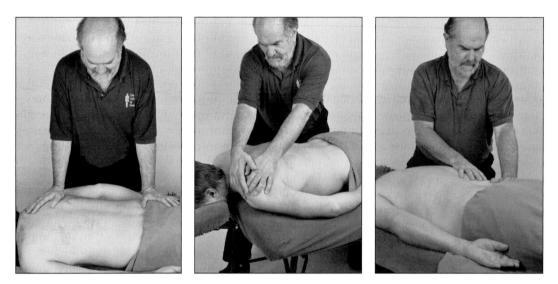

Figure 1.14: Moving your body behind your hands – the massage 'dance'.

Move *around* the table, regularly changing position so that you keep your body aligned behind your hands, like a snooker player lining up for successive shots. At first, your massage may be disjointed as you stop the massage to move your body. With practice, you can learn to smoothly reposition yourself. Ultimately, you can develop this into a fluid, continuous *'dance'* around the massage table as you move between strokes and also within strokes (see Chapter 4), like the moving 'dance' of a tennis player.

This is not easy to communicate in a book. And, this book focuses on one aspect of bodyuse at a time, extracted from the flow of the massage, in order to highlight each one. However, once each one is familiar, it needs to be integrated back into the continuity of the massage 'dance'.

Why 'Dynamic'?

What is meant by 'dynamic' when referring to the massage practitioner's bodyuse? The interwoven aspects, which are summarised below, can only be hinted at in a book. To experience them, you will need to search out massage treatments that encompass them and teachers who can help you to bring them alive in your work.

Physically, the ideal in massage is to work with a balance between strength (when necessary), ease and precision. This requires the development of power in an integrated fashion throughout the body, not just relying on the relatively small muscles of the arms and hands, but also harnessing the power of the larger muscles of the legs and lower trunk. Then, as the practitioner moves, s/he ideally uses natural body strength in a *dynamic* way that is neither hard nor stiff, so that s/he can work with ease and fluidity whilst being able to apply firm pressure when it is needed.

Working too hard can lead to tensing up and inflexibility, whilst being too relaxed leads to sloppiness and a lack of energy. The balance of strength and ease, fluidly combined into rhythmical action and backed up by the development of an attitude that balances enthusiasm and concentrated focus, is the ideal of many solo activities such as skiing, figure skating and high diving, and martial arts such as judo, aikido and Tai Chi. Skilled exponents of these activities are graceful in action. Similarly, this blend of elements can give a dynamic grace to the massage practitioner's work.

In massage, it is not just the techniques that matter, but also *how* they are delivered. The way that the practitioner works will be transmitted to the client via the body-to-body level of communication that is part of massage. Working in a stiff, leaden way will not evoke the same response in a client as working in a *vital, dynamic* way that incorporates energy and alertness.

This, of course, is enhanced by moving fluidly around the massage table/chair in the *massage 'dance'* (see Chapter 4). Applying good 'body mechanics' by aligning your bodyweight behind your working tools is essential. However, it can be done in a stiff, mechanical and disjointed way. Ideally, a massage treatment is a moving, dynamic 'dance', in which the practitioner moves fluidly to continually reposition themselves.

Practitioners can then pace themselves. Massage is a demanding physical activity. Although practitioners may be pleasantly tired at the end of a day's work, this dynamic way of working will enable you to use each massage session as a 'workout' to energise yourself, rather than approaching it as a grinding chore that will wear you out.

Preparing your body to back up your hands in this way also enables you to respond and adapt the massage to suit the client's build, the tensions that you palpate, and the micro-responses in their tissues that you feel directly under your hands. So the massage can also be dynamic in the sense of not being preordained but able to change as dictated by the needs of the moment.

Self-monitoring

This book presents *general* guidelines for looking after your body and using it well for massage. In order to work out how techniques work best *for you*, you need to develop the ability to constantly pay attention to *your own body* (see Chapter 5). This enables you to assess the effects on your body of doing each stroke, and to work out how to adapt it or to find alternatives that suit you.

If the process of self-observation while massaging is unfamiliar, you will probably find it difficult at first to keep your attention both on yourself and on the client, and to coordinate this into a fluid massage. However, with practice, you will find that this can become an integral part of your way of working, so that you are automatically taking care of your body.

It is a useful practice to take a few moments at the end of each session to observe your body and reflect on the overall session. This can be a time to assess which techniques may have contributed to any cumulative strains and which were most effective and least strainful.

In the process your massage style may undergo changes. You may find yourself relying more on some types of techniques and using others less. You may even begin to leave out techniques that seem too demanding on your hands or the rest of your body, or use them only with certain clients.

You will hopefully find your massage becoming a living, developing process, due to *your own* changing needs, comfort and aptitudes as well as varied needs of different clients. Ideally, you will develop the perceptions and ideas that can save your body so that you have the chance of a long and interesting career, rather than having it cut short by strains and injuries that could also limit the rest of your life.

Review

In massage, the practitioner's ease of working is just as important as any specific stroke or technique.

The *cumulative* effects of poor working habits can cause stresses and strains to the practitioner's body.

Do not continue doing strokes that strain your hands or your body. Try to find other ways of doing these strokes, or other techniques.

If you can't find satisfactory alternatives, consider changing the way that you work, and, if necessary, the range and type of clients that you treat.

However effective you are, there are *limits* to everyone's abilities, determined by your build, level of fitness, and the pressures in your life.

Problems in the hands mostly arise from overusing the thumbs and fingers for applying pressure, and by working with them bent back or sideways.

Save your fingers and thumbs by supporting them, and conserve them, whenever possible, by using larger tools such as your knuckles, fist, forearm or elbow instead.

Wrists problems can arise by regularly applying pressure through them when they are bent.

Shoulder stiffness and backache can arise from stiff or awkward working postures, or through relying on upper body muscle power for massage.

Good bodyuse practices:

- Reduce the strain and wear and tear on your body;
- Help you to be more efficient in using your energy, and more effective in the precision and the power that you can deliver;
- Enable practitioners with a small build or small hands to increase the power that they can bring to massage sessions;
- Make it easier for you to *monitor* the *responses* in the client's tissues under your hands, and to adapt to them, and;
- Benefit the recipient, who experiences the massage as less 'attacking' and therefore easier to respond to.

Good bodyuse involves:

- Keeping your hands relaxed and using them skilfully;
- Generating the power for pushing, pulling or sustained pressure techniques from your lower body;
- Aligning your body behind your working hands (or forearms etc.);
- Bending from your hips when you are leaning forward, and not just in the lower back;
- Moving behind each stroke for the power and movement, rather than standing still;
- Continuously repositioning yourself around the massage couch to keep your body aligned behind your working tools;
- Developing this, with practice, into a fluid, continuous 'dance' around the massage table.

The ideal is to cultivate an attitude of 'relaxed alertness' which balances enthusiasm with calm concentration, and to work in a *dynamic* way that combines natural body strength with ease and precision, and fluid movement with power.

CHAPTER 2

Common Problems in Doing Massage

The strains of massage often escape our notice. Occasionally there will be a single dramatic trigger for practitioners straining themselves, such as attempting to lift a client's large, heavy leg, especially if it is done awkwardly. However most problems arise from the *cumulative* effects of awkward, physically stressful and/or repetitive ways of working, *particularly when you are applying pressure.*

Moments of strain or overwork that may be of little concern in *one* massage can build up into problems if they are repeated over weeks and months. The cumulative effect of these small strains can ultimately equal the effect of one moment of great strain. For example, regularly applying pressure that causes a slight discomfort in your thumb can produce the same effect as suddenly spraining it. Therefore you need to consider techniques not just in terms of one moment during a massage, but how you are going to feel at the end of a full day's/week's massage.

This chapter looks at common massage practices which can lead to aches and strains for the practitioner. It focuses on five aspects:

- The potential problems in the rigid application of massage;
- Problems that can arise from common massage techniques;
- Some common massage beliefs that may lead to awkwardness and strain in action;
- Problems due to poor positioning and use of the practitioner's body, and;
- Postural habits that practitioners bring to the table.

Following descriptions of common problems, some ways of reducing or avoiding them are suggested. The next chapter contains further ideas for addressing many of these problems, and the rest of the book looks at these in more detail. Chapter 46 has a checklist of pointers to consider if you find that you are regularly feeling strain in particular areas of your body.

Addressing Poor Practices

Some problems, such as reaching too far over the massage table, have relatively straightforward remedies – 'Stop doing it!' – although it takes time to become conscious of habits and to change them, especially deeply ingrained postural habits. And you may find yourself reverting to them in times of stress. Therefore you will need to give them regular attention for some time.

Other potential problems need addressing in a more general way to reduce the likelihood of them building up – for example, using other parts of your hand (or your forearm), whenever possible, to reduce the workload on your thumbs and fingers.

Knowing of these potential problems enables the practitioner to monitor and to modify unhelpful ways of working, or replace them with other, less strainful techniques. However, by the time that physical problems arise, the contributing habits have often been established for some time. Therefore it is important to learn to *monitor your own body* as you massage (as well as the client's responses) and adapt your massage accordingly, until this becomes an automatic part of your way of working (see Chapter 5).

As you read through this chapter, bear in mind that changes in your working situation, such as an increase in your workload, can also effect your ease in your body and your resilience. Changes in the rest of your life can also affect your energy for doing massages. Chapter 43 offers ideas on addressing some common work stresses and suggestions on rebalancing activities outside of work to reduce your stresses and maintain your energy.

Rigid Application of Massage

Sticking to a Set Massage Routine

Many massage teachers are obliged by their syllabus to teach a set routine. Or they may teach their own specific way of working, without any adaptations to suit the build and capabilities of individual massage students. So the techniques and the way of applying them that you originally learnt may not suit you; in any case they won't fit every client.

Although most of us initially learnt a massage routine, you do not have to stick rigidly to it, or use strokes that do not work well for you. *There is NO set massage routine that must ALWAYS be followed, and there are NO must-do techniques.* Treat the massage strokes and sequence that you originally learnt as basic building blocks from which to create adaptations. Vary the parts of your hands and arms that you use for each technique. Reshape your massage repertoire around *what suits you*, the practitioner, as well as the client's build, needs and responses.

Find ways of working that are *easy* and *comfortable* for you, the massage practitioner, in order to reduce the wear and tear on your body. A range of techniques from massage traditions from all over the world are readily available these days to learn and choose from, so no technique is absolutely indispensable. Choose those that work best for you in the situation.

Not Monitoring Your Energy and Comfort

The energy and abilities that you have available for massage can vary according to your health and fitness, your previous strains or injuries, your workload, and events in the rest of your life. For example, you may need to be careful of your fingers after doing extensive computer work, or of your wrists after doing a lot of driving. You may need to conserve your fingers after an injury. You may be in the process of moving house, or doing DIY, gardening or other activities that make demands on your hands and on your energy. And at times, events in your personal or family life may also limit the energy that you have to offer clients.

It is important to adapt your way of working according to these factors, rather than feeling that you must 'soldier on' even when you are unable to deliver the massage without strain on your body.

Women, of course, have additional factors to take into account. They are often not as strong as men, often have more family demands placed on them, and have regular energy fluctuations due to hormonal cycles.

Limiting Massage Myths

There are some beliefs that are common in massage circles which lead practitioners to put unnecessary stresses on their bodies, as well as reducing the effectiveness of the massage session.

Believing That Deep Work Has to be Painful to be Effective

A common myth is that deep massage must be painful for the client to be effective. This often leads practitioners to strain *their own* bodies to deliver this pressure. It is likely to lead into a vicious cycle of working harder and harder as the client tenses against the discomfort of the massage.

Of course, this is not to say that all massage must be wimpy. Once you have established a level of trust in a massage, it is possible to challenge the client for periods of time by slowly increasing the pressure *at a rate that is manageable* for the client (taking them into the realm of 'good pain'). The deeper that you work, the more slowly you need to go, in order to give the client's body time to get accustomed to the pressure and let you in. Therefore, it is essential for you to be in a comfortable position, leaning your bodyweight while staying relaxed in your own body, so that you are able to *wait* for the client's tissues to 'melt' and let you through.

Believing That You Must be Able to Massage Every Client

Some people have been led to believe that they must be able to massage every client – no matter how much it strains *their own* bodies. However, there are absolute limits to everyone's abilities due to their build. *There is no client that you MUST be able to treat,* irrespective of your build or the client's build and the pressure that they want.

Some practitioners can find it hard to accept these limitations. They have an image of themselves helping the whole world through massage, and being able to provide the pressure that every client demands. And practitioners can be embarrassed or ashamed about referring clients on to other people who are more suited to deal with them.

However, if you regularly push your body beyond your comfortable limits, you will strain yourself. If you persist in doing this, you will cause yourself permanent damage and become unable to pursue your career, which is of no use to yourself or to your clients. Sometimes, it can be essential to refer clients on to colleagues whose build and strength is more suited to the massage that the client wants.

Denying Strains in Your Own Body

It can be difficult to admit that we are having problems. It is a potential threat to our livelihood and our identity. Professionally it doesn't look good. Clients often feel that a health practitioner should *never* have any health problems. And we may not feel safe admitting such problems to our colleagues, especially those who disparage any sign of 'weakness'. We can also feel that we are letting the profession down. These factors can lead to an attitude of shame about having problems.

Practitioners can come to feel very alone and even helpless with a problem when they have no opportunity to talk it over with others without fearing disapproval. It is important to find situations in which you can confidentially discuss professional problems, get understanding and support, and begin to look for solutions. This may be with a trusted colleague or friend, an individual supervisor or in a supervision group.

Potential Problems in Common Massage Techniques

Most massage training in the English-speaking world is based on *Swedish Massage* which was put together by Per Henrik Ling early in the 19th century as a small part of the *Swedish Movement Cure*. Massage was not seen by Ling as a full-time career in its own right, and the techniques were not envisaged for prolonged everyday use. Ling and his followers didn't initially use massage often enough for problems to emerge. However, by the end of the 19th century when some people began to focus just on massage, there were already reports of practitioners straining their hands.

Practitioners need to be careful of relying on and overusing some common techniques. A number of techniques in common currency such as kneading with the thumbs, which are appropriate for occasional use or for working lightly, are not adequate for prolonged use or for applying firm pressure. So practitioners can run into problems when attempting to use them for deeper work. They are not particularly effective for the client and can often lead practitioners to work too hard to deliver the pressure, usually by tensing their shoulders which adds to the pressure on their hands and increases the likelihood of straining them over time.

And Swedish massage has often been taught as a hands-only activity, with no sense that the rest of the body could be involved. This leads to the practitioner relying on upper body power, and consequently overusing the shoulders, which also puts unnecessary pressure on the practitioner's hands.

Overusing the Thumbs and Fingers

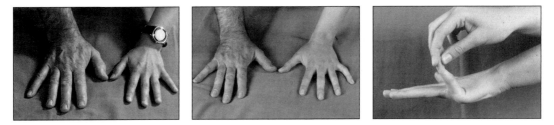

Figure 2.1: Fingers and thumbs at risk; a) average / small hands, b) average / long slender digits, c) hypermobile digits.

Massage techniques that involve extensive use of the fingers and thumbs are the most likely to cause problems. Practitioners with small hands, and long slender fingers and thumbs and/or hypermobile fingers and thumbs need to be especially careful about using these types of strokes.

The smallest parts of the hands are the least effective and most at risk when you are applying pressure. So, as a general principle, try to use the largest (appropriate) areas of your hand whenever you can.

Because the tips of the fingers and thumbs are the most sensitive for palpating the client's structures, there is a great temptation to overuse them. To save these vulnerable structures, use them for initially palpating an area, and then, if possible, use larger areas of your hands (or forearms) for massage techniques that require pressure. While these other areas are not as sensitive, you will find that you can learn to feel more than you might expect with them through practice. And, while you are learning, you can use the fingertips of your supporting hand for more discriminating palpation.

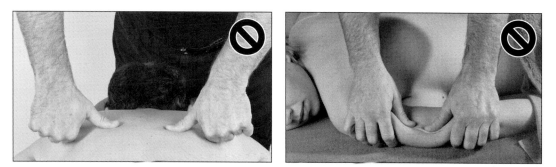

Figure 2.2: Strokes which put the thumbs at risk; a) applying pressure through the thumbs, b) firm kneading with the thumbs hyperextended.

The thumbs are the most commonly strained part of the hand in massage. Regularly applying pressure through them is the most common cause of cumulative problems in the thumb joints, especially if they are hyperextended when you are doing this (see Chapter 13). People with hypermobile thumbs need to be especially careful about this.

Save them by using your knuckles, especially for kneading strokes, and your elbow for deep pressure.

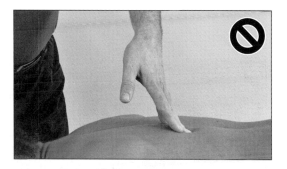

Figure 2.3: Fingers at risk; applying pressure through hyperextended fingers.

As with the thumbs, using the fingers to apply pressure is the most common way of straining them, especially if they are hyperextended (see Chapter 12). If you have long, slender fingers, using them too much for kneading or for squeezing large, firm muscles can also strain them.

Overusing Other Parts of the Hands

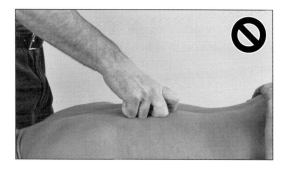

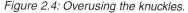

Figure 2.4: Overusing the knuckles.

While other parts of your hands are less vulnerable than your thumbs or fingers, they too can be overused. This applies especially to your knuckles (proximal interphalangeal joints, see Chapter 15). Supporting them in action with your other hand will reduce the pressure on them (see figure 2.6). And, whenever possible, use your fist instead (see Chapter 16), which is a stronger, less vulnerable tool, or learn to use your elbow (see Chapter 19).

Straining the Wrists

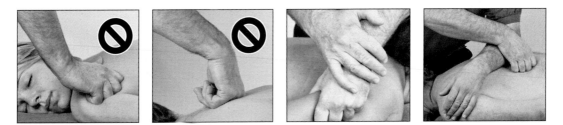

*Figure 2.5: Looking after the wrists; a) overextended, b) overflexed,
c) stabilising the straight wrist, d) supporting under the straight wrist.*

Practitioners can strain their wrists, usually through working with the wrist consistently hyperextended. So keep your wrist relatively straight (but not stiff) and, if possible, support it with your other hand (see figure 17.17).

Use Both Hands Whenever You Can

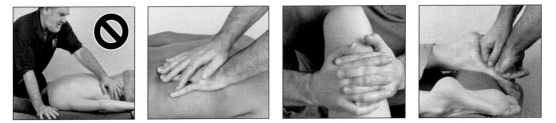

Figure 2.6: Using your hands; a) leaving one hand idle, b), c), d) using the hands together.

Many practitioners regularly work with one hand only, often while resting the other hand on the table or on the client's body. However, if your other hand is not involved in another essential activity, it is better to use it to support your working hand instead (see figure 11.23), or to use both hands equally (see figure 11.25). This shares the workload between your hands, which reduces the pressure on each hand, makes the techniques easier to apply and gives you greater control over them.

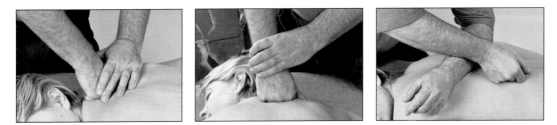

Figure 2.7: Having one hand support the other.

Overusing the Dominant Hand

This is a related problem. The majority of the population are right-handed and tend to overuse the right hand and underuse the left. One of the challenges and excitements of massage is learning to be relatively ambidextrous.

Observe what you are doing with your dominant hand and teach your slower hand to replicate the strokes. This takes practice, but it is something that you can work on during massage sessions. Even though you may never become quite as skilful with the non-dominant hand, this will spread the workload more evenly between your hands. This is often easier for left-handers who are used to accommodating to a right-handed world.

In two-handed strokes, such as percussion strokes, it is quite important to work at a pace that suits your non-dominant hand (see figure 37.2). You are likely to tense up if you try to drive your non-dominant hand to match the more skilled one.

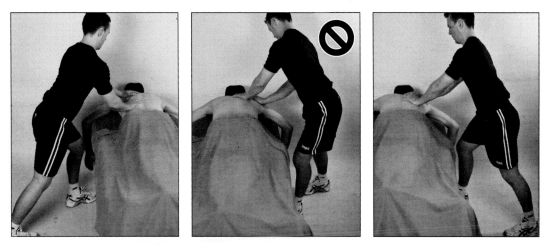

Figure 2.8: 'Mirroring'; a) left foot forward, b) left foot forward on opposite of table, c) right foot forward.

Overusing your dominant hand doesn't only make extra demands on the hand, it also forces uneven use of your body. People will usually position their bodies to support the dominant hand. Therefore, when using your non-dominant hand, 'mirror' your usual stance so that your body positioning then supports your non-dominant hand. This is crucial for doing the equivalent stroke on each side of the massage table.

Overusing the Hands Generally

However, no matter which part of your hand that you use, your hands won't be particularly effective if you are working extensively on clients with large builds and/or well-used muscles. You need to be especially careful about this if you have small or slender hands. Learn to use your forearm and elbow (see Chapters 18 & 19) to save your hands.

Problems of Positioning and Bodyuse

Having the Table Too High

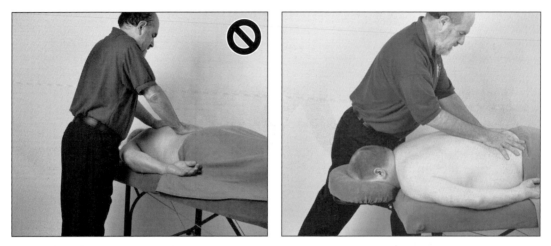

Figure 2.9: Massage table height; a) table too high, b) table at a good height.

If the table is too high for a practitioner, he will be unable to effectively use his bodyweight behind his hands, and will therefore overuse the upper body. A lower table enables the practitioner to involve the whole body, which reduces the demands on his shoulders, arms and hands. Chapter 7 looks at how to gauge the ideal height and width of a table for the individual practitioner.

Standing Still

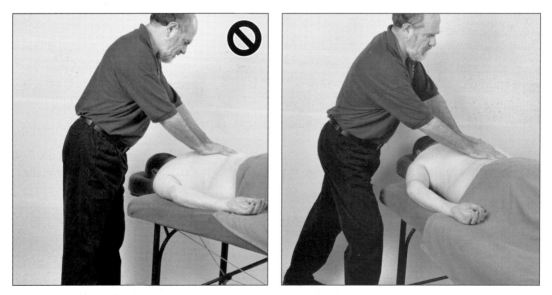

Figure 2.10: Standing still; a) working stiffly, b) moving around.

Standing still at the table can lead to problems. It reduces the involvement of your bodyweight for power and fluid movement. This leads practitioners to rely on the upper body only and thus overuse their shoulders and arms. Moving around the massage table or chair in order to reposition yourself for each stroke takes the pressure off your arms and back.

Leaning Against the Side of the Table

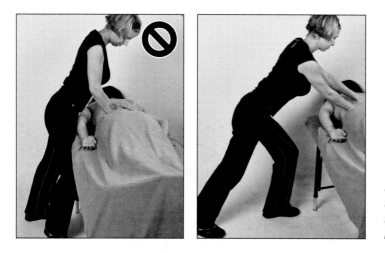

Figure 2.11: Distance from the table; a) leaning against the side of the table, b) using more space.

Standing against the side of the table has similar consequences. It limits the movement of your body in the same way that standing against the table would restrict your ability to play table tennis. It also puts pressure on your lower back when you are doing sliding effleurage, kneading, wringing or pressure strokes, or trying to reach very far.

Overreaching

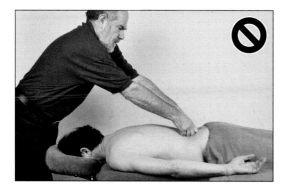

Figure 2.12: Trying to reach too far from the end of the table.

It is easy to strain the lower back through trying to reach too far down from either end of the table or trying to reach too far across from the side of the table. Obviously tall practitioners can comfortably reach further than shorter practitioners.

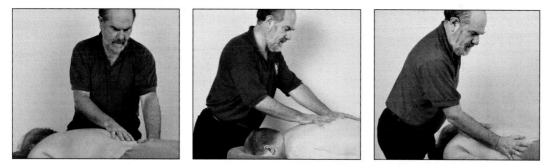

Figure 2.13: Moving to cover the client's back; a) at the far side of the table, b) at the head of the table, c) on the close side.

Shorter practitioners should not try to reach so far. Instead, they can reach down each side of the client's back in turn by moving to one side of the table and then to the other.

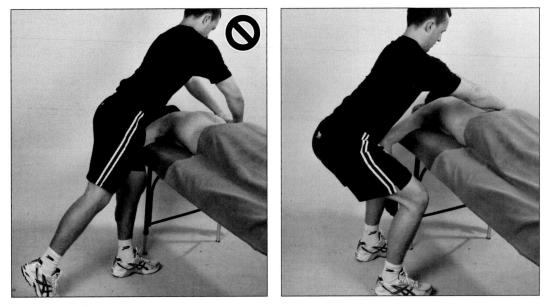

Figure 2.14: Reaching across the table; a) going up onto tiptoes,
b) dropping down to reach across.

Some practitioners try to extend their reach by rising up onto tiptoes. This is not a good position to maintain for any length of time, as it requires continuous tensing of your hamstrings and calf muscles, and isn't as balanced or as powerful as pushing with the whole foot planted firmly on the floor. Instead, lower your body slightly by bending your legs as you reach. This takes the strain off your lower back, particularly when you are reaching across the table.

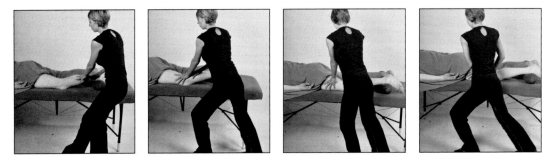

Figure 2.15: Stepping up alongside the table for long strokes; a) starting position,
b) stepping up with the back foot, c) transferring weight onto the back foot and stepping forward,
d) new position.

In a long stroke, step up alongside the table to maintain the sweep of the stroke. To do this, bring your back foot up behind your front one, and let the weight move onto it as you step forward with the front one. This is particularly important for short practitioners working on tall clients.

Trying to Apply Pressure on the Client's Far Side
When you are standing at the side the table, it is relatively easy to do pushing and pulling strokes (such as kneading and wringing strokes), on the far side of the client's body *provided* that your arms are long enough for you to be able to reach across without straining your own back.

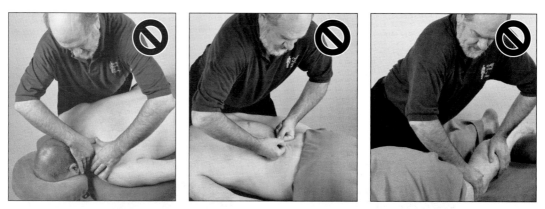

Figure 2.16: Working too far across the client's body; a) across to the opposite shoulder, b) applying pressure on the far side, c) on the leg.

However, it is difficult to apply pressure on the far side of the client's body from the side of the table. You are likely to be putting pressure on your back and tensing your shoulders, and you still won't be very effective. Instead, cross to the other side of the table to apply pressure.

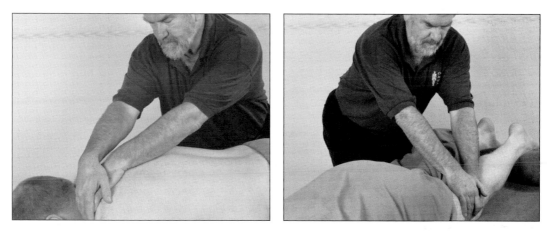

Figure 2.17: Working comfortably; a) on the opposite shoulder, b) on the far leg.

If your arms are long enough, you can comfortably reach across to push or pull on the far side of the client's body. Or you can cross to the other side of the table to apply pressure.

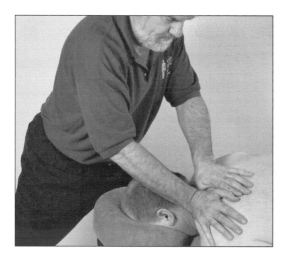

Figure 2.18: Applying pressure on the shoulder.

Trying to Work Symmetrically From the Side of the Table

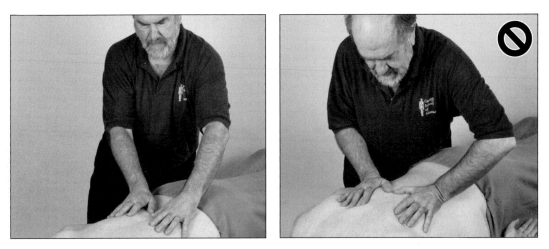

*Figure 2.19: Working symmetrically from the side of the table; a) light stroking,
b) trying to apply pressure on both sides.*

This follows from the last point. It is impossible to apply pressure equally on both sides of the client's back from the side of a massage table, and you are likely to be straining your shoulder as you attempt to reach across. It is only possible for the practitioner to comfortably apply symmetrical pressure from the head or the foot of the table (remembering not to reach too far, see figure 2.12).

Trying to Maintain Continuous Contact

Most massage practitioners are familiar with the idea that, once you have established connection with the client, it shouldn't be broken until the massage is complete. This is a good idea, akin to a dentist giving you full and continuous attention during a dental treatment.

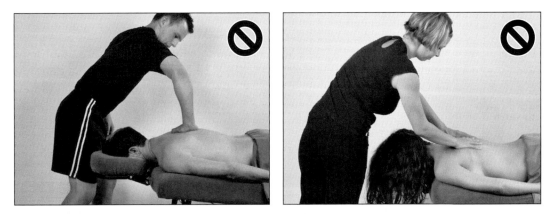

*Figure 2.20: Maintaining physical contact as you move around the table;
a), b) crossing awkwardly.*

However, the idea of 'maintaining contact' can be rigidly interpreted to mean that continuous *physical* contact should be maintained at all times. This leads the practitioner to move awkwardly and with unnecessary strain in the attempt to maintain this contact while moving from one part of the client's body to another, no matter how difficult this is. (It also denies the practitioner the opportunity for a momentary break from focusing on the client in order to regather energy and focus).

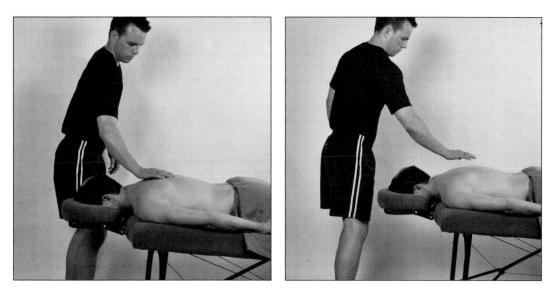

Figure 2.21: Getting around the table easily; a) with light contact, b) lifting the hands off.

Of course it is disruptive if the practitioner *abruptly* breaks contact without warning, or continually makes and breaks contact. However, once an atmosphere of trust and ease has been established in a massage session, you can take your hands off the client's body for a few seconds before the client starts to feel 'abandoned', *as long as* making and breaking contact are *gradual* and *unhurried*, rather than abrupt or heavy handed. As the client relaxes into the massage, you can make these contact breaks longer without losing continuity.

These short contact breaks enable you to fluently finish massaging one part of the body and move on to another area, and/or to cross from one side of the table to the other. Lift your hands smoothly from the client's body on one side of the table, take a few moments to cross to the other side, and then remake contact in a fluid, relatively 'seamless' way.

This is also useful if you need to leave a client during a massage session, for example when getting extra equipment or dealing with an interruption. Slowly break contact with the client so that there is minimal disturbance, tell them (in a calm, unhurried way) that you will be back in a moment, do what you need to and then resume contact with minimal disruption.

Postural Habits
People bring their familiar postural habits, which are often unconscious, to the massage table. Over time, poor posture can put great strain on the practitioner's body, even if s/he is only doing light massage.

A number of bodywork disciplines can help you to become conscious of your postural habits and offer you ways of changing them. Deep tissue massage modalities such as Rolfing® work directly on the body to release and rebalance restrictive muscle patterns. 'Exercise' systems such as Yoga, the Alexander Technique, the Feldenkrais Method®, and Pilates offer instruction that can help you to change postural habits (see Chapter 44).

These will get you started on dealing with these problems. If you are addressing a familiar, long-held posture, remnants of it can remain for a long time so it will need regular attention. You may find it useful to have a video made of yourself working, or have a teacher or colleague watch you in action and give you feedback. Learning to move around the table is also crucial rather than spending long periods standing in one place.

Hunching Over

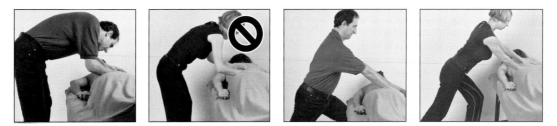

Figure 2.22: Leaning over the massage table; a) tall person hunches over, b) 'beginner's crouch', c), d) leaning without slumping.

Hunching over the massage table is a common habit. Massage novices are often so focused on what they are doing with their hands that they do not realise that they are hunching over (in a 'beginner's crouch'). This stance can easily become ingrained as part of the practitioner's habitual, unconscious working posture, so experienced practitioners need to monitor themselves for this too. Hunching over can lead into a cycle of back strain and/or a rigid slumped posture, which further reinforces this way of working. Practitioners are likely to tense their shoulders and to work too hard with the hands and arms with the possibility of straining these areas as well. This physical posture may be reinforced by an attitude that you as a professional should give his/her complete attention to the client *only*, and ignore your own comfort (or discomfort).

Tall people, who are used to stooping to accommodate to the world around them, need to be particularly careful about not falling into this habit at the massage table. It's also a major problem for visually impaired massage practitioners, who are accustomed to bringing their faces close to any object for maximum visual input.

The ideal is to have your trunk both 'straight' and *supple* (see figure 25.14). A practitioner needs to be able to lean towards the table with the whole trunk (whilst maintaining its full length) by bending the knees, rather than crumpling in the back.

Standing Stiffly Upright

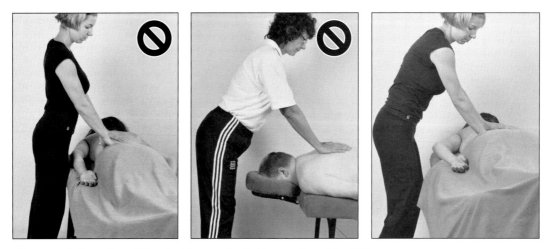

Figure 2.23: Standing stiffly; a) stiff upper body, b) standing with stiff knees, c) bending the knees to lean forward.

Some people are accustomed to standing stiffly upright. At the massage table, this posture also forces the practitioner to work almost entirely with the shoulder muscles, and arms and hands. It can create shoulder aches, stiffness and pain and sometimes neck and back aches. If this is a familiar posture to you, widen your stance, bend your knees slightly and focus on swaying forward and back with your massage strokes. And reposition yourself behind each stroke.

Old Injuries

Many people have restricted ways of moving due to old injuries. These are often unconscious and may no longer be necessary. Work out how to move around the massage table/chair as much as you can without causing yourself discomfort. Also try attending some exercise classes or individual treatments that focus on flexibility (see Chapter 44) to see if the limitation is still essential to protect a weakness or has just become an unnecessary habit.

Review

The strains of massage and their slow accumulation often escape our notice.

Problems can arise through the rigid application of massage, such as:

- Sticking to a set massage routine, even if it strains you;
- Not monitoring your energy and comfort, and modifying the massage accordingly;
- Believing that you must be able to massage every client, no matter your own build or their demands, and;
- Denying strains in your own body.

The most widespread problems that arise from using common massage techniques are:

- Relying too much on the thumbs and fingers;
- Overusing other parts of the hands, and overusing the hands generally, which can be addressed by learning to use the forearms and elbow;
- Straining the wrists, by applying pressure through them when they are bent;
- Overusing your dominant hand;
- Working with one hand only when you could use both.

There are two common myths in massage that can lead to awkwardness in action and possible strain:

- Trying to keep continuous physical contact with the client, even when this puts you into strainful positions, and;
- Believing that deep work must be painful to be effective, and consequently straining your body to deliver this.

Problems can arise from having the massage table too high, which can cause you to overuse your shoulders and arms and to strain your back.

They can also arise from poor positioning of your body, such as:

- Standing still, instead of moving around the table;
- Standing against the table, which restricts your ability to involve your lower body;
- Trying to reach too far along or across the table, instead of changing position;
- Trying to apply pressure on the far side of the client's body, which is difficult to do and likely to strain your back;
- Trying to work symmetrically on the client's back from the side of the table, which is similarly difficult and will overtax your shoulders and is also likely to strain your back.

The practitioner's postural habits can also cause problems. The most common are due to:

- Hunching over;
- Standing stiffly upright, or;
- Moving awkwardly because of unconscious protective habits relating to old injuries.

CHAPTER 3

Good Working Practices

This chapter summarises some useful principles to bear in mind when doing massage, and provides examples of putting them into practice. It expands on the basic principles of looking after your body covered in Chapter 1. Many of the ideas covered in this chapter address the problems outlined in the previous chapter. The aim is to reduce the wear and tear on your body, and to make your work easier, more efficient and more effective. Later sections of the book cover specific applications of many of these principles in more detail.

The principles covered are useful when doing light massage strokes. They are crucial to minimise strain and avoid damage to your hands and body when you are *applying pressure*, as it is the *slowly accumulating effects* of doing many massages that cause problems, which often go unnoticed. This is particularly important if you have a small or light build, small or slender hands and/or hypermobile thumbs and fingers.

The ideas presented here may feel strange at first because of unfamiliarity. So take time to try them out fully in order to find out how they can work best *for you*. Modify or adapt them as you need to. It will take practice to incorporate them into your massage work. Bear in mind that one principle of bodyuse is described at a time for clarity throughout this chapter and much of rest of the book. However, they need to be blended together into a moving, flowing massage 'dance' (see Chapter 4), like the graceful, fluid 'dance' of a champion skater or a skilled sports player.

This chapter looks firstly at some of the rebalancing activities and other ways of replenishing yourself that can be done outside massage sessions. These are covered in detail in Chapters 43 & 44.

The central part of the chapter covers ways of reducing the pressure on your working tools in massage sessions. Your hands are the most vulnerable of the practitioner's common tools and the most commonly damaged. Detailed guidelines on making the work of your hands easier are presented in Section 3 of the book (see Chapters 11–17). The *'Hands-free' Massage* section (see Chapters 18–21) looks at using your forearm, elbow and other parts of your body to take the pressure off your hands.

The last part of this chapter covers some general ideas on using your body to support your working tools. The section on *Using Your Body* (see Chapters 22–28) has further information on the effective use of each part of your body. The *Integrated Bodyuse* section (see Chapters 29–32) looks at positioning and moving your body to generate the power and movement to support your working hands/forearms and reduce the strain on them. Sections 7 & 8 (see Chapters 33–42) look at how to apply these principles to particular types of strokes and various working situations.

Outside of Massage Sessions

Use Warming-up Exercises and Have Winding-down Time
Because massage is a physically demanding activity, you need to warm-up your body in preparation for a day's work, and to take some time to wind-down at the end of the day (see Chapter 10). Warm-ups can range from a few minutes of quick stretches to a more extensive routine to prepare you for a full working day. Similarly, it is good to take a few minutes at the end of your working day to mentally and physically wind-down, or have a longer winding-down time if you can, for example by having a long soak in a hot bath.

Rebalance Your Bodyuse Outside of Massage Sessions
Applying pressure is a large part of many massage sessions. This puts compressive pressure throughout the joints of the practitioner's body. *Doing stretches* is a useful antidote for this. Stretches can also be used to maintain general flexibility (see Chapter 10).

If you are doing a lot of massage, be careful *not to overuse your hands* in other activities outside of massage sessions. Problems can arise through the cumulative pressure of spending considerable time on computers, mobile phone texting, doing extensive DIY, gardening or craft work, or playing a musical instrument.

Because massage is a demanding physical activity, you need to *look after your body* as sports players do, for example by eating nourishing food, and getting enough good quality rest. You also need to *replenish yourself* by doing things that nourish your spirit or you could find yourself heading in the direction of 'burnout' (see Chapter 43). What nourishes each person is different, of course, and can vary from time to time for each individual. It can include receiving bodywork yourself, having social time with friends and family, involvement in activities to let off steam, hobbies and leisure activities, attending sports and arts events, time to yourself, time in nature, and meditative and/or spiritual practices.

And be realistic about your energy. Have regular days off and holidays. And, if you can, take time out when you are undergoing stressful times yourself. I took a month off work when my mum died, for example, because I knew that I had no energy to give to other people.

General Principles in Massage Sessions

Take Care of Your Hands When Doing Repetitive Activities and/or Applying Pressure
It is the cumulative effect of doing *repetitive movements* and *applying pressure* that wears practitioners down and causes them strain. Therefore try to avoid doing the same sorts of techniques over and over, especially if you find them difficult or tiring. And give your hands and arms a rest from the compressive effects of applying pressure by doing light stroking, rhythmical movements, or applying stretches, when appropriate.

Be Guided By Your Own Comfort
Work *within your personal comfort limits*. This book provides guidelines and suggestions, but you need to work out how to apply them in ways that are most useful *for yourself*. Therefore it is crucial to *monitor* your body and energy as you massage (see Chapter 5), and to adapt your massage accordingly. Do *not* keep doing things which strain or overwork your body.

What is comfortable for you can change from day to day. For example, on some days you might feel full of energy and happy to work beyond your usual capacities; on other days you may find that you need to focus on conserving your energy.

There are *no* techniques that absolutely must be done. There is now an abundance of available techniques from massage traditions from all over the world, so choose ways of working that best suit you – those that are most effective with the least strain to yourself.

If there are techniques that you would like to use but find uncomfortable to do, try adapting them so that they're less stressful on your own body. Alternatively, experiment to see if you can find other ways of achieving the same effect.

Respect Your Limits

It is also important to understand and respect your limits, which will be determined by your build, natural strength and fitness, the stresses in your life and your workload (see Chapter 43). Do not try to work beyond these. Refer clients on if necessary.

Involve Your Whole Body in Massage Strokes

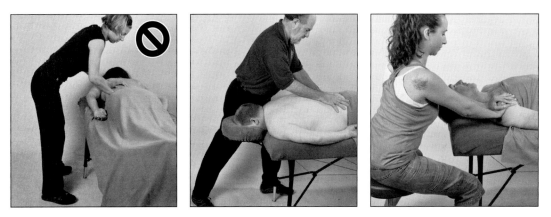

Figure 3.1: Ways of doing massage; a) standing still and just using the hands, b) using the whole body, c) using the body when seated.

Massage is sometimes taught as an activity in which practitioners stand still and just use their hands. The ideal, however, is to involve your whole body in moving with the massage strokes. This is looked at in more detail later in this chapter (see figures 3.20–3.36). The next chapter focuses exclusively on this massage 'dance', and Chapters 22–28 look at how to integrate each part of your body into this 'dance' to support your working hands/forearm, etc. Even when you are seated, you can provide a powerful impulse for your working hands by swaying forward (see figure 3.25).

Aligning your body behind your working hands/forearm backs up your working tools (hands, forearm or elbow) with the power of your bodyweight. Your hands contain small, relatively weak muscles compared to the large muscles of your trunk and your legs. Using your lower body as much as possible for power conserves the small arm muscles for fine-tuning the massage techniques.

This has a number of benefits. It reduces the strain on your hands, arms and shoulders, and spreads the workload throughout your whole body. It increases your effectiveness, and provides more power and fluidity to the application of massage techniques.

It also engages the practitioner more in the session not only physically but, as a consequence, *mentally* as well. It is much easier to let your attention wander if you are only using your hands, and the rest of your body is not 'committed' to the massage.

Stay Relaxed in Your Body

Keeping your body appropriately relaxed as you work has two benefits. It conserves your energy and it supports the powerful but relaxed use of your hands.

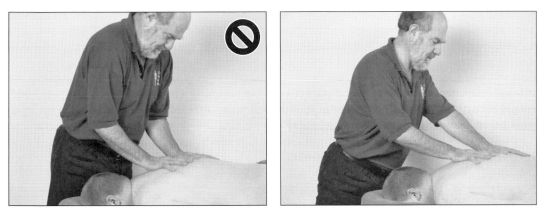

Figure 3.2: Physical attitude for massage; a) tensing up, b) appropriately relaxed but dynamic.

Novices often tense up and hold their breath as they try to pay attention to all of the elements of a massage session. With experience, practitioners learn to relax their shoulders, arms and back, to breath easily and to not stiffen their knees. The ideal is not to be too 'laid back', but to establish a balance between ease and action, like a skilled skater. You can also see this attitude of 'relaxed alertness' when watching skilled practitioners of many eastern martial arts.

If you tense your shoulders, for example, you will feel how this also tends to stiffen your arms and hands, reducing your power and ease of working and also your sensitivity to the receiver's responses. You may also find yourself unconsciously stiffening other parts of your body, standing more stiffly and/or holding your breath.

Reducing the Pressure on Your Working 'Tools'

When you have mastered using the rest of your body in an appropriately relaxed fashion, fine-tune this approach by focusing on your hands.

Relax the Non-working Parts of Your Hand

In each stroke that you do, work out which parts of your hand are essential and which parts are not being used and can therefore be relaxed.

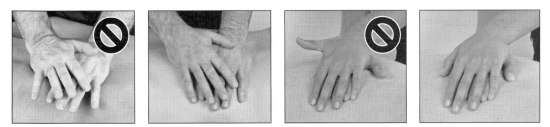

Figure 3.3: Relaxing the non-working parts of the hands; a) stiff fingers when using the hand,
b) relaxed fingers when using the hand, c) stiff thumb when using the fingers,
d) relaxed thumb when using the fingers.

For example, it is a common habit to stiffen the thumb when using the fingers, but it is quite unhelpful. And when using your hand, have your fingers relaxed rather than lifted up, which tends to stiffen your whole hand.

Relaxing the non-working parts of your hand is emphasised many times in Chapters 11–16. It conserves your energy, makes the delivery of the massage strokes more effective, and also makes it easier for you to feel the receiver's responses. Practice will enable you to master the ability to maintain this relaxation even when you are applying pressure.

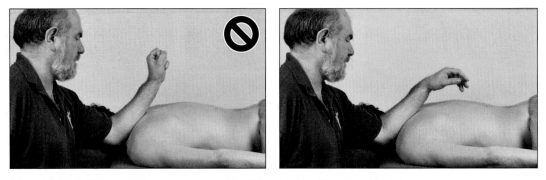

Figure 3.4: Working with the forearm; a) with stiff hand, b) with relaxed hand.

For the same reasons, relax your hand when using your forearm or elbow (see Chapters 18 & 19).

Conserve Your Fingers and Thumbs

Unfortunately, massage training can overemphasise using the fingers and thumbs, which are the smallest, weakest and most often damaged of the available tools for the delivery of massage techniques. They are fine for light massage, and they are often essential for the initial palpation of an area and the identification of tensions. However, they are the least effective massage tools and the most vulnerable for techniques that involve pressure. It is rather like trying to hammer in the pegs of a circus tent with a pin hammer – you are likely to damage the tool with little or no useful results.

Bear in mind that learning to use your body well increases the effective force that you bring to bear through your hands. So this can cause more problems if you just rely on your thumbs and fingers for the delivery of massage strokes.

Therefore, as far as possible, reduce the amount that you use your fingers and thumbs. This is especially important for practitioners with small hands or long, slender and/or hypermobile thumbs and fingers. Save them for the situations in which you can't use anything else because of the delicacy needed or the lack of working space, for example when working on the client's face.

Use Kneading Sparingly

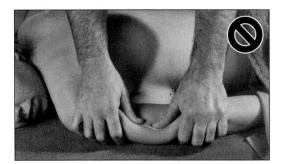

Figure 3.5: Kneading with hyperextended thumbs.

Many kneading strokes are quite demanding on your thumbs. On large muscles, use larger areas of your hands instead, to achieve the same effect without the pressure on your thumbs. For example use your knuckles to move the muscles around or your fists or elbow to dig in more.

Use the Largest 'Tools' Possible

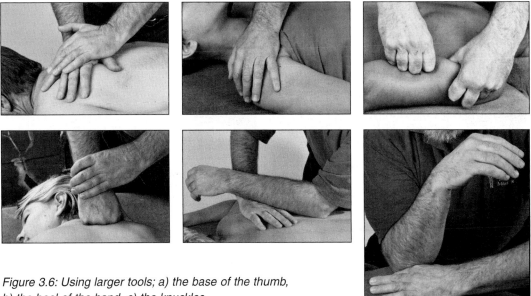

Figure 3.6: Using larger tools; a) the base of the thumb,
b) the heel of the hand, c) the knuckles,
d) the soft fist, e) the forearm, f) the elbow.

Use the largest working tools that are appropriate in order to minimise the strain on your digits, and to maximise your effectiveness. If it is possible, use;

• The base of your thumb (see figure 14.4) or the 'reinforced thumb' (see figure 13.15) instead of the point of your thumb;
• Your knuckles (proximal interphalangeal joints, see Chapter 15) or your fist (see Chapter 16) in place of your fingers or thumbs, and;
• The heel of your hand for larger spread pressure (see figure 14.7).

While other parts of your hands are less vulnerable than your thumbs or fingers, they too can be overused. This applies especially to your knuckles. Use your fist instead whenever you can; it is a stronger, less vulnerable tool. And get training in the skilful use of your forearm and elbow (see Chapters 18 & 19) to substitute for your hands entirely for firm strokes. And, whatever tool you are using, support it in action with your other hand to reduce the pressure on it (see figures 3.7–3.8).

Of course, none of these areas are as sensitive for palpation as the finger and thumb tips, but with practice, you will learn to feel more with them than you would expect. And you can also use the fingertips of your supporting hand to help you palpate the tissues.

However, no matter how efficiently you work, there are limits to *everyone's* abilities, so don't try to regularly work beyond these. Refer clients on and/or cut down your workload if necessary.

Use Both Hands Together Whenever You Can

Whenever you are using one hand on its own for doing massage strokes, you have to rely substantially on your shoulder and arm muscles to control it. If your other hand is available, use both hands together – either using one hand to support and guide your working hand or using both hands together in the action. This reduces the workload on your hand whilst giving you greater control and power, in the same way that a tennis player uses both hands together for a backhand stroke.

Using your hands together enables you to control the power and the movement of your strong massage strokes primarily through positioning and moving your body. This provides greater stability in delivering your techniques, particularly when you are applying pressure, which makes them more even and fluid. It also enables you to use your hands with greater precision.

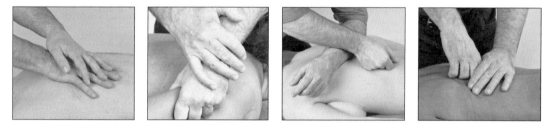

Figure 3.7: Using both hands together; a) hand-on-hand pressure, b), c) supporting the working hand, d) guiding the working hand.

Placing one hand on the other is a simple way to increase the pressure in a stroke. You can easily increase it further by leaning your bodyweight forward. Or you can use your other hand (or forearm) to passively support your working hand or to actively guide it.

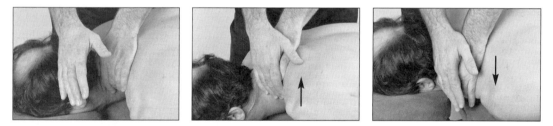

Figure 3.8: Pushing and pulling with a double-handed grip; a) the hands, b) pulling with the fingers, c) pushing with the heels.

Pushing and pulling strokes can also benefit from a double-handed grip. Take hold of the muscle with one hand. Use your covering hand to move the under-hand, alternately pushing and pulling across the muscle. Push more with the heel of your under-hand, and 'grab' with your curled fingers in pulling. This spreads the load between both hands, and allows the main effort of pushing/pulling to come from swaying forward or leaning back. It is especially effective across the top of the shoulders (on the upper trapezius) and for working across large back muscles or the large muscles of the legs.

You can use both hands together to squeeze and stretch the client's calf muscles. Interlock your fingers, 'clamp' the muscle with the heels of your hands, and then move this 'grip' around to stretch the muscle.

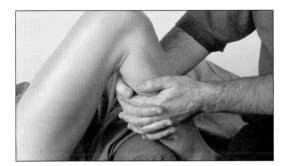

Figure 3.9: Interlocked fingers grip.

Look After Your Wrists
The wrist is the second most commonly strained area of massage practitioner's hands.

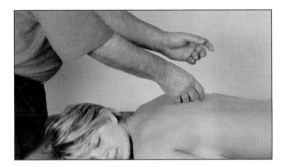

Figure 3.10: Having a bent wrist – percussion.

Many massage techniques involve varying the angle of the wrists within the stroke. If you are working lightly, for example 'brushing' across the tissues, this is unlikely to cause problems. And, in most percussion strokes, you need to keep your wrist loose or the technique will be jarring to you and the client.

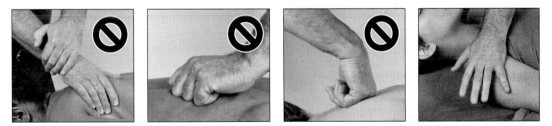

Fig 3.11: Applying pressure; a), b), c) bent wrist, d) straight wrist.

However, if you are applying pressure, try to keep your wrist relatively straight. Even if you are only applying light pressure, it is a good habit to cultivate. And it is crucial when you are applying sustained pressure. If your wrist is bent, the transfer of power from your arm to your hand will be inefficient, which often leads you to apply more force. In addition, part of your effort will be used in maintaining the stability of your wrist. These effects together put considerable pressure on the wrist which doesn't work well at an angle, and can strain it (see figure 17.8).

Learn to be Ambidextrous

This has two facets in massage.

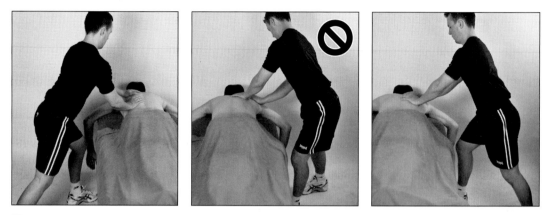

Figure 3.12: Mirroring strokes on each side of the table; a) leading with one hand, b) using the other hand with body still positioned to support the dominant hand, c) mirroring body posture to support the non-dominant hand.

Massage practitioners, particularly those who are right-handed, often rely on their dominant hand and consequently overuse it. So it is important to learn to use your non-dominant hand (and forearm) to mirror the skills of your dominant one. This not only saves your dominant hand/arm but it also enables you to do the equivalent stroke from each side of the massage couch. Bear in mind that this involves mirroring the position of your whole body to support your non-dominant hand, not just changing the hand that you use.

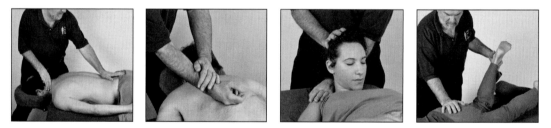

Figure 3.13: Using both hands simultaneously in different ways.

There is another aspect of ambidexterity to be aware of in massage – learning to simultaneously do different but related activities with each hand (see figure 11.27 – 11.29). And, of course, it is important to teach yourself to mirror this way of working also.

Balance Pressure With Stretching

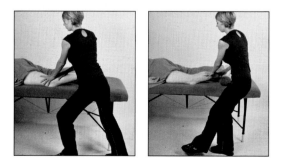

Figure 3.14: Relaxing during light stroking; a) stroking forward, b) stroking back.

A large part of massage involves applying pressure of varying amounts on the client's muscles. This also consistently compresses the practitioner's joints, particularly those of the upper body. Doing stretches outside of the massage session will go some way to rebalancing this (see Chapter 10). There are also ways of relaxing and opening out many of the joints of the upper body in massage sessions to give yourself a break from constant compression strokes.

You can relax your whole upper body when you are doing light stroking. As you sway forward you will be putting some pressure on the joints, of course. As you sway back to pull your hands back, focus on letting your hands 'drag' so that each joint opens out to its fullest capacity.

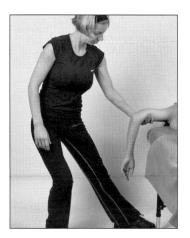

It is hard to totally relax your wrists and hands in massage sessions, except by learning to use your forearm and elbow (see Chapters 18 & 19). However, you can stretch out the rest of your upper body joints by incorporating stretches of the client's body into your treatments. When doing a stretch, sway back to utilise your bodyweight and take the time to relax your upper body as much as you can to take advantage of this (see Chapter 39).

Figure 3.15: Stretching one's own body while stretching the client.

Using the Table and Cushions (or Your Own Body) for Stability When Applying Pressure

When you are applying pressure or doing concentrated work on a small area, resting the area of the client's body on which you are working on the massage table (or chair) will stabilise it. You can also use cushions on the table for this. This reduces the pressure on your own arms and hands to provide the stability as well as delivering the pressure. It enables you to use both hands together, which takes pressure off your upper body (see figures 3.7–3.9). It also makes it easier to move and to reposition yourself for each stroke.

Use the Massage Couch or Chair for Support

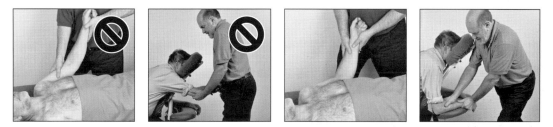

Figure 3.16: Applying pressure on the client's forearm; a), b) while holding it in the air,
c) with it resting on the table, d) resting it on the arm rest of a massage chair.

For example, rather than holding a limb in the air when you are applying pressure, use the couch or chair to support it whenever you can. This saves you considerable effort and enables you to be more precise and effective.

Use Cushions and Bolsters to Support the Client

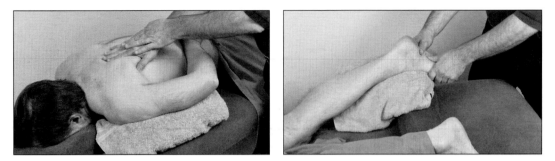

Figure 3.17: Using supports on the table; a) cushion under the client's shoulder, b) cushion under the client's foot.

It is standard practice to use bolsters and cushions to help make the client comfortable on the massage table. However, you can also use them to support the specific area that you are working on, such as the sole of the prone client's foot, or the side-lying client's leg.

And you can use a pile of cushions to build up supports for parts of the client's body. For example, supports under the prone client's ankle will relax the hamstring muscles, enabling you to work more deeply into them. A cushion under the prone client's shoulder lifts up the scapula for you to massage under it.

Use Your Own Body to Support the Client

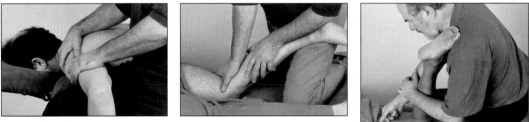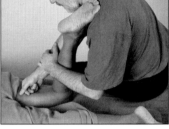

Figure 3.18: The practitioner uses their own body as a support; a), b) the practitioner's thigh, c) the practitioner's shoulder.

You can also use your own body to provide this support (see Chapter 21). For example, you can position your thigh or your bent leg as a support for parts of the client's body, or rest the client's ankle on your shoulder. (Use a small towel to keep oil off your clothing when doing these).

Backing Up Your Working Tools With the Rest of Your Body

When we first learnt to massage, many of us concentrated just on our hands in order to get the strokes 'right'. However massage is more than just using your hands. The delivery of massage strokes needs to involve your whole body (see figure 3.1), not just the part of your hand (or forearm) that is the focus of your techniques. Skilfully positioning and moving your body enables you to use your bodyweight for the power and fluidity of the massage, rather than standing still and using only the muscle power of the upper body. This gives you maximum effectiveness with minimal effort and strain.

Move Your Arm to Support Your Hand

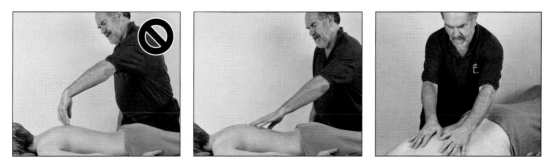

Figure 3.19: Moving your arm with the stroke; a) with stiff, unmoving hands, b), c) with hands and arms involved.

Even for strokes in which you are just using your fingers, such as small kneading and squeezing strokes, your delivery will be stiff, more awkward and tiring if you don't involve your arm in the movement. When doing squeezing movements, for example, have your hand moving a little, rather than held stiffly. Move it forward to initiate the squeeze, and pull back once you've taken hold of the tissues. And, if you are supporting it with your other hand (see figure 3.7), have your hands moving together.

Move Your Body to Support the Movements of Your Hands

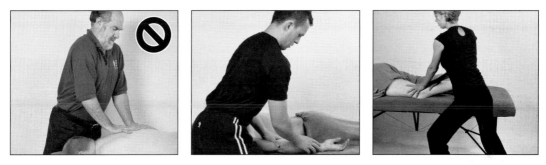

Figure 3.20: Moving your body with your hands; a) standing stiffly, b), c) swaying with effleurage strokes.

However, just moving your hands is not enough. Whenever possible, generate power and fluidity for massage strokes by swaying your body rather than standing still and just relying on your shoulder and arm muscles. Sway forward to slide your hands forward and/or apply pressure. Sway backwards for pulling. Using your body in this way, even for small movements, will enable you to keep your shoulders, arms and hands relatively relaxed. This makes it easier to monitor the client's responses. Monitor your breathing also. Breathing out as you push or lean forward will reduce the likelihood of tensing up.

Be especially attentive when you are doing small, finely focused techniques. Even after learning to massage 'with the whole body', many of us revert to stiffening up without realising it when we are just using our fingers and/or thumbs. You also need to make sure that you're not remaining rigid when doing percussion or vibration strokes (see Chapters 37 & 38) or pressure point techniques (see Chapter 35).

Even when you are seated or kneeling (see Chapters 31 & 32), you can underpin the work of your hands by swaying forward and backwards. This need only be a small sway of your trunk, but it has a very different effect from staying still and just using your arms.

Align Your Body Behind Your Working Tools

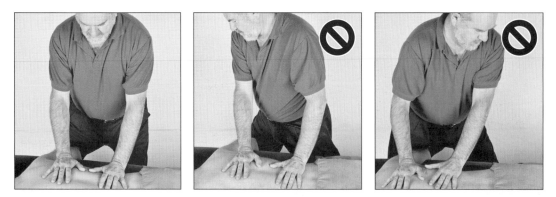

Figure 3.21: Bodyweight behind your hands for pressure; a) hips behind the hands,
b), c) hips turned away from the hands.

You can only effectively harness the power of your bodyweight when it is positioned behind your working tools (your hands or forearm). In practical terms, you can monitor this by making sure that your hips face directly towards your working tools (see figure 27.9–27.13).

If your hips are not aligned with your working tools, the power of your bodyweight will be directed elsewhere and will thus be lost to your hands/forearms – causing you to tense your arms and shoulders to provide the power. You will probably find that you are twisting your trunk as well, which increases the likelihood of strain.

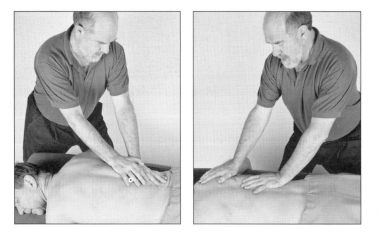

Figure 3.22: Changing position to change the direction of force applied.

Changing your orientation changes the direction in which you are able to apply pressure. If you try to change the direction of pressure without reorienting your body, you will be twisting your body and losing effectiveness. Even when you are just focusing on one area of the client's body, you need to change your position to change the direction of the force that you are applying.

Generate Power by Leaning Your Body

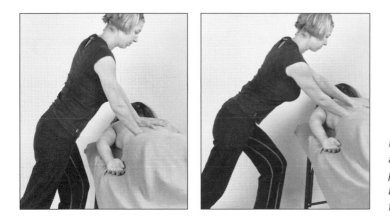

Figure 3.23: Applying pressure;
a) leaning a little for small pressure,
b) leaning forward to increase the force.

Lean towards the massage table to sustain the force in sliding strokes or to apply stationary pressure on one area. You can regulate the amount of pressure by how much you lean forward.

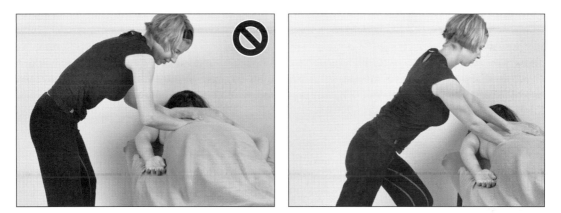

Figure 3.24: Leaning; a) bending in the lower back, b) leaning the whole trunk as a unit.

Bend your knees to initiate the movement so that you can lean with your whole trunk. If you were to lock your knees, you would have to bend over in your lower back (see figure 28.4). This would interrupt the transmission of power from your legs to your trunk and cause you to overuse your upper body. Over time it would also be likely to strain your lower back.

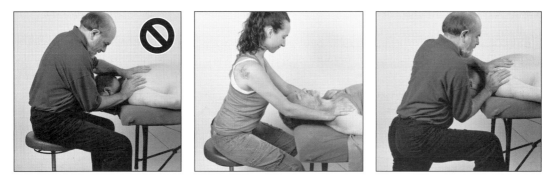

Figure 3.25: Leaning while seated and kneeling; a) crumpling the trunk, b), c) leaning with the whole trunk.

When you are seated, for example while massaging the receiver's head, you can still lean and sway to provide the power and initiate the movement of your massage strokes. Take care not to hunch over, but to lean with your whole trunk. Have your feet comfortably planted on the floor to support this (see Chapter 31).

Swaying for Sliding Movements or to Apply Pressure

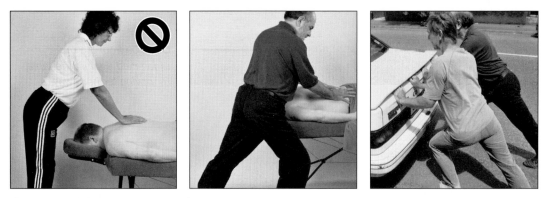

Figure 3.26: Initiating movement; a) standing still and overusing the arms and shoulders, b) swaying forward for pushing, c) pushing a car.

Sway your body for sliding strokes, rather than standing still and overusing your shoulder and arm muscles. This delivers power to your hands and fluidity to the movements. Using your body in this way enables you to keep your shoulders, arms and hands relatively relaxed, which helps you to monitor and adapt to the client's reactions.

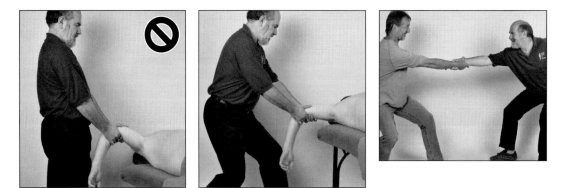

Figure 3.27: Pulling strokes and stretches; a) pulling with the upper body only, b) swaying backwards for a stretch, c) tug of war.

Sway backwards to apply stretches, pulling as people do in a tug of war team.

Do not stand against the table, as this will restrict your ability to sway and cause you to work with your upper body only. Move in closer to the table or further away from it as your massage techniques dictate.

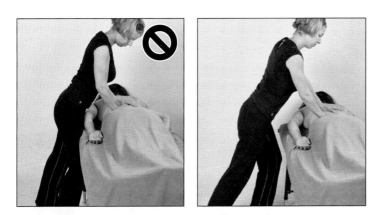

Figure 3.28:
Distance from the table;
a) jammed against the table,
b) moving further away.

Move Your Body in the Direction of the Stroke

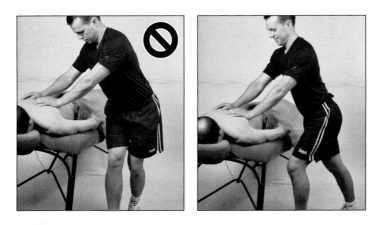

Figure 3.29: Swaying with
sliding strokes;
a) turned away,
b) facing the movement.

This follows fairly obviously. When you are doing a sliding stroke, do not just position yourself to face in the direction of the force that you are applying. Orientate yourself so that you can also move in the direction of the movement.

Use Your Body to Balance Between Pressure and Movement

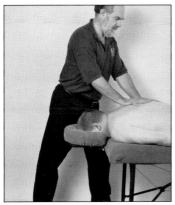 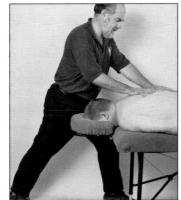

Figure 3.30: Incorporating
pressure in a sliding stroke;
a) rising up to increase the
pressure,
b) sinking lower to push
forward more.

When you are sustaining pressure in a sliding stroke, there are two components to balance – the pressure and the movement of the stroke. By rising up or sinking lower with your body, you can balance between how much pressure you are applying and how easily you can slide forward. If your weight is *above* your working hand (or forearm), you can press down firmly. Stepping back and sinking lower makes it easier to slide the stroke forward by swaying forward from your lower body. Of course, the more that you lower your body to push forward, the less pressure that you will be able to bring to bear. Moving between these two extremes enables you to regulate the balance between them according to how much of each is appropriate.

Only Apply Pressure Where You Can Involve Your Bodyweight

Therefore it is obvious that it is easy to apply pressure in some positions and more difficult or even impossible in others. Your position will determine how possible it is to apply pressure and in which direction. This is covered in more detail in Chapter 30.

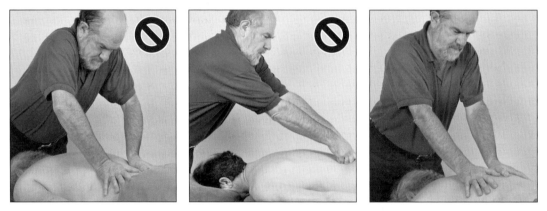

Figure 3.31: Applying pressure on the client's back from the head of the table; a), b) straining, c) reaching a comfortable distance.

For example, you can easily press down on a prone client's shoulders from the head of the massage table. However you can't effectively continue this pressure very far down the client's back. Even if you have long arms, it is difficult to get your weight above your hands to press down onto the client's lower back. Trying to do this puts pressure on your own lower back.

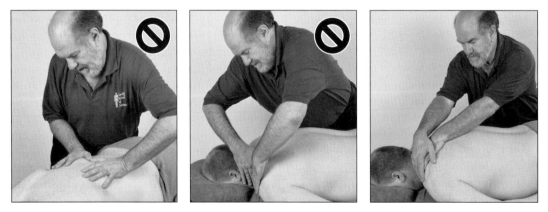

Figure 3.32: Working across the table; a), b) straining on the far side, c) working comfortably on the opposite shoulder.

It is also impossible to apply pressure on the far side of the client's back from the side of the table. And you are likely to be tensing your shoulders and putting pressure on your lower back without being effective if you try to do this.

Move From an Aligned Position to Do Stretches and Lifting Movements

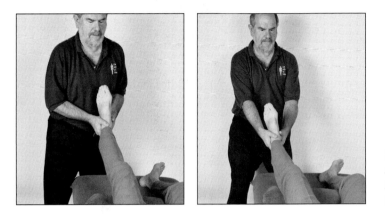

Figure 3.33: Doing stretches; a) the beginning alignment, b) the orientation of applying the stretch.

The alignment of your body is also important when you are doing a stretch, for example of the client's leg. Prepare yourself by facing the client's limb with your back in the direction in which you intend to move. Do the stretch by taking hold of the limb and moving in this direction, which usually involves stepping or 'sitting' back.

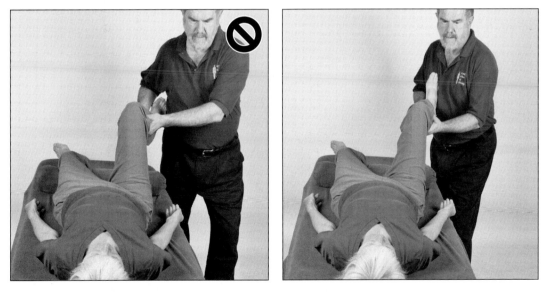

Figure 3.34: Lifting the client's leg; a) out of alignment, b) facing the direction of the lift.

Orientate yourself too for lifting a limb. Face the limb and your intended direction of movement. It would put more pressure on your body not to align yourself in this way. It would also reduce the ease and effectiveness of the movement (see Chapter 39).

Use the Client's Position to Best Advantage

Every position in which you can put the client has its advantages and limitations. You will find that you can work effectively on certain parts of the client's body when s/he is in one position that are difficult or impossible to get at in other positions. Strokes, which are very difficult when working on the floor for example, are quite feasible at the table (and vice-versa).

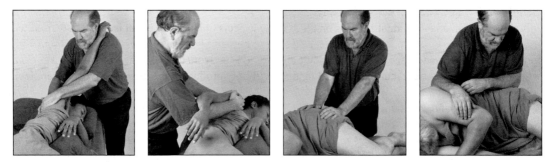

Figure 3.35: Working with the client lying on the side; a), b) working on the client's shoulder, c), d) working on the client's hip.

And, having the client lying on the side gives you 360° access to the shoulder and the hip, compared to the more restricted access when the client is prone or supine.

Integrating Your Bodyuse Skills into Massage Treatments

'Dance' Around the Massage Table/Chair

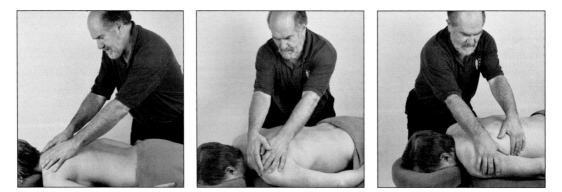

Figure 3.36: Moving around the table – the massage 'dance'.

With practice, massage practitioners can learn to blend all of the elements covered in this chapter together into their work. Skilled practitioners reposition themselves for each successive stroke, like a snooker player. As they become practiced, the massage treatment can become a more fluid continuous 'dance' in which the practitioner constantly moves appropriately both between and within strokes, like the 'dance' of a skilled tennis player (see Chapter 4).

Use Your Breathing to Help Your Pacing and Energy

Monitor your breathing. When sliding forward with pressure or applying sustained pressure, there is a temptation to unconsciously hold your breath or else to inhale sharply. Both of these breathing patterns feed into the vicious cycle of tensing the upper body to apply the pressure. It is best to exhale gently when applying pressure.

Work With Your Eyes Shut At Times
Shutting your eyes is a useful way of reducing the external stimuli, so that you can focus on the sensations of the client's responses under your fingers, palm or forearm, etc. and the feelings of how you are using your own body and your breathing. This will help you to avoid stiffening up in your sliding strokes. Even just defocusing your eyes can be useful in this way (see figure 25.2).

Blend the Art and the Science of Massage
Initially, as the massage student focuses on all of these aspects of bodyuse, it can lead to a rather stilted massage. Massage which is only based on the *science* of massage (on anatomical knowledge, the ability to identify tensions, and a technical understanding of good 'body mechanics' for applying strokes) and which is done in a 'correct' but mechanical manner will only produce a stiff massage-by-numbers feel.

Through practice and experience, a practitioner can learn the feeling of massage. This involves blending in the essential qualities that make up the *art* of massage – rhythm, fluidity, evenness, continuity and appropriate pacing. These are hard to describe in a book. You can develop them through watching demonstrations and receiving treatments which incorporate them through working with music, and through good coaching and practice.

Review

Outside of massage sessions:

- Use warming-up exercises and have winding-down time, and;
- Do things to rebalance your bodyuse.

In massage sessions:

- Take care when doing repetitive activities and/or applying pressure;
- Be guided by your own comfort;
- Respect your limits;
- Involve your whole body in massage strokes, and;
- Stay appropriately relaxed in your body.

Reduce the pressure on your 'working tools' by:

- Relaxing the non-working parts of your hand;
- Using kneading sparingly;
- Using the largest 'tools' possible;
- Using both hands together whenever you can;
- Supporting and guiding your working hand/forearm with your other hand;
- Looking after your wrists, by not having them bent when you apply pressure;
- Learning to be ambidextrous;
- Balancing pressure with stretching.

When applying pressure, get stability by supporting the client's body:

- On the massage table or chair;
- On cushions and bolsters which are on the table, or;
- On your own body.

Back up your working tools with the rest of your body by:

- Moving your arms and body with your hands;
- Aligning your body behind your working tools;
- Generating power by leaning your body;
- Swaying your body to initiate massage movements;
- Moving your body in the direction of the stroke;
- Balancing between pressure and movement in your massage strokes;
- Only applying pressure where you can involve your bodyweight;
- Moving from an aligned position to do stretches and lifting movements;
- Using the client's position to best advantage.

Integrate your bodyuse skills into massage treatments by:

- Moving around the massage table, rather than standing too long in one position;
- Using your breathing to help your pacing and energy;
- Working at times with your eyes shut;
- Blending the science with the art of massage.

CHAPTER 4

The Massage 'Dance'

This book focuses on two aspects of delivering massages – effective ways of using the 'tools' of massage (your hands, forearm and elbow etc.), and how to use your body to support them. Good body 'mechanics' involves positioning and moving your body so that you can use your bodyweight to give power and fluidity to the massage. However, just focusing on this can lead to a rather stilted massage.

Fluid movement involving the 'musical' qualities of massage – rhythm, fluidity, continuity and evenness – is another aspect of good massage. With experience, the continuous repositioning *between* and *within* strokes can become a coordinated, fluid '*dance*', like the moving '*dance*' of a skilled tennis player. The client then experiences an integrated, effective massage. The massage is also more satisfying to the practitioner instead of being a disjointed, tiring grind.

This chapter summarises the main elements that contribute to this moving 'dance':

• Integrating your whole body to deliver the massage;
• Swaying and leaning your body to give power and fluidity to your strokes;
• Aligning your body behind your working tools;
• Repositioning yourself for successive strokes;
• Moving within and between strokes in a fluid, coordinated 'dance'.

Obviously, the printed word and illustrations can only present ideas as a starting point for your own explorations. Watching and receiving massages from other people, and getting coaching from skilled practitioners and teachers are all helpful in this process. And then, of course, *practice* is essential in developing experience in applying these principles to your work.

General Principles of Good Bodyuse

When people first learn the techniques of massage, they inevitably focus intently on what they are doing for the client, often at the expense of their own bodies. However, with experience, practitioners come to appreciate that paying attention to their own bodies is also essential for working effectively and maintaining stamina. The ideal presented in this book is to develop the feeling of how to best use your body as an integral part of delivering any technique (see Chapter 29). This involves developing the connection between what you are doing with your hands and how you position and move your body to support them until this coordination becomes instinctive. The goal is to work in a way that is simultaneously *dynamic* and *relaxed* in order to apply force without strain.

Good bodyuse enables you to work with ease and fluidity. Even if you have a small build, this enables you to give a relatively firm massage when it's appropriate. It lets you work firmly *and sensitively* at the same time. You can focus on *coaching* your client to release tension (see Chapter 6), instead of gritting your teeth, tensing your body, and trying to 'force' them into relaxing. As you work more effectively with less strain and tension in your own body, your client will feel less 'attacked' and find the massage easier to respond to.

Of course it takes time to change unhelpful habits, especially as newer practices often feel strange at first and demand the use of unfamiliar muscles. However it's worth persevering in order to make your massages easier and, in the long term, to maintain your career. Bear in mind that this book only offers general guidelines for looking after your body as you massage. You need to experiment to discover how the ideas presented *work best for you* by monitoring yourself and making adjustments as you massage (see Chapter 5). Practice will enable you to learn to move your attention between the receiver and yourself so that this dual focus becomes familiar and automatic.

Over time, you will also learn to relax the areas of your body that you are not presently using, and to keep the working areas as relaxed as possible. You will also start to notice how various strokes work for you. You can then adapt them (or substitute for them) to suit your build and the size of your hands (see Chapter 9) and evolve your massage style accordingly.

Use Your Whole Body
As is emphasised throughout this book, standing still and only using your arms and hands for the massage is tiring and ineffective.

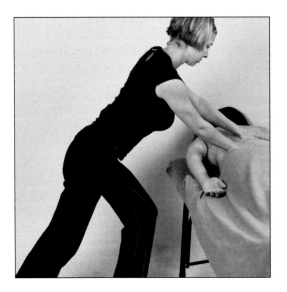

Figure 4.1: Dynamic bodyuse – overall posture – legs provide power; length in the trunk; hips behind the hands; shoulders relaxed.

Instead, position and move your whole body to generate the power and fluidity of your massage techniques. Your legs act as your base and are the source of your power, in the same way that a good golf drive or tennis swing is powered by the movement of the lower body. Bending your knees as you sway, push or pull from your legs also makes it easier to incorporate the essential massage ingredients of fluidity, continuity and evenness, and to maintain a comfortable rhythm.

When this power is then transferred up through your trunk, it takes the pressure off your upper body, which is so often overused in massage. This enables you to keep your shoulders relatively relaxed (see figure 22.13), and to deliver power through your hands (or other working tools such as your forearm or elbow) without stiffness or strain. You can then be probing, sensitive and adaptable in your hands / forearm.

Working Stances

Two stances are commonly used for leaning your weight and moving with your massage strokes.

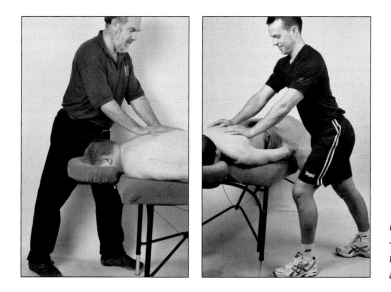

Figure 4.2: The 'lunge' stance – one foot forward – for sliding strokes and for applying pressure.

The 'lunge' stance, in which the practitioner has one foot forward and one back, is the most often used. It is the best position for applying pressure or for movements that travel forward and back. It uses the momentum of your lower body to deliver power, fluidity and evenness to your hands. When you are standing alongside the massage table or at the head of the table, you can use this stance for applying sustained pressure on one area, for effleurage strokes along the client's body, including sliding pressure strokes, and for leaning your weight behind travelling kneading strokes. At the side of the table, this stance is also used for double-handed 'wringing' strokes across the client's trunk or leg (see figure 28.16).

(Make sure that your back foot is turned towards your hands in the lunge stance, so that your lower body is not turned away from the stroke, see figure 28.20).

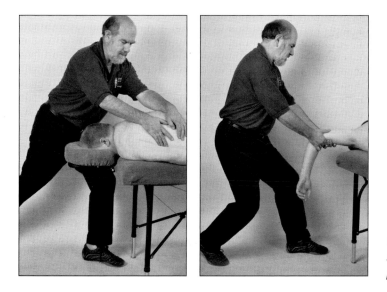

Figure 4.3: The 'lunge' stance; a) for a pulling stroke, b) for a passive stretch.

The 'lunge' stance is also useful for applying passive stretches.

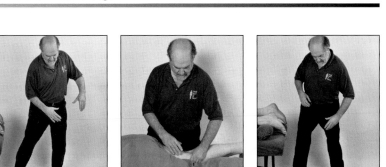

Figure 4.4: The 'horse' stance – feet side by side – swaying sideways for large kneading strokes.

In the 'horse' stance (named for the horse-rider), the massage practitioner stands with the feet side by side to face across the table. This stance is used for swaying from side to side when doing large kneading strokes such as on the client's thigh.

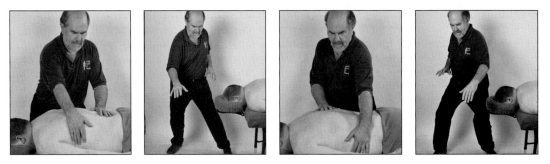

Figure 4.5: The horse stance; twisting the body for wringing strokes.

It is also used for wringing strokes in which you twist from side to side to propel each arm in turn across the client's back or leg.

Moving Your Body With Your Hands

It is important to move for each stroke so that you deliver continuous power to your hands. Your hands can then be strong, when it's appropriate, while remaining relatively relaxed and sensitive to the client's responses. Even when you are only using light pressure in sliding strokes, swaying forward and back will give evenness to the strokes.

(Many people find that positioning and swaying the body in the way that is described here can also be applied to daily activities, such as ironing, sweeping, using the vacuum cleaner, and sawing wood. It helps you to be more effective with less expenditure of energy, while taking pressure off your back. Even washing the dishes at the sink can be enhanced by softening your knees and swaying a little, rather than standing stiffly).

Lean Forward for Pressure

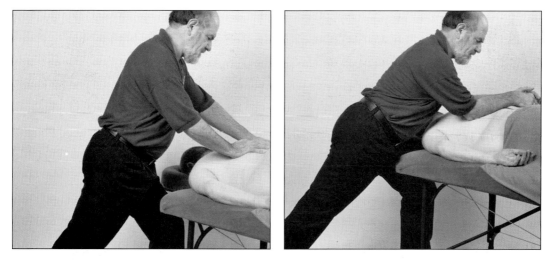

Figure 4.6: Applying pressure by leaning; a) on the hands, b) on the forearm.

To apply sustained pressure on one area, lean forward to deliver the power of your bodyweight to your working hand(s) or forearm. When using your forearm, widen your stance in order to lower your weight (see figure 18.24). This reduces the potential for straining your lower back by hunching over.

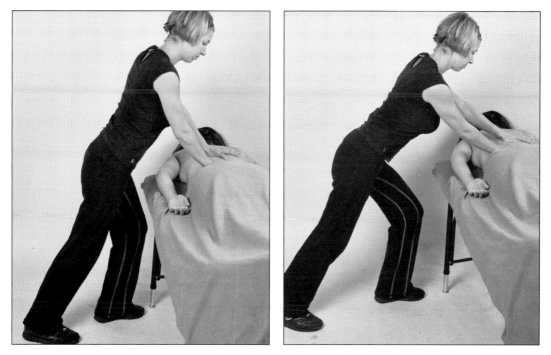

Figure 4.7: Regulating the pressure; a) leaning a little for light pressure, b) leaning more for heavy pressure.

Regulate the amount of pressure that you are applying by how much you lean. Lean forward more to deliver heavier pressure.

Sway Forward for Fluid Sliding or Pressure Movements

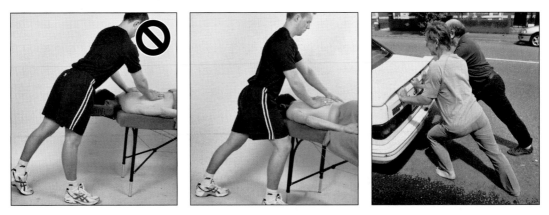

Figure 4.8: Pushing; a) not bending the front knee when pushing, b) bending the knee to push forward, c) pushing a car.

Sway your body for sliding strokes. Bend your front knee as you sway forward to keep your whole body involved. This helps you to push from your legs, in the same way that you would naturally do when pushing something large and heavy, such as a car.

If you find yourself stiffening up each time you apply pressure and/or sway forward, check out whether you are inhaling or holding your breath, both of which reflect and reinforce stiffening up in these strokes (see figure 26.2). Try a rhythmic *exhalation* with the stroke instead to stay more relaxed.

Sway Back for Pulling

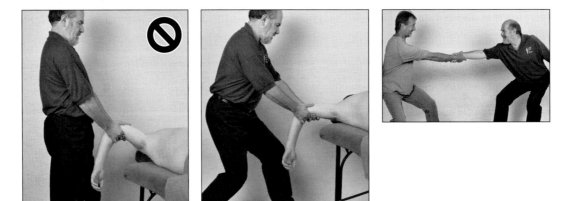

Figure 4.9: Pulling; a) standing and pulling only with the upper body, b) pulling by 'sitting' back, c) pulling a partner.

Practitioners sometimes try to do pulling stretches by standing still and merely using the upper body. However, the pull is much stronger with considerably less strain on your body if you involve your bodyweight to pull your arms by 'sitting' back. If you need to increase the power of this movement, sink your weight lower by bending your knees more as you sway back and/or step back with your back leg. (You can practice this with a partner, pulling by sitting back rather than just with your upper body, like a tug of war game for two).

Sway While Seated

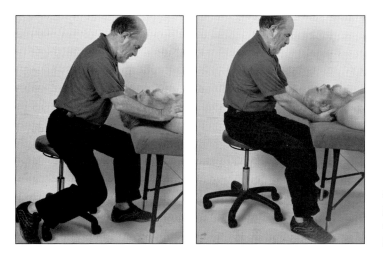

Figure 4.10: Pushing and pulling while seated; a) pressing forward, b) pulling back.

Even when you are seated you can still sway to initiate the power and movement of your massage strokes. Lean with your whole trunk rather than hunching over, even for small movements of your hands. Have your feet comfortably planted on the floor to support this movement (see figure 31.13).

Positioning Yourself and Moving

Aligning Your Body Behind Your Working Tools

Massage beginners often stand with their feet planted in the same place for a number of strokes. However, you need to reposition your body behind your working tools for each successive stroke so that you can deliver the power of your bodyweight to your hands / forearm. This applies whether you are focusing the pressure on one area or doing sliding strokes.

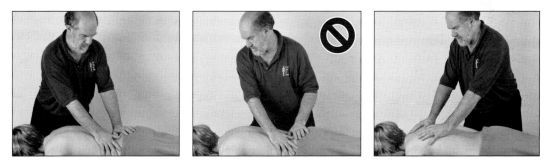

Figure 4.11: Aligning the body and hands; a) hands in front of hips, b) body twisted, c) hands in front of hips.

Have your hips *directly* behind your working tools. Face in the direction of your intended application of pressure or movement. Otherwise your upper body will be twisted, which can cause strain and will reduce the effective transmission of force.

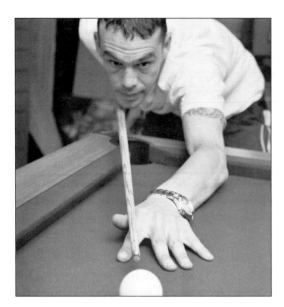

Figure 4.12: Snooker player lining up for successive shots.

Initially, novices need to practice repositioning themselves for each technique, like a snooker player lining themselves up for each successive shot. With experience, you will learn to integrate this into a coordinated, fluid '*dance*', like the moving 'dance' of a skilled tennis player (below).

Changing Position to Avoid Overreaching
So far, this chapter has focused on working from a single position for each stroke. However not all strokes can be comfortably done without changing your position. This is particularly important when trying to work from a single position would lead to overreaching, which can put pressure on your lower back and is likely to make the movement disjointed.

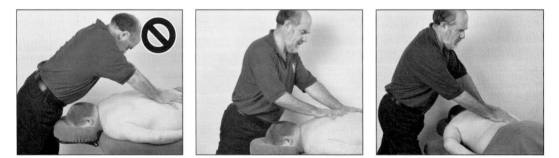

Figure 4.13: Working on the client's back; a) trying to reach too far from the end of the table, b), c) moving to the side of the table.

For example, it is easy to strain the lower back by trying to reach too far down the client's back from the top of the table. Instead, reach down each side of the client's back in turn by moving to one side of the table and then to the other.

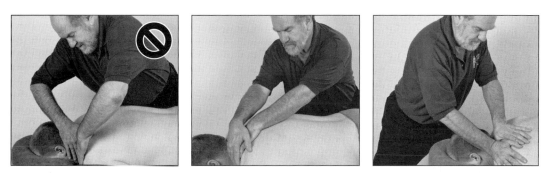

*Figure 4.14: Working on the client's shoulders; a) trying to reach too far, b) comfortable reach,
c) moving to face the shoulder.*

Do not try to reach too far from the side of the table onto the client's opposite shoulder. Do what is comfortable for you from this position, and then move to face the shoulder to apply pressure on it.

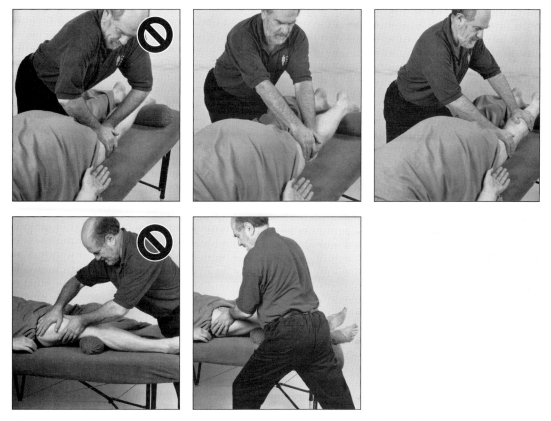

*Figure 4.15: Working on the client's legs; a) trying to reach too far, b), c) comfortable reach,
d) trying to reach too far, e) moving to an easier position.*

Similarly, do not try reaching too far across or along to work on the client's leg. Do what is comfortable and then change position to work more comfortably.

Changing Position Within Strokes

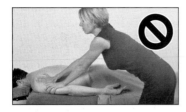

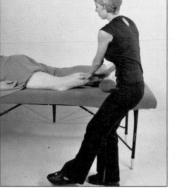

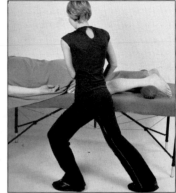

Figure 4.16:
Long effleurage strokes;
a) overreaching from a single
position, b), c) shorter strokes
from two positions.

Similarly, you may not be able to comfortably cover the full length of a tall client's arm, leg or back with a single effleurage stroke, especially if you, the practitioner, are short. There are two simple solutions to this. One is to do two (or more) short overlapping effleurage strokes, stepping up to a new position for each one.

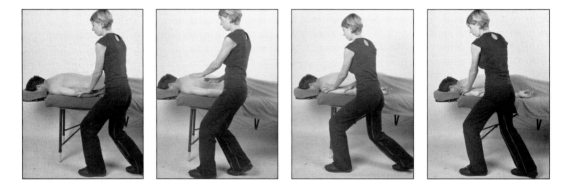

Figure 4.17: Stepping forward alongside the table for long strokes; a) starting position,
b) stepping up with the back foot, c) transferring weight onto the back foot and stepping forward,
d) new position.

Another option is to step forward alongside the table during the stroke to maintain the sweep of a single long stroke (and to step back on the return stroke). To step forward, bring your back foot up behind your front one, and then let your weight move onto your back foot as you step forward with the front one (somewhat like a waltz step).

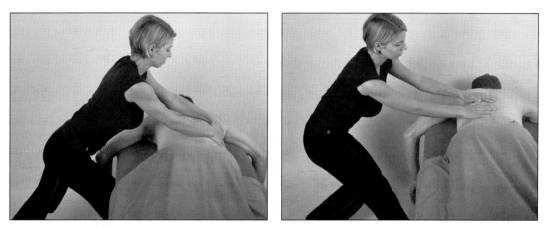

Figure 4.18: Double-handed wringing across the client's back;
a) stepping towards the side of the table, b) stepping back.

You may find that you need to move in a similar way when you are doing a double-handed wringing stroke across a client's back, stepping in towards the side of the table when you are pushing and then stepping back for pulling.

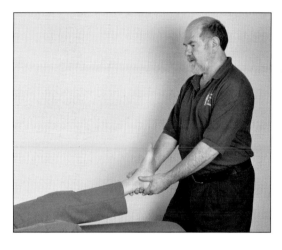

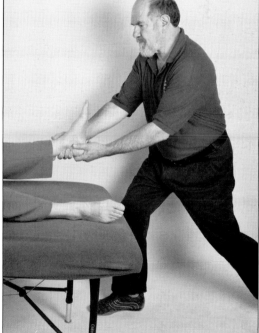

Figure 4.19: Changing position when
stretching the client's leg.

You may also find it necessary to step back when you are applying a stretch.

The Massage 'Dance'

Obviously it takes practice to learn to reposition your body smoothly for consecutive strokes so that the power of your bodyweight is consistently behind your working tools. It requires similar practice to be able to change position smoothly while maintaining a stroke. Practice stepping forward, back or sideways and turning without disruption to the massage.

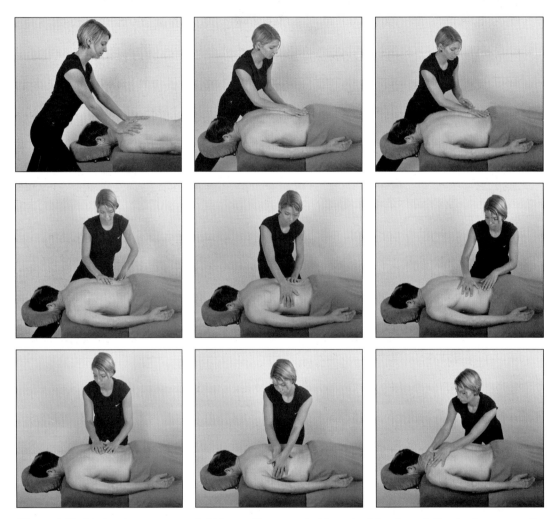

Figure 4.20: Strokes in sequence; a), b) long effleurage stroking, c), d) turning, e), f) wringing across the back, swaying sideways for large hand kneading, g), h) sweeping across the back, i) sweeping across the shoulders.

For example, you could begin a massage on the client's back in the lunge position with long effleurage strokes. Then turn to face across the table in the 'horse' stance for wringing strokes across the back. In the horse stance, you could then sway side to side for large hand-to-hand kneading strokes.

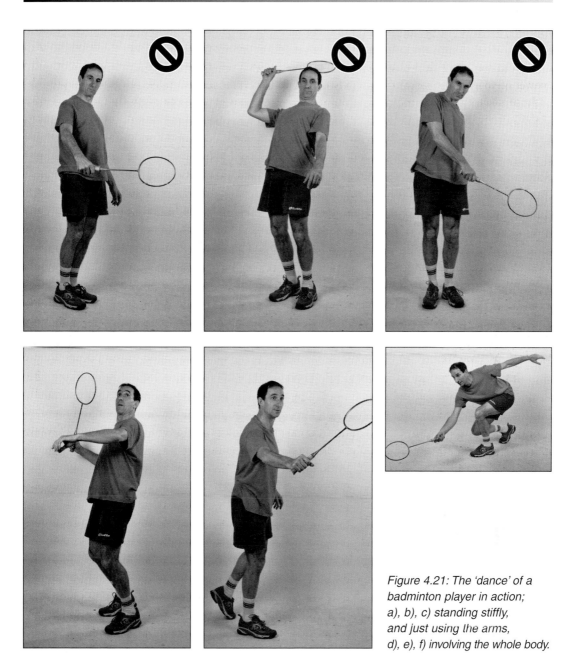

*Figure 4.21: The 'dance' of a
badminton player in action;
a), b), c) standing stiffly,
and just using the arms,
d), e), f) involving the whole body.*

When it all comes together, the massage can develop into a coordinated 'dance' around the massage table in which the practitioner moves fluidly within and between strokes, like the moving 'dance' of a skilled tennis or badminton player moving to position themselves for each consecutive hit.

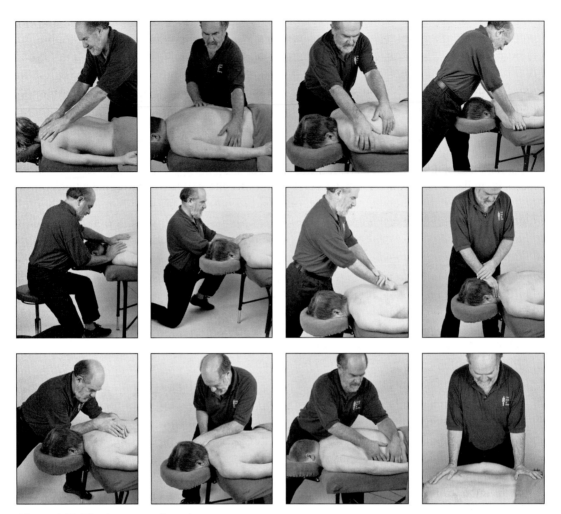

Figure 4.22: The 'massage dance'.

Being able to move fluidly from one position to another is crucial in making each massage into an integrated experience for the recipient, rather than a series of disjointed techniques. It is also more satisfying for the practitioner than slogging away at a disjointed, tiring grind. It will help you to avoid getting locked into stiff working patterns, and keep you lighter, more energised and supple in your body. It will also help you to develop your stamina for doing massage. So it is important to put in the practice necessary to master this.

Practising the 'Dance'
Initially, it is best to exaggerate the movements of the 'dance' until moving your body behind your hands becomes second nature. Coordinating this with your breath (see Chapter 26) will help you to keep the massage easy and fluid. As you develop this coordination into an organic part of your massage style, you can make the dance smaller and quieter, more like the relaxed but dynamic coordination of a practised athlete or dancer. As this way of working becomes more familiar and comfortable, you will appreciate that not only is it less tiring, but it can, in fact, be energising. Developing your general stamina will enable you to increase the number of massages that you do in a day without exhaustion or straining your body.

You may find yourself stiffening up again in the future, particularly when you are stressed or learning new strokes. If you feel this happening, deliberately exaggerate the movements associated with each stroke until you've re-established the fluid, relaxed feeling of the 'dance'.

Working in this way will enable you to be more versatile. It makes it easier to 'experiment' within massage sessions, expanding the range of techniques that you call upon and using them in a variety of ways.

Ultimately, the ideal is to be so at home with how you work, including how you use your body, that you don't have to think about it. You can 'get out of your own way', and just get on with working thoughtfully and intuitively, simultaneously moving your body and applying massage techniques. The process is similar to how skilled footballers craft their skills into instinctive 'poetry in motion'.

Review

Do not stand stiffly, hunch over, tense your shoulders, or just use your upper body for massage.

Generate the power and fluidity for applying pressure, or pushing and pulling techniques from your lower body.

Transmit this power up through your trunk so that your shoulders and arms can be relatively relaxed to deliver it to your hands.

Whether you are pushing, pressing or pulling, align your body behind your hands to use your bodyweight effectively.

Lean forward to push or to apply static pressure, bending your front knee.

Regulate the amount of pressure that you are delivering by how much you lean.

Sway your body to provide the power and fluidity for a movement.

'Sit' back for pulling strokes and stretches rather than just pulling with your upper body.

When you seated, sway forward and back, even for small hand movements.

Use the lunge stance for effleurage strokes, for applying pressure and for pulling strokes and stretches.

Use the 'horse' stance for facing across the table. Sway sideways for large kneading strokes. Twist your body for wringing strokes across the client's leg or back.

Change position within strokes to avoid overreaching and consequently straining your back.

Reposition yourself for successive strokes to get your body behind your hands.

Integrate these changes of position into a fluid, continuous 'dance' around the massage table / chair.

Exaggerate the movements of the 'dance' at first until moving your body behind your hands becomes second nature.

CHAPTER 5
Self-monitoring

The ideas presented in this book, which focus on how to do massage with the least strain on your body and with maximum efficiency and effectiveness should not be applied *rigidly*. They are intended as general guidelines to help you to find out *what works for you* – what causes you strain and what suits you.

This can only be done by paying attention to *how* you are using your body as you massage, assessing the effect on your body of doing each stroke, and adapting them to suit yourself or finding better alternatives. Bear in mind that it is the *cumulative* strains that develop over the course of doing many massages that are the main cause of problems. So monitoring how you use your body will enable you to make adjustments *before* small strains develop into major problems.

The long-term aim is for you to develop the ability to *continuously* pay attention to your own body and breathing throughout the massage. With practice, the process of self-monitoring and adjustment then becomes an automatic part of the application of every massage stroke.

Developing Self-monitoring

At first, this may seem quite demanding when there are so many other aspects of the massage session to focus on at the same time. Do not be alarmed if this initially disrupts the familiar continuity of your massage. It is important to persevere; changing habits takes attention and practice over time. Catching the early stages of strain and then changing poor practices will pay off by enabling you to maintain your career with your hands intact. It is essential for anyone who hopes to work in the field for more than a few years, and is especially important for those with small builds.

While this chapter focuses on monitoring your body *during* massage sessions, bear in mind that your body can also be affected by events in the rest of your life. In times of stress, for example, you will need to monitor that you are not unconsciously tensing your body. And you will also need to watch out for this when you are working in difficult situations or with clients who you find hard to get on with.

Distribute Your Attention Between Yourself and the Client
Learning to move your attention between your own body and the recipient takes time. Initially, you are likely to find yourself forgetting the client as you focus on your own bodyuse, and then ignoring your own body when you turn your attention back to the client. It takes practice for it to become comfortable and familiar to focus on how you are delivering techniques and, at the same time, on how the client is receiving and responding to them, while also keeping track of the other elements of the massage session. In fact, you may initially feel that you are 'cheating' the client and have disengaged from them by not giving them your complete attention all of the time. However, this is ultimately a healthier (and necessary) balance of attention in order for you to sustain your career.

Assess Techniques

Ideally, in assessing each technique, the practitioner focuses not only on the best way of applying it but also considering its role in the overall massage, whether it is essential to the massage, and if there is an easier way of creating the same effect by using a different sort of technique. In this process, your massage style may change. You may find yourself relying more on some types of techniques and using others less or even discarding them. You will hopefully find your massage becoming a living, developing process, rather than an unchanging routine. Ideally, you will also develop the perceptions that will help you to look after your body so that your career is not cut short.

Do not continue doing strokes that strain your hands or your body. Find options, such as other ways of doing the relevant techniques, or other techniques. Discuss this with colleagues who may have solutions or suggestions for alternative techniques. If you can't work out what you're doing that is contributing, or how to remedy the problem yourself, get an experienced colleague to watch you and give you suggestions or have yourself videoed. Or find a bodywork practitioner who can help you, such as a skilled sports coach, a martial arts teacher, or a practitioner of the Feldenkrais Method® or the Alexander Technique. If you can't find satisfactory alternatives, consider changing the way that you work and, if necessary, the range and type of clients that you treat.

Common Problem Areas

Practitioners most commonly strain *the base of the thumb* and *the wrist*, so watch out for early warning signs such as persistent niggles or aches. The danger signs that indicate the development of serious problems in these areas are:

- Pain that persists *after* massage sessions;
- Waking in the night with pain;
- Hypersensitivity to bumping these areas;
- Sudden weakness or loss of control of your hands, such as dropping things.

Practitioners can also develop strain in the back, especially the *lower* back. And tension can slowly build up here and in the shoulders and neck.

Responding to Problems

It's important to address these strains, as they can lead to long-term problems if they are left unchecked. As you monitor and deal with the direct strains of how you use your body in massage sessions, bear in mind that they can also be aggravated by stresses at work or in the rest of your life, so you may need to think about how to reduce these as well (see Chapter 43).

If you are experiencing pain in your hands, either sharp shooting pain or dull aching pain, look at the suggestions in Chapter 45 for ways of dealing directly with the problem. At the same time, consider how to change your way of working to reduce the pressure on these areas. Chapter 13 has information on protecting your thumbs, and Chapter 17 on looking after your wrists. Also look at Chapters 15 & 16 for ideas on using your knuckles and fist to save your thumbs, and Chapter 35 on applying pressure techniques. To further save both of these areas, find a trainer who can teach you the skilful use of your forearm and elbow (see Chapters 18 & 19).

Tension in the practitioner's shoulders, neck and the back are initially likely to produce general soreness and stiffness with restricted movement. This can be eased by receiving massage and by exercises that enhance your suppleness (see Chapter 10). Regular massage and stretching are the most effective ways of mobilising your shoulders. Back problems may need additional attention from an osteopath, chiropractor or physiotherapist. Chapter 43 has further suggestions about how to deal with back strain if it develops.

Individual Strengths and Weaknesses

Each person will have their own strengths and weaknesses to take into account according to their build, their habits, and their previous activities and injuries. You may find, for example, that you need to be careful about specific ways of using your body because of old injuries. Or you may discover that your body has been unnecessarily guarding a long healed injury. Hopefully the wide scope of this book will give each reader useful ideas to apply to their own situation.

Self-inventory Procedures

In addition to monitoring your body during massage sessions, it is useful to spend time at the beginning and end of a working day, and, if possible, between clients, to take stock of your energy and how your body is. This will help you to work out what physical and mental preparations you need for the day ahead, how to maintain and rebalance your body and your energy during the day, and what you need for winding-down after your day's work.

And, of course, developing your ability to tune in to your body in this way makes it easier to monitor your body during massage sessions. The more that you can fine-tune your sensing of your body, the more you will be able to pick up early feelings of awkwardness and strain and adjust your working practices to minimise the toll on your body.

At the Beginning of the Day

In the early years of practice, many practitioners find it useful to begin the working day with a systematic check through each part of the body and of their energy and frame of mind for the day. This is easiest if you can find some time when interruptions are unlikely and there are the least distractions, for example by arriving early at work.

Sit or lie in a comfortable position, and, as far as possible, put other concerns out of your mind. Focus your attention on your body and systematically 'scan' your way from your head to your feet and down your arms, assessing each area in turn, to sense:

* Where in your body you feel most relaxed and where you feel more tension;
* Where you feel supple and where you are stiff;
* Which parts of your body feel ready for action and which areas feel like they need more waking up;
* Areas of niggling, aching or soreness;
* Areas that you will need to be careful of during the day due to weaknesses, knocks and bruises, or injuries (old or recent).

Check in also on your overall energy:

* Whether you are in a state of high or low physical energy;
* Whether you find it easy to work or you feel tired, sluggish or drained;

and your state of mind:

* Whether you feel mentally preoccupied or able to be attentive, scattered or focused, ruffled or calm and centered, 'wound up' or relaxed, or sluggish or alert, and;
* How background events in your life are affecting you.

(Separating one's being into body, energy, mind and emotions is helpful for thinking about them, but obviously in real life, they overlap and interrelate).

This checking in may sound time consuming. However, with practice, it can be condensed into a brief routine 'scan' of your body and energy that becomes a standard part of your working day, in the way that any professional checks their equipment before, during and after the day's work. Therefore, it is useful to spend the time developing this self-assessing procedure in the early years of your practice so that it becomes instinctive to consistently monitor your body and your energy, before and after you work as well as when you are doing massages, and to make consequent adaptations to the way that you work.

Preparations That Arise Out of 'Stocktaking'

Taking stock of your body and your energy at the beginning of the day will enable you to work out what sort of physical and mental preparations you need on any given day. Depending on your needs, these could include general 'limbering up' or specific stretches for suppleness, exercises for energising, calming and centering yourself, and self-massage (see Chapter 10). This check-in will also alert you to any areas of your body that need special care during your massage sessions in order to take pressure off them.

Knowing which areas of your body are stiff at the beginning of the day can also indicate what stretches you could usefully incorporate into the massage session to help relax and loosen yourself up in these areas. For example, you can stretch your legs back, in turn, while you are applying static pressure on the client (see figure 10.3). Or you can exaggerate the movements of your shoulders to loosen them when you are doing wringing or kneading strokes.

During the Working Day

The primary focus of self-monitoring will be on how you are using your body as you massage. However, it's also useful if you can regularly take a few minutes throughout your working day, for example between clients, for a quick check in and rebalance of your body and energy. This is an opportunity to reflect on how the techniques that you've been using may have contributed to any cumulative toll on your body. This can be particularly helpful in the early years of working when you are first learning to assess the effects on your body of different techniques. In any case, it's good practice to take a minute to mentally 'let go' of the last client, and re-centre yourself in preparation for the next one.

Checking your energy between clients can also be important when your energy is fluctuating due to hormonal changes or events in the rest of your life. If you don't have time between clients, you can still take a few moments for a quick 'self-inventory' while your client is changing and getting on the table.

At the End of the Day

Check your body again at the end of a working day, for any specific discomforts, soreness or strains that you've developed (beyond the general feeling of having had a good physical workout) or that have been aggravated. These observations will highlight what sort of winding-down stretches and self-massage would be most useful to finish your working day. They will also alert you to the areas of your body that may need special attention in the future and to the working habits that may have contributed. Refer to Chapter 46 to point you towards possible causes.

It is also important to consider the bigger picture of how your body is at the end of each working week and how you are in your body over longer time periods, for example throughout your working year and over years.

Pacing Yourself

As you develop your effectiveness through self-monitoring and consequent adjustment, bear in mind that there are *limits* to every person's abilities. If you are regularly exceeding what you can easily do by consistently working beyond your comfortable physical capabilities – regularly doing too many massages in a day, or not taking enough breaks during your working day – you will begin to wear yourself out. And if you consistently work in this way, you are likely to damage your body.

Therefore it is also important to pay attention to pacing yourself during the working day to make allowances for your energy cycles. Some people are morning people and others only come to life in the afternoon or evening. Many people experience a low energy time directly after lunch or in the mid afternoon. If you start the morning fresh but are flagging later in the day, think about how to conserve your energy for this part of the day. If you are sluggish at the beginning of the day, you could ease yourself gently into your first massage session and then use the physical activity of the session to gradually move more and wake up your body. If it is in your control, you might even consider not booking clients for the low energy parts of your day.

Pacing yourself is also very important when your energy is fluctuating, for example when you are undergoing a stressful time, affected by hormonal cycles, or recovering from a cold or illness. So, as well as monitoring how you feel after each session, consider the bigger picture of how you get through each working day and each working week, and the importance of having breaks and doing other activities that nourish you. Chapter 43 looks at these factors in more detail.

Review

Using your body well needs constant attention *throughout* massage sessions, taking account of your own ease and comfort in delivering techniques.

Adapt techniques, and discard or expand your use of techniques to suit your build and comfort.

Pay particular attention to the commonly strained areas (the thumbs, fingers, wrists, shoulders and back), to your own specific weaknesses and to the areas of your body that you tend to overuse.

Take stock of your energy, your body and state of mind at the beginning of the working day, to work out what you have to offer and what physical and mental preparations you need for the day ahead.

During the day, monitor your body and make adjustments as you work. In breaks between clients, check in on your body and energy to determine how to maintain and rebalance your body and your energy during the day.

At the end of the day, check your body again to work out what you need to wind-down after your day's work, and also to reflect on techniques and working habits that may have stressed your body during the day and will therefore need attention in the future.

Monitor yourself to work out how to pace yourself in each massage session and throughout your working day, taking account of your overall workload and other events in your life.

CHAPTER 6

Feeling Your Way

Ideally a massage treatment combines effective ways of delivering the massage with the ability to *'listen'* with your hands (or forearm or elbow) to the client's responses and to adapt to them.

The way of using your body that is presented in this book is not only important for effectively delivering massage strokes with power, evenness and fluidity. It is also essential for the equally important task of *feeling* (palpating) with your hands or other massage tools. If you are standing still and tensing your shoulders and arms to generate power, your whole upper body will be stiff, which makes it more difficult for you to feel the client's build, tensions and responses.

This chapter focuses on palpating with your hands, which are the common tools of massage (see Chapters 11–16) and the most sensitive for feeling. However palpation can also be done via whichever part of your forearm or elbow that you are using (see Chapters 18 & 19).

Palpation

In the strictest medical sense, *palpation* refers to using touch to examine and identify body structures and problems. In this book, I use the word in its broader meaning, to cover *any* perceptions of the client that you gain through the medium of touch. In massage, this can include identifying:

- The thickness and pliability of the skin and variations in temperature;
- Individual muscles, bones, tendons and ligaments;
- The client's build, especially the size and proportions of the bones and muscles, and whether the musculature is soft, hard or sinewy;
- How tension is distributed through the body, and the quality of each area of tension – which can vary from the 'dynamic' tension of overuse (which can often be felt in the right upper trapezius of a right-handed client) to the 'sluggish', un-energised tension of underuse (often evident in the left shoulder of the same client) and the hardened tension of long-set postural habits (which is common, for example, in the lumbar section of the erector spinae muscles);
- The client's 'energy' which is particularly palpable in the muscles, ranging from flaccidity to a 'lived-in' or well-used quality, and;
- The client's responses that you feel during the massage in the tissues that you are working on, such as tensing against the massage when the pressure is too much, or the slow softening as you 'tease' the tissues into relaxation.

The ability to palpate these qualities develops through practice.

Massage practitioners can develop other perceptions by undertaking training in bodywork which focuses on other qualities. For example, shiatsu practitioners are concerned with the flow of energy or stuck points along the meridians of the body, and cranio-sacral therapists learn to perceive the rhythms of the cerebrospinal fluid.

Backing Up Palpation With Other Perceptions

Your ability to monitor the client will be enhanced by looking and listening for non-verbal cues, such as changes in breathing, facial expressions and signs of relaxation such as slowed down verbal responses to your requests for feedback. These can confirm and extend the perceptions gained through palpation and also provide you with extra information. For example, you may hear subtle changes in the client's breathing, such as a deep sigh of release or notice a gradual slowing down as they relax. Or you may pick up a flicker of movement at the periphery of your vision that indicates a reaction against your touch, such as tensing the jaw or a sudden holding of breath.

These can often be perceived unconsciously. You may be focusing so much on your hands, for example, that you don't realise that a 'hunch' about how to work is actually based on a perception gained through another sense. Over time, experience in trying out these educated hunches in a critical fashion (by applying them carefully and monitoring the client's responses, including getting verbal feedback if necessary) will contribute to the development of your intuition.

People who have spent time with babies or animals become accustomed to picking up and responding to non-verbal communication. If this is unfamiliar territory for you, massaging animals such as dogs or cats will quickly give you practice in this area – feeling the responses under your hands, while monitoring their breathing and level of relaxation. If they like what you are doing, they will stay for it, or even lean into your hands and go glazy-eyed. If they do not like it, they will bristle, bite you and/or run away. You can also practice pacing the rate at which you increase pressure, not pushing them too fast, but, once they've relaxed and trust you, feeling how they will tolerate a gradual increase in pressure (*see* 'good pain' and 'bad pain' below).

Feeling With Your Hands

Learning to use your hands well is a necessary step in the development of the ability to feel with them at the same time.

As You Gain Experience, Focus on Relaxing Your Hands

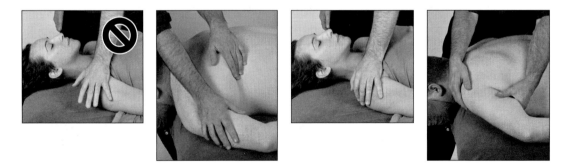

Figure 6.1: Using the hands; a) stiff working hands, b), c), d) relaxed, 'alive' hands.

Massage novices often use their hands in stiff and awkward ways as they initially struggle to master the techniques. It takes time to learn to work effectively in a coordinated way without unnecessary tension, especially if you are unaccustomed to using your hands. However, through instruction and practice, you can learn to use your hands more skilfully, more effectively and with less strain and more ease (see Chapter 11). The ideal is to work with a balance of power, ease and sensitivity.

Learning to use your bodyweight to provide the power for your hands is an essential part of saving you from tensing them in an attempt to 'muscle through'. Using warm-up exercises to relax and enliven your hands and get them supple can be an important preparation for this (see Chapter 11).

However, merely using your hands well is not enough. It needs to be allied with feeling your way as you massage. The ideal is to combine ease and sensitivity so that your hands are relaxed but not limp, active but not tense, searching but not prodding, and able to respond and adapt to the client's build and responses.

Let Your Hand 'Melt' As You Make Contact

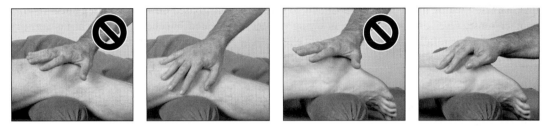

Figure 6.2: Making contact; a) stiff hand, b) relaxed, 'melting' hand, c) stiff hand, d) soft 'melting' hand.

When you place your hands on the client's body, let them relax so that they 'melt' like liquid chocolate and take on the shapes of the surface contours. Relaxing your shoulders and not holding your breath will help you to soften your hands which makes it easier to 'listen' with them and respond to any changes. If your hands are on the client's back, for example, have them resting lightly enough to be moved by the client's breathing (but not so 'wispy' as to be irritating), rather than impeding it by being heavy-handed.

This feels better for the client too. Stiff and unresponsive hands tend to invoke an instinctive wariness in the client rather than inviting them to relax. Making contact too abruptly or forcefully is likely to produce a similar reaction. For most people, it is also more acceptable to receive full palm contact rather than poking fingers. With practise, the practitioner learns to feel with the whole palm.

Let Your Hands be Moulded by the Client's Body Contours in Sliding Strokes

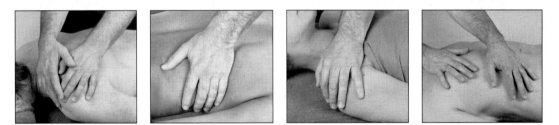

Figure 6.3: Sliding your hands over contours of the client's body.

Try to retain this relaxed quality as you glide your hands over the client's body, letting them be continuously moulded by the surface contours. If you do this with familiar effleurage strokes (with oil), this light 'skin stroking' will enable you to gain a sense of the surface texture of the skin, its temperature and energy.

Bear in mind that it is difficult to slide your hands smoothly if you are standing rigidly. Swaying your lower body provides fluidity, evenness and power (when appropriate) to your massage strokes. The more even your delivery, the easier it is to notice even small variations in the client's tissues, in the same way that driving a car at constant speed makes it easier to feel variations in the road surface under the car wheels.

Increase the Pressure Without Tensing Your Hands to Feel the Underlying Tissues

By increasing the pressure as your hands slide you will also be able to sense the thickness and density of the skin and the subcutaneous connective tissue, and something of the underlying structures, especially the bones, muscles and tendons. With practice you will be able to identify conditions such as the stringiness, softness or hardness of the muscles. You will learn to distinguish the thickness and texture of the muscle layers, and the tensions and energy in them, which indicate differences in their development and use.

These sensations can be used as a guide to how much pressure to apply. Increase it, for example, where the muscles are thickest and tightest, and decrease it where the bones are close to the surface. You will also be able to feel and adapt to reactions in the client's muscles, such as the softening of release or small flickers of tensing up if the pressure is too much or you are applying pressure too abruptly (or if you are working stiffly or jerkily). Reactions to your touch can also be due to body conditions such as ticklish or sensitive areas or to bruising.

Some strokes involve lifting your hands off and then re-establishing contact. As you remake contact, focus on reactivating the capacity for sensing through each part of your hand as you settle it back onto the client.

Don't Overuse Your Sensitive Fingertips

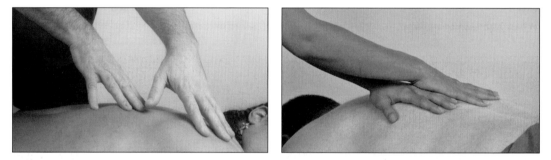

Figure 6.4: Conserving the fingers; a) using fingertips only, b) using your palm.

There is a temptation to rely solely on your fingertips for feeling your client's build and responses because of their great sensitivity. This can lead to overusing them and consequently underusing other parts of your hands. It is initially useful to palpate the area with your fingertips and then search for the same landmarks and qualities with other parts of your hands, especially the front of your fingers and your whole palm. With practice, you can train all of the areas of your hands to pick up more information. You can also palpate with the fingers of your supporting hand at the same time as you are using it to guide your working hand or forearm. Section 4 (see Chapters 18–21) contains ideas on using and simultaneously palpating with other massage tools such as your forearms, elbows, knees or feet.

Be careful also not to fall into the common tendency to stand still and stiffen your hands when focusing the massage on a small area, as this reduces your ability to feel with your hands as well as putting more pressure on them.

Relax the Non-working Parts of Your Hands

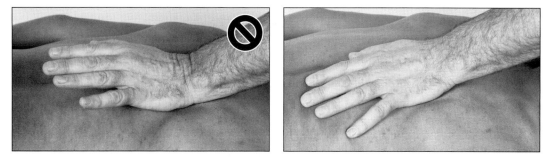

Figure 6.5: Relaxing the non-working parts of the hand; a) using the palm with stiff fingers, b) with relaxed fingers.

Whichever part of your hand that you are using, try to keep the rest of your hand relaxed. This enables you to feel more, and makes your touch more acceptable to most clients. For the same reasons, keep your hand as relaxed as possible when you are using other massage tools such as your forearm (see figure 18.10).

When Squeezing or Kneading Tissue, Use as Much of Your Digits as Possible

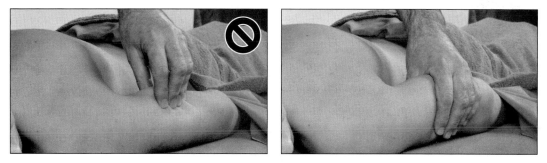

Figure 6.6: Taking hold of tissues; a) with fingers and thumb only, b) with a larger part of the hand.

Keeping your hands relaxed in this way so that you can feel as much as possible with the whole front surface is also important when you take hold of the tissues to stretch them with kneading, squeezing and wringing techniques. Use as much of your hands as you can for these strokes to conserve your fingers and thumb.

Do not stand stiffly and just use your upper body. Initiate the movements by moving your arms and keep your body aligned and moving behind your hands to deliver power and evenness. This saves you from working too hard with your hands, and thus stiffening them, which would reduce your ability to feel the client's responses.

Keep Your Hands Relaxed When You Are Applying Pressure

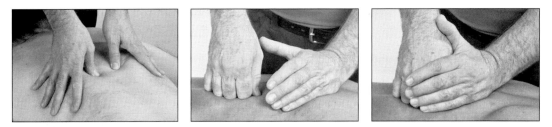

Figure 6.7: Compression strokes; a) applied with stiff hands, b) relaxed, active hands.

Try to retain the same combination of ease, effectiveness and 'listening' when you apply firm compression strokes. The deeper the pressure that you are applying, the more carefully that you need to monitor the client's responses. Instead of trying to force the tissues into submission, apply pressure that is manageable for your client, and wait for the tissues to soften (to 'melt') and allow you to move through – in the way that a hot knife gradually cuts through frozen butter. Taking time is important; if pressure strokes are done too fast, the client will tend to tense against them, and the practitioner's capacity to feel tissue reactions under his hands is reduced.

It is crucial to this process to position and sway your body to provide the power, when appropriate, so that you can keep your hands relatively relaxed. This enables you to sustain *consistent* pressure without strain, which gives the tissues time to 'trust' and accommodate to the pressure.

Support Your Thumbs When You Are Using Them to Apply Pressure

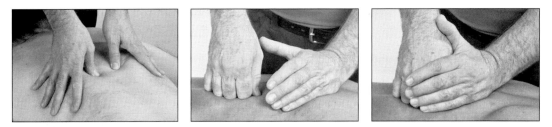

Figure 6.8: Working on pressure points; a) with unsupported thumbs (use sparingly), b), c) supporting your thumb.

Positioning yourself and leaning your bodyweight behind your working tools is also essential when you are applying pressure on one spot. Not only does this enable you to sustain the force evenly for a period of time while keeping your shoulders, arms and hands relatively relaxed, it also makes it easier for you to feel. This is especially important when you are using your thumbs, which are often strained in massage. If you find it essential to use your thumb, support it with your other hand.

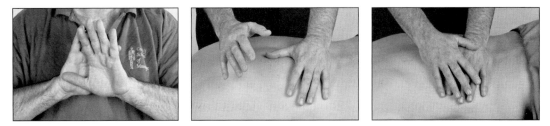

Figure 6.9: Using a 'reinforced thumb'.

Or use your thumb as a passive sensing tool 'reinforced' by your other hand which provides the control and pressure (see figure 13.15). If possible, learn to use and feel with larger areas of your hand or your elbow.

Keep Your Hands and Wrists Relaxed in Percussion Strokes

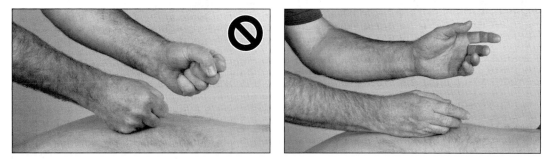

Figure 6.10: Percussion; a) with stiff hand, b) with relaxed hand.

Because the contact with the client is intermittent when you are doing percussion strokes (see Chapter 37), it is a little harder to palpate the client's structure and monitor responses. However, by this stage of the massage, you will generally have covered the area with other strokes and have a good sense of it. If not, do some more sliding strokes with pressure. Then, when you do the percussion strokes, use the moments of contact to feel for the familiar structure and the responses in the tissues. This is like making sense of a radio broadcast through static or of a scene viewed under strobe lights.

A few percussion strokes, such as pounding, require a relatively firm hand (but not rigidly tensed, see figure 36.10). However, most are best done with a relaxed hand and a relatively loose wrist, which makes monitoring easier. With practice you will learn to sense with whichever part of your hand that you are using for the percussion technique. Do not stay in one place but keep your body moving, even if it is just swaying from side to side. This will remind and help you to keep your shoulders and breathing from tightening up which, in turn, would lead you to tense your hands unnecessarily (which would reduce your ability to feel with them).

Watch for the Effects That Travel Through the Client's Body in Stretches and Body Rocking

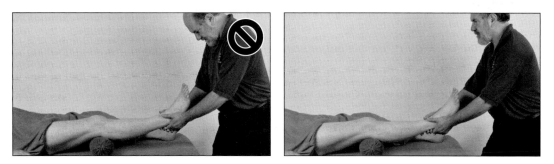

*Figure 6.11: Monitoring effects when stretching the leg; a) only watching the client's foot,
b) looking at follow through effects in the client's trunk.*

Monitoring the effects of passive stretches (see Chapter 39), and body rocking and limb rolling (see Chapter 40) is different from monitoring the responses to other types of strokes. You are seeking to track the effects in the client's body *at some distance* from the point of application. For example, when you are stretching the client's leg, you want to see the follow through effects in the hips and trunk.

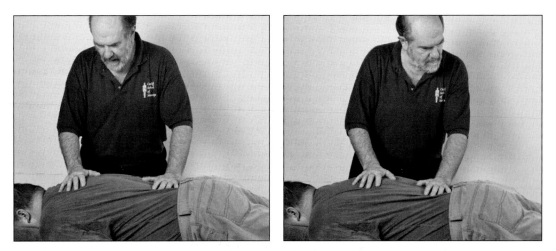

Figure 6.12: Monitoring the effects of rocking the client's body; a) watching the immediate effects, b) looking at the effects in the client's lower body.

Similarly when rolling the client's body from side to side, the practitioner is interested in the follow-through and the restrictions in the rest of the body, as well as the immediate effects. People sometimes find that *watching* rhythmical movement interferes with their ability to *feel* it through their hands. So, in order to feel more, try shutting your eyes, defocusing them or looking away at times (see figure 24.2). And, of course, positioning your body so that you can lean in and keep your hands relaxed makes it easier to sense through your hands.

Massage as a Dialogue

Even if you were originally taught an unwavering 'massage-by-numbers' routine, there are simple ways of tailoring the massage for each individual. In talking with the client, you will have gained some sense of how they want you to work, the depth of pressure that they want, and the types of massage strokes to use. This gives you a broad sense of how to put together a massage to suit each person's needs and the level of pressure that is most appropriate for them – whether to do light stroking for nurturing or to operate with greater pressure, depth and specific focus for a sportsperson, and whether to apply calming strokes for a tense or nervous client or to use energising techniques.

Involving Your Body for Power Makes it Easier to Feel the Client's Structure and Responses
This book emphasises aligning and moving your bodyweight behind your working tools to make it easy to deliver the appropriate power with fluidity and evenness. If, instead, you were to stand still, stiffen your legs and tense your shoulders or hunch over, you would be likely to be working stiffly. As well as putting strain on your body, this would reduce your ability to feel the client's responses. And the tenser that you are in your own body, the more that your attention would be occupied with the effort of how hard you are working and any associated feelings of strain in your body. So these would be the main things that you would sense. This would make it difficult to notice responses in the client's tissues, unless they are large and very obvious. You would also have less leeway to adjust your techniques.

However, if you are using your body in ways that reduce the effort (while still being effective), this will claim less of your attention. It is then easier for you to notice responses in the client's tissues – even small, subtle micro-responses – and to adapt to them. And, because your body is more relaxed, it is not such an effort to change or vary what you do. At times, it can be helpful to shut or defocus your eyes to help you to focus on the sensations under your hands. Learning to move your attention between the recipient and your own body takes time and practice (see Chapter 5).

Monitor the Client's Responses and Adapt Your Massage Techniques Accordingly
Your general sequence of strokes gives you a structure within which to feel your way. The motor-sensory 'loop' – of delivering the massage and simultaneously feeling how the client responds – enables you to adjust your massage techniques *moment-by-moment*. Even with a limited repertoire of strokes, working in this way enables you to personalise the massage treatment for each client. In fact, even within a single stroke, you can vary the part of your hand/forearm that you are using and the pressure, direction and speed of the stroke for a rich effect. You can apply a technique, feel the response and modify the technique, and then adapt to the response that this modification evokes, and so on. The massage can develop into a wordless 'dialogue' between you and the client, which is carried via your hands and backed up by asking for verbal feedback from the client when necessary.

Encourage Release, But Don't Try to Force It
You can't *make* someone relax, but you can 'tease out' the tension from his muscles by encouraging and coaching him. Of course, you can't guarantee that a client will let go of tensions, but he is more likely to do so than if you just increase the pressure regardless of his reactions. Rather than trying to *force* the client into submission, you can gradually apply more pressure when you sense that it is appropriate and within his comfort range. If you press too suddenly or too heavily, the recipient will instinctively tense against this intrusion, and, if you continue to push through this reaction, you are quite likely to bruise him. However, if you take more time, patiently maintaining the pressure, he is more likely to respond with a gradual relaxation of his muscles. And, of course, using your body well enables you to maintain an even pressure with minimal strain as you wait for the tissues to 'melt'.

Blending rhythm and fluidity into massage movements can bring out a dynamic grace in the massage practitioner's work. Incorporating these qualities into the massage is more likely to give the client a good feeling about his/her own body than if you are working stiffly or awkwardly. This is similar to the feeling that you can gain when a skilled golf professional guides you in a golf stroke or a skilled dancer leads you in a couples dance, even if you are inexperienced.

Working in this way also encourages the client to get in touch with his/her own body, which they are less likely to do if the massage session is painful and uncomfortable. So there is more of a chance for them to learn about their own tensions and what relaxation feels like. This opens up the opportunity for them to think about the habitual ways that they use their body that create stiffness and tension and about how to change these habits.

'Good Pain' and 'Bad Pain'
This is not to imply that you should just work very lightly and hesitantly for fear of provoking a negative reaction. You can work strongly as long as it remains within the client's manageable limits, which you can monitor via your hands and, if necessary, by asking. When you have established an atmosphere of trust, for example, you can work firmly within the client's comfort zone, and also try nudging the edge of this comfort zone. For the sake of longer term ease, most clients can manage short periods of 'good pain' – pressure which is challenging but remains tolerably within their comfort zone. The practitioner's job is to 'read' the responses in order to judge the manageable amount of pressure, working out when to challenge the client and when they need breathing space.

The amount of pressure that can be comfortably managed will vary from person to person. It will also be different for different areas of the body, and can vary for the same person on different occasions. However, if the pressure is too much, or is applied too suddenly or too early in the massage, or is continued for too long, the client is likely to tense against it ('bad pain'), which is counter productive. So reduce the pressure when the body responses clearly indicate that your client needs a respite from the level of pressure that you've been using.

Bear in mind that what the client says may be different than what his body indicates. He may tell you that he wants more pressure, but when you press more firmly, his body reacts against it. This needs some talking through with the client to agree on how you handle it.

Pacing Massage Sessions

Monitoring and adapting to the client's responses will determine the appropriate pacing and 'shape' of a massage session. From the client's body reactions, you will discover her tolerance for an increase of pressure, the rate of increase with which she is comfortable, how her preferred level of pressure varies in different areas of her body, and her preference for particular types of strokes and for more attention being given to particular parts of her body. You will also find that different areas of her body need different sorts of attention.

In the early years of practice, it is good to regularly check out your impressions by asking the client for verbal feedback on these points. With experience, you won't need to ask as often. Monitoring the body responses (and asking when necessary) will also enable you to work out the appropriate overall level of pressure that will satisfy your client, rather than not being firm enough to address her tensions or being too heavy handed and leaving her feeling bruised.

The Quality of Your Touch

Your working tools (your hands, forearm and elbow) carry another related responsibility, in addition to being the instruments for the interrelated activities of 'diagnosing' and delivering the massage. They are the vehicles for *communication* with clients, conveying our mood and our attitude to them.

Attitudes Are Conveyed Through the Hands

In our everyday lives, we regularly have the experience of responding instinctively to different types of touch. Whenever we shake hands, for example, we gain an impression of the person, which influences our attitude towards them. The manner in which they take your hand hints at their temperament and/or their attitude towards you. For example, the handshake of the flaccid, 'limp fish' variety generally feels like it offers you nothing. Are you having your hand crushed by an over-hearty person who is also likely to ride roughshod over any of your opinions that differ from his? Does the handshake convey disapproval, or that the person isn't really interested in you? Is it smothering or over-solicitous? Or is the handshake friendly and welcoming? Does it indicate someone at ease with herself, and able to put you at your ease?

In the professions that involve touch, the quality of contact, which is often quite unconscious, can affect the recipient in a similar way. What are your reactions, for example, when a hairdresser yanks you about in the course of washing or cutting your hair? How does it feel when an inexperienced, anxious nurse prepares to give you an injection? Or when a doctor gives you an examination as if you were an insensitive lump of meat? Or a gym instructor pushes you through exercises as if you were a malfunctioning machine that just needed more force to get it into shape? On the other hand, how does it feel when a professional adopts a good 'bedside manner' to treat you in a calm, friendly, interested way?

How You Touch / Massage Clients is Important

In massage too, it is important to consider *how* you touch your clients, and what the quality of your touch communicates? Does your way of touching encourage your clients to disengage from the massage, or to react against it? Or does it encourage them to relax and 'go' with it? Whether they are conscious of it or not, clients respond to the *quality* of your touch. You cannot expect to lull a client into relaxation, for example, if you are handling them awkwardly, disjointedly, with irritation or unnecessarily forcefully.

So our hands convey attitudes to clients, which help them to feel welcomed and relaxed or make them wary. So the quality of touch is one of the significant elements of massage. Touching clients in ways that are tentative, anxious, disjointed, disinterested, disapproving or disdainful are counterproductive. Those types of touch encourage clients to feel wary, or even to tense against our touch and to become 'resistant'.

Thus the *way* that we touch clients is as significant in creating an atmosphere of trust, and therefore encouraging relaxation, as the techniques that we use. Whether we are conscious of it or not, our working tools (our hands, etc.) convey our professional 'bedside manner' (calm, friendly, interested, and giving each client our attention) which will help put the client at ease. Or they convey our lack of ease if we are nervous, uncertain, hurried, or scattered. They also carry our attitudes, such as interest in each individual client, preoccupation with other concerns or the bored delivery of an indifferent routine.

So, it's worth working on developing a friendly, firm (when appropriate) but relaxed touch, not only to conserve our hands and to be able to feel more, but also to help put clients at their ease.

Creating a Trustworthy Atmosphere
So touching clients in a way that establishes an easy, trustworthy atmosphere, which encourages them to relax, is part of the job. This is not always easy to do, especially when you are new to massage. It takes practice and experience to reduce one's unfamiliarity/clumsiness and disjointedness. And it is harder if the client is nervous or anxious.

You can't expect clients to automatically feel relaxed with you; you have to earn their trust by your manner, and the way in which you talk to them and touch them. If you, the practitioner, develop a way of working that is simultaneously powerful, dynamic and relaxed, and incorporates the essential massage qualities of rhythm, fluidity and continuity, you can communicate these qualities via your hands to the client. This creates an easy, relaxed atmosphere for the client that encourages him to trust you. This makes it easier for him to relax and to let go of his tensions.

The way that you use your body is an essential ingredient, of course, in the way that you use your hands. Before massage novices learn to be fluent with their own bodies and the techniques, they are often hesitant and disjointed in both body and hands, which doesn't inspire confidence in the client. If you are working too hard with your upper body, you are likely to be working stiffly with your hands. If you are stiff in your body, your massage strokes are unlikely to be fluidly executed. The client is likely to pick up on this, often quite unconsciously, and is less likely to relax. Conversely, being too 'laid back' leads to sloppiness and a lack of energy.

Combining Strength and Calmness
By contrast, using your body in a way that is simultaneously relaxed and dynamic, which is the ideal of this book, opens the possibility of keeping your hands both powerful and relaxed. Working in this way creates a relaxing atmosphere.

Because the communication in a massage session is not just verbal but is physically transmitted body-to-body, a good 'bedside manner' requires you to be physically calm and centered, but with energy. So, in order to convey a quality of *calm strength*, you need to *embody* this quality in the way that you use your whole body as you massage.

This harnessing of energy in action in a centered way, which combines power and ease, is the ideal of many physical sports. You can see it in the concentrated activity of champion skaters, skiers, high divers and golfers. Balancing power and ease in a state of 'relaxed alertness' is also a goal in many Eastern martial arts such as judo, aikido and Tai Chi. In fact many Eastern massage trainings include training in yoga or martial arts of this type to help the practitioner to learn how to embody these qualities.

If embodying this combination of power and ease is unfamiliar, you might consider training in one of these disciplines, as it is a great asset to the dynamic work of massage. Once you have incorporated these qualities through practice, you can take them into massage sessions. Make sure that you focus on your hands as part of this learning, so that you learn how to direct these qualities into your hands and through them to the client, rather than impeding its passage by holding your hands stiffly.

Some people find it easy to incorporate this frame of body/mind into their work. Others find that it requires quite an effort, as it is very different from how they are in the rest of their lives. Practitioners can find that it not only enhances their approach to massage sessions, but is also an enriching experience in itself. For some practitioners, doing massage with these qualities is an essential regular grounding experience, which balances out the demands and stresses of the rest of their lives.

Review

As you do a massage, monitor the client's body responses to gauge the moment-by-moment reactions and adapt your techniques accordingly.

Back up your palpation by looking and getting verbal feedback from your client.

As you gain experience, focus on relaxing your hands so they are more available for sensitive palpation, by:

- Letting your hands 'melt' onto the client's shape as you make your initial contact;
- Letting your hands be moulded by the contours of the client's body in sliding strokes;
- Increasing the pressure to feel deeper tissues by leaning your bodyweight more to avoid tensing your hands;
- Keeping your wrists and hands relaxed in percussion strokes.

Use as much of your hands as possible for squeezing ands kneading to conserve your sensitive fingertips.

Support your thumbs when using them to apply pressure.

Don't just look at where your hands are, but watch for the effects that travel through the client's body in stretches and body rocking.

Position, lean and sway your body to make the work of your hands easier, which makes it easier to feel with them.

Encourage release in the tissues rather than trying to force it.

It can be appropriate to challenge the client with some periods of 'good (manageable) pain' in a massage session, but avoid 'bad pain' (too much pressure, too suddenly applied or for too long).

Talk with the client about differences between the pressure that he says he wants and the contrary reactions that you feel in his body.

Monitoring and adapting to the client's responses to different types of strokes, pressure and attention to each part of the body will determine the appropriate pacing and 'shape' of a massage session.

Bear in mind that *the way* that we touch the client is as significant in creating an atmosphere of trust, and therefore encouraging relaxation, as the techniques that we use.

A good 'bedside manner' requires you to be physically calm and centered, but with energy. Learning to use your body with a balance of energy and ease will help you to embody the quality of *calm strength*.

Preparations

There are a number of things to think about in preparing to do massage which will affect how you are able to work:

- Your build and aptitudes;
- The clothing that you wear and your massage equipment, and;
- The way that you prepare yourself physically and mentally for massage sessions.

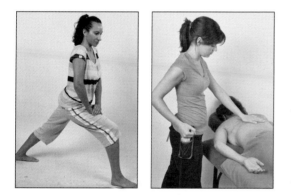

Your build and abilities will determine the clientele that you are able to work with and what you are able to do in massage sessions. Your clothing needs to be suited to dynamic physical activity. Your working environment and massage table need to be set up to suit your build. There are also pointers on using the rest of your massage equipment in ways that enable you to move around easily and use your body well.

Massage is a demanding physical activity, which also requires a concentrated focus of your attention. So it is useful to spend time at the beginning of each working day doing physical and mental preparations for the day ahead, to do mini-exercises to maintain your energy and suppleness during the working day, and to wind-down at the end of the day.

CHAPTER 7

Massage Equipment

The equipment that you use in massage affects how you work. It is important that your working environment and massage table / chair are set up to suit your build, and that you can use your equipment in a way that enables you to move around easily and use your body well. This chapter looks at the factors that will affect how you use your body when setting up and using massage tables and associated equipment, and using massage oil containers.

Later chapters cover seating for the massage practitioner (see Chapter 31) and using a portable massage chair (see Chapter 39).

The Massage Studio / Treatment Room

Before looking at the equipment in your studio, there are a few points to bear in mind about the treatment room itself:

- Try to get some natural light and fresh air into your room if possible.
- If this isn't possible, try to make time to go outside during your working day.
- Most heating, which is necessary to keep the client warm, dries out the air. So keep your room a little humid, for example by having a pot of water on or near heaters. And make sure that you drink enough water.

The Massage 'Table' / 'Couch' / 'Bench' / 'Plinth'

These names are used interchangeably for this piece of equipment. In this book I will mainly refer to the massage table.

The standard length of around 180 centimetres (6 feet) works well for most people (unless your main clientele is world standard basket players). However, your height and the length of your arms will influence your decision on the best *height* and *width* of table for you to work on. Spend some time working on different tables to find out what works best for you. When you've established the best table dimensions for yourself, adapt your strokes so that you are working in the way that's most comfortable for you, for example not trying to reach further than is comfortable across the table.

Working Whilst Seated
Sitting will give you the best control of small massage movements, for example when you are massaging the client's head. How you are able to sit and work at the head of a massage table will be affected by the structure of the table legs and the nature of your stool or chair. These are covered in detail in Chapter 31.

The Height of the Table

The height of the massage table is crucial. The table either needs to be adjustable, or to be built to suit the individual practitioner. An adjustable height table enables you to share it with someone who needs a significantly different height to work on, or for you to adjust if you have a large client or intend working with the client lying on the side, or for you to do other types of bodywork that require a different height working surface. It is ideal if you can work on an electrically or hydraulically adjustable table, so that you can change it mid-session if you need to. This also enables you to lower the table for clients who have difficulty climbing onto it because of their abilities or because you are a tall practitioner.

Avoid Working on a Table That's Too High or Too Low

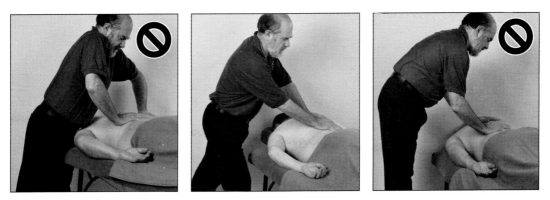

Figure 7.1: The height of the table; a) working on a table that's too high,
b) working on a table that suits the practitioner, c) working on a table that is too low.

Working on a table that's too high forces you to overuse your upper body, without being able to involve your bodyweight for power and fluid movement. If the table is too low, you are likely to hunch over. The ideal height enables you to position yourself so that you can lean your bodyweight for power and sway your body for moving strokes.

A Good Maximum Table Height is Measured by Sweeping Your Fist Along the Top of the Table

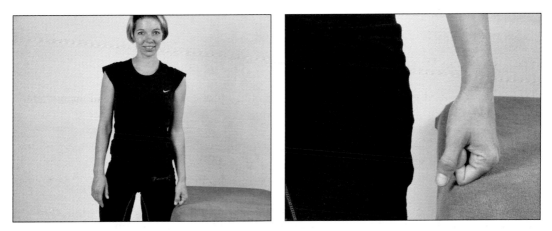

Figure 7.2: Measuring the height of the table.

To find out the best height for you to use for massage, stand next to the table, wearing your usual working footwear. Adjust the height until you can brush your lightly closed fist along the surface of the table *with your shoulder relaxed*. This gives you a good starting height to work from. Try working on the table set at this height using the bodyuse principles covered in this book, and also with it a little lower, to discover the specific height that best suits you. If you do not have a hydraulic or electric table that would enable you to adjust it mid-session, have it set low enough that you can comfortably use your bodyweight – even when you have a large person on it or when your client is lying on the side.

Try To Have a Table That's Wide Enough for Large Clients and for Applying Stretches

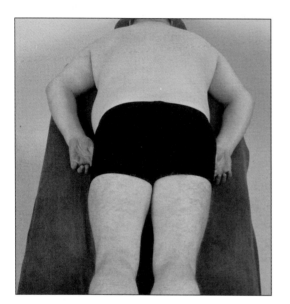

Figure 7.3: The width of the table; wide enough for a large client.

Ideally, your massage table will be wide enough for large clients to lie with their arms comfortably by their sides. Tables that are between 71 and 74 cms wide (28 to 29 inches) accommodate most people.

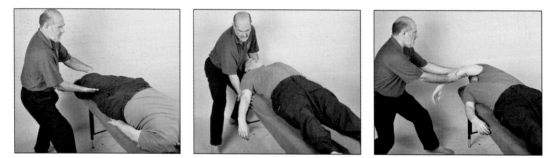

Figure 7.4: Using a wide table for applying stretches.

Practitioners who use large amounts of stretching and rhythmical techniques generally like a wide table so that they can work without fear of pushing or pulling the client off the table.

An 'Hourglass' Shaped Table Will Enable Short Practitioners to Get Closer to the Client

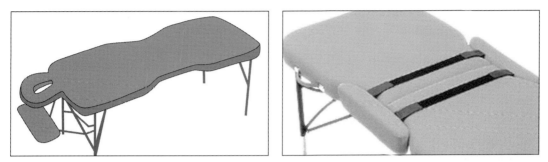

Figure 7.5: a) an hourglass shaped table, b) table with a clip-on arm rest.

However, the table width also needs to suit the practitioner's build. Practitioners with short arms need a narrower table to work on than those with a longer reach. 'Hourglass' shaped tables provide extra width for the client to comfortably rest their arms whilst giving the practitioner maximum access to the client's back. Or some narrow tables have clip-on arms rests for extra width.

The practitioner also needs to think carefully about the width if they intend to carry the table around. A wide table is harder for a short practitioner to carry without it dragging on the ground or on stairs.

On Narrow Tables, Tuck the Client's Arms Under the Drape to Stabilise Them

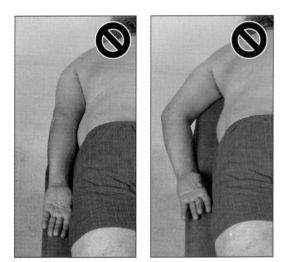

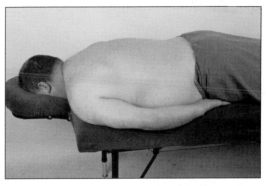

Figure 7.6: The client's arm by his side;
a) held in, b) falling off the table,
c) tucked under the client's hips.

It can be difficult to finds a comfortable place for the large client's arms, especially on narrow tables. The client has to hold it by his side otherwise it is in danger of falling off the table if he relaxes. Some people get the client to tuck his hand under his hip, but while this stabilises it, there are drawbacks. This pressure on the hand can be uncomfortable for some clients. And it is a disruption for both you and the client if you want to move his arm and then put it back in place.

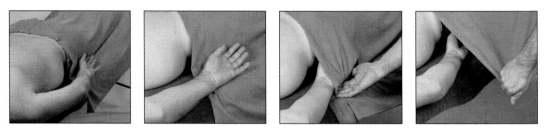

Figure 7.6 (cont.): d), e) the hand on the drape, f) tucking the hand under the drape, g) releasing the drape to move the arm.

A better option is to tuck the client's hand under the drape to stabilise his arm. Slide his hand under the drape, and push the drape in under his hand to tuck it in. Then, when you want to move his arm, it's a simple matter to pull out the edge of the drape to release his hand, and later to tuck it back in when you want to return his arm to his side.

Setting Up and Carrying Portable Tables

Practitioners who look after their bodies *during* massages can still strain their backs by not being careful when they are *setting up* or *carrying* portable massage tables.

It's Easiest for Two People to Lift a Table

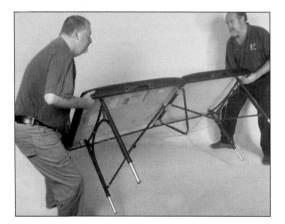

Figure 7.7: Putting portable tables up and down with two people lifting – bending the knees to avoid straining the back.

Putting a table up or down requires care to avoid straining your back. If you can get help, it is easy for two people to lift and lower it, as long as you coordinate the movement and *bend your knees* to save your backs.

Save Your Back When Lifting Up a Table on Your Own
You can raise and lower a portable table on your own, if you are careful. *Don't* bend over the table and grab it, as this will put strain on your back.

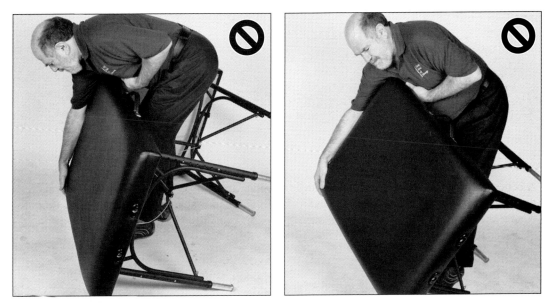

Figure 7.8: Putting a portable table up and down on your own;
a), b) reaching over and straining the back.

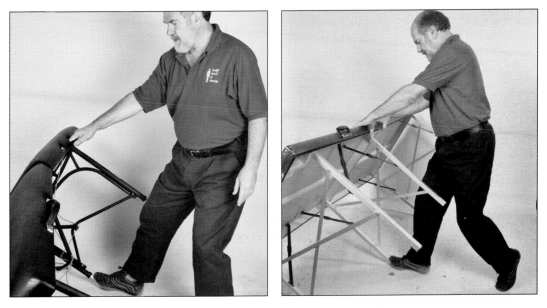

Figure 7.8 (cont.): c) foot against the end leg, d) foot against the centre leg.

Instead, place your foot against one of the far side legs and 'sit' back to pull the table towards yourself to lift it. Even then, take care of your back in this slightly twisted position. Gently lower the table by moving forward to reverse this process. If the table has a centre leg for you to put your foot against, this is easier.

Look After Your Back When Moving Portable Tables
Carrying tables can be strainful on the practitioner. If you move your table around a lot, think about getting a light table. And, if you don't have to go up stairs very often, get a trolley or a cover with wheels to save carrying the table.

Take Care of Your Back When Getting a Table in or Out of a Car

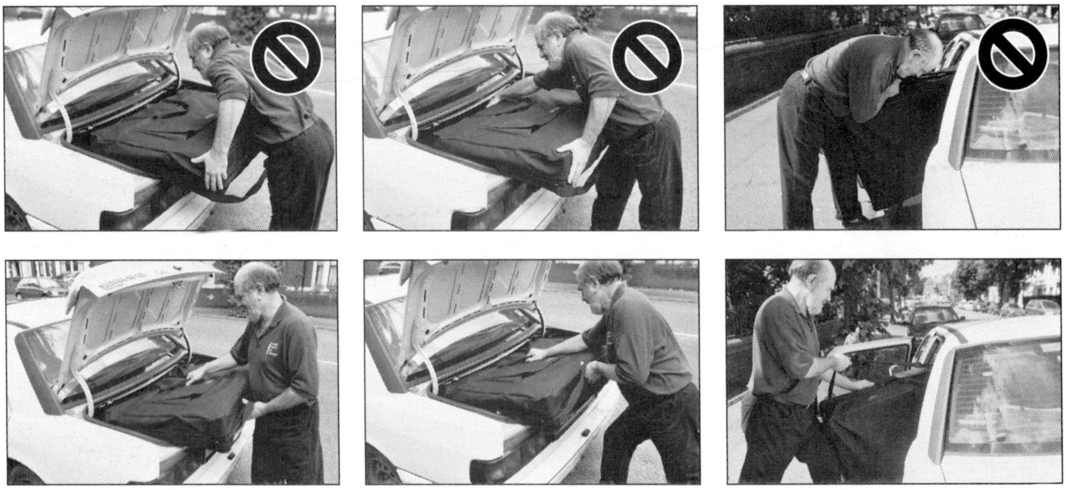

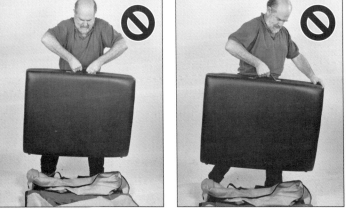

*Figure 7.9: Getting a table in and out of a car; a), b), c) potential strain on the back,
d), e), f) moving the table comfortably.*

Getting a table in and out of a car also needs care to avoid straining one's back. Side straps on the carry
case will help you to do this. Even then, be careful not to hold the table horizontally out from your body
for any length of time, especially when you are leaning forward to get it into the car. And take care not
to hunch over as you get the table in or out.

Take Care of Your Back When Getting a Table into the Table Cover

*Figure 7.10: Lifting and dropping
the table into the cover.*

Getting a table in and out of the carrying cover also needs care. Lifting the folded table to drop it into
the cover can be a strain, especially for short people.

It is much easier to tilt it onto one end and slide a section of the cover onto the exposed end. Then roll
the table back onto the cover and tilt up the other end to get the cover over this end. Then you can drop
it back centrally and zip up the cover. Reverse this process to get the table out of the cover.

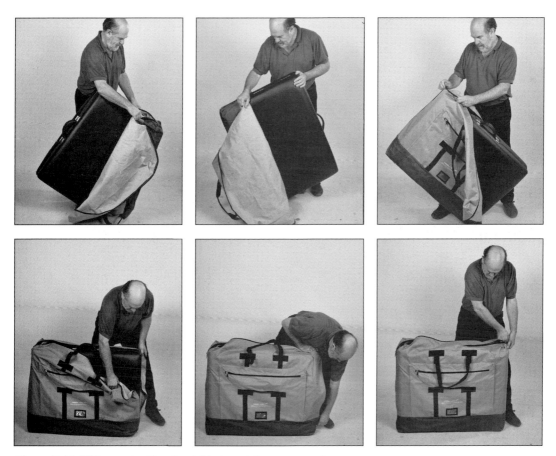

Figure 7.10: Tilting and rolling the table to get the cover on it.

Space Around the Massage Table (or Chair)

Have Enough Space Around the Table to Avoid Feeling Cramped or Hemmed in as You Work

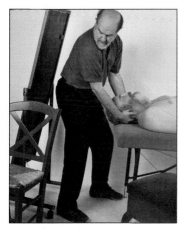

If you feel cramped or restricted as you move around the massage table (or chair), you are likely to stiffen up and work awkwardly. So it is crucial to make as much space as you can around the table (or chair) so that you can move easily and reposition yourself most effectively for each stroke. This includes stepping in close to the table for some strokes and stepping further away for others, and also changing the direction that you are facing.

If your working space precludes doing certain strokes easily, you will need to either modify those strokes or leave them out of your massage entirely. If you have less space on one side of the table, take extra care of your body on the restricted side.

Figure 7.11: Restricted space.

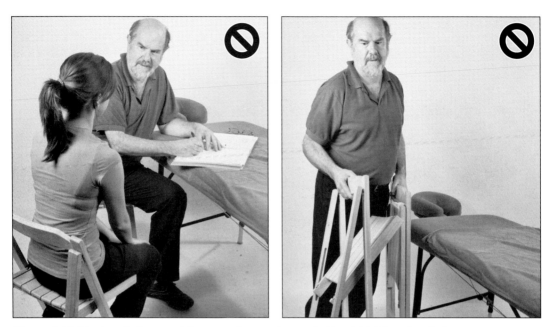

Figure 7.12: Moving chairs out of the way; a) seated consultation, b) folding the chairs away.

If you sit with the client for the consultation, you may need to move the chairs out of the room for the treatment, or have chairs that you can fold up and store out of the way.

Don't Let Your Equipment Impede Your Ability to Move Around the Table

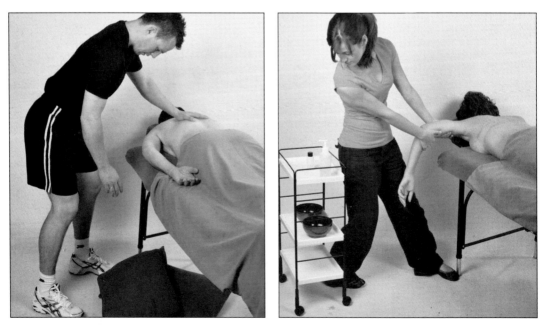

*Figure 7.13: Equipment in the way; a) spilling out from under worktable,
b) working around a trolley.*

Do not let your support equipment restrict your movement around the massage table. For example, if you store spare cushions, bolsters or linen under your table, make sure that they don't spill out into your way. Place your oil bottles/dishes where you won't restrict your movements in order to avoid them. If you use a trolley for your oils and other equipment, move it so that it doesn't get in your way as you work your way around the table.

Using Bolsters and Cushions for Support

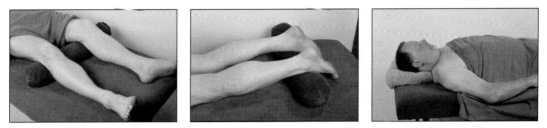

Figure 7.14: Bolsters under the legs for support; a) at the back of the client's knees, b) under the client's ankles, c) cushion under the client's head.

Cushions and bolsters are used in a range of ways for the client's comfort. For example, a bolster under the back of the supine client's knees takes pressure off their lower back. It also enables you to apply pressure around the joint without fear of overstretching or straining it. A cushion under the front of the prone client's ankles serves a similar purpose there. Many clients need a cushion under the head to lie comfortably supine. And cushions will help the client lie comfortably on the side, for example because of leg or back problems or when the client is pregnant.

Using Cushions to Support the Client Will Free You Up to Move More

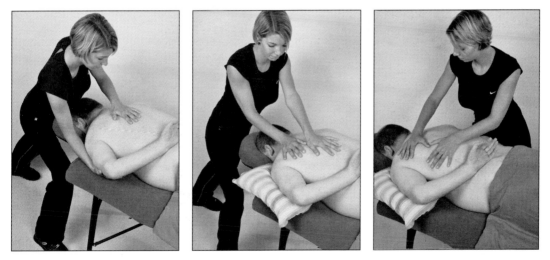

Figure 7.15: Supporting the client's shoulder; a) by hand, b), c) with cushions.

However, you can also use them to conserve your energy by providing support for the client that you would otherwise have to provide yourself. This will save you from having to hold up the client's limb, and it will enable you to move and reposition yourself around the table with both hands free to massage. You can put a cushion under the prone client's shoulder to support it, for example, so that you can work around their scapula from a range of angles.

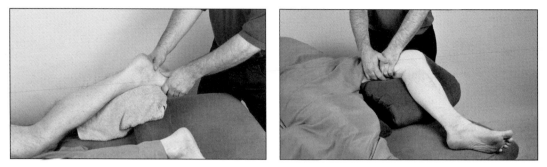

Figure 7.16: Other cushion supports; a) under the prone client's foot – for sole work,
b) under the knee – knee bent wide for adductor work.

In a similar way, you can build up cushions under the prone client's foot to do extensive work on their sole. Supports under the supine client's bent knee will enable them to relax it as you work on the adductor muscles of the inner thigh.

Use Cushions to Save Your Knees in Kneeling

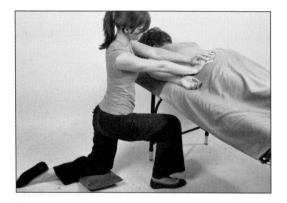

Figure 7.17: Cushions for the practitioner to kneel on.

Cushions are also very useful to save your knees when you are kneeling.

Using Massage Oil

Massage oil is generally used for working on a client on a massage table, although massage treatments can be done without oil (see Chapter 36). Massage in a portable massage chair (see Chapter 41) is generally done without oil, due to the difficulty of keeping the client adequately draped and the likelihood of dribbling oil over the structural parts of the chair. Massage with the client on a futon or mat on the floor can be done with oil, although this position makes it harder to maintain the fluidity of the massage. Many traditional styles of floor massage such as shiatsu and Thai massage are done without oil.

Oil Dispensers
When using oil, use containers that give you the greatest control over dispensing your oil, and minimise the spillage (and consequent disruption) if they are knocked over. The easiest to use are a pump dispenser bottle or a plastic squeeze bottle with a small outlet nozzle. When you put the bottle down, place it where it won't get in your way and restrict your movements.

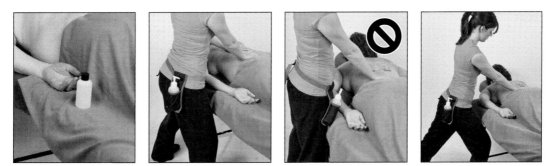

*Figure 7.18: Oil dispensers; a) squeezable oil bottle, b) pump bottle in holster,
c) holster in front gets in way, d) holster at the back out of the way.*

Some people put the squeeze bottle in their pocket, although this can stain their working clothes over time. An alternative is to use a holster, which particularly suits the pump dispenser bottle. When you are not in the act of dispensing oil, push the holster around to your back so that it doesn't get in the way of your movements.

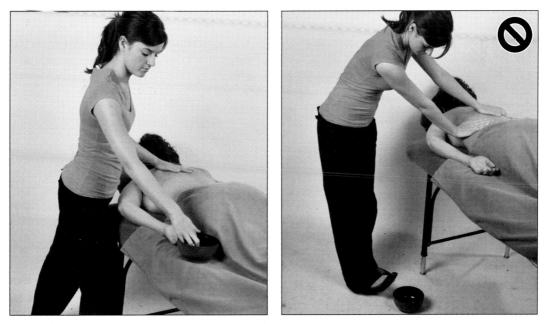

Figure 7.19: Oil dish; a) on the table – at risk of spillage, b) in the way on the floor.

Aromatherapists who mix up a different blend of oils for each client sometimes use an open dish. This requires more attention to ensure that you aren't restricting your movements to avoid knocking it over if it is on the table, or kicking it when it's on the floor. If you put the oil dish on a trolley, make sure that the trolley doesn't impede your movement around the table (see figure 7.13).

Another solution is to use a different oil bottle for each client, and then to clean them out at the end of each working day.

Try to Apply Oil Without Disrupting Your Massage

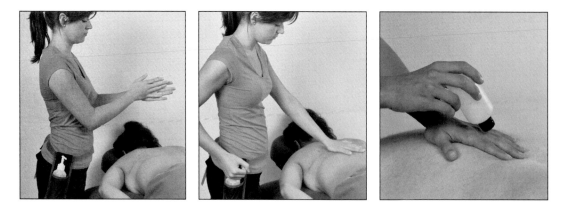

Figure 7.20: Applying oil; a) stopping to rub hands together (try to avoid),
b) small amounts from the dispensing bottle, c) pouring it onto the back of sliding hand.

Many massage novices stop the massage in order to rub the oil between their hands each time that they apply fresh oil (often to warm the oil). Using a pump bottle will enable you to apply small amounts of fresh oil directly onto the client at intervals which won't be substantial enough to make the client feel cold (i.e. to do it with minimal disruption to the massage), Another way of maintaining the continuity of the massage is to pour the oil onto the back of your moving hand and then gradually stroke it onto the client with your other hand. Have your working hand sliding slowly enough to make this easy to coordinate without jerkiness. Of course it takes practice to learn to do these oil applications smoothly and to not stop your working hand while you focus on dispensing the oil with your other hand.

Review

Make sure that the massage table is not too high for you, which would force you to overuse your upper body, or so low that you have to hunch over.

Short practitioners might consider having a narrow table, perhaps with clip-on arm side arm supports, in order to be able to get close enough to work easily on the client's back, or an 'hourglass' shaped table.

Take care of your back when putting up or taking down portable tables by putting your foot against the leg of the table and raising or lowering it, rather than reaching over to lift it.

Take care also when getting the table in or out of a car.

Make as much space as possible around the massage table so that you're not cramped or restricted in your massage.

If your space is restricted, modify or leave out strokes which you can't easily do.

Use bolsters or cushions to support the part of the client's body that you are working on in order to free you up to use both hands and to move around the massage table.

As you massage, position your oil bottle or dish where it will least restrict your movements.

Try to apply the oil with minimal disruption to your massage.

CHAPTER 8

Clothing

Your working clothes need to look professional. This chapter focuses on how they also need to serve you in dynamic physical activity, not impeding your massage strokes and enabling you to move freely. Although the information in this chapter may seem obvious, I have seen people working without taking these things into account.

Some people favour a simple uniform; others prefer neat exercise clothes or smart casual clothing.

Dress

Wear a Short-sleeved or Sleeveless Top

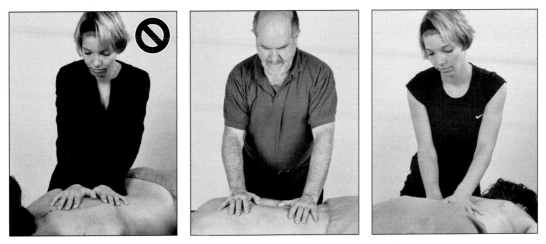

Figure 8.1: Practitioner's top; a) long-sleeved, b) short-sleeved, c) sleeveless.

Wear a short-sleeved or sleeveless top, so that there are no long or puffy sleeves to get in the way.

Tie Back Long Hair

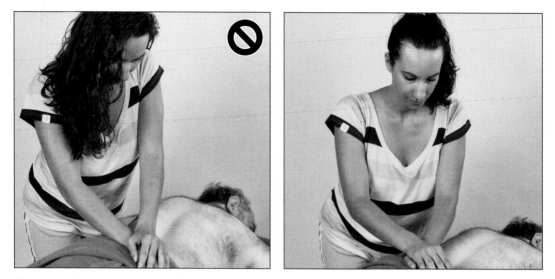

Figure 8.2: Long hair; a) loose, b) tied back.

Tie back long hair so that you do not restrict your movements, either to see and/or to keep it out of the way.

Wear Trousers or Shorts That Allow You to Move Easily

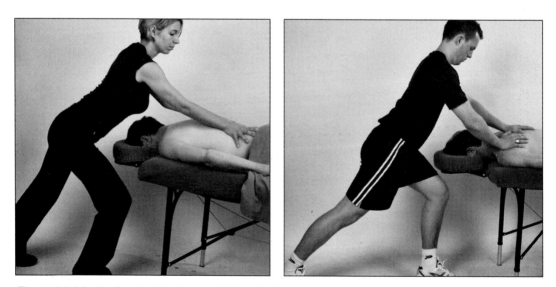

Figure 8.3: Moving freely; a) in trousers, b) in shorts.

Whatever you wear, make sure that your trousers / shorts / culottes do not restrict your ability to sway, squat and stretch as you move around the massage table or chair.

Wear Footwear That Moves With Your Feet

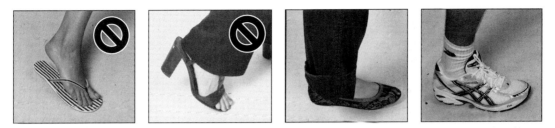

Figure 8.4: Working footwear; a) open heeled footwear, b) high heels, c) flat-soled shoes, d) trainers.

If you wear footwear while massaging, it is crucial that it moves with your feet. Wearing open heeled footwear would restrict your ease in moving around the table/chair as you make sure that they stay on your feet. And being restricted in the movements of your feet will also restrict the movement of the rest of your body.

High heels are no more appropriate for massage than for sports activities. Flat-soled footwear enables you to bend your knees and to move in the ways that are essential to massage. If you are not accustomed to wearing flat-soled footwear, you may need to regularly stretch your calf muscles and quite possibly your hamstrings too (see figure 28.41).

Glasses and Jewellery

Do Not Wear Loose Glasses
If you need to wear glasses, make sure that they don't impede the movements of your head, which in turn would restrict how much you move your body. You might try out contact lenses instead. Or, if you do wear glasses, make sure that they fit tightly to your head, or keep them in place with a sports band.

Wear a Wrist Support if Necessary

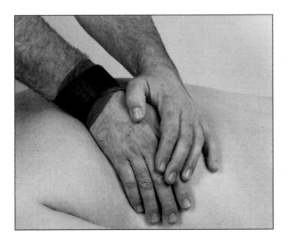

Figure 8.5: Wrist support.

If you have trouble with your wrists, you may want to wear a wrist support to protect it and to remind yourself to keep it relatively straight as you work. However, don't just rely on that support to solve the problem. Be careful about the way that you use yourself wrist in massage (see Chapter 17) and look after your wrists in everyday life and seek professional advice to help them recover (see Chapter 46).

Don't Wear a Watch

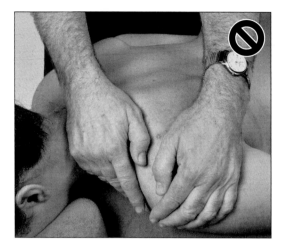

Figure 8.6: Wearing a watch restricts hand use.

Wearing jewellery restricts the way that you are able to use your hands. Remove any jewellery that you can so that it doesn't impede you. Keep your hands and arms as free as you can of rings, watches, bracelets and bangles.

If You Can't Remove Rings, Turn the Projecting Parts Away from the Client and Be Very Careful When Applying Pressure

If you wear rings that are impossible to remove, turn any projecting parts away from the client. And, wherever possible, press down with the other hand. For example, if you applying hand-on-hand pressure, place the ringless hand underneath. If you have irremovable rings on both hands, be very careful when applying pressure on thin muscle areas, such as pressing on the client's forehead.

Take Off Dangling Neck Scarves, Pendants and Long Necklaces

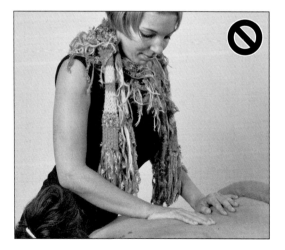

Figure 8.7: Dangling neck scarf that gets in the way.

Take off anything that dangles from your neck and would get in the way and stop you from moving freely, such as long necklaces, pendants and scarves.

Review

Wear light, loose, comfortable clothing for massage that enables you to move easily without getting hot.

Have a short-sleeved or sleeveless top, and wear trousers / shorts / culottes that allow you to move easily.

Tie back long hair.

Wear contact lenses or make sure that your glasses are firmly in place so that they don't restrict your head movements.

Wear wrist supports if you need them.

Take off your watch and hand, wrist and neck jewellery so that they don't restrict you or scratch the client.

If you can't remove rings, turn the projecting parts away from the client, and be careful when applying pressure.

Wear flat-soled shoes / trainers that will move your feet.

CHAPTER 9

The Practitioner's Build and Aptitudes

Massage is sometimes taught as if all practitioners are a standard size and can do the same strokes in the same way. The techniques taught are often best suited to the student of average size and strength, or to those whose build is most like that of the teacher. (Massage can also be taught as if all clients are the same and need the same treatment, which reinforces the teaching of a 'one-size-fits-all' massage formula). However, massage techniques don't work equally well for those with different builds.

The way that practitioners work needs to suit their build and aptitudes. This chapter looks at factors that practitioners of different builds need to keep in mind in choosing a massage table and using a range of massage techniques. It also looks at adaptations that may be necessary to accommodate to other factors in practitioners' lives.

General Factors: Build, Strength and Stamina

The Practitioner's Build

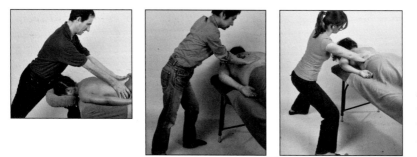

Figure 9.1: The practitioner's build; a) large, strong body and hands, b) short, stocky build, c) slender.

Practitioners with a large, strong body and hands are the least likely to encounter problems through doing massage. (This is the build of many masseurs / masseuses in the baths / saunas / hamams in North Africa and the Eastern Mediterranean). Having a stocky, robust build (which is common amongst practitioners in Eastern and Southern Europe and in China) is also likely to sustain a practitioner through years of doing massage without problems. So does the short, wiry build of many South Asian massage practitioners. Practitioners with these builds will find the information in this book helpful in reducing the wear and tear on their bodies through their work, and maintaining their energy for doing massage and ease in working.

However, practitioners with a small, light frame or a tall, slender build will need to be most vigilant throughout their careers about how they use their bodies and hands. They are the ones most at risk of straining their bodies through doing massage. While the information in this book is for everyone, it is written especially to help these people avoid damaging their bodies.

The Practitioner's Strength

While this book covers effective ways of using your body so that even those with small builds can deliver firm massages, there are *limits* to the strength that each practitioner can develop. This will be an important factor in determining the practitioner's ability to do certain strokes, the amount of pressure that they can consistently apply, and the number of clients that they can comfortably deal with in a working day and working week. The main points to bear in mind are to make sure that you are not straining your hands or your body by the particular strokes that you do, and that you are not regularly working beyond your comfortable capacity.

Ideally, the practitioner's strength will match their choice of clientele – whether to work with the light massage techniques of aromatherapy, for example, or to work in the more physically demanding area of sports massage. And if the practitioner is interested in the nurturing side of massage, s/he may decide to work in the areas of baby or geriatric massage, or with people with health or mental problems, which are generally less physically demanding (while often being more emotionally involving).

The Practitioner's Stamina

People with a background in sports, building work or general nursing are likely to be accustomed to sustained physical activity, and usually have some developed stamina. Those without this type of background need to allow time, if possible, to build up a clientele and develop this. Or they need to think about how to look after themselves if they take on a massage job or if their workload suddenly increases. Developing your massage stamina needs to be supported in a similar way to training for a sports event. Make sure that you get good rest and replenishment outside of work, eat nourishing food, and receive massages yourself (see Chapter 43).

Many people pace themselves by only doing massage part-time. Some people do quite different sorts of activities in the other part of their working life. Others do associated activities such as teaching community massage classes, exercise or flexibility classes, yoga or martial arts classes, or stress management.

Another option, particularly for those who are self-employed, is to offer treatment sessions that combine massage with other less physically demanding skills such as muscle testing, assisted stretching methods (see figures 39.29 & 39.30), flexibility coaching or personal yoga teaching, relaxation coaching and stress management, life coaching or counselling, or other 'alternative' therapies such as acupuncture or naturopathy.

The Practitioner's Height and Reach

Ideally a practitioner's equipment should be adaptable to suit your height. Your height will also influence the sort of strokes that work best for you and how you apply them, and the aspects of massage work that you need to be most careful about.

The Height and Width of the Massage Table

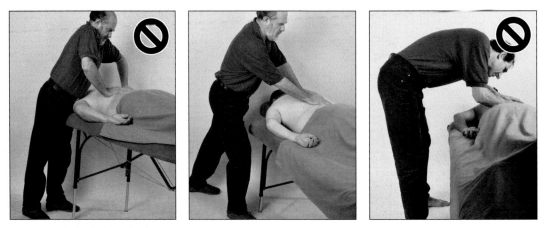

Figure 9.2: The height of the table; a) working on a table that's too high,
b) working on a table that suits the practitioner, c) working on a table that's too low.

Practitioners need a table that works for their height and the length of their arms or one that can be adjusted to suit them (see figure 9.1). Working on a table that's too high forces you to overuse your upper body, without being able to involve your bodyweight for power. A practitioner with short arms will need the table to be a little higher than someone of the same height with longer arms.

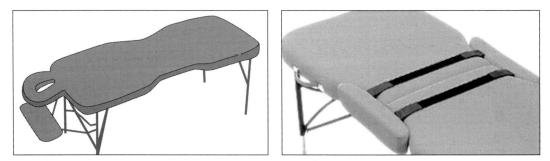

Figure 9.3: Massage table width; a) 'hourglass' shape, b) table with side clip-on arm.

Practitioners with short arms could think about using an 'hourglass' shaped table to maximise their reach across the client. Or to use a narrow table with clip-on arm rests in order to get in close while enabling the client to rest their arms comfortably.

The Height of the Massage Chair

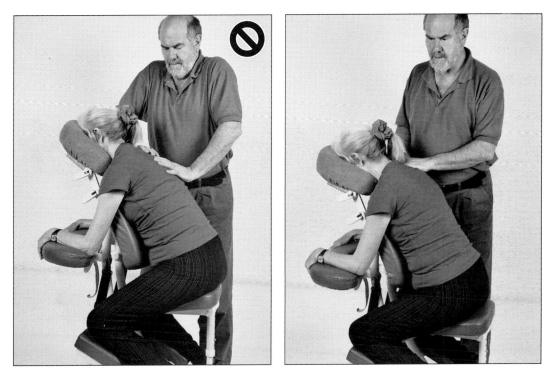

Figure 9.4: The height of the massage chair; a) chair too high for practitioner, b) comfortable height for practitioner.

Most portable massage chairs can also be adjusted to accommodate to practitioners of different heights.

The Practitioner's Reach

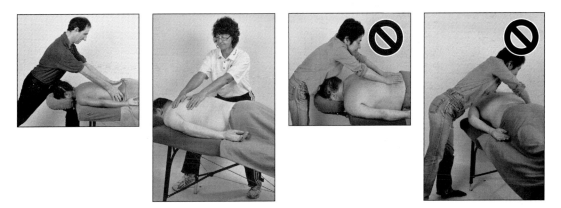

Figure 9.5: The practitioner's reach; a), b) tall practitioner reaching comfortably, c), d) short practitioner trying to reach too far.

The distance that each practitioner can comfortably reach will depend on his/her height and arm length. For example, tall practitioners can reach further down or across the client's back without strain than shorter practitioners.

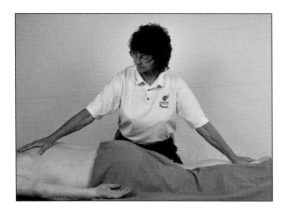

Figure 9.6: Tall practitioner reaching comfortably from one position.

Practitioners with long arms can comfortably reach a larger area and do longer continuous strokes from one position. Those with short arms need to change position more often to avoid straining their backs by trying to reach too far.

Doing Equivalent Strokes

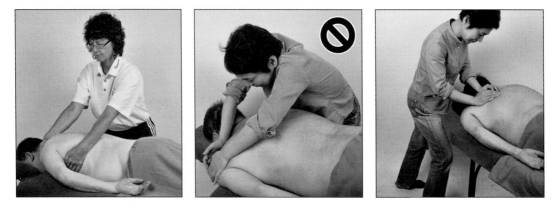

Figure 9.7: Lifting the client's shoulder; a) tall practitioner reaching across,
b) short practitioner trying to do the same stroke, c) short practitioner working on the close side.

When there is a choice, tall people may find it easier to reach across the table to do certain strokes on the far side of the client's body. Shorter people will find the equivalent strokes more comfortable and effective to do on the close side. For example, it is easiest for the shorter practitioner to work on the close side of the client's shoulders. And a short practitioner might do a pushing stroke, which a tall person would find easiest to replicate by reaching across the client and pulling.

Tall Practitioners

Looking After Your Back

Tall people need to be careful of the lower back when doing massage. The lower back muscles (the lumbar section of the erector spinae group of muscles and the quadratus lumborum) provide an important postural support for the lumbar spine. Because of the distance between the top of the pelvis and the lower ribs in tall people, these muscles have to work harder and there is more potential for problems here compared to people with a shorter, more compact build.

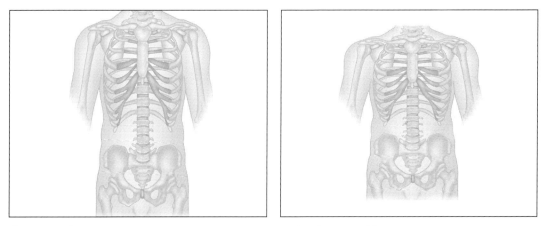

Figure 9.8: Lower back musculature; a) tall practitioner, b) short practitioner.

In addition, tall people are often accustomed to hunching over to fit into a world that is made for people shorter than themselves, which puts further pressure on the lower back. This habit can be worsened by bending over the massage table or chair to look closely at their work.

If you are tall, you will therefore need to take special care to maintain length in the back without holding it stiffly (see figure 25.14). Pilates work is very good for developing strength and stability in the lower trunk muscles. Yoga, the Alexander Technique, and the Feldenkrais Method® also offer ways of developing length and uprightness in the trunk without rigidity.

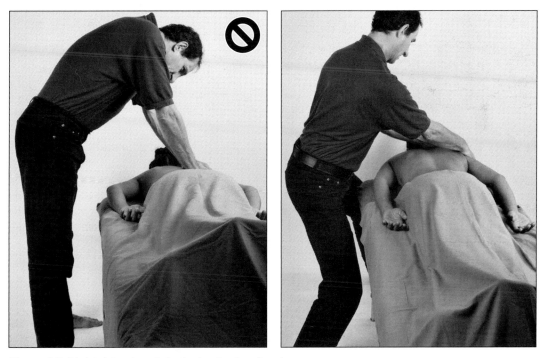

Figure 9.9: Maintaining length in the back when leaning;
a) hunching over, b) bending the knees to lean forward.

When you are leaning towards the massage table, bend your knees instead of hunching over or 'collapsing' the chest. You may also need to take up a wider stance.

Having Enough Space

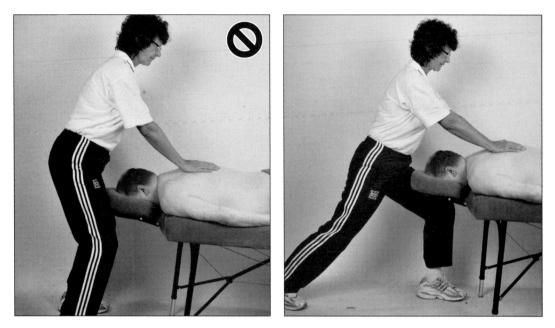

Figure 9.10: The tall practitioner working around the massage table;
a) working in a cramped way, b) taking more space.

In order to ensure that you can maintain the length of your back, have enough space around the massage table/chair to work comfortably, rather than being cramped in.

Bending Your Knees to Save Your Back When Reaching

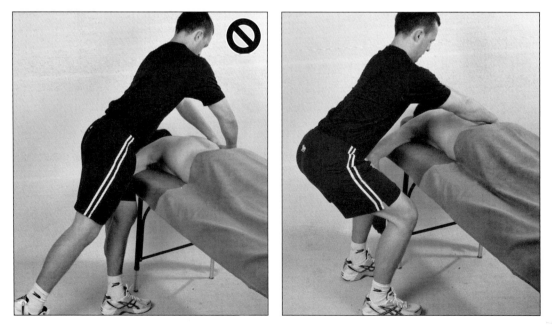

Figure 9.11: The tall practitioner reaching across the table; a) standing up and reaching too far,
b) bending the knees while reaching.

Tall people with long arms can easily reach across the table to the far side of the client's body. This also requires a small bend of the knees, instead of standing straight-legged and putting pressure on the lower back.

Moving Your Body

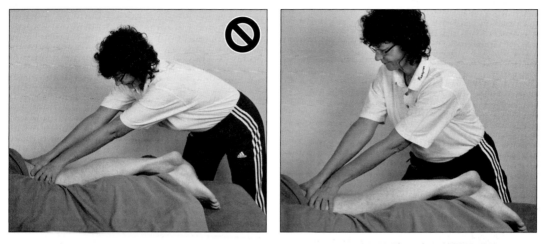

Figure 9.12: Involving the body; a) just reaching with the arms, b) swaying the body with the hands.

Because of the ease and extent of your reach if you are tall, there is a greater temptation to just use your arms for massage strokes. So tall practitioners may need to regularly remind themselves to involve their whole bodies by swaying with the movements of their hands.

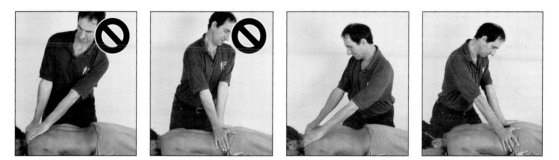

Figure 9.13: The direction of reaching; a), b) twisting the body,
c), d) changing position to stay behind the hands.

And remember to change position in order to change the direction of your massage strokes, rather than just twisting your body.

Short Practitioners

Not Working Too Hard

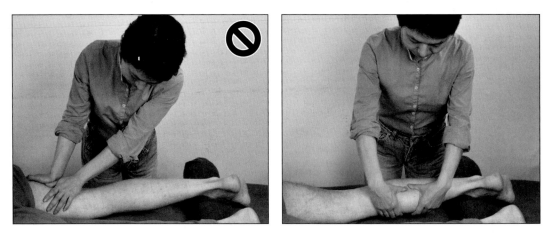

Figure 9.14: Bodyweight behind hands for power; a) not behind, b) weight behind hands.

Because of their build, short people can develop the belief that the only way that they can create force is by pushing hard. So, if you are short, bear in mind that positioning your body well and leaning forward is the way to generate effective, sustainable power without straining. You may be surprised at how much power you can comfortably deliver in this way.

However, bear in mind that there are limits. Rather than wrecking your body in an attempt to deny this, consider referring on clients who are too big and/or whose muscles are too tight for comfortable handling on a regular basis.

Avoiding Overreaching

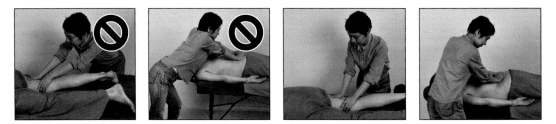

Figure 9.15: Short practitioner; a), b) trying to reach too far, c), d) moving up to avoid overreaching.

Because you cannot reach as far as a tall practitioner, you will need to move around the table/chair much more to avoid straining your back.

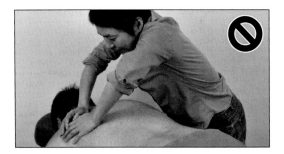

Figure 9.16: Short practitioner trying to work on the far side of the client's back.

It is particularly important to avoid trying to reach across the client's back on the far side.

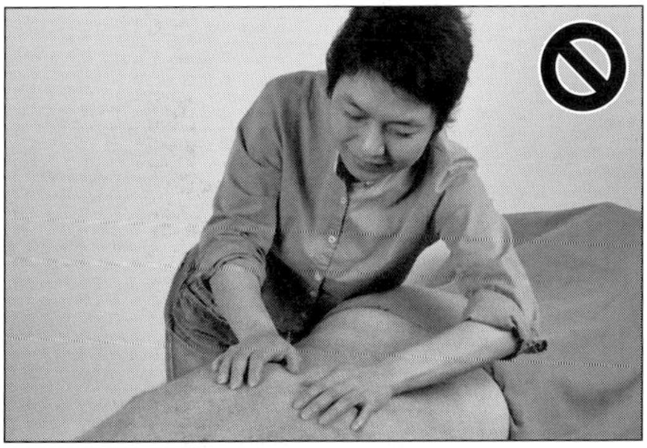

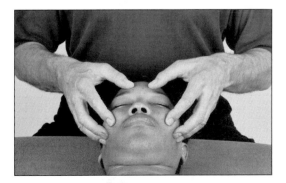

Figure 9.17: Short practitioner trying to work on both sides of the back simultaneously.

Working simultaneously on both sides of the client's back is not easy for any practitioner to do without strain. Short practitioners need to be especially wary of this. Work on the close side and then cross to the other side of the table to work on the other side of the client's back.

The Practitioner's Hands

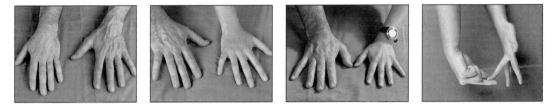

Figure 9.18: The practitioner's hands; a) average hand/large, strong hand, b) average hand/slender hand, c) average hand/small hand, d) hypermobile fingers.

The size of practitioners' hands, particularly of the thumbs and fingers, varies considerably. You need to take the size of your hands into account when deciding what types of massage strokes to use and how to apply them. Practitioners with large hands are least likely to have problems in applying pressure. Problems are much more likely to arise for those with small hands, or with long, slender and/or hypermobile thumbs and fingers.

Large Hands
Practitioners with large hands can generally apply firm pressure and knead and squeeze tight muscles without strain, even on large-framed, active clients.

Figure 9.19: Practitioners with large hands – working on the client's face.

The main problem is working sensitively on small areas such as the client's face, using the fingertips where the practitioner with small hands would need to use the whole hand.

Small Hands

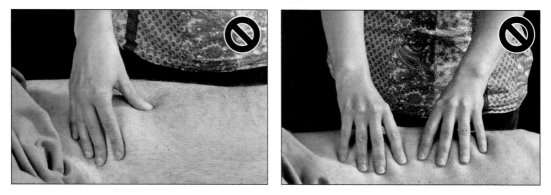

Figure 9.20: Small hands; a), b) straining on large muscles.

Practitioners with small hands can work with great finesse on small areas. However, if you have small hands, you won't find it easy to do effective kneading or squeezing on large muscles or to apply pressure on large areas without strain. It is important for you to switch to using your knuckles or fist whenever you can, and to save your hands entirely by learning to use your forearm and elbow.

Small, Slender and/or Hypermobile Digits
Using your whole body effectively for massage, as covered in this book, brings considerable power to bear through your hands. So you need to monitor carefully that you are not putting too much pressure through your hands.

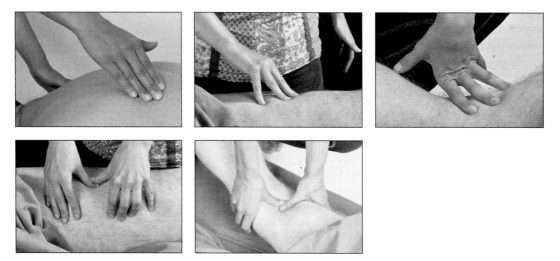

Figure 9.21: Digits at risk when applying pressure; a) long slender fingers, b) small fingers, c) hypermobile fingers, d) small thumbs working on big muscles, e) hypermobile thumbs.

Practitioners with long and slender and/or hypermobile thumbs and fingers are most at risk of straining them when applying pressure. Those with small hands also need to be careful not to strain them on clients with large, tight muscles. Pressing with the digits puts pressure on the joints, especially hypermobile digits which readily bend under pressure. (And the digits don't transfer much power when they are bent back, so it is not an effective way of applying pressure anyway).

Incidentally, these are not good builds for doing shiatsu, pressure point work or reflexology. I would encourage these people to think very carefully before embarking on a career based in these modalities. These styles of bodywork are much more suited to people with larger, stronger hands or those with short, stocky digits which are not hypermobile.

Try to reduce the amount of pressure point work that you do with your digits, and learn to use your forearm and elbow instead for firm work.

Conserving Your Fingers and Thumbs

Ways of conserving your fingers and thumbs are covered in detail in Chapters 12 & 13. These include:

- Avoiding using them too much for applying pressure;
- Not hyperextending them when applying pressure, and;
- Supporting them with your other hand.

You can also save them by:

- Switching to using your knuckles and fist whenever possible (see Chapters 15 & 16);
- Learning to use your forearm and elbow (see Chapters 18 & 19) to save your hands entirely, and;
- Reducing the amount of deep massage that you do in treatments by incorporating more stretches to release muscle tensions, including stretches that involve the client such as muscle energy techniques, etc. (see Chapter 39).

You could also consider:

- Referring large, active people on to colleagues;
- Focusing your work on the lighter, nurturing side of massage rather than on remedial, sports or structural massage, and;
- Learning complementary skills to offer clients in treatment sessions such as personal training or counselling.

Practitioners at Different Ages

Practitioners obviously need to work differently at different ages.

Young Practitioners

When you are younger, you can rely on your stamina and resilience to carry you through heavy workloads of physically demanding massages. Some people are lucky enough to have a background gained through sports or exercise classes that give them skills to use their bodies well. For a certain time, you can even get away with not doing warm-up preparations, not worrying about how you are using your body in sessions, not getting enough sleep and/or drinking too much.

However, by their thirties, many practitioners start to notice strains and the need to take more care of their bodies, both within and outside of massage sessions. By this stage, it's crucial to begin focusing on your bodyuse in treatment sessions if you going to sustain your career. It takes time and persistence to change ingrained habits and to develop consistent self-monitoring if it's new to you, so you might want to make this the primary focus of your professional development for a year or two.

Older Practitioners

This will enable you to continue to work into your forties and fifties. By then, working effectively with the least strain needs to be an instinctive part of your massage work. Of course, you will have developed a certain stamina if you have been massaging for years. However, you no longer have the resilience of youth to call upon.

Monitoring your bodyuse (see Chapter 5) needs to be one of the factors that helps you to develop your own idiosyncratic style of working that suits your build, strength, abilities and interests – developing the techniques that you have an affinity for and find least tiring, and adapting or discarding those that don't work well for you. And self-monitoring also remains important as you are more likely to have injuries and wear and tear that you need to adapt to and compensate for as the years go by.

The focus of massage work often changes as well. Many of us entering the field initially learn to do a general all-over massage or a sports 'rub down' for clients, perhaps including some special techniques on the way. However, over time, practitioners often want to go further. This may start with spending more time on a client's specific problems, and training in a wider range of techniques that give you a bigger repertoire for doing this. Having more techniques to choose from not only increases your skills and effectiveness. It also enables you to look after your body. Most importantly, you no longer have to repeat the same limited set of actions which would repeatedly stress parts of your body in particular ways (which is a major factor in most repetitive strain problems). You can use different techniques for varied effects with different clients. And you can choose the techniques that work best for you and develop them, and adapt or relinquish others or only use them with certain clients.

Developing Wider Skills

Many practitioners become interested in addressing the causes or contributing factors of client's stresses and/or offering clients ways of looking after themselves. This could include training in muscle testing techniques, and counselling, or in exercise or health guidance that you can offer clients. These avenues also reduce the amount of hands-on work that you do. Obviously it's easier to incorporate these changes if you work for yourself.

Some practitioners become involved in working with specific client groups. Working with babies, pregnant women, senior citizens, those with learning difficulties or people with particular medical problems is often less physically demanding – although it can make more emotional demands of you. The physical demands of working with particular sporting groups need to be monitored carefully.

Over the years, many practitioners also reduce the workload on their bodies through the natural changes of career development – through experience, training and practice, and following their interests. This may include cutting down on the hands-on side of massage by doing other related professional activities, or leaving it entirely. Some people find it important to pass on their knowledge and experience through coaching and teaching. Other common avenues include moving into management (for example of a spa or health centre), running health programmes (including individual coaching and exercises classes), and making and/or selling massage and related health products.

Life Factors

The practitioner's energy and their ability to apply themselves can be affected by many other factors. People may need to adapt their way of working to accommodate longstanding physical problems or recent injuries. Your energy can fluctuate depending on your workload and events in your work situation and in the rest of your life. Most people have times during the day when they function better than others. And, of course, women's energies will be affected by hormonal cycles and changes. All these need to be taken into account in determining what energy you have to offer each client, and how best to deliver it while conserving yourself.

The Practitioner's Physical Background

As mentioned earlier, the practitioner's previous background will affect their preparedness for sustained physical activity. Those with a sports background will generally have some stamina, although your sport may have made quite different demands on your body. Depending on your sporting experience, you may also have to learn to pace yourself rather than constantly pushing yourself to the limit.

On a daily basis, most practitioners find it useful to do warm-ups to prepare for the working day, or to do mini warm-ups during the day to re-energise themselves or to move back into action after desk work (see Chapter 10).

Practitioners with small hands and those who are unaccustomed to working with their hands may find it useful to do supervised workouts in the gym to build up the strength of their hands. Those with a sedentary background may initially need extra activities such as martial arts, dance, skipping, skating or skiing, in order to energise and strengthen their legs. Doing these or other types of movement to music may also be a necessary preparation in order to learn to incorporate fluidity and rhythm, which are such essential qualities for massage.

Visually Impaired and Blind Practitioners

People who are partially sighted or totally blind often stand stiffly and are stilted in their movements because the world is full of objects which they can bump into without warning. Learning to move freely (in an uncluttered space) around a massage table/chair is important for these people and can be very liberating for them.

Learning exercises for suppleness (see figures 10.1–10.13) plays an essential part in this. It is also very useful to learn to move to music and/or to do exercises that involve continuous fluid movement such as swimming, aquarobics or Tai Chi. This is especially important for those born without sight as they have often missed out on doing activities that would enable them to develop a sense of rhythmical or fluid movement. Horse riding (through *Riding for the Disabled*) can also help people gain a feeling for continuous, rhythmical movement. So can being led by a partner in a couples' dance such as salsa or a waltz or in activities such as skating.

Obviously, if you have visual restrictions, you need to have set positions for your equipment, and to make sure that anything stored under the table doesn't spill out into your way. If you have a table permanently set up and there's room underneath it, a shelf under the table is very useful.

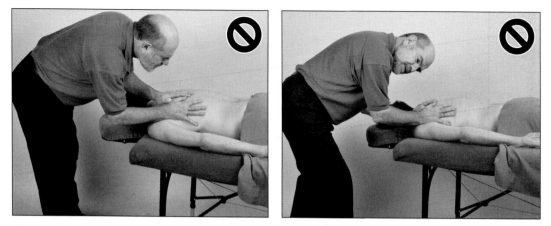

Figure 9.22: Looking; a) hunching over to see better, b) leaning closer to hear the client's responses.

If you are partially sighted, watch out for the tendency to hunch over in order to see as much as possible. Bend your knees in order to lean forward with your whole trunk.

Hearing Impaired Practitioners
Practitioners with hearing problems often rely on the client's facial expressions and maybe also lip reading to understand the client's responses. When the client is prone, these practitioners often find themselves hunching over as they strain to hear the client's feedback.

If you have restricted hearing, even if you use hearing aids, it can be useful to arrange beforehand with the client to give you simple visual signals, which create the minimum disruption for them when you ask for feedback. 'Thumbs up' and 'thumbs down' are probably the commonest gestures used for this. These can be used for gaining a variety of information, as long as you can work out a way of asking questions that only require 'yes/no' answers. These can include questions about the pressure, whether the client wants more work on an area, if they are comfortable with a stretch and whether you could take it further, and if they feel some release in their muscles.

When you and the client are used to one another, you will be able to work out ways of signalling that require less effort from the client, such as a small turning up or down of their palm. You may also develop other signals between you that help them to communicate with the least effort, disruption or shouting. This could include a specific signal that indicates that they want to get your attention, such as a particular finger movement. You might also develop a shorthand for them to indicate that they want to communicate about particular aspects of the massage. Don't overload the client with lots of signals to remember, of course, but work them out with each client when the need for communicating about a particular aspect of the massage regularly arises.

These could include signals that indicate that they are getting cold, that they want you to increase the pressure (for example by pointing down) or to lighten off (brushing away), that they feel muscles releasing (for example by letting their hand flop open), or that the pressure is too much (for example through a 'grabbing' hand gesture).

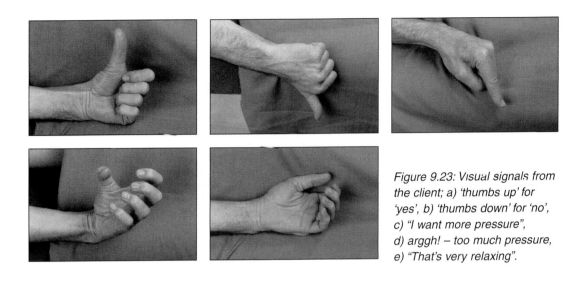

Figure 9.23: Visual signals from the client; a) 'thumbs up' for 'yes', b) 'thumbs down' for 'no', c) "I want more pressure", d) arggh! – too much pressure, e) "That's very relaxing".

The Pregnant Practitioner and the New Mother

This last section of the chapter looks at how the common experiences of pregnancy and early motherhood can affect your ability (and desire) to do massage. It is important to bear in mind that being pregnant affects each person in different ways, and can change during the pregnancy. For some women, it doesn't require much adjustment apart from compensating for the way that the growing baby affects weight bearing and posture. Other people experience big changes in their energy and comfort, which will affect how they are able to work. These will determine how much massage you can comfortably do during your pregnancy and when you feel the need to stop.

The overall intention of this section is to encourage you to listen to your body and to make decisions based on this, rather than feel that you must plough on regardless. I think it is important to emphasise this, because you may have to go against the expectations of your workplace in order to look after your own health or to safeguard the pregnancy, or because you no longer have the energy or desire to give to other people. For example, in today's work-driven culture, people are often expected to work 'as normal' until just before the birth and then be back at work very shortly afterwards. Even if you have more say about the timing of this, your work situation may require you to make decisions about winding-down, stopping work and how soon you return to work (and whether part-time or full-time) long before you have a clear idea about how the pregnancy, the birth and the new baby will affect you. If you are lucky enough to work for yourself, or have an understanding work situation, you may be able to make your decisions as you see how things develop.

Incidentally, fathers-to-be need to consider how to manage their workload so that they can support their pregnant partner, be involved in the birth and parenting, and maintain their own energy for this.

The Stages of Pregnancy
For many women, the first trimester is the most challenging as their bodies adjust to changes, low or fluctuating energy, and effects such as morning sickness. This may mean cutting back on work or even, for some people, stopping work altogether at this stage.

The middle trimester is the best for many women. Often, your body will settle into the pregnancy. And, even after a difficult first trimester, energy often returns. At this stage, many women find that they can handle a reasonable workload. However, it is important not to push yourself too much. And, if you are already getting large, take care of your back and legs in the ways described below.

There is considerable variation of comfort in the third trimester. Some women continue to feel comfortable and energised. Others experience the discomforts of hormonal side-effects such as water retention, for example in the wrists, and varicose veins. As the growing baby takes up more abdominal space, it can affect your physical energy by restricting your breathing and putting pressure on your stomach and digestive tract (causing you to eat little and often). Unless the baby is very small, there will be changes in your lower back posture, and the amount of weight that your legs have to carry. The implications of these for your bodyuse are described below. Your legs may also be affected by the baby pressing on abdominal blood vessels and nerves which feed them.

In any case, you are quite likely to be feeling more tired as you go through this stage And there will be a time when you will want to turn your energy away from other people and just focus on your family, preparing your 'nest' for the birth and looking forward to the new life.

Massaging Whilst Pregnant
The growing baby can affect your lower back posture, the weight that your legs have to support, and how close to the table that you can get. Obviously this needs more attention in the later part of your pregnancy.

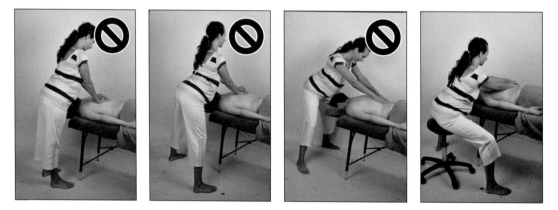

Figure 9.24: Managing the extra weight; a) standing stiff-legged, b) sway back, c) trying to reach too far, d) sitting down.

As the baby grows, you will find yourself standing and walking a little differently to accommodate the extra weight. Make sure that you don't stiffen your legs in order to support the extra weight. (This would put even more pressure on your lower back). Remember to sway your body for strokes and to move around the massage table so that you get your bodyweight behind your working hands (or forearm, etc.). Work sitting down whenever you can to take the weight off your legs (see Chapter 31).

It is also important to monitor how the extra weight is affecting your lower back. Try to keep your lower back from collapsing forward into a swaybacked shape. This would put considerable pressure on your lower back during massage treatments. Avoid the other extreme too of hunching over to try to compensate. If necessary, do exercises to maintain more length in your lower back and strengthen your lower back and abdominal muscles. A midwife may be able to give you some exercises for this, or to direct you to appropriate classes. Some yoga and Pilates teachers run special pregnancy classes, and some do individual coaching as well.

The size of your growing 'bump' will also affect how close to the table you can get. As it gets larger, take care of your back by not trying to reach so far and by moving around the table more instead.

Conserving Your Energy

As well as reducing the number of massages that you do as your pregnancy progresses, think about how you can conserve your energy within each massage session. Whenever possible, try to use easier hands-on skills in preference to more physically demanding ones. For example, you might increase the amount of pressure techniques that you apply by leaning your bodyweight and reduce the amount that you use petrissage or friction techniques. And you might get the client to assist you in stretches instead of lifting their heavy limbs yourself.

You can also try to reduce the hands-on element of treatments (with the client's agreement). For example, you might spend more time guiding clients through exercises or talking them through relaxation procedures. Or you might call on other skills that you have, such as muscle testing or counselling. This is obviously easier to negotiate if you work for yourself.

Cutting Down and Stopping Work

You will need to monitor your energy carefully, so that you can sustain it. This will determine how many massages that you feel you are able to do. You might also begin to refer on more of your large clients and/or those with the tightest muscles as your pregnancy progresses.

It is essential that you don't jeopardise the pregnancy or your own health. This may mean cutting down (or even stopping) earlier in the pregnancy than you had expected.

In any case, there will be a time in the later stage of your pregnancy when your physical energy for doing massage is likely to reduce and you don't have much attention to give other people.

It is important that *you* decide as far as possible when to start winding-down your work, the pace of doing this, and when you need to stop.

Complications in the Pregnancy

Difficulties in the pregnancy can potentially affect your health and energy and/or the safety of the pregnancy and the growing baby. You will need to give these time and attention. You may need to cut down on your massage work to accommodate to them.

Three other events – miscarriages, voluntary terminations and stillbirths – also need time for physical and emotional adjustment. You will probably need some time out from massage work for this.

After the Birth

How soon you consider massaging again will depend on many factors. Some people want to stay at home as long as they can to enjoy their new baby, especially with a first baby. Others soon miss the stimulation of social contact and the routines and the physical activity of work. The support (both emotional and practical childminding) that you have from a partner (or not), and from family and friends will also affect your energy for work. And obviously your finances will affect decisions about when to start work again.

As far as you are able, try not to return to work until you feel ready to engage with the outside world again. This is often longer with a first baby, as you and your family have to make bigger adjustments to the parenting role. And, of course, in addition to the factors mentioned above, it will depend on the baby's temperament and how your relationship with the baby develops.

When you do start back to work, monitor your energy carefully. If possible, start part-time so that you can ration your energy and redevelop your stamina.

For some people, this is a time to reflect on their work, and perhaps to consider a change of emphasis or even a change of career.

Review

The practitioner's way of working needs to suit their build and aptitudes.

Choose a clientele that you can handle without working beyond your comfortable capacity.

The massage table and massage chair need to be set up to suit the practitioner's height and the length of their arms.

Practitioners with short arms may find it best to use an 'hourglass' shaped table, or a narrow table with clip-on arm rests.

The distance that each practitioner can comfortably reach will depend on their height and arm length.

Practitioners with long arms can reach a larger area and do longer continuous strokes from one position. Those with short arms are often better at delivering concentrated pressure.

Tall people will find it easier to reach across the table, while it is easier for the shorter practitioner to work on the close side of the client.

Tall practitioners need to:

- Be careful of the lower back when doing massage, by keeping the back 'straight' (and supple) and bending from the knees;
- Avoid hunching over;
- Avoid standing stiffly to reach across the table;
- Give themselves enough space to work comfortably around the table, rather than cramping themselves in, and;
- Be sure that they are involving their whole body, and not just relying on their reach.

Short practitioners need to:

- Make sure that they are not tensing up to push instead of positioning their body well and leaning their bodyweight forward;
- Move around the table to avoid overreaching;
- Work on the close side of the client rather than trying to reach across;
- Step up alongside the table during a long effleurage stroke rather than trying to do it all from one position;
- Refer on clients who they can't comfortably handle.

Practitioners most at risk of straining their hands are those with long, slender fingers and/or hypermobile thumbs and fingers. They should avoid:

- Putting too much pressure through them;
- Bending them back in the process, or;
- Doing too many thumb or finger pressure techniques.

Use the knuckles or the heels or the backs of the hands instead, or learn to use the forearm and elbow.

Practitioners with large hands are least likely to have problems in applying pressure. They may only be able to use two or three fingertips when working on small areas.

People with small hands need to be wary of overusing and straining them.

You need to monitor your physical energy and your ability to apply yourself in relation to how you are affected by:

- Injuries or physical problems;
- Your workload;
- Events in your work situation and in the rest of your life;
- Your daily energy fluctuations;
- Hormonal cycles.

Practitioners with a sporting background will have stamina. They may need to learn to pace themselves.

Those with a sedentary background may need to undertake specific exercises and/or gym work to develop stamina, energise and martial arts, skating, etc. to strengthen their legs in action.

Blind and partially sighted practitioners may need to learn to move fluidly, and to avoid hunching over in order to see as much as possible.

Practitioners with hearing problems can organise to get feedback through hand gestures from clients in order to avoid hunching over to hear the client's comments.

Pregnant practitioners need to look after their backs when massaging, by avoiding trying to reach too far or hunching over, and sitting down when they can. They also need to monitor themselves carefully and reduce or stop work to avoid jeopardising their health or that of the developing baby.

CHAPTER 10

Warming-up and Winding-down

Massage is a demanding physical activity, which also requires a concentrated focus of your attention. As with other concentrated physical activities, it's best to warm-up rather than going into it cold. It's useful to spend time at the beginning of each working day doing physical and mental preparations for the day ahead. Even for a single massage, a few minutes of self-preparation are helpful.

Warm-ups can range from set exercise routines, to systematically working through each area of the body, or doing what feels essential in the moment. Depending on your needs, these could include:

- Stretches to release stiffness and increase your suppleness;
- Energising exercises to wake up your body for action, or;
- Calming and centering procedures.

This is an integral part of massage training in many parts of the world, in which students learn stretching routines, a martial art or yoga routines as part of their daily preparation for their work.

> **Note:** I strongly advise you to have a general health check before undertaking a new exercise programme. This is *absolutely crucial* if you have any physical problems or health concerns, or if you are unaccustomed to physical exercise. It is also strongly recommended if you are over 40.

What This Chapter Covers

This chapter covers simple ways of preparing yourself physically and mentally for massage, maintaining your energy and suppleness during the working day, and winding-down at the end of the day. For ease of description, the preparations are divided into physical exercises, breathing exercises and mental preparation, but bear in mind that each affects the other. For example, energising exercises will wake both your body and your mind, and also affect your breathing. Doing mental relaxation and/or breathing focused relaxation will also relax your body.

The chapter begins by looking at the range of qualities that physical warm-ups can encompass such as suppleness, strengthening, energising, relaxing, and developing coordination. These are the ideal qualities that are presented in this book for doing massage – combining power and energy with ease in action.

The next section looks at breathing exercises, mental preparation, and preparations such as calming and centering which combine mental and physical components. Then there is a look at the role of exercises during your working day for maintaining your flexibility and sustaining your energy and focus. Finally there is a brief look at ways of winding-down at the end of the day.

Doing Exercises

You may already have an established exercise routine that incorporates the sort of exercises covered in this chapter. If not, the exercises described here offer you a simple, general warm-up that covers the main areas of the body. If you initially find them difficult, persevere – with a little practise they will become easier. However, if you feel, after a time, that you are still trying too hard and causing yourself stress with the exercises, get coaching from a sports trainer, or a yoga or martial arts teacher.

If you don't have prior experience of doing warm-ups from exercise classes or sports activities, it's good to attend a class to get started under supervision. This will give you a practical sense of exercises, and a range of experience so that you can choose what suits you.

Developing Self-monitoring

As well as preparing you for doing massage treatments and helping you to keep in shape and to maintain your vitality, doing regular warm-ups has other benefits. These preparations will prime you for monitoring yourself during massage sessions (see Chapter 5). They will help you to develop the ability to observe your postural habits, including those that are developing through your massage work, and to feel which areas of your body need attention each day and what sort of attention.

This will enable you to develop your own exercise routines to address these and to work out how to maintain your energy during your working day. (Chapter 43 looks at the longer term aspects of looking after yourself and maintaining your energy for massage over time). It will also give you practical experience of a range of stretches and other exercises that you can offer to clients for 'homework'.

Part 1: Stretches and Mobilising Exercises for Suppleness

If you are stiff in your body at the start of a massage, you are likely to begin working too hard until you warm-up into the massage, and your massage will probably be stilted and disjointed. Even a few preliminary stretches to limber up your body will make it easier to give a powerful, fluid massage in a relatively relaxed way.

When you don't have much time before a massage or between clients, stretches are generally the most useful exercises.

Principles of Stretching

Basic warm-ups for most activities involve stretching and mobilising joints to reduce body stiffness and tension and to increase suppleness. In any case, it's good to begin a warm-up with stretches, especially first thing in the morning and particularly if you wake up stiff or it takes you time to get into your day.

Try to do them in a relaxed fashion, in the way that a cat stretches on waking. This gently wakes up the muscles, rather than jumping straight into more active exercises, which can be jarring for muscles if you do them cold. As you stretch, watch that you're not either breathing in forcefully or holding your breath, both of which tend to make you stiffen up.

Start with the most comfortable stretches. Then gradually challenge your body more as the muscles warm-up into action. Once you've warmed-up a little, stretches can be followed by energising / 'waking up' exercises.

Quick Stretches

Whole Body Stretches

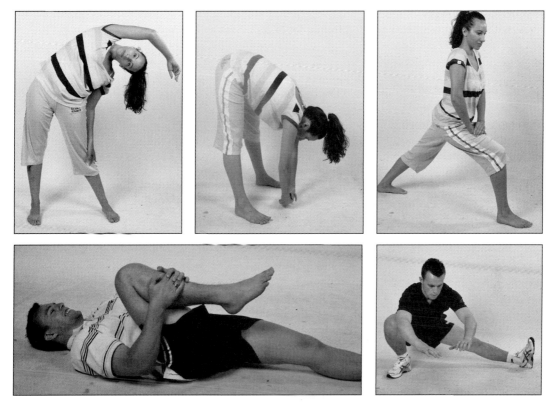

Figure 10.1: Whole body stretches.

If your time is quite limited, do some whole body stretches.

Rebalancing Stretches

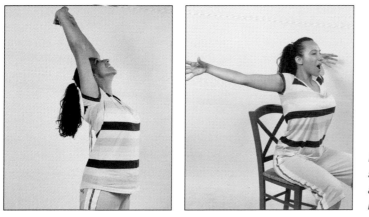

Figure 10.2: Rebalancing stretches; a), b) stretching the arms and hyperextending the trunk.

If you have the time, do stretches for each area of the body. If not, focus on those that rebalance your body from the tendency to hunch over the massage table. For example, stretch your arms up and back to open your chest combined with hyperextending your trunk.

Stretches Whilst Massaging

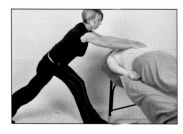

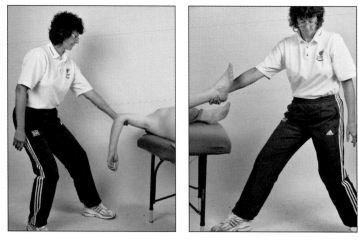

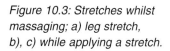

Figure 10.3: Stretches whilst massaging; a) leg stretch, b), c) while applying a stretch.

If you don't have time to do stretches before a massage session, you can use the massage itself to stretch yourself. This is also useful if you notice yourself stiffening up during the massage. For example, you can stretch your legs while you're doing effleurage strokes or applying pressure. And you can do releasing stretches for yourself when you are stretching the client (as long as this doesn't disrupt the massage or divert your attention completely away from the client).

Stretches and Mobilising Exercises for Each Area of the Body

These or similar exercises can be used as part of your preparations at the beginning of the day, for releasing tensions between clients, and for winding-down at the end of the working day. Their use can vary from brief 'tune-ups' to an extensive daily routine. Adapt them to suit yourself. For example, you may need to modify them because of old injuries. You might find that, by giving more attention to certain areas, you can begin to release some long-held tensions. And some days you will be stiffer than others and need to start into exercise more slowly.

For simplicity, the stretches and mobilising exercises are described from the top of the body downwards. Use them in whatever order suits you, and vary them to keep them interesting for yourself. Once a basic set of exercises is familiar, pay more attention to the areas of your body where you regularly get stiff and those areas that are tight or sore at that particular moment. There are more exercises for many areas of the body in later chapters, which focus in detail on how you use each area of your body in massage.

The elbow and knee fold up and straighten. There is a greater range of movement in the shoulder, wrist and hip joints, and the ankle. This is the basis for the exercises described below for these joints, beginning with stretches forward and backwards (flexion and extension) and sideways (abduction and adduction), and then incorporating these into a circular movement (circumduction), which mobilises the complete range of movement of the joint. The leg and arm can also be rotated. Trunk and neck movements include side-bending, forward and back-bending, and rotation.

Begin these movements slowly and evenly so that you don't jar the muscles or the joint structures (the capsule and ligaments) before they are warmed-up. Once each movement has become familiar, focus on executing it more smoothly and easily, which fine-tunes your control of the relevant muscles and your ability to switch easily between using and relaxing them. This enables you to apply this in the massage – to use them with minimal appropriate effort when they are needed for an action, and to let them relax when they are not.

As you mobilise each joint, spend more time on re-establishing movement in the range that is less used in massage, or not used at all, in order to rebalance your body. For example, massage techniques (along with most everyday activities) require you to hold your arms forward at the front of your chest, so focus on stretching them backwards to open up your chest.

Neck Movements

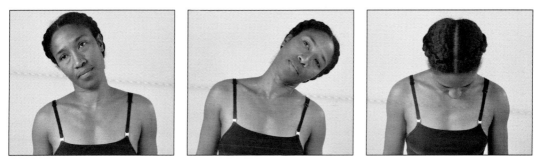

Figure 10.4: Neck movements – dropping the head to the sides and forward.

When doing massages, there is a tendency to stiffen the neck as we watch our work. Release neck tension by doing head movements. Tilt your head from side to side, and drop it forwards. (These days, it is not recommended to drop your head backwards, as people can have undiagnosed cervical spine problems which this can aggravate).

Arm Stretches

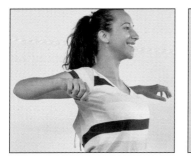
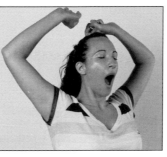
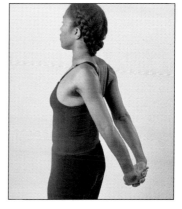

Figure 10.5: Arm stretches to open the chest;
a) stretching arms up, b) stretching your arms back,
c) with interlocked fingers.

Arm stretches help to open up your chest and also to mobilise your shoulders. They are useful to rebalance having your shoulders and arms reaching forward for long periods, which is required in so many everyday activities and in most massage strokes and can easily become an unconscious habit.

These stretches can be done either standing or seated. Stretch your arms up and/or back, so that your shoulders are pulled back and your chest is opened and widened. This stretch can include some hyperextension of your trunk to open and release the front of the chest. People often find themselves yawning with the stretch to gather air into the expanded chest.

This stretch can be enhanced by interlocking your fingers behind your lower back, with the palms facing each other, and straightening your arms. Then, if it's not a strain, lift them a little to take it even further.

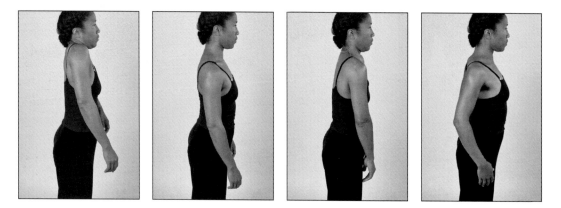

Shoulder Movements
Figure 10.6: Mobilising the shoulders; a) lifting the shoulders,
b) releasing the shoulders to drop down and widen, c) taking the shoulders forward,
d) taking the shoulder blades back.

Unless we monitor our shoulders carefully, most of us unconsciously tighten them (including as we massage), so they need attention in any warm-up. Stand with your arms relaxed and hanging down by your sides or sit in a chair that allows you to let your arms hang. Raise your shoulders up towards your ears, breathing in fully as you do so, and then let them widen and drop gently down onto the top of your chest while also letting your breath release. Next, bring your shoulders forward around the front of your chest, and then take them backwards so that your shoulder blades move towards your spine.

When you've repeated each of these movements a few times, combine them into shoulder circles in which your shoulders move through each of these four directions. Try to keep your arms relaxed and dangling throughout these movements.

People can find it hard to retain this suppleness in activity. You may find it helpful to undertake activities which incorporate shoulder movements in action, such as rowing, martial arts, or juggling/circus skills.

Mobilising the Hands
Because your hands are used so much in massage, it is crucial to give them attention in warm-ups and also during and at the end of your working day. There are a series of exercises for the hands and the wrists at the end of the next chapter (see figures 11.46–11.50). These include alternately clenching your hands and then opening them into a stretch, shaking them out, stretches for your fingers and wrist mobilising exercises. As you do hand exercises, focus on keeping your shoulders and breathing relaxed.

Hand exercises are useful in the development of manual dexterity and coordination, especially if you are unaccustomed to skilled manual activity. Learning a musical instrument or undertaking craft activities or playing computer games that develop hand/eye coordination can also be helpful.

Mobilising the Trunk

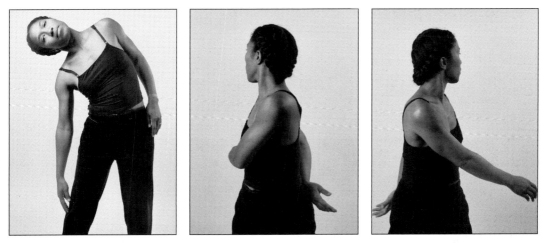

Figure 10.7: Mobilising the trunk; a) side-bending, b), c) rotation.

Simple stretches to mobilise the trunk include side-bending and twisting (rotation) from side to side. Ways of maintaining spinal suppleness are covered in more detail in Chapter 25 (see figures 25.16–25.18).

Mobilising the Hips and Lower Back

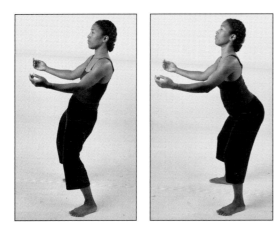
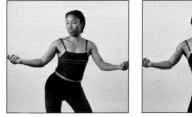
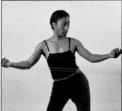

Figure 10.8: Mobilising the hips; a) swaying the hips forward, b) swaying the hips backwards, c), d) swaying the hips from side to side.

For hip movements, stand with your feet at least as far apart as the width of your hips. Sway your hips from side to side, and then forward and back. Then take them in a circle as if you were keeping a hoop spinning with your hips. Of course, as you do these movements, you are simultaneously mobilising your lower back and also getting movement in your knees, your ankles and your feet. So this is a good way of getting movement throughout your lower body.

Leg Stretches

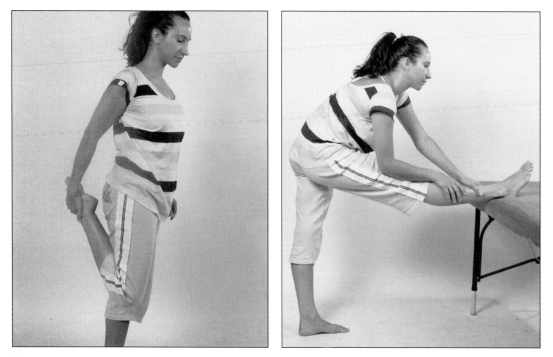

Figure 10.9: Leg stretches; a) quadriceps stretch, b) hamstrings stretch.

Many people will be familiar with leg stretches from sporting and martial arts activities. The commonest stretches involve bending the leg back to stretch the quadriceps and leaning forward with your foot resting on a high surface to stretch the hamstrings and the gastrocnemius.

Side-bending (see figure 10.7a) will also stretch the muscles at the side of the hips, particularly gluteus medius and the tensor fasciae latae.

Mobilising the Ankles

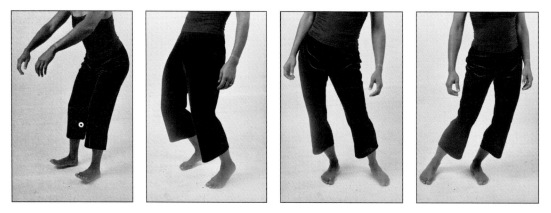

*Figure 10.10: Mobilising the ankles; a), b) swaying forward and back,
c), d) swaying from side to side.*

It is crucial to have supple ankles for swaying smoothly and easily as you massage. To mobilise your ankles, stand and sway your weight forward and back, bending your knees and hips to avoid overbalancing. Next sway from side to side, and then extend this into a circular movement, continuing to use your bodyweight and your arms as a counterbalance. Not only do these movements activate each part of your ankle; they also awaken each part of your foot in turn as your weight moves through it.

Rebalancing Your Body

No matter how good our self-monitoring, we all tend to tense up and hunch over a little as we focus on doing a massage. So exercises which balance up the postural habits that commonly arise from doing massages are important. These follow very easily and naturally from the stretches and mobilisations described above.

Some exercise systems teach a rigid, inflexible idea of posture which can lead to stiffness in everyday activities and when doing massage. However, when disciplines such as yoga, Pilates and the Alexander Technique (or combinations of these approaches) are well taught, they offer an experience of flexible posture. Other systems look more directly at dynamic posture. Maintaining strong, flexible posture in action is the focus of the Feldenkrais Method® and of many martial arts. Studying them will help you to appreciate the difference between stiff posture and a way of moving that is both dynamic and supple.

Balanced Posture – a Checklist
Of course, it is much easier to find a balanced posture, when you're not involved in activity. Regularly taking a few minutes to re-establish this using the checklist below will remind you of the qualities that are good to maintain as you work. The main things to focus on are:

- *Relaxing your shoulders* to counter the tendency to unconsciously tense them 'around your ears', and *widening your shoulders* rather than having them rounded because of the need to constantly reach forward in massage techniques (see figure 22.1);
- *Relaxing your arms and hands* (see figure 23.8);
- Keeping *your neck long and supple*, with your head 'floating' lightly upwards to rebalance the tendency to bend your head over to look closely at what you're doing (see figure 24.1);
- Having your *trunk long and supple* to counteract the tendency to hunch over at the massage table (see figure 25.14);
- Keeping your *breathing easy and full*, rather than restricted by hunching over (see figure 26.1), and;
- *Softening your knees* so that you have enough 'give' in them to allow you to sway a little, rather than having them stiffly locked back (see figure 25.14).

Part 2: Other Physical Preparations

Depending on your needs of the moment, there is a range of other types of warm-ups. Of course, many of them incorporate more than one quality. For example, many other exercises include elements of stretching. Many martial arts exercises and some styles of yoga are designed for the simultaneous development of strength and suppleness.

And many of the warm-up and release activities described below can be used in a variety of ways. For example, self-massage can be used for the release of deep tensions through deep pressure techniques, or you can use percussion strokes to focus on energising yourself.

Strengthening Exercises

Strengthening the Hands

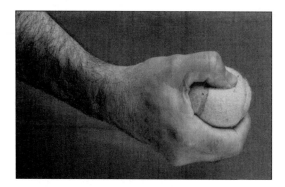

Figure 10.11: Strengthening the hands – squeezing a ball.

Novice practitioners often feel the need to build up the strength of their hands and arms. You can strengthen your hands by regularly squeezing a rubber ball outside of work, for example when watching television. Don't overdo it at the beginning, but build it up gradually.

Strengthening the Whole Body

Practitioners may also want to strengthen the whole upper body. This can be important for those who come to massage without much of a physical background and/or those with a small build and soft muscles. In fact, you may feel the need to work on your whole body in this way. A personal trainer will be able to guide you in developing an appropriate gym routine or home programme for this.

When focusing on building strength, incorporate exercises that also keep you supple. The focus of many types of yoga, martial arts exercises, the Pilates system and the Feldenkrais Method® is to combine strength and flexibility in action, which is an ideal combination for doing massage.

Dynamic Exercises for Energising Yourself

However, being able to combine strength and suppleness in static exercises is not enough. It is important to be able to incorporate these qualities into activity. This can be done by following your stretching and mobilising warm-up (and strengthening exercises) with more dynamic activities as long as you're not tensing up to do them. This enables you to begin your day with vigour and to renew your energy throughout the day, particularly during the mid-afternoon blues.

In addition to enlivening your body, these exercises will help your cardiovascular and respiratory systems, and also help you to develop stamina.

Energising Exercises

Ways of energising yourself between clients include:

* Shaking and vibrating your hands, feet, limbs, trunk and your whole body, and;
* Vigourous self-massage, especially self-percussion and muscle vibration.

Other ways of increasing your physical energy include:

* Skipping, dancing, swimming, running, cycling and aerobic exercises, and;
* Jumping up and down, or bouncing on a 'rebounder' trampoline.

Another aspect of energising yourself is to use breathing and meditative techniques to raise your inner energy (see below).

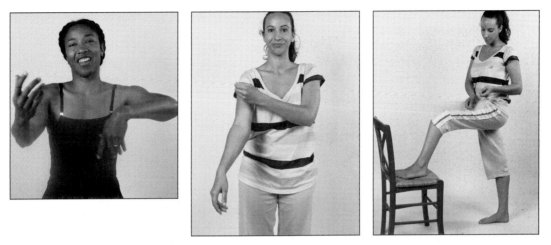

Figure 10.12; Energising exercises; a) shaking out the arms and hands, b), c) self-percussion.

Lightening and Energising Your Legs

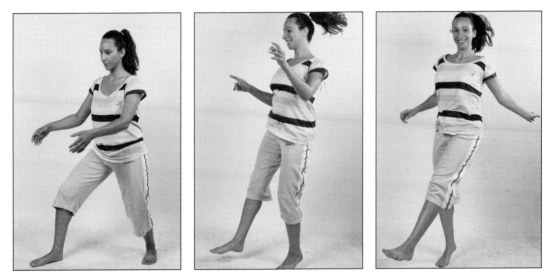

Figure 10.13: Legs; a) grounded in massage, b), c) energising legs through other activities.

It can be especially important to focus on dynamic exercise for your legs. A central theme of this book is using your whole body for the massage, particularly pushing from your legs to generate the power behind massage techniques (see Chapter 28). However, if this is the only way that you use your legs, it may lead to a sense of heaviness and sluggishness in them. So a healthy balance for this, outside of massage sessions, is to lighten and energise them by activities such as running, swimming, jumping, skipping, dancing or trampolining.

Physical Relaxation

It is important to be able to relax your body in order to prevent a slow accumulation of tension, which often happens unnoticed. Physical relaxation can also be used in conjunction with mental relaxation procedures such as meditation, or as preparation for them.

Most exercise routines incorporate elements of relaxation through stretching and mobilising parts of the body. However it can be useful at times to focus purely on relaxation.

Tensing and Relaxing

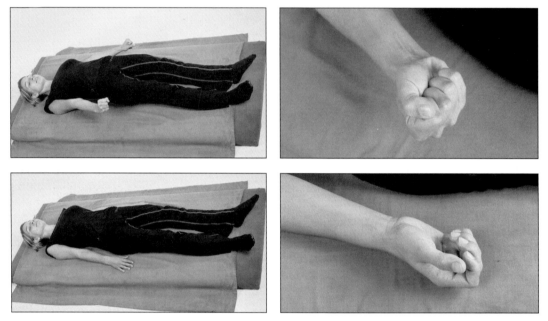

Figure 10.14: Tensing and relaxing the body; a), b) tensing the body, c), d) relaxing.

The classic relaxation procedure involves *tensing and then relaxing* each part of the body in turn. The simplest way of doing this is while sitting or lying in a comfortable position. If you only have a short time, you can tense and relax your whole body a few times.

If you have enough time, focus on each area of your body in turn – your feet and legs, buttocks and abdomen, chest and breathing, hands and arms, shoulders and neck, and face and jaw. Breathe in strongly and then hold your breath as you tense each area for five to ten seconds. Then release your breath and simultaneously let the tension go. Take enough time to allow yourself to relax as completely as possible in that area. Work your way systematically through your body, doing this a few times for each area in turn. Spend more time, if necessary, on the areas where you are tightest and/or those areas where you find it most difficult to let go.

Relaxing the Areas Most in Need
Once the feeling of relaxing has become familiar in each area of your body, it can be applied just to whichever part most needs it. This can be done between clients, for example, while you are sitting or standing. A quick body scan will reveal where you are holding most tension (which, for most people, is in the shoulders much of the time). Tense up that area while holding your breath in, and then let your breath go as you focus on relaxing the area.

Relaxing While Massaging

In fact, once this process is familiar, you can apply it when you are doing massages. With practise, you will learn to notice areas of tension in your body and relax them as you work. This also enables you to notice when a massage technique causes you strain and needs to be either changed or replaced by a technique that is easier on your body. This is a basic part of developing the process of self-monitoring and adjustment that will enable you to look after your body and maintain your career in massage (see Chapter 5).

Developing your ability to stay relaxed in action can be helped by studying many martial arts systems, the Alexander Technique or the Feldenkrais Method®.

Massage

Self-massage

Regular self-massages of 5 to 10 minutes throughout your working day can help to counteract the build up of tension in your shoulders, arms and hands which are used so much in massage. These can be done firmly using strong kneading and pressure techniques to release tensions, or vigorously with percussion techniques to 'wake up' and energise your muscles. You may also be able to organise to exchange short 'pick-me-up' massages with colleagues in your workplace.

Receiving Massages

At the end of the day, you may feel the need for a more extensive self-massage or massage exchanges with colleagues. Bear in mind that receiving regular massage / bodywork treatments is important for massage practitioners for general self-maintenance (see Chapter 43).

Part 3: Physical-Mental Warm-ups

Many physical warm-ups have a mental component. In fact, some physical preparations, such as relaxation and energising exercises, are often used as much for their mental effect as for their physical effect. And some mental attitudes can only be established partly or wholly through physical preparation. This section briefly covers two qualities that are both physical and mental and therefore need a combined preparation in order for you to embody them – centering and grounding.

Centering

Centering yourself involves gathering your energy and mental faculties to focus them towards an activity, rather than approaching it in a scattered, unfocused way. In massage, there needs to be a physical component to centering as well, so that it is not just a mental attitude but is also *embodied* in the way that the practitioner delivers the massage. (It also requires regular self-monitoring throughout the massage session to ensure that you are staying focused, relaxed and even in your breathing and in your delivery of the massage). Centering that is both mental and physical can be observed in the preparations of a skilled high diver for an exacting dive or of a professional golfer for making a difficult shot.

Centered Movement

In many activities that involve movement, including massage, there is also a more specific meaning to physical centering – centering movement around the pelvis, the body's centre of action (see figure 27.3). This is crucial to activities such as skiing, skating, surfing and skateboarding and also to Eastern martial arts such as judo, aikido and Tai Chi. In shiatsu also, practitioners learn to centre themselves in the *hara* (the energy centre of the body) in order to move from there. Learning one of these activities can be particularly helpful for practitioners who have come to massage from a sedentary background, which tends to disengage people from the lower body and the potential power to be gained through the coordinated use of the legs and the pelvis.

Centering Exercises

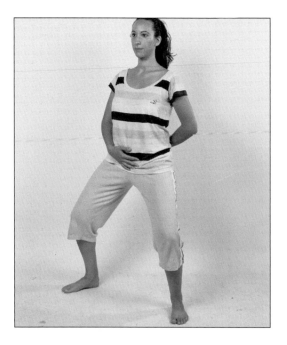

Figure 10.15: Centering exercises
– breathing into the 'hara'.

Simple ways of centering are:

• Breathing deeply into the 'hara', perhaps with your hands on the front and back of your lower abdomen to help you to focus here, and/or:
• Standing in a wide stance and swaying to give you the feeling of how to centre movement around your hips and pelvis.

Grounding
Most activities that involve centered movement also incorporate grounding – feeling the connection of one's lower body to the floor/ground, and the consequent power and energy that can flow up through your lower body. Therefore the same sorts of activities can be a good preparation for getting grounded in your body. In many Asian styles of massage, practitioners learn martial arts as part of their preparation and self-maintenance. This enables them to move in a centered, grounded way – pushing from the legs and swaying smoothly – rather than standing or sitting still and just working from the upper body.

Part 4: Breathing

Suiting your breathing patterns to activity is an essential part of the physical warm-ups and the physical-mental preparations described above. It is also integral to the mental preparations described below. In addition, breathing can be used in preparation on its own in two important ways.

Calming Breath

If you are nervous, for example about meeting a new client, it can be useful to take a few *calming breaths* to calm and help prepare yourself. If you have two or three minutes to focus on this, sit comfortably, 'switch off' from your surroundings, and focus on deepening and slowing your breathing (see Chapter 26).

Energising Breath

Strong and slightly faster breathing can be used to *energise yourself* by raising your inner energy. Do not make it too fast or jerky to avoid winding yourself up.

Part 5: Mental Preparations

As mentioned above, there is a mental component to many physical warm-ups, and some physical warm-ups are used primarily for their mental effect – these effects can be enhanced by focusing on mental procedures. The aim of mental preparation is to help you to bring your attention to bear on the massage, focusing on the client and on monitoring and dealing with anything that arises, rather than being scattered or preoccupied.

Calming and Centering Yourself

Forms of *meditation* such as using a mantra or 'watching' your breath can be helpful to calm and centre yourself as part of your preparations at the beginning of a working day. *Visualisations* (of relaxation, wellbeing and/or healing,) can be both relaxing and replenishing. *Yoga, Tai Chi* and many other *martial arts* are directed as much towards centering yourself mentally as towards physical wellbeing. Many of the other physical preparations such as *gentle stretches, breathing exercises* and *relaxation procedures*, also have a calming mental effect.

Having a Mental Checklist

In preparation for working with clients, it can be useful to go through a quick mental checklist, reminding yourself of anything that you need to be vigilant about during the massage. This can include habits that you're trying to change, particular ways of working or strains on your body to monitor, and general reminders to yourself such as keeping your body moving and your shoulders relaxed.

Time Out – Switching Off

During the working day, it can be useful to *mentally 'switch off'* when you have a few minutes between clients or during your meal break to relax and refresh yourself. Ways of doing this include:

*   Taking some *deep calming breaths* or a *'cat nap'*,
*   A few minutes of *daydreaming*, or;
*   Doing *mini meditations*.

It is also important to finish thinking about the last client, so that you can be ready for the next one.

Mentally Finishing Your Working Day

At the end of the day, there are two main aspects to mentally finishing the day – thinking through any residual concerns from the day, and then winding-down. Many people find that they can do this on a bus or train or while walking, doing exercise or playing sport. Some people can do it whilst driving. It can be quite important to have space between work and a busy home life or social activities to separate them.

Part 6: During the Working Day

Brief versions of many of the extended morning warm-ups can be used during the working day for releasing any developing tensions, and for maintaining flexibility, rebalancing your body, and maintaining and renewing your energy and focus. If you only have very limited time between clients, a few stretches for your whole body, a quick relaxation of tight body areas or a few calming breaths are useful. It's also good to take a minute to mentally finish with the last client, and to re-center yourself in preparation for the next one.

When you have a longer break between clients, you may feel the need to do more extensive stretches, energising or self-massage.

Part 7: At the End of the Working Day

Physical Release and Replenishment
Many of the morning warm-ups such as the stretching and flexibility maintenance exercises are also helpful for winding-down and re-centering at the end of the day. It is also important to check through your body and note any tensions, stiffness and discomforts that have developed through your working day. You can then focus on these in your exercises to avoid them building up into major problems. This can also be the focus of any self-massage or 'pick-me-up' massage swaps that you organise with colleagues. And this will also alert you to what you need to monitor in the future as you work.

Winding-down
Try to have some 'breathing space' in which to separate yourself mentally from work before you re-enter the rest of your life. If they have time, many people like to wind-down at the end of the day by having a warm shower or taking a long soak in a bath / hot tub, by taking a walk, doing some exercises, or by having some winding-down social time with friends or colleagues. As part of their mental switch off from the working day, many people find it useful to have a short catnap on a bus or train, or to have some daydreaming time while walking or exercising.

Review
Warm-ups can help you to:
- Prepare yourself physically and mentally for doing massage;
- Maintain your energy and suppleness during the working day, and;
- To wind-down at the end of the day.

Stretching and mobilising exercises reduce body stiffness and tension and increase suppleness. They can be used between clients to rebalance your body.

Start with comfortable stretches. As your muscles warm-up into action, extend them and add in more energising / aerobic exercises.

If your time is limited, do some whole body stretches.

If you have more time, work through each area of your body, or focus on those areas that need it more.

You can also include stretches while you are doing massages, e.g. stretching your legs.

Stretching and mobilising exercises include:
- Neck movements;
- Arm stretches to open up the chest;
- Mobilising your shoulders;
- Clenching and relaxing your hands;

- Mobilising your wrists;
- Trunk movements;
- Leg stretches for the hamstrings and calves;
- Side-bends for the lateral hip muscles;
- Hip circles, and;
- Movements to mobilise the ankles.

Regularly squeeze a rubber ball to strengthen your hands.

When focusing on building strength in your body, also incorporate exercises that keep you supple.

Use dynamic exercises, such as aerobic exercises, running, skipping or dancing to:

- Energise your body;
- Build your cardiovascular endurance;
- Develop stamina, and;
- To renew your energy throughout the day.

To release tension, tense and then relax your whole body a few times.

If you have time, tense and relax each part of the body in turn.

Short self-massage during or at the end of your working day can help to counteract the build-up of tension in your body, particularly your upper body.

Centre yourself in your body by standing in a wide stance and swaying to give you the feeling of how to centre movement around your hips and pelvis. Or breathe deeply into the 'hara' (the energy centre of the body) with your hands on the front and back of your lower abdomen to help you to focus here.

Activities which help the practitioner to feel 'grounded' – feeling the connection of one's lower body to the floor/ground, and the consequent power and energy that can flow up through your lower body – include skiing, skating, surfing and skateboarding and Eastern martial arts such as judo, aikido and Tai Chi.

You can use your breathing to calm yourself by taking a few calming breaths, or, if you have a few minutes, by sitting comfortably and focusing on deepening and slowing your breathing.

Forms of meditation such as using a mantra or 'watching' your breath can be helpful to calm and centre yourself as part of your preparations at the beginning of a working day.

Strong and slightly faster breathing can be used to energise yourself.

When you have time during the working day, it can be useful to mentally 'switch off' for a few minutes to relax and refresh yourself.

At the end of the working day, check through your body and note any tensions, stiffness and discomforts that have developed. Focus on these in your stretching exercises. This will also alert you to what you need to monitor as you work.

At the end of the day, think through any residual concerns about your clients and your work.

Then mentally finish the day by doing some mental and/or physical winding-down. This could include:

- Having a warm shower or taking a long soak in a bath/hot tub;
- Taking a walk;
- Playing sport or doing exercises, or;
- Having some social winding-down time with friends or colleagues.

If possible, have some space between your work and your home life.

Using the Hands: the Traditional Tools of Western Massage

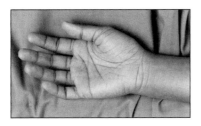

This section of the book focuses on how you to use your hands skilfully – reducing the strain on them while simultaneously using them effectively. Chapter 11 looks at the common causes of straining the hands in massage and offers general ideas on reducing these strains. Chapters 12–16 cover each part of the hand in turn, and Chapter I7 focuses on looking after your wrists when you are using your hands. (The next section of the book (Chapters 18–21) looks at saving your hands altogether by using other massage tools, particularly your forearm and elbow).

Potential Problems

More than most other activities, massage requires you to consistently apply compressive pressure for extended periods through all of the joints of your upper limb from your shoulders down to your digits. This puts considerable pressure on your hands which are the most commonly used working tools for massage, and, until recent decades, were the *only* tools used in Western massage. Compared to the other tools that can be used for massage such as the forearm and elbow, your hands are relatively small, weak and vulnerable.

It is the *accumulation* of strain in your hands over the course of a number of massages that causes problems. So, although you can safely do the occasional massage that puts pressure on your hands, *regularly* working in a strainful ways can cause problems. If small discomforts in these areas are not addressed, they can accumulate and lead to long-term damage. The thumbs and wrist are the most commonly strained areas in massage through poor use and/or putting too much pressure through them. The fingers are sometimes also strained in this way.

The aspects of massage that put the greatest pressure on your hands are:

- Doing repetitive movements;
- Consistently applying pressure through your digits;
- Hyperextending your thumbs, fingers and/or wrist when applying pressure through them;
- Using your thumbs and fingers when you could use larger, less vulnerable parts of your hands, such as your palm, knuckles and fist;
- Not supporting them with your other hand whenever you can in order to reduce the workload on them;
- Overusing your hands, including applying more pressure than they can comfortably handle, and;
- Standing still and only using your shoulder and arm muscles for massage strokes rather than generating the power through leaning and swaying your body.

The Limits of Using Your Hands

As you work through these chapters, it is important to bear in mind that there is a *limit* to what each person can comfortably do with their hands. While using your body effectively enables you to relax your shoulders, arms and hands, it also increases the power that you are delivering to your hands. So make sure that this doesn't put too much pressure on them. And learn to use your forearm and elbow in order to save them whenever you can.

Using Your Body to Support Your Hands

The way that you use your whole body is crucial to delivering power, control and fluidity to your massage techniques, in the same way that a hammer or a surgeon's knife are no good without somebody wielding them skilfully. Some basic guidelines on using your body to support your hands and reduce the strain on them are presented in Chapter 11. This involves positioning your body behind your hands and leaning or swaying your bodyweight to power your massage strokes. This enables you to keep your shoulders, arms and hands relatively relaxed. The ideal is to have your hands simultaneously relaxed and strong with the power transmitted to them. Information on bodyuse that is pertinent to using each part of your hand is included in the chapter on using that part, and detailed information on bodyuse is covered in Section 5 of the book (Chapters 22–28).

Monitoring With Your Hands

Channelling the power generated by your body through your hands has further useful consequences. Your hands are the most sensitive tools for palpating the client's structure and tensions, and being able to keep them relaxed makes it easier to feel with them. Being able to monitor and respond to your client's responses in this way enables you to personalise your massage for each individual. You will be most effective if you teach yourself to palpate with each area of your hand, so that you are able to feel with whichever part that you're using. The ideal in massage is for your hands to be 'alive' – channelling and directing the power generated in your body, and feeling and responding to the client's build, tensions and responses to the massage.

Communicating Through Your Hands

Your hands are also the vehicles of your communication with the client (see Chapter 6). If you are tense and awkward, for example, you are likely to be conveying this through your hands. Your clients are then less likely to relax into the massage, whether or not they are conscious of the cause of their wariness. By contrast, using your bodyweight enables you to keep your hands more relaxed and therefore able to deliver a massage that can be firm (when appropriate) without stiffness. This encourages clients to respond more positively and 'go with' it more easily.

Hand-brain Coordination

The hand uses more brainpower than any other part of the body. Researchers into comparative anatomy generally believe that, via the adoption of upright posture, which freed the hands from supporting the body, the development of the human brain has gone 'hand-in-hand' with the development of using the hands (in tandem also with the development of speech and language). The rise of interest in practising bodywork over recent decades has been partly due to the need to rebalance the effects of an increasingly sedentary and cerebral lifestyle by reconnecting with this hand-brain coordination (as well as meeting the needs of clients to rebalance their own lives by reconnecting with their bodies and looking after them). Many other popular activities such as doing arts or crafts, gardening, DIY, physical exercise, sports, martial arts and dance also reflect the human need to engage in activities that have immediate physical results.

Experiment, Discovery and Learning

For most people, the satisfaction of such activity is not only in achieving results. It comes directly from the physical, mental and expressive enjoyment of the activity itself. And it also comes from the associated process of learning, in which new connections are established in the brain through mastering skills, refining them and applying them in new ways, and through the development of insights and intuition that come through practice and experience. Learning is, of course, an uneven process with times of stagnation and setbacks as well as periods of slow incremental development, steep learning curves and periods of levelling out.

In massage sessions, some practitioners just expect to slog through a familiar routine, or else to give all of their attention to the client at their own expense. However, you can approach massage as a potential laboratory for developing your skills while attending to the client and simultaneously looking after yourself. Hopefully, the suggestions in this section of the book (and the next section on 'hands-free' massage) will give you more than just methods of saving your hands. As well as steering you away from potential problems, this offers you ways of expanding your massage repertoire by incorporating new ideas and by using familiar tools and techniques in new ways. Initially, you'll need to practice outside of massage sessions to become proficient with these. However, once you have confidence and a reasonable level of skill, you can also begin to experiment with variations and extensions within sessions with clients.

CHAPTER 11

Looking After Your Hands

The hands are the common working tools of massage. This chapter looks at the commonest causes of straining them in massage and offers ideas on reducing this strain. The chapter includes exercises for keeping your hands supple and for developing your dexterity for massage.

The rest of the chapters in this section of the book (Chapters 12–17) cover each working area of the hand in turn, looking in more detail at how to use them most effectively with the least strain. Using your body well to support your hands is covered in detail in Chapters 22–28.

Although the general principles covered in this chapter apply to most strokes, each type of stroke has its own special challenges. Chapters 33–40 cover commonly used massage strokes in detail, including how to use your body to support them.

Hands Most at Risk

All practitioners need to be aware of the potential risks of overusing and straining their hands. However, it is particularly important for those with small hands, and those with long, slender and/or hypermobile thumbs and fingers to take extra care as their hands are the most vulnerable to injury, especially when applying pressure.

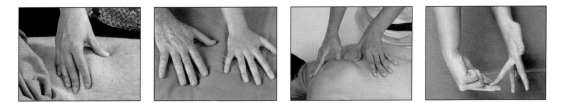

Figure 11.1: Hands most at risk; a) small hands, b) long, slender fingers, c) hypermobile thumbs, d) hypermobile fingers.

The Accumulation of Strain

The majority of hand problems develop from the *accumulation* of strain over the course of doing many massages. This generally arises from using your hands awkwardly, doing repetitive movements and/or through overusing them to apply pressure. The joints of the thumb and the wrist are the most commonly strained areas. It is less common to strain the fingers by overusing them for applying pressure but it can occur.

The main ways of reducing the strain on your hands are to:

• Vary the techniques that you use and the areas of your hand that you use to deliver them;
• Use the largest part of your hand that is appropriate with techniques that involve pressure;
• Support your working hand with your other hand;
• Use both hands together, whenever possible, to reduce the workload on your solo hand;
• Use cushions and bolsters to support the client's body in order to free up your hands, and;
• Save your hands entirely by using your forearm or elbow.

Signs of Strain

Watch out for early warning signs of strain, particularly in your thumbs and your wrists. Common symptoms of *repetitive strain* are intermittent or persistent pain when you're not using your hands, including waking at night with sudden pains through the affected area, and sensitivity to bumping your hands. Wrist problems can also lead to tingling or numbness in parts of your hands, and weakness or even loss of control in the hands.

Rest your hands whenever you can. Regular massage can help as a preventative measure. It can also provide some relief from the pain/tensing cycle if you already have problems. If you have persistent pain, especially if it persists when you are *not* working, seek specialist help (see Chapter 45). Many people find that acupuncture, deep massage and/or osteopathy / chiropractic / physiotherapy can help to reduce an established problem.

Poor Working Practices

Massage novices often use their hands in stiff and awkward ways as they initially struggle to master the techniques.

Flaccid Hands

Some massage novices are totally unused to using their hands. A few years ago, when I first met a student who was totally blind, she stood absolutely passively, waiting to be given permission and told what to do. I was shocked by the flaccidness of her hands, which hung down, looking lifeless and 'empty' as if she'd never used them for anything. I learned that she had always been pushed to the background in her family and had developed a totally passive attitude to life. By the end of a year's training, her hands were lively. Even in repose they held some vitality. She had begun to 'inhabit' them, learning to use them and get her body moving to support them. And she had simultaneously 'taken hold' of her life – making decisions of her own about her direction in life, which was a new step for her.

Stiff Hands

In contrast, some students grab clients as if they were stubborn pieces of meat, who can only be 'tenderised' through brute force. This is generally done with stiff, hard hands, usually backed up by rigidity in the body and a grim, determined jaw. I once had a student who had worked for years with her dad who was a horse trainer. In the beginning she needed to be regularly reminded that her fellow students didn't need or want the same pressure as horses.

Tense Shoulders

When people are first learning to massage, they often unconsciously tense their shoulders and arms, and consequently use their hands stiffly. Hopefully, through practice and instruction, practitioners learn to use their bodyweight so that they can use their hands in a relaxed way instead of trying to 'muscle through'. However, even after learning to massage 'with the whole body', many of us revert to tensing our shoulders without realising it when we are using our fingers or thumbs to focus on small areas, when we are doing percussion strokes, when we are applying sustained pressure, or when we have to deal with a well-built client with well-used muscles.

There is a strong connection between how we use our hands and how we hold our shoulders. If you are stiffening or straining your hands, you are also likely to be instinctively tensing your shoulders. You may also be holding your breath and stiffening your back. In fact you could be unconsciously tensing throughout your body, which is likely to feed back into this cycle of pain and tensing. Conversely, being tense in your shoulders, which is an unconscious habit for many of us, is quite likely to lead to unnecessary tension in our hands. This is often reinforced by unconsciously holding one's breath. So, in monitoring your body as you massage, check your shoulders whenever you notice tension in your hands, and vice-versa. And, when you are changing the way that you use your hands, consciously relax the rest of your body as well (particularly your upper body) to ensure that these associated tensions don't draw you back into old habits.

The Relationship Between Your Shoulders and Hands

Check the connection between your hands and shoulders for yourself. Rest your relaxed hand on your partner's body. Tense your shoulders and note how difficult it is not to tense your hand as well. (You may also find that you are tensing other parts of your body, standing more stiffly and/or holding your breath too).

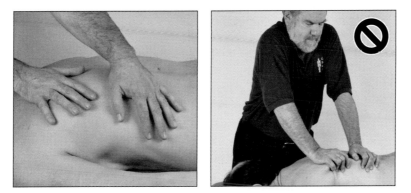

Figure 11.2: Connection between the shoulders and the hands;
a) relaxed hand, b) tense shoulders and hands.

Then relax your shoulders and hands again. Tense your hands this time and notice the instinctive tightening of your shoulders.

Straining the Digits and the Wrist

Take care not to overuse your fingers or thumbs. Only use them for a small part of each massage session, unless the massage is mainly light stroking. Save them for the situations in which you can't use other parts of your hands (or forearm) because of the lack of working space or the delicacy needed, for example when working on the client's face.

Straining the Thumbs

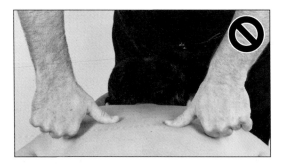

Figure 11.3: Using pressure with a hyperextended thumb.

Straining the thumbs is one of the two most common work related injuries for massage practitioners (the other being straining the wrist). Thumb problems primarily arise from:

- Putting too much pressure through them;
- Working with them hyperextended, and;
- Overusing them, for example to knead large, well-used muscles.

Chapter 13 covers ways of looking after your thumbs.

Straining the Fingers

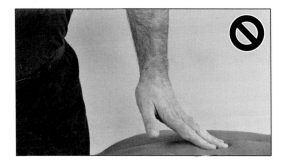

Figure 11.4: Using pressure with hyperextended fingers.

The fingers can be strained too, though it happens less often. There is a temptation to rely solely on your fingertips because of their great sensitivity in feeling the client's build and responses. This can lead to overusing them when firm pressure is needed in a massage treatment. They are not particularly effective for this, and are vulnerable to strain if they are used too much for delivering pressure (see Chapter 12). And, like the thumbs, the fingers are especially at risk if they are hyperextended when you are applying pressure.

Overusing the Knuckles

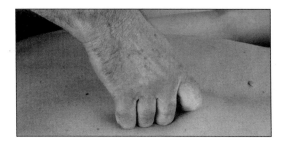

Figure 11.5: Using the knuckles for circling pressure strokes.

It can be useful to initially palpate the client's tissues with your fingers, and then use larger, stronger parts of your hand (or forearm) for firm massage strokes. While other parts of your hands are less vulnerable than your thumbs or fingers, the 'knuckles' (the proximal interphalangeal joints, Chapter 15) can also be overused for pressure strokes. Only use them for a small part of each massage. Whenever possible switch to using your fist or elbow to save your knuckles.

Working With Your Wrist Bent

Most wrist problems develop from regularly applying pressure with the wrist bent backwards (hyperextended). Bending your wrists forward (flexion) or to the side are less common problems, but will also strain your wrist if they are done too often.

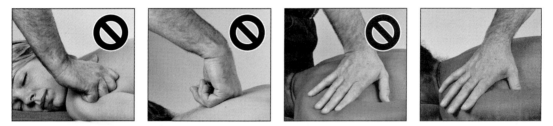

Figure 11.6: Bending the wrist; a) hyperextended wrist, b) overflexed wrist, c) wrist bent to the side, d) having a straight wrist.

Bear in mind that using your wrists awkwardly will cause you to work harder than necessary with your hands. In fact, any strain on your wrists will cause you to tense your hands, and very often your shoulders as well. Of course this all puts extra pressure on your wrists, which sets in motion a vicious cycle of strain and tension.

Conserving Your Hands and Wrists

The Ideal – Balancing Power, Ease and Sensitivity

The ideal presented in this book is to position yourself and to use your bodyweight so that you can conserve your hands while working effectively, instead of trying to 'muscle through'. This enables you to combine power, ease and sensitivity so that your hands are relaxed but not limp, active but not tense, searching but not prodding, and able to adapt to the client's build and responses. This section of the chapter covers practices that will help you to work effectively with the least strain on your hands.

Minimise Thumb Kneading

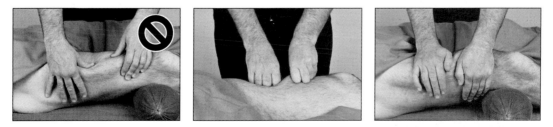

Figure 11.7: Alternatives to thumb kneading; a) kneading with your thumbs – hard work, b) knuckle kneading, c) wringing between your hands.

It is particularly important to minimise the amount of kneading that you do with your thumbs. While thumb kneading is fine for small areas of soft muscle, it is hard work and not particularly effective on large, tight, well-used muscles. It is a common source of strain in the thumbs. Practitioners with small hands or long, slender thumbs need to be particularly careful, and may need to discard this stroke entirely to save their thumbs. There are other ways of achieving the similar effects, such as kneading with your knuckles, 'double-handed' wringing (see figure 11.14), circling fist pressure or using your elbow.

Use the Largest Appropriate Part of Your Hand

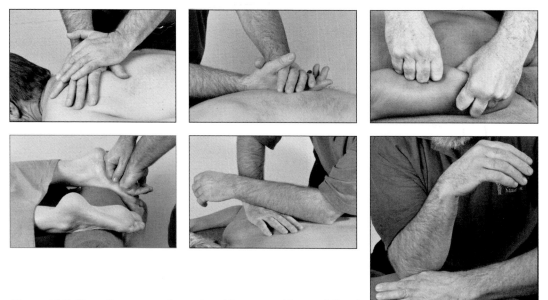

Figure 11.8: Use other areas of your hand/forearm; a) base of thumb, b) back of hand, c) knuckles, d) fist, e) forearm, f) elbow.

In fact, it is always worth considering whether there is a larger, less vulnerable part of your hand that could do the massage job required, particularly when you are increasing the pressure that you are applying or you want to sustain the pressure for some time. For example, you can conserve your fingers and thumbs by using the heel or the back of your hand (see Chapter 14), your knuckles (see Chapter 15), or your fist (see Chapter 16). With practice, as you get accustomed to using other areas of your hands, you will also develop the ability to sense more through these areas. And, whenever you can, save your hands entirely by learning to use your forearms for large sliding movements (see Chapter 18), or your elbow for focusing pressure more precisely on a small area (see Chapter 19).

Vary Your Massage Techniques
Vary the massage techniques that you use (see figures 11.22–11.24), so that the pressure is not constant and not always on the same part of your hands.

Use Your Other Hand Rather Than Leave it Idle

Whenever you use one hand alone, you have to use your shoulder and arm muscles more for control than when your hands are together. Additionally, whenever you are keeping one hand stationary, for example resting it on the receiver's body or on the massage table, there is a temptation to also stay still, rather than moving with your working hand.

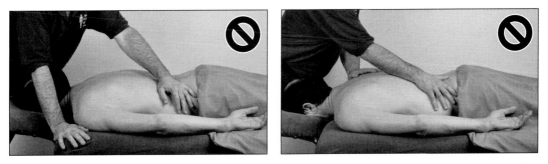

Figure 11.9: The non-working hand resting idly.

So, whenever possible, use your 'spare' hand to support your working hand, rather than leaving it idle. This spreads the workload between your hands. It is particularly important when you are applying pressure. Moving your hands together also makes it much easier to get your body moving behind your strokes.

Support Your Wrist With Your Other Hand

Supporting your wrist will help you to keep it straight and also reduce the pressure on it.

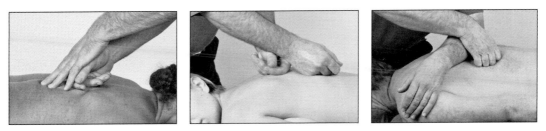

Figure 11.10: Resting the working hand over the supporting hand.

One method of doing this is to rest your wrist over your supporting hand/forearm. In these strokes, resting your *supporting hand* on the client's body provides stability for your working hand.

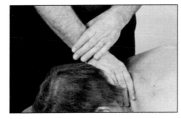
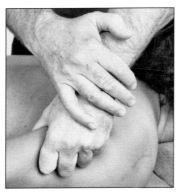
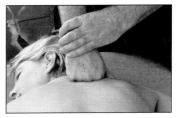

Figure 11.11: Holding the working wrist; a) for squeezing, b) for 'knuckle kneading', c) using the fist.

You can also hold your wrist and guide your working hand, for example, when squeezing the client's neck. And use your other hand to support 'knuckling' strokes (see figure 15.5). When doing this, take care to keep your *supporting hand* (as well as your working hand) as relaxed as possible.

Work 'Double-handed' to Increase Power and Precision
In fact, it is often easier to do 'double-handed' strokes. Whenever the twin tasks of applying force and of controlling the stability and precision of application can be shared between your hands, it takes the strain off both hands and consequently off your arm and shoulder muscles.

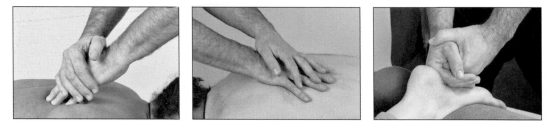

Figure 11.12: Double-handed strokes for pressure; a) increasing finger pressure, b) hand-on-hand, c) one fist inside the other.

It is quite important for those with small hands to work with one hand on the other when applying pressure. In fact, working hand-on-hand is useful for all practitioners when you are attempting to concentrate pressure on a small area through your fingers, especially when you are working on well-developed, tight muscles. Position your body and lean forward to deliver the pressure.

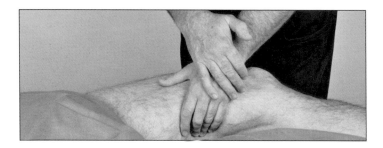

Figure 11.13: Hand-on-hand kneading, on the adductors.

Working double-handedly also conserves your hands in large kneading strokes, for example when you are working on the adductors on the inside of the thigh.

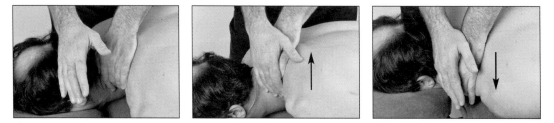

Figure 11.14: Two-handed 'wringing'; a) hands together, b) pulling with the fingers, c) pushing with the heels.

And you can save your thumbs by working double-handed. For example, instead of trying to knead with your thumb on well-used shoulder muscles, use a double-handed 'wringing' stroke. Have one hand on top of the other, with the underhand taking up the shape of the shoulders and the upper hand directing the movement. Push forward with the heels of your hands, and pull back with slightly hooked fingers.

Have Contact Between Your Hands for Mutual Support When You're Using Them Together

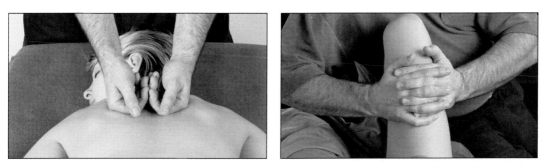

Figure 11.15: Using your hands simultaneously; a) with contact between your hands for mutual support, b) interlocked fingers for stabilising heels of the hands pressure, around the thigh.

Whenever you are using both hands at the same time for firm pressure strokes, try to have contact between them so that they act as mutual supports for each other. This reduces the overall workload as well as reducing the work of each hand, and makes it easier to deliver power directly by leaning and swaying your body instead of just relying on your shoulder and arm muscle strength. The movement is then more fluid and even.

Keep Your Hands as Relaxed as Possible

Most people unknowingly carry a level of tension in their hands. This applies to massage practitioners too – we often hold our hands 'in readiness' for work. Massage beginners often use their hands in stiff and awkward ways as they struggle to master the techniques, and practitioners can get into the habit of working too hard with their hands when clients want more pressure.

So it is important to take time to regularly relax your hands and to monitor them during massages in order to keep them as relaxed as possible. This breaks the slow, unconscious build-up of tension, which would tie up energy and make your massage disjointed and less effective. Using your hands stiffly also tends to evoke a wariness in the client (often unconscious) instead of encouraging them to relax. This is not to imply that you should have floppy hands for massaging, but use them with an *appropriate* effort, rather than maximum force.

Reducing unnecessary tension in your hands will also help you to be more effective by diverting less of your effort to tightening your hands and delivering more of it directly to the client. In addition, when your hands are relaxed, clients feel less 'attacked' and therefore are more likely to 'let you in' more and to 'go with' the pressure that you apply, i.e. to relax their muscles. And because your brain is not occupied with how hard *you* are working, you will be more able to feel subtle responses in the *client's* muscles that tell you when the pressure is acceptable, when you can sustain the pressure and wait for the tissues to soften (to 'melt'), when you can proceed to increase the pressure or when they need you to back off.

Feeling the Difference Between a Relaxed Hand and a Stiff Hand

It can be useful to regularly take a few minutes to relax your hands as completely as you can. You can do this in your warm-ups, during your working day and at the end of the day. It is particularly important if you feel that tension is slowly accumulating and/or you wake up with stiff hands. It gives your hands a rest and recovery time.

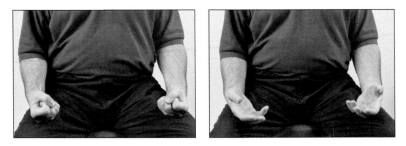

Figure 11.16: Tensing and relaxing the hands; a) tensing the hands, b) letting them relax.

If you find it hard to relax your hands, begin by tensing them, holding them clenched for about ten seconds, and then let them gently uncurl and soften.

Try to relax your hands in treatment sessions too, for example whenever you are resting your hand for a few moments on a client. Over time, with practice, you'll develop the ability to relax them even when you're using them during treatments. And then focus on only engaging the areas that you need to use at the moment and then relax that part when you're not using it (see figure 11.18).

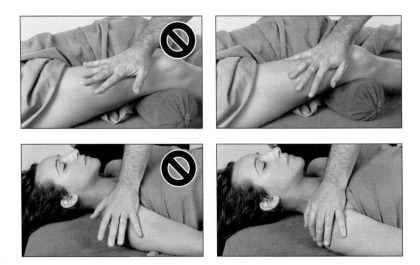

Figure 11.17: Placing the hand on partner's body; a) stiff hand, b) soft hand on thigh, c) stiff hand, d) soft hand on shoulder.

For many people it takes time to learn to monitor and relax their hands. You may need to practice this outside of professional massage sessions to get used to relaxing them. One way of doing this is place your hand on your partner's body, deliberately stiffen it, and then focus on relaxing it so that it 'melts' onto the contours of your partner's body, wrapping around it with maximum contact like cheese melting onto toast under a grill.

You will feel how your relaxed hand uses less energy and enables you to give more of your attention to palpation. If your partner then does the same thing to you, you will appreciate from the receiving side how the stiff hand feels harder and less trustworthy, while the relaxed hand feels more acceptable and easier to respond to.

As you practice this, bear in mind that it is essential to move your arm (see figure 11.37) and to position and lean and/or sway your body (see figure 11.38) to initiate the power and fluidity of massage strokes. If you don't do this, you are likely to be tensing your shoulders for the power, which makes it very hard to relax your hand.

Relax the Non-working Parts of Your Hand

It is relatively easy to relax your whole hand when you are just resting it on your client's body, in sliding strokes or when you are applying stationary pressure. However, the challenge in massage is often to use part of your hand while staying relaxed in the areas of your hand that are not essential to the technique. This takes more practise.

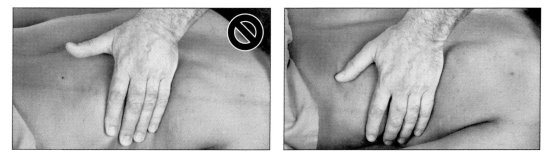

Figure 11.18: Focusing on the non-working parts of your hand; a) tense thumb, b) relaxed hand.

Some practitioners have the unconscious habit of stiffening their fingers when they are using the heel of the hand, or of stiffening the thumb when using their fingers. This uses unnecessary energy, tends to stiffen your hand and reduces your ability to palpate the client's responses.

It takes time to get used to simultaneously monitoring the working *and* the non-working parts of your hands. However it is important, not just for powerful strokes but also when you are focusing on small, precise techniques, in which situation many of us unconsciously tense up.

Applying Pressure Without Tensing Your Hand

Practice with a partner outside of massage sessions to get used to relaxing the non-working parts of your hand. Place your hand on a large area of a partner's body, such as the back, and relax it as much as possible so that it takes on the shape of the body area.

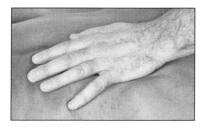

Figure 11.19: Keeping your hand relaxed when applying pressure through different parts.

Then increase the pressure that you are applying through each part of your hand in turn – through the heel of your hand, the base of your thumb, the centre of your palm or your fingers. At this stage of the exercise, change the part of your hand through which you are delivering pressure ONLY by leaning your body differently, not by tensing your shoulder or arm. The greatest challenge for most people is to do this without stiffening their hand. If you find this difficult, it is worth persevering. Not only will it save you energy and feel better to your clients, it will also help you to learn to use your hands with more precision. Make sure to practice with your non-dominant hand, which is likely to need more attention.

Once you are familiar with selectively using and relaxing parts of your hand while it is stationary, then slide it along in an effleurage stroke. Take it slowly enough that you are able to let your hand mould to the contours of your partner's body and, at the same time, to selectively vary the amount of pressure and the area of your hand with which you apply it according to the thickness of the muscle and the amount of tension that you feel under your hand.

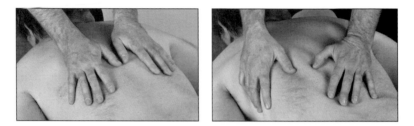

Figure 11.19 (cont.): keeping both hands relaxed.

Then do this simultaneously with both hands. You might want to start by doing this symmetrically, for example doing sliding strokes down each side of your partner's back from the head of the table. Then simultaneously focus on doing different things with each hand, while keeping the non-working parts of each hand relaxed.

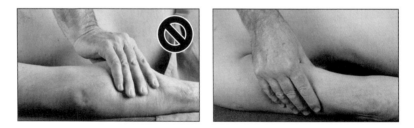

Figure 11.20: Relaxing the hand for squeezing; a) squeezing with an unnecessarily tense hand, b) squeezing with a relaxed hand.

If you feel that you regularly tense your hands unnecessarily in other types of strokes, it is also worth practising outside of massage sessions to keep your hand relaxed when doing them. The easiest way to practice this is to initially do it with your hand stationary by stopping for a moment in mid-stroke. In a squeezing stroke, for example, take hold of an area of muscle and maintain this grip while feeling out what is the least effort that is essential for executing the squeeze. Relax the parts of your hand that are not necessary to the stroke. Then practice doing this as you do the stroke at your normal pace. Apply the same principles to other types of strokes.

Use Mechanical Massage Tools to Save Your Hands

Using a mechanical tool for focused pressure will also save your fingers and thumbs, but you won't be able to monitor the client's responses so well. Take care, when pressing on the tool, that your wrist is not bent. Firm but slightly yielding tools such as a compressible ball are easier to use as they approximate your hands more than solid tools.

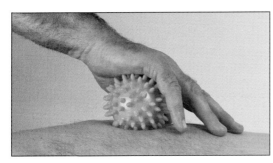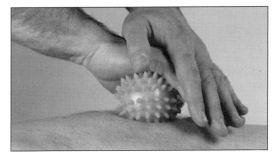

Figure 11.21: Using a spiky ball.

Save Your Hand and Wrist Whenever You Can

Using your body effectively behind your hands, as described in this book, will increase the pressure that you can bring to bear. No matter your build and how effectively that you use your hands, there is a limit to how much pressure you can comfortably apply through them. So it is important to learn to use the forearm and elbow (see Chapters 18 & 19) whenever you can.

If Necessary, Reduce Other Hand-intensive Activities in Your Life

Take account of the rest of your life activities as well. With the rise of computers and digital technology, we are constantly called on to press with our thumbs and fingers. Monitor how much you use your hands. If in addition to doing massage you are also spending time doing hand-intensive activities such as computer work or games, house decoration or maintenance, gardening, sports in which you use a bat, racquet or club, or playing a musical instrument, you may need to cut down on some of these activities to give your hands a rest.

Develop Your Dexterity and Coordination

The mobilising exercises for your hands and fingers at the end of this chapter or similar exercises are useful preparations for developing dexterity and coordination. Other activities which will also give you this grounding include arts or craft work, learning magic tricks or juggling, doing woodwork or metalwork, or playing a musical instrument. The following ways of developing your dexterity in massage will also enable you to spread the workload throughout your hands, which reduces the pressure and potential strain on each part.

Vary the Strokes That You Do

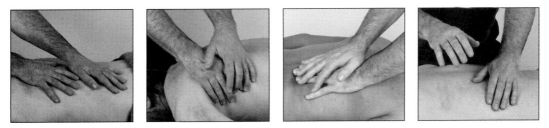

Figure 11.22: Vary strokes; a) stroking, b) doing a stretch, c) applying pressure, d) percussion.

During a massage session, try to vary what you do, rather than doing one stroke for any great length of time. For example, intersperse techniques that involve applying pressure, which compresses your joints, with effleurage strokes that let your hand relax, stretches which open out your joints, and percussion that enables you to shake out your hands.

Vary the Areas of Your Hands That You Use

To take the pressure off your thumbs and fingers, try using other parts of your hands in a variety of ways whenever you can. You could give yourself the challenge of finding as many different parts of your hand that you can use for a given technique. For example, use your fingertips for light stroking ('feathering'), and your whole hand for broad effleurage strokes. Switch to your fist for deep sliding pressure ('stripping' the muscles, see figure 16.19). (And use your forearm or elbow for the deepest pressure, see Chapters 18 and 19).

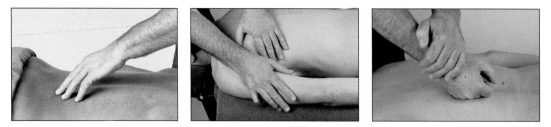

Figure 11.23: Using varied areas of the hands for stroking; a) 'feathering' with the fingertips, b) stroking with the whole hand, c) 'stripping' a muscle with the fist.

Vary How You Use Your Hand Within a Stroke

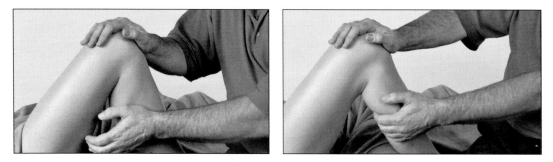

Figure 11.24: Variety in a wringing stroke; a) pushing forward with the heels of the hands, b) pulling back with the fingers.

You can also vary how you use your hands within a stroke. For example, in wringing strokes, push forward with the heel of your hand, and pull back with your fingers.

Exploring Using One Area of Your Hand in a Variety of Ways

To expand your repertoire of possibilities, focus on one area of your hand and experiment to see how many different techniques you could adapt and use it for. When you are using your whole hand for an effleurage stroke, for example, you could put more pressure through the heel or the outer edge of your hand as you push away from yourself, and dig in a little with your fingers as you slide back with your hand.

Experimenting to find new possibilities with the less commonly used parts of the hand such as the back of the hand (see figure 14.13) or the outside edge (see figure 14.11) can also be helpful in opening up a range of possibilities while also taking pressure off the most (over)used areas.

Balance Your Hand Use – Teach Yourself to be Ambidextrous

Take care not to overuse your dominant hand. This is especially important for right-handed people, who are much more unbalanced in their hand use than left-handers who have to adapt to a right-handed world. If it seems necessary, do extra strengthening exercises for your weaker hand.

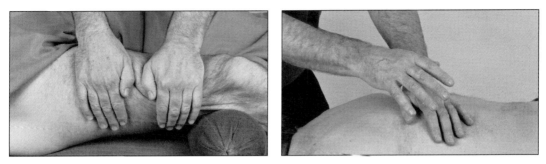

Figure 11.25: Using the hands evenly; a) for wringing, b) for percussion.

Learning to be ambidextrous is one of the essentials of massage. It can be challenging at first, but it is crucial to avoid overusing your stronger / more skilful hand. Practice using your hands as equally as you can for techniques such as wringing and percussion. At first, you may find this frustrating if your non-dominant hand is weaker, slower and less skilful. Take time to teach your less-used hand to copy the dominant one, and do techniques at a pace and pressure that suits your non-dominant hand. Perseverance and practice will bring it towards the level of your dominant hand. Otherwise you will end up in a vicious cycle of continuing to overuse your dominant hand and underusing the other one.

Mirror Your Hand Use (and Bodyuse) on Opposite Sides of the Table

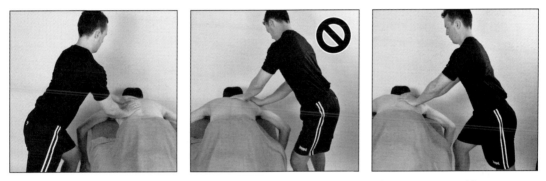

*Figure 11.26: Mirroring hand use and body position on opposite sides of the massage table;
a) on one side, b) not mirroring on the other side, c) mirroring on the other side.*

Learning to use both hands relatively equally is also important for applying the same technique on opposite sides of the massage chair/table. When doing this, take care to mirror the whole stance that you use to support each hand.

Learn to Simultaneously Use Each Hand in Different Ways
Increasing your ambidexterity also underpins the development of another essential coordination skill for massage – learning to simultaneously use each hand in a different way. Learning to use both hands actively in different ways at the same time will develop your ability to focus on each hand, and therefore accustom you to using them more equally.

Two ways of doing this have been covered above – having one hand support the other (see figures 11.10 & 11.11), and double-handed strokes (see figures 11.12–11.14). In both of these types of strokes, it is important not to slip into using one hand to do most of the work.

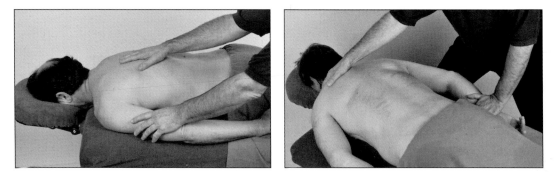

*Figure 11.27: Simultaneously doing the same technique on different areas;
a) stroking down the back and arm, b) squeezing the shoulder and wrist.*

Another way of developing this is to apply the same sort of technique at the same time on two different areas of the client's body. For example, you can simultaneously stroke down the client's back, arm or leg, or squeeze the client's shoulder and wrist. This helps you to get used to simultaneously working with different scales of size and pressure. (Incidentally, these sorts of strokes can give the client interesting experiences of the interconnection of his/her body. This can be especially helpful for clients who are out of touch with their bodies).

Vary What You Are Doing With One or Other Hand

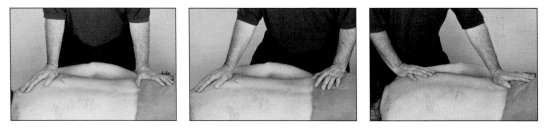

*Figure 11.28: Making the same strokes more different; a) pressing equally on the scapula and hip,
b) pushing the scapula more, c) pushing the hip more.*

A variation on this idea is to gradually make the two strokes more different. For example, begin applying equal pressure on the scapula and hip to push them apart. Then turn your body and lean more towards the scapula to increase the pressure and encourage it to stretch up the back of the ribs (while keeping the hip stabilised). Or to turn the other way and push the hip more.

Try Doing Different Strokes at the Same Time

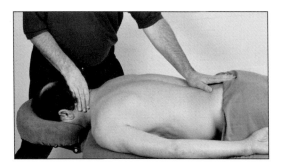

*Figure 11.29: Sliding one hand down the back
while squeezing the neck.*

It is a small step from this idea to doing different strokes with each hand at the same time. For example, gradually slide one hand down the prone client's back while squeezing the neck muscles.

It takes time but it is worth the practice that's needed to make these sorts of stroke comfortable and easy. Experimenting further with combining two familiar strokes in this way will not only develop your dexterity, but will also provide you with ways of expanding your repertoire.

Use Supports to Save Your Hands

Supporting the client's body or finding ways of supporting your working hand(s) whenever you can, reduces the pressure on your hands.

Use the Recipient's Body to Provide Support

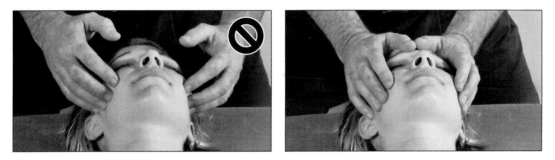

Figure 11.30: Using the fingers to apply pressure; a) with no support,
b) with other parts of the hand providing support.

When using the tips of your fingers for delicate work on small areas such as the client's face, you will be able to work with greater precision if you rest the heels of your hands on the face. Clients often find this greater contact on the face quite soothing. (When you are doing finely-tuned techniques on small areas such as the face, sitting down will help to reduce the pressure on your shoulders and arms to provide stability while enabling you to work with greater precision, see figure 31.1).

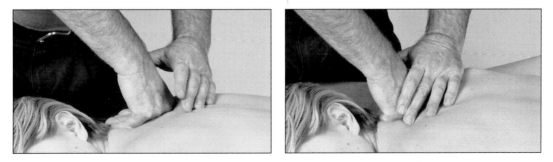

Figure 11.31: Resting the supporting hand on the client's body.

Similarly, in firmer strokes, you can rest your supporting hand on the client's body to take pressure off your working hand.

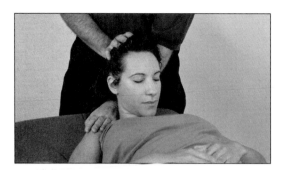

Sometimes, you can also use the client's body to give you support or pivots for applying a stretch.

Figure 11.32: Using the receiver's body for support in a neck stretch.

Use the Massage Couch for Support

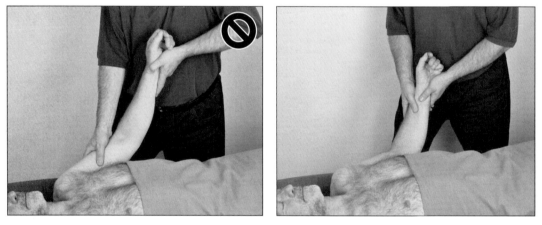

Figure 11.33: Applying pressure on the client's forearm; a) while holding the arm in the air, b) using both hands with the limb supported on the table.

Whenever you can, use the massage couch or chair for support when you are applying pressure, rather than holding a limb in the air. This saves you considerable effort. It also enables you to use both hands together while simultaneously controlling the limb.

Use Cushions and Bolsters for Support

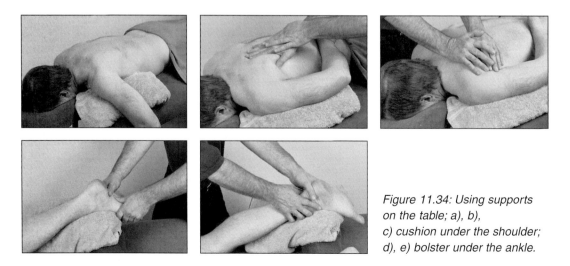

Figure 11.34: Using supports on the table; a), b), c) cushion under the shoulder; d), e) bolster under the ankle.

Similarly, you can use bolsters and cushions to support parts of your client's body when you are applying pressure, particularly when you are concentrating on a small area. This provides greater stability, while reducing the pressure on your hands to provide this stability. As well as allowing you to use both hands together for the massage strokes, this frees you to move around the table / chair to best position yourself for each stroke.

Use Your Own Body to Support Your Work

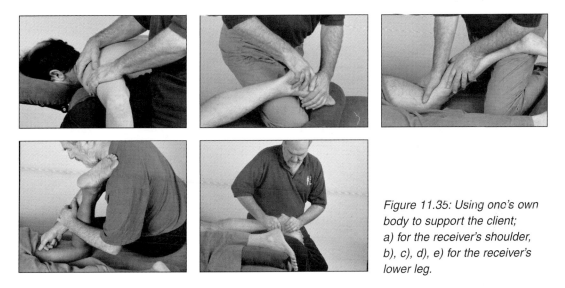

Figure 11.35: Using one's own body to support the client; a) for the receiver's shoulder, b), c), d), e) for the receiver's lower leg.

Bear in mind that you can also use your own body, particularly your leg, to support parts of the client's body. Sometimes this support can also act as an effective third 'hand' (see Chapter 21) to move a part of the client's body as well as to support it.

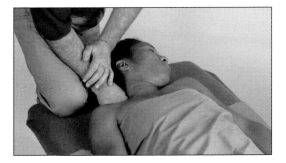

You can also use your leg to support your working tools. For example you can put your knee on the table to support your arm across your thigh when doing strong, finely-tuned work on the client's neck. It is also very useful to use your leg to brace your working arm when you are doing a floor massage (see Chapter 42).

Figure 11.36: Using the thigh to support the working hand.

Involving Your Body to Support Your Hands

Bear in mind that the skilful use of your hands alone is not sufficient for good massage practice. How you use the rest of your body to support your hands (see Chapters 22–28) has a major effect on how you are able to use them. The ideal is to have your hands relaxed and simultaneously strong with the power transmitted from your body. This section of the chapter touches on some important aspects, which are covered in more detail in Chapters 22–32.

Move Your Arms With Your Hand Movements

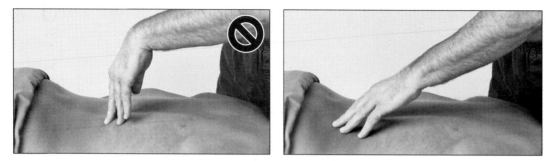

Figure 11.37: Using the hand; a) just moving the hand, b) moving the arm with the stroke.

Even for small strokes in which you are just using your fingers, your delivery will be stiff, awkward and tiring if you do not also involve your arm in the movement. Move your arm for sliding strokes, for example, not just your hand.

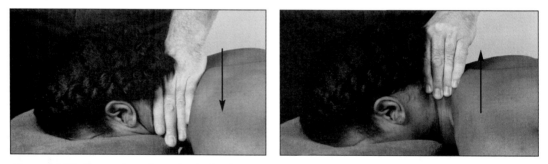

Figure 11.38: Squeezing; a) moving in for the squeeze, b) stretching the muscle.

And, when you are doing squeezing movements, move your arm forward to take hold of the muscle and back to stretch it.

Get Your Body Behind Your Working Tools

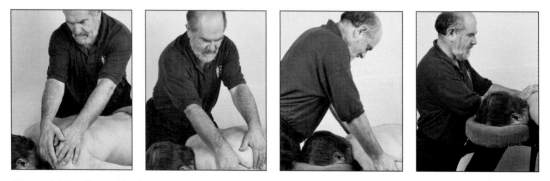

Figure 11.39: Repositioning oneself to face the hands.

Position your body directly behind your hands for each stroke.

Lean Forward for Power

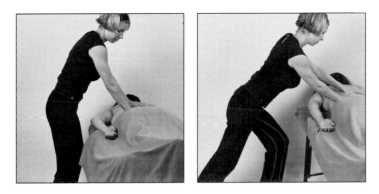

Figure 11.40: Leaning to apply pressure; a) a little pressure, b) leaning further for more pressure.

Lean forward to create the power for each stroke. Regulate the pressure by how much you lean your bodyweight.

Avoid Standing Still and Overusing the Upper Body

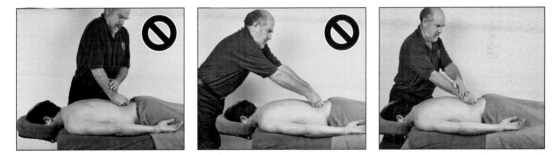

Figure 11.41: Standing still; a) working stiffly, b) overreaching, c) moving into a comfortable position.

Standing still and just using your upper body makes unnecessary demands of your hands and shoulder muscles.

Whenever Possible, Move Your Body With Your Massage Strokes

Swaying your whole body with a massage stroke will give fluidity and evenness to the movements of your arms and hands, and deliver power when necessary. This reduces the need to rely on your arm, hand and shoulder muscles to generate power.

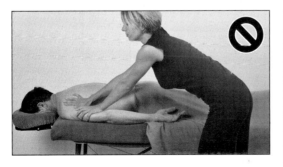

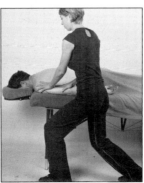

Figure 11.42: Swaying with massage strokes; a) not moving, b) swaying for effleurage.

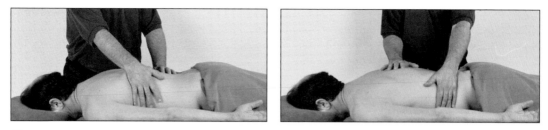

Figure 11.42 (cont.): c), d) twisting for wringing strokes.

Swaying forward and back for effleurage strokes is fairly obvious.

However, it is also important to move for other sorts of strokes. For example, twist your body for wringing strokes by swivelling one hip forward to push one hand forward and let the other hip pull the other arm back.

Hand Maintenance

Strengthen Your Hands

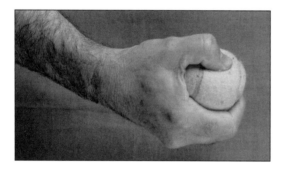

*Figure 11.43: Strengthening the hands –
squeezing a ball.*

It can be helpful to build up the strength of your hands and arms. You can strengthen your hands by regularly squeezing a rubber ball outside of work, for example when watching television. Do not overdo it at the beginning, but build it up gradually. Those with small hands may also find it useful to get coaching from a fitness trainer to develop an exercise routine for strengthening their hands and wrists.

Get Regular Massages for Your Hands and Forearms
Getting your hands regularly massaged and/or massaging them yourself is helpful in keeping them from getting too tense. Do not neglect the muscles of your forearms that control your hands – the flexor muscles at the front of your forearm and the extensor muscles at the back.

Self-massage Your Hands and Forearm Muscles

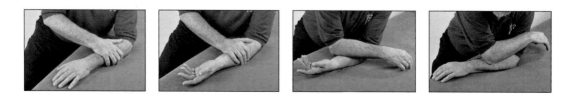

Figure 11.44: Self-massage on the forearm muscles.

It is good to regularly massage your own hands and also the forearm muscles, which control your wrists and fingers and thumbs. Rest your forearm on your massage table for this rather than a hard surface. Try not to tire your hands while doing it – learn to use your forearm in order to save your hands. Use the 'soft' forearm (the bellies of the flexor muscles, see figure 18.1) to massage, keeping the hand of your working forearm relaxed and palm down (see figure 18.3). Work firmly on the muscle bellies in your forearm, ease the pressure at your wrists, and then apply pressure across your hand, including your fingers, putting more pressure on the front of your hand than the back.

Do not sit stiffly and just use your shoulder muscles to power your forearm, but lean and sway your weight to deliver pressure (see figure 18.26). If you're not using oil, maintain the pressure and sway forward to stretch the skin in order to get moving pressure over the underlying muscles.

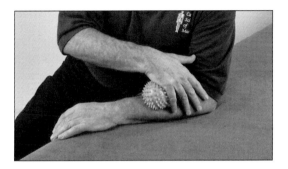

Figure 11.45: Massaging the forearm with a spiky ball.

You can also use yielding mechanical massage tools such as a spiky ball, particularly to get into the extensor muscles.

Stretching and Mobilising Exercises for Your Hands

Being able to relax and enliven your hands and to get them supple are important preparations for massage work. Warm-up exercises that help you to do this also form the basis for developing manual dexterity (see figures 11.22–11.29). And, after doing a massage, simple stretches of your hands and fingers will help to release tension. As you do these exercises, focus on keeping your shoulders and breathing relaxed.

Clench and Stretch Your Hands

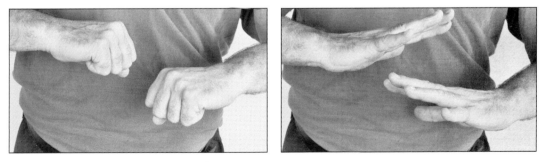

Figure 11.46: Mobilising the hands; a) clenching the hands, b) opening them into a stretch.

Alternating between clenching your hands and opening them out into a stretch is a simple way to release stiffness and get your hands moving.

Shake Out Your Hands

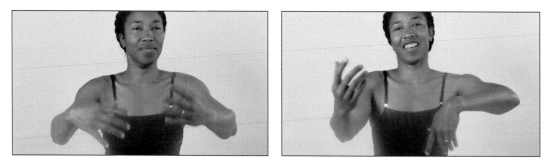

Figure 11.47: Shaking out the hands.

Shaking out your hands will simultaneously relax and energise them. Don't make the shaking too forceful or jarring. Vary the way that you shake your hands so that you can direct the shaking to as many parts of your hands as possible. For example, you could imagine that you are trying to shake something sticky off your hands. Imagine that it is stuck to your thumb at first, and then to each of your fingers in turn, then to the back of your knuckles, the side of your hand, and so on.

Stretch Your Fingers

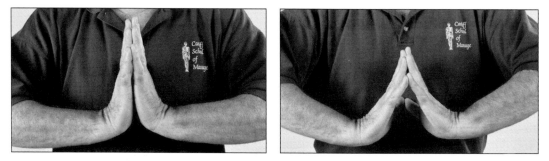

Figure 11.48: Lowering the hands in the prayer position to stretch the fingers.

Because our fingers are so often a little flexed in everyday life, it is useful to stretch them back, as long as it is not done too forcefully or they are already hypermobile. An easy way of doing this is to place your hands together in the prayer position in front of your body, and slowly lower them.

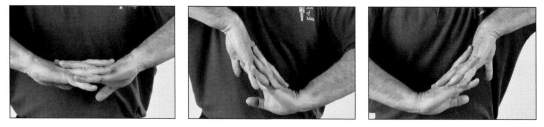

Figure 11.49: Stretching interlocked fingers.

Another way is by interlocking the fingers of both hands and gently stretching them back, or by interlocking the fingers of one hand through the other and using this grip to stretch your fingers, as you would for a client.

Mobilise Your Wrist

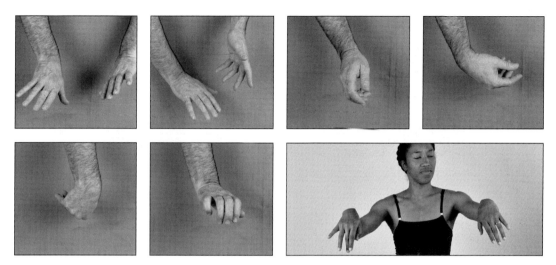

Figure 11.50: Wrist stretches.

Give your wrists attention too. Stretching your hands forward, back and sideways is an easy way to promote suppleness in your wrists. You can extend this by joining these movements into a smooth wrist circle that incorporates pronation and supination of your forearm. Do not stiffen your shoulders, which would restrict the movement.

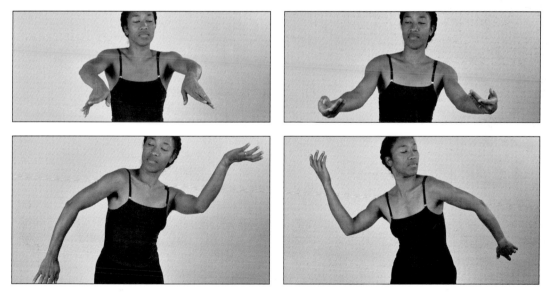

Figure 11.50 (cont.): Involving the shoulders.

In fact, it is useful to extend the movement to include your shoulders so that you mobilise the whole of your arm and shoulder girdle.

Develop Fine-tuning Finger Control

Having stretched the parts of your hands, specific mobilising exercises that focus on your fingers will help you to develop your dexterity, particularly if you're not used to using your hands.

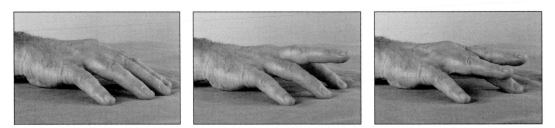

Figure 11.51: Fine-tuning finger control; a) relaxed fingers, b) lifting a single finger, c) lifting fingers in pairs.

One way of doing this is to place your hand prone on a flat surface and lift your fingers one by one, while focusing on keeping the others down. Then lift them in pairs, for example simultaneously lifting your index and ring fingers, or your middle and little fingers. Then vary the combinations. Next, try lifting the matching fingers on both hands at the same time. If you've mastered this and want a challenge that will help you to develop your dexterity further, try using other combinations or simultaneously lifting different fingers on each hand.

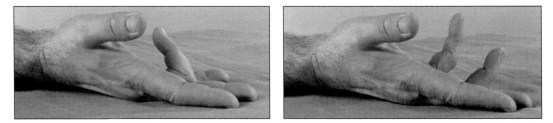

Figure 11.52: Further finger control; a), b) curling the fingers.

You can also do similar exercises for your fingers in flexion. One way is to curl your fingers alone and in various combinations without moving the other fingers. Most people find this hardest to do with the ring finger.

Review

Most hand problems develop from the *accumulation* of strain through using your hands awkwardly, doing repetitive movements and/or through overusing them to apply pressure.

Practitioners with small hands or long, slender thumbs and fingers, or hypermobile fingers and thumbs need to be especially careful about how they use their hands.

Watch out for early warning signals of strain in your hands, especially in your thumbs and wrists, such as intermittent or persistent pain when you're not using your hands, sensitivity to bumping them, tingling or numbness in them, and weakness or loss of control.

Do not overload your hands by using them extensively for physical tasks in your spare time as well as working hard at massage.

Rest your hands when you can. Get regular massages and/or give yourself regular self-massage for your hands and the muscles of the forearm.

Stretch and shake out your hands before and after massages to relax and enliven your hands and to help keep them supple.

Learn to relax them during treatment sessions, especially the parts of your hand that are not being used in a technique.

Do mobilising exercises for your wrists. Strengthen you hands if necessary, by regularly squeezing a rubber ball or through supervised exercises and gym work.

Mobilising exercises for your fingers will help to develop your dexterity, which increases your massage skills while spreading the workload throughout your hands.

Avoid overusing your fingers and thumbs or straining them by having them hyperextended when applying pressure.

Do not let your wrist bend when applying pressure.

Minimise the amount of thumb kneading that you do.

Use the largest, most appropriate area of your hand for applying pressure.

Vary your massage techniques.

Rather than leaving your other hand idle, use it for:

* Supporting the wrist of your working hand, or;
* Working double-handedly (using both hands together for strokes).

Keep your hands as relaxed as possible, and learn to relax the non-working parts of your hand.

Whenever you can, save your hands by using:

* A tool such as a rubber ball, or;
* Your forearm or elbow.

If necessary, reduce the amount of hand-intensive activities in the rest of your life.

Develop your dexterity and coordination by:

* Varying the strokes that you do;
* The areas of your hand that you use;
* How you use your hand within a stroke;
* Learning to be ambidextrous;
* Learning to simultaneously use each hand in different ways.

Reduce the pressure on your hands by supporting your hands, by:

* Using the recipient' s body to provide support for your hands;
* Use the massage couch for support;
* Using cushions or bolsters on the table for support, or;
* Using your own body to support your work.

Involve your body to support your hands by:

* Moving your arms and your body with massage strokes;
* Positioning your body behind your hands and leaning your body to deliver power;
* Swaying your body for the movement and fluidity of the strokes.

CHAPTER 12

Taking Care of Your Fingers

The fingers are the most delicate part of the hand. They are quite vulnerable to strain and are often overused in massage. This chapter focuses on the commonest risks to your fingers in massage and ways of reducing these. It also looks briefly at other parts of your hand and arm that you can use to conserve your fingers.

Caution!

The main practices which put pressure on your fingers and can strain them if they are done too often are:

- Applying firm pressure with your fingers;
- Hyperextending your fingers when applying pressure through them;
- Not supporting your fingers when pressing with them, and;
- Using your fingers when a larger part of your hand or arm would be more effective for applying pressure.

Be aware of the temptation to stiffen your shoulders when pressing with your fingers, which in turn is likely to lead to stiffening your hands (and therefore your fingers) more. And, if you are *straining* your fingers, you are very likely to be unconsciously stiffening other areas of your body, particularly your shoulders and your back.

With the rise of digital technology, we regularly call upon our fingers to press buttons, although less so than the thumbs. This can compound any strains that you develop from overusing them in massage.

Fingers Most at Risk!

Bear in mind that there are limits to the amount of pressure that a practitioner's fingers can take. *All practitioners* need to watch that they are not putting too much pressure through their fingers at any moment in a massage session, and to monitor the cumulative effects over time of using the fingers to apply pressure.

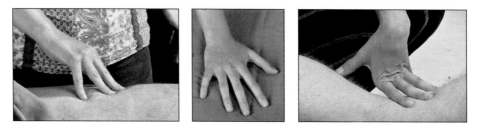

Figure 12.1: Fingers at risk; a) small fingers, b) long slender fingers, c) easily hyperextended.

However, practitioners who have small hands, long, slender fingers, and/or hypermobile fingers, need to take special care of their fingers, particularly when applying pressure (and also of their thumbs, see Chapter 13). The cautions and suggestions in this chapter are *particularly relevant* for these practitioners.

Substitutes for Your Fingers

The fingertips have a sensitivity that is unsurpassed for initially palpating areas of the body. This can lead to overusing them, especially for applying sustained pressure. So it is good to get into the habit of conserving your vulnerable fingers whenever possible. Once you have palpated an area with your fingers, consider whether another, larger part of your hand or forearm would better do the massage job required. Many of these alternative tools can also be used to save your thumbs (see Chapter 13).

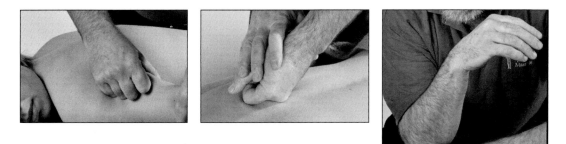

Figure 12.2: Saving the fingers in pressure strokes;
a) knuckle kneading, b) using the fist, c) using the elbow.

When you are focusing pressure on a small area, you can save your fingers by using your knuckles instead (the interphalangeal joints, see figure 15.1). On larger areas, use your fist (see Chapter 16) or the back of your hand (see figure 14.13) if possible. The medial wrist bones can also be used to apply pressure (see figure 14.17) and so can the bony areas around the elbow (see Chapter 19).

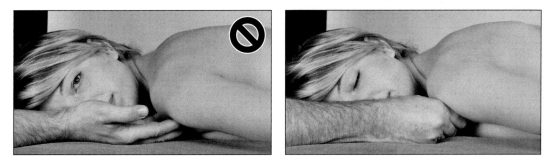

Figure 12.3: Pressing up; a) fingers pressing up, b) using the soft fist on the side.

Be careful when pushing up under a client's body. Be especially wary of letting too much weight press down onto your fingers for any length of time. Use a soft fist instead. (Even then, be aware that there are limits, depending on the size of your hand and the weight of the client).

Protecting Your Fingers When Using Them

It is not always feasible to use substitutes for your fingers because of the precision or delicacy required, for example when you are working on the client's head or applying very precise pressure right next to the spine. So the rest of this chapter looks at ways of reducing the strain on your fingers when you cannot avoid using them.

It is useful to prepare your hands with the type of exercises covered in the previous chapter for suppleness (see figures 11.46–11.50) and developing coordination (see figures 11.27–11.29). These exercises can also be useful for releasing tension between treatment sessions and at the end of the working day. If you have small or slender fingers, you may also find it helpful to do strengthening exercises for them (see figure 11.43).

Use as Much of Your Fingers as Possible

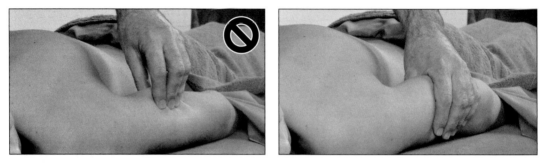

Figure 12.4: Taking hold of muscles; a) overusing the fingertips, b) using more of the hand.

There is common tendency to overuse the fingertips in massage strokes such as kneading and squeezing muscles. Instead of just using the tips of your fingers and thumbs for these techniques, try using more of your hand – your palm and the base of your fingers and thumbs.

Relax Your Hands
Massage novices tend to stiffen their hands as they focus on learning strokes. This uses unnecessary energy and often leads to tensing other parts of the body. It is relatively easy to learn to relax your whole hand when you are just resting it on the client's body. It takes practice to learn to relax the non-working parts of your hand in each stroke (see figure 11.19).

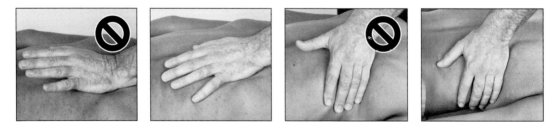

Fig 12.5: Relaxing the non-working parts of the hand; a) tensing the fingers when using the heel of the hand, b) using the heel of the hand with relaxed fingers, c) tensing the thumb when using the fingers, d) using the fingers with the thumb relaxed.

Take care not to stiffen your fingers when using other parts of your hands such as the heel. Another common habit to watch out for is stiffening your thumb when using your fingers. Both of these make an extra demand on your fingers.

Don't Hyperextend Your Fingers When Applying Pressure
When you are applying pressure through your fingertips, make sure that your fingers do not hyperextend. This puts considerable strain on them and is not effective in transmitting power. Practitioners with long, slender or hypermobile fingers need to be especially careful about this. Even if you straighten your fingers, take care not to let the last section of them hyperextend.

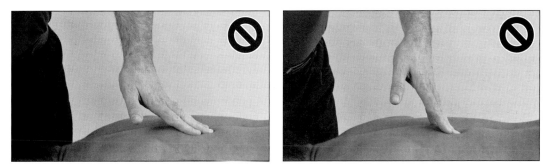

Figure 12.6: Hyperextending the fingers when applying pressure through them;
a) hyperextending the fingers, b) hyperextending last section of fingers.

Be careful too when you are pressing sideways with the flat surface of your fingers, for example when massaging a client's scalp. It is very easy for your fingers to hyperextend in this situation, which puts unnecessary pressure on them.

However, if you do a lot pressure work with them, it is good practice to regularly stretch them back briefly to release the flexor muscles from stiffening into one position (see figure 11.48).

Finding the Best Angle for Applying Pressure Through Your Fingers

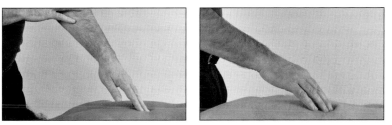

Figure 12.7: Finger angles; a) straight fingers, b) slightly curled.

Straightening your fingers is better when you are applying pressure with the tips or the flat surface of the last section. However, although this doesn't strain them like hyperextending them, it is a hard position to maintain when you press firmly. Try this position and then compare it with curling your fingers *slightly*. Most people find that having them slightly curled, which engages the strong flexor muscles, is the strongest position for applying pressure. It also enables you to keep your fingers more relaxed as you apply the pressure.

Use Your Fingers Together

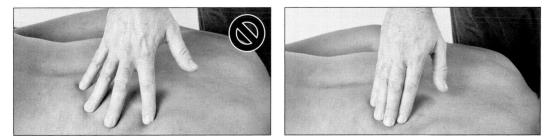

Figure 12.8: Using the fingers together for firm strokes; a) fingers spread and pressing separately,
b) together as a unit for applying pressure.

Try to only use your fingers separately for small movements that do not involve much pressure, such as light stroking movements on the client's face. When you are applying pressure with your fingers, use them together as a single group, to reduce the force on each one. And also keep them together for other firm strokes such as wringing.

Supporting Your Working Fingers

In addition, try to support your fingers whenever possible. This is crucial for reducing the pressure on them.

Support Them With Other Parts of Your Hand

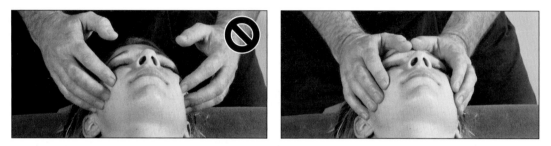

Figure 12.9: Support with other parts of your hand; a) with no support,
b) with other parts of the hand providing support.

When using the tips of your fingers for delicate work, for example on the client's face, rest the heels of your hands on the client if you can. As well as relaxing your hand, this gives you more support, which takes pressure off your fingers and enables you to work with greater precision. Clients often find this greater contact on the face quite soothing.

Use Your Other Hand to Support and Guide Your Fingers

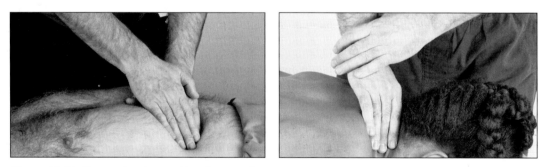

Figure 12.10: Supporting the working fingers; a) light circling on the abdomen,
b) squeezing the client's neck.

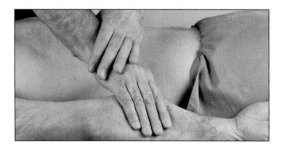

Figure 12.11: Maintaining the squeeze and
stretching the muscles.

Whenever you can, using your other hand to guide your working hand provides greater control and fluidity, even in light sliding strokes such as a circling movement on the client's abdomen. It is helpful in stronger actions such as squeezing the client's neck muscles. It is crucial when you want to work more firmly, for example squeezing the client's forearm muscles or the large muscles of the thigh.

In firm squeezing strokes, you can further reduce the work of your fingers. Instead of rhythmically squeezing and releasing the muscle, take hold of the muscle with one hand and maintain this grip. While maintaining the squeeze, use your supporting hand to move it so that you stretch the muscle. Sway back to provide the impetus for this.

Use Your Other Hand to Add Pressure to Finger Strokes

When it is appropriate, you can also use your supporting hand to add pressure to your finger strokes, *as long as it is not too much for them.*

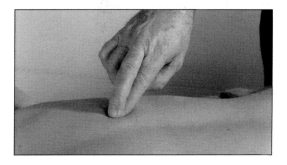

Figure 12.12: Adding pressure to finger strokes; finger on finger pressure – use with caution.

Pressing on your fingers enables you to focus pressure on a small area. A common way of doing this is by pressing the middle finger on the index finger. However, this is hard work on your fingers unless they are large and strong. Even then, use this technique sparingly and monitor your fingers carefully for any sign of strain developing.

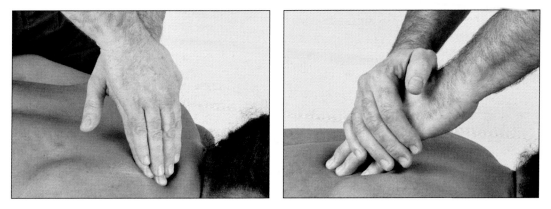

Figure 12.13: Using the other hand to focus pressure; a) using the other hand to focus pressure, b) increasing and spreading the pressure.

It is less strainful to focus the pressure by pressing onto your working finger(s) with your other hand. To increase the pressure and spread it across your fingers, press your other hand across all of your fingers.

Support Under Your Working Fingers

However, if your fingers still have to provide the stability because they are the only point of contact with the client's body, they will be taking a lot of pressure.

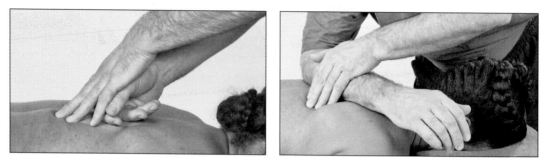

Figure 12.14: Stabilising the working fingers by resting the support on the client's body; a) resting on your other hand, b) resting on your other forearm.

One way to reduce the pressure on them is by resting your working hand across your supporting hand or forearm, which is resting on the client's body. (However, if you want to apply more pressure, switch to other tools such as your fist or your elbow).

Support Your Fingers in Pulling Strokes

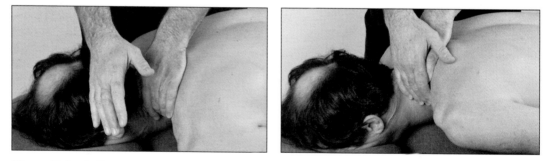

Figure 12.15: Pulling with the hands together; a) the under-hand 'hook' shape, b) pulling with the fingers.

Use your hands together to conserve your fingers in firm pulling strokes as well. Curl the fingers of your working hand into a 'hook' and then 'wrap' your supporting hand around this 'hook'. This divides the work between your hands – the underhand holds the shape while the top hand does the pulling. Pull back with your whole body so that you don't tense your shoulders and arms, and consequently your hands.

Involving Your Body

Move Your Hand and Arm With Your Finger Movements

Even when you are using your fingers for light sliding strokes, such as a light 'feathering' effleurage, keeping your arm still would make the movement awkward and stilted. It would also put extra pressure on your wrist. So move your whole arm for the sweep of the movement (and sway your body with it too).

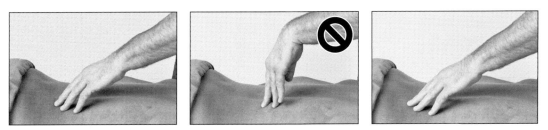

Figure 12.16: Using the fingertips for 'feathering' towards oneself; a) the starting position,
b) with the arm held still, c) moving the arm with the stroke.

Moving your arm with other types of strokes also delivers more power when it is appropriate, as well as evenness. When you are rhythmically squeezing and releasing muscles, for example of the client's forearm, it would be much harder work on your fingers (and your wrist) if you were to keep your hand stationary, and your delivery would be less fluid and powerful.

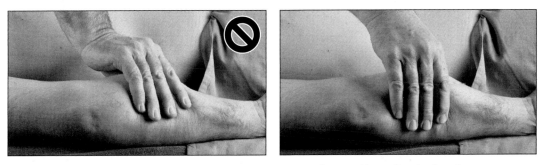

Figure 12.17: Squeezing forearm muscles; a) just using the fingers, b) moving the hand.

Review

Be careful of your fingers in massage if you have small hands, slender fingers or hypermobile fingers.
Whenever you can, use larger tools such as your knuckles, fist or elbow to save your hands, especially when you are applying pressure.
When you can't avoid using your fingers, protect them by:
- Using as much of your fingers as you can;
- Relaxing the non-working parts of your hand;
- Not hyperextending your fingers when you are applying pressure;
- Using your fingers together;
- Stabilising your hand for very small finger movements by resting the heel of your hand on the client's body;
- Using your other hand to support your working hand and to add pressure to your strokes;
- Using both hands together for firm pulling strokes, and;
- Moving your arm and swaying your body for large movements.

CHAPTER 13

Protecting Your Thumbs

The thumbs are probably the area of the body that massage practitioners most commonly strain. They are stronger and more mobile than the fingers while providing a similar sensing ability, and are therefore used in many 'classic' massage techniques. So it is easy to overuse them, particularly in kneading and for applying pressure. This chapter focuses on the best ways of using your thumbs while keeping the pressure on them to a minimum. It also looks briefly at substitutes that you can use to save your thumbs.

Caution – Thumbs at Risk!

It is important to monitor how you use your thumbs, as it is easy to put pressure on them in massage strokes. Most thumb strains develop over time through:

• Putting too much pressure through them;
• Having them hyperextended when applying pressure, and;
• Not supporting them so that they take all of the pressure.

Be particularly careful not to hyperextend your thumbs when you are kneading (see figure 13.3), wringing (see figure 13.4) or applying pressure (see figure 13.5).

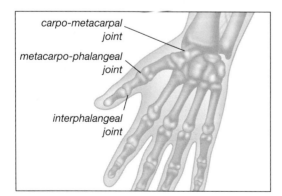

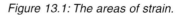
Figure 13.1: The areas of strain.

Problems most commonly arise at the base of the thumb (the carpo-metacarpal joint), or sometimes at the metacarpo-phalangeal joint. Working with the thumbs regularly hyperextended also puts pressure on the interphalangeal joint.

The common warning signs of strain are pain in the thumb joints, and/or sharp pain in the lower forearm – in the bellies of the forearm muscles which control the thumb.

Initially, the feeling of strain will only occur when the practitioner is actually doing massage. However pain that persists outside of massage sessions or sudden pains that wake you at night are indications of serious problems developing. These require attention:

- Switching to using your knuckles, fist or elbow whenever possible;
- Changing the way that you use your thumb (covered in this chapter);
- Massage and other treatments to ease the strain, and;
- Maybe adjustments in the rest of your life to reduce how much you use your thumbs.

Monitor Your Thumbs
Bear in mind that using your body effectively, as *covered in this book, will bring more power to bear on your thumbs. So monitor that it is not too much for them, and switch to other tools such as your knuckles, fist or elbow whenever you can.*

Thumbs Most at Risk

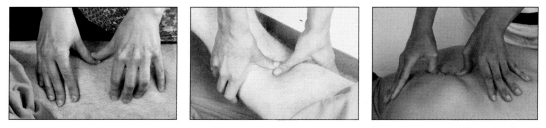

Figure 13.2: Thumbs most at risk; a) small hands, b) long, slender thumb, c) hypermobile thumb.

Practitioners most at risk of thumb strain are those with small hands, long, slender thumbs, and/or hypermobile thumbs. These practitioners therefore need to be particularly careful about how they use their thumbs (and also of their fingers, see Chapter 12).

Tensing the Shoulders Puts Pressure on the Thumbs
There are some other things to be aware of. When you are focusing your massage work on a small area, there is a great temptation to stand still and unconsciously tense your shoulders compared to when you are doing large sweeping strokes. Tensing your shoulders, arms and hands puts more pressure on your thumbs.

Monitor How Much You Use Your Thumbs for Other Activities
As well as taking care of the thumbs in 'classic' Swedish massage strokes, practitioners need to be careful if they also use them in other ways in treatment sessions, for example in doing reflexology and trigger point work.

And you also need to pay attention to how much you use your thumbs in everyday life. Thumb strain in massage sessions can be aggravated by extensive mobile phone texting, for example.

Alternatives to the Thumbs

Your thumb and fingers are irreplaceable for the initial palpation of the tissues, and for light massage strokes. Because of this, there is a great temptation to overuse them for pressure strokes. This chapter focuses primarily on the safest and most effective ways of using your thumbs in massage *when you can not avoid using them* for working firmly.

However, it is important to consider using other, larger parts of your hands and arms for applying pressure whenever you can. You can be more effective while conserving your vulnerable thumbs (and also your fingers, see Chapter 12). Initially, you will probably need to regularly use your fingers or thumbs to monitor any changes in the client's tissues, or to use the fingers of your supporting hand (see figure 13.13). With practise, you will find that you can develop the sensitivity of these other massage tools.

Another Way of Kneading

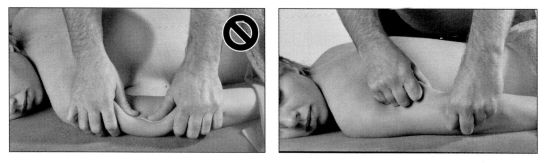

Figure 13.3: Kneading large muscles; a) hyperextending the thumbs, b) knuckle kneading.

Kneading forms a significant part of the 'classic' massage repertoire. However, kneading with the thumbs is hard work and not particularly effective on large, tight muscles such as well-used quadriceps or hamstring muscles. A better alternative is 'knuckle kneading' (see figure 15.4).

Another Way of Wringing

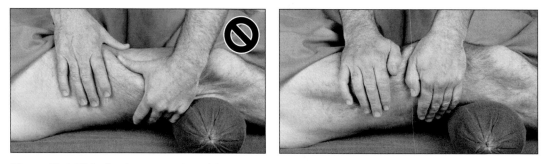

Figure 13.4: Wringing large muscles; a) hyperextending the thumbs,
b) wringing with just the heel of the hands.

Wringing strokes also put pressure on your thumbs and you are also quite likely to hyperextend them to push across muscles. So use the heel of your hand for pushing instead, and have your (relaxed) thumbs move with your fingers.

Alternatives for Pressure Strokes
The base of your thumb (see figure 14.4) is a good substitute for delivering general pressure over a wide area, but, whenever you can, switch to your fist (see Chapter 16) or your elbow (see Chapter 19) for focusing firm pressure on a small area.

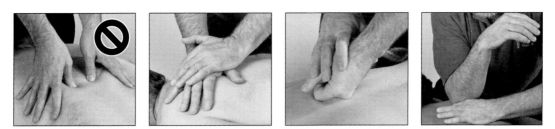

Figure 13.5: Alternatives for applying pressure; a) hyperextended thumb, b) the base of the thumb (thenar eminence), c) the fist, d) the elbow.

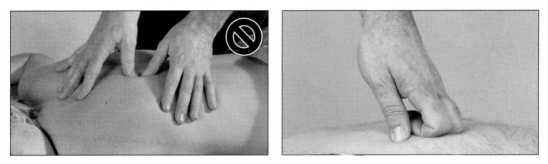

Figure 13.6: Friction strokes; a) thumb friction, b) knuckle friction.

In 'friction' strokes, in which the thumbs are moved in small intersecting pressure circles, they are even more at risk of hyperextending and maybe even buckling as you press down through them. These strokes can also be done with your knuckles instead (but take care not to strain them through overuse, see figure 15.7). For larger areas, your fist (see Chapter 16) or your elbow (see Chapter 19) will provide you with stronger, more effective and less vulnerable tools for moving pressure strokes.

Mechanical Tools

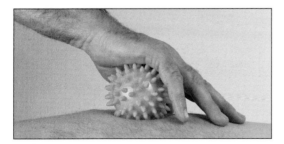

Figure 13.7: Mechanical tools – spiky ball.

Some people use yielding mechanical tools for focused pressure to save their thumbs, although you can not feel the client's responses through them as well as you can directly through your hands. However, with practice you can learn to be relatively sensitive with them.

Protecting Your Thumbs When Using Them

The rest of this chapter looks at reducing the pressure on your thumbs by:

• Keeping your hand relaxed;
• Making sure that your thumb is not bent back;

- Supporting it with your other hand whenever possible, and;
- Using your body well to support your thumb.

Keep the Non-working Parts of the Hand Relaxed

Many people tend to unconsciously stiffen up the non-working parts of their hands, especially when they are first learning to massage. Holding your hands stiffly as you massage will affect your thumbs.

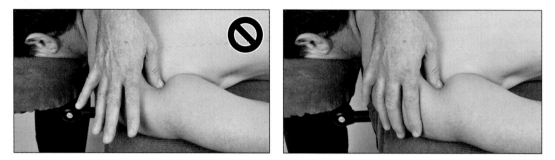

Figure 13.8: Relaxing the non-working parts of the hand; a) stiff fingers when using the thumb, b) relaxed fingers when using the thumb.

Stiffening your fingers, for example, is a common habit when using the thumb. This puts extra pressure on your thumb and will tend to lead you into unconsciously stiffening it.

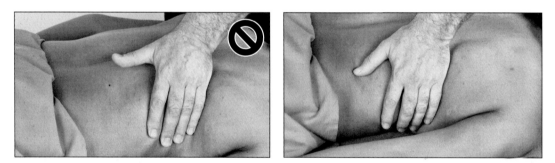

Figure 13.9: Using the thumb unnecessarily; a) stiff thumb when using the fingers, b) relaxed thumb when using the fingers.

Another common habit is to stiffen your thumb when using your fingers. This also uses the thumb unnecessarily. Instead, work out which parts of your hand are essential for a technique, and relax the rest.

Don't Hyperextend Your Thumb

It is crucial to avoid hyperextending your thumb when you are pushing with it, for example in kneading or wringing strokes, or using it for pressure strokes. Having your thumb hyperextended puts considerable pressure on the joints, and reduces the effective transmission of power from your body. You would be constantly overworking the forearm and hand muscles that control your thumb. Regularly working in this way can easily strain your thumb and could lead to long-term problems.

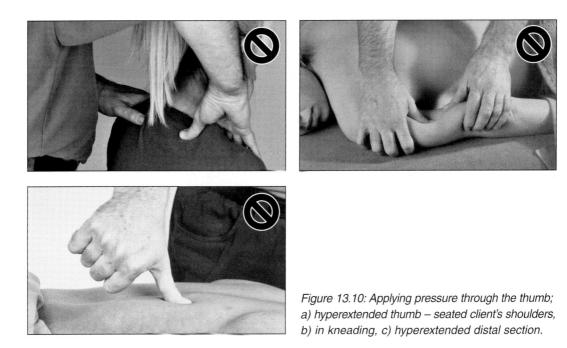

Figure 13.10: Applying pressure through the thumb;
a) hyperextended thumb – seated client's shoulders,
b) in kneading, c) hyperextended distal section.

When you need to apply pressure through your thumb, keep it in line with your forearm as much as possible, so that the power comes directly to it from your arm. Even then, watch that the last section of your thumb (the distal phalanx) doesn't hyperextend, which would put great pressure on the interphalangeal joint. Supporting it with your other hand (see figure 13.13) will help you to avoid this.

Supporting Your Thumb

Even when your thumb is in line with your arm, there is considerable pressure on the joints when you are applying pressure through it. Supporting your thumb will reduce this pressure on it. The more support that you give it, the more effective and less vulnerable it will be. Even so, bear in mind that there are limits to how much force your thumb can take, so monitor what is comfortable for you, and switch to your knuckles, fist or elbow whenever possible.

Support it With Other Parts of Your Hand

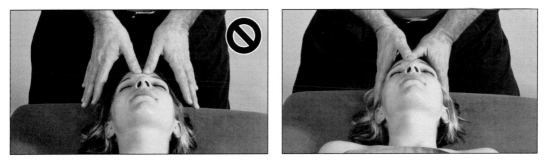

Figure 13.11: Stabilising thumb pressure; a) the unsupported thumb,
b) resting your fingers on the client for stability.

When pressing with your thumbs on a small area, rest other parts of your hand on the client's body for stability, whenever possible. When pressing on the crown of the client's head, for example, stabilise your hand by resting your fingers on another area of the client's head.

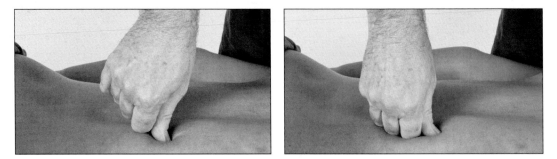

Figure 13.12: Supporting your thumb with your fingers; a) curled behind it, b) knuckles resting on the client's body.

Another way of supporting your thumb is to curl your fingers and press them behind it. However, your lone thumb still has to provide the stability. So rest your curled knuckles on the client's body to reduce the pressure on your thumb.

Use Your Other Hand to Support Your Thumb

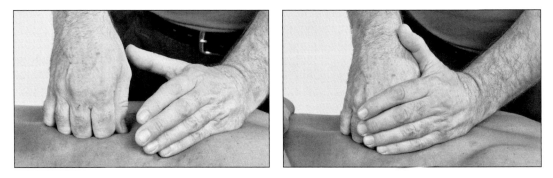

Figure 13.13: Guiding the thumb; a) the containing hand, b) the 'contained' thumb.

Use your *other hand*, whenever you can, to support and control your working hand, focusing particularly on taking even more pressure off your thumb. 'Wrap' your supporting hand around your working hand (in which your thumb is already supported by your curled fingers).

If this containing hand is not in contact with the client's body, your working thumb would still have to provide stability, which puts substantial pressure back onto it. So rest your supporting hand on the client's body for the greatest stability, which will enable you to keep it relatively relaxed. This further reduces the pressure on your thumb, which is then *only* applying the pressure. You can now guide your working thumb with much greater precision.

Be Careful About Pressing on Your Thumb to Apply Pressure
Some people apply thumb pressure by pressing the tip of the other thumb on it. This is hard work for both thumbs, and you have to take care not to hyperextend them. Unless you have large, strong thumbs, you are in danger of straining them if you do very much of this. The other common practice of using your fingers for the pressure also needs care to avoid hyperextending them and to make sure that the pressure is not too much for your thumb.

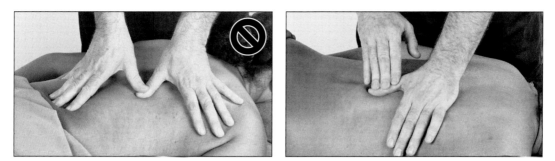

Figure 13.14: Pressing on the thumb; a) thumb on thumb,
b) fingers pressing on the thumb (use sparingly).

Use a 'Reinforced Thumb' for Applying Pressure

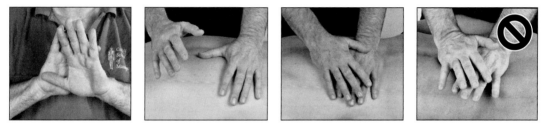

Figure 13.15: The reinforced thumb; a) how the thumb fits into the heel of the hand,
b), c) pressure applied through the thumb, d) having stiff fingers.

A much more effective option is to use a 'reinforced thumb' – pressing the heel of your supporting hand onto your thumb. Rest your thumb on the client's body, and place the heel of your other hand on it so that the middle joint of the thumb (the interphalangeal joint) lies snugly in the gap between the two pads (the thenar and hypothenar eminences) of your supporting hand. The pressure is therefore applied on the two phalanges of the thumb, and not on the joint. Take care to keep both hands relaxed, especially your thumb. Control the technique by directing the power from your bodyweight through your top hand, using your thumb as a passive tool.

The advantage of this technique is that:

• The pressure is still concentrated precisely on a small area;
• You are able to palpate the effect through your sensitive thumb;
• You generate and direct the force by swaying your body so that your thumb can *remain relaxed*.

It takes practice to master this way of working. For many people, the hardest aspect is to *totally* relax the thumb and not try to use it in the technique. Monitor that you are staying within the pressure range that is comfortable for your thumb.

Leaning your body more over your hands will enable you to increase the pressure that you are delivering. You can tilt your supporting hand to press more on the tip of your thumb for single point pressure, or press down through the length of your thumb to spread the pressure. Alternatively, you can push more horizontally to slide your thumb along or across muscles, such as the erector spinae muscles of the lower back.

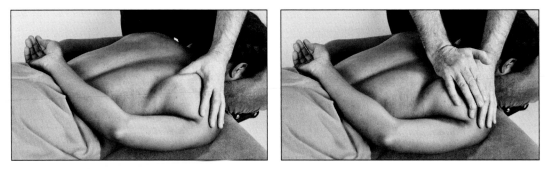

Figure 13.16: Getting under the edge of the scapula.

The reinforced thumb is also useful for working firmly in small areas, such as alongside the spine or under the medial edge of the scapula.

Lean Forward for Power
As is emphasised throughout this book, do not stand still and just use your upper body muscles to apply pressure. Because this is tiring, it is likely to cause you to stiffen your hands, including your thumbs. Instead, lean slowly forward so that the power comes from your bodyweight, and you are able to stay relatively relaxed in your body (and your hands).

Review

Be careful of your thumbs if you have small hands, slender thumbs, and/or they are hypermobile.

Monitor any strains that arise in your thumb joints or your forearm muscles, receive treatments, and make changes in how you use your thumbs to prevent strains developing further.

Use your thumbs sparingly for firm kneading strokes and for applying pressure on small areas.

Save your thumbs in wringing strokes by just using the heel of your hand and your fingers.

Whenever you can, use alternatives such as your knuckles, fist or your elbow.

Keep the non-working parts of your hands relaxed to avoid putting unnecessary pressure on your thumbs.

Don't hyperextend your thumb when applying pressure.

Support your thumb when you are applying pressure by:
- Curling your other fingers behind it;
- Resting those curled fingers on the client's body, and;
- Using your other hand to support and guide your working hand.

Use the 'reinforced thumb' to focus pressure on a small area – pressing with the heel of one hand on your relaxed thumb.

Position your body and lean forward for applying stationary pressure with your thumbs.

Sway forward and move your hands for travelling thumb strokes such as kneading.

CHAPTER 14

Using Other Parts of Your Hands

Massage practitioners can come to rely too much on their fingers and thumbs because of their great sensitivity in palpation. This and the following chapters look at spreading the workload to conserve your vulnerable digits by using other massage tools, which are more effective, especially when you are applying pressure.

This chapter focuses on using other areas of your hand and wrist. The fleshy areas of your hand – the base of the thumb, the heel of the hand, the palm and the side of the hand – can be used for delivering general pressure across a wide area. Although the wrist bones are not strictly part of the hand, they are covered in this chapter because they are used in a similar way to the other parts of the hand. They can be used to apply harder, bony pressure focused on a small area. The back of the hand can be used for 'raking' pressure over a wider area.

The next two chapters look at the use of the largest bony tools of the hand – the knuckles and the fist – for delivering firmer pressure than is possible with the areas covered in this chapter. And the next section of the book looks at ways of saving your hands entirely by using other parts of your body, particularly your forearm and elbow.

Before looking in detail at each of these areas, it is worth focusing on three elements that are common to all of them.

Palpation

When you are first learning to use these tools, you may feel the need to regularly return to your fingers or thumbs to palpate any changes in the client's tissues, or to continually monitor the client's responses with the fingers of your supporting hand. However, you will find that you can develop the sensitivity of these other tools through practice.

Variation Within Strokes

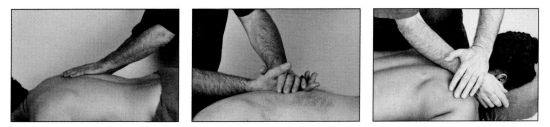

Figure 14.1: Consecutive strokes; a) palm effleurage, b) the back of the hand, c) the medial wrist bone.

Try varying the areas of your hand that you use in consecutive strokes.

For example, you could do a sliding effleurage stroke with your palm, then a 'raking' stroke with the back of your hand once or twice, and then use your medial wrist bone on the next pass over the same area to focus the pressure more precisely.

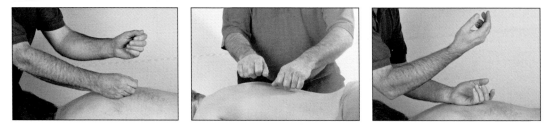

Figure 14.2: Percussion strokes using varied parts of the hands; a) the side of soft fist, b) the knuckles, c) the back of the hand.

And many parts of the hand can be used in percussion strokes to reduce the common reliance on the fingers and the cupped hand. For example, the knuckles can be used for 'rapping', or the side of an open hand or a soft fist. Some people also like using the back of the hand, although this doesn't work for everyone. To avoid overusing any one area when doing percussion, change gradually from one part of your hand to another while maintaining your rhythm and the level of pressure (see Chapter 37).

Using Your Body

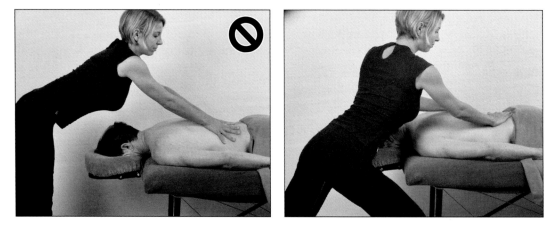

Figure 14.3: Using your body; a) standing still and just using your arms, b) swaying forward.

Whichever part of your hand that you are using, do not stand still and just use your arms. Position your body behind your working hands, and apply pressure by leaning your bodyweight forward, regulating that pressure by how much you lean. Swaying forward provides power and evenness to sliding strokes.

The Base of the Thumb

The thumbs, which are the most overused and the most often strained massage tools, are commonly used for applying firm pressure on small areas (see previous chapter). Whenever the pressure can be spread a little, save them by using the base of your thumb (the thenar eminence) instead.

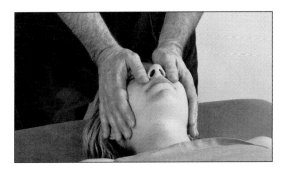

Figure 14.4: Applying pressure with the base of the thumb.

The base of the thumb works well on areas such as the client's forehead, for example, for both stationary and sliding pressure.

Relax the Rest of Your Hand

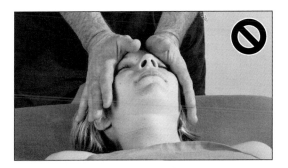

Figure 14.5: Stiffening the thumb and holding the fingers stiffly.

Keep the rest of your hand relaxed, particularly your fingers, and make sure that you are not bending your wrist too much in the process, which would put pressure on it. Relax your shoulders and position yourself so that you can lean your bodyweight to provide the power, rather than tensing your upper body.

Use Your Other Hand to Increase the Pressure

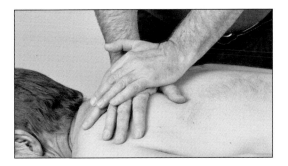

Figure 14.6: Pressing with the other hand on the base of the thumb.

Press on top with the heel of your other hand to increase the pressure, rather than stiffening your hand. Press on the central part of the metacarpal bone, and not on the joints at either end of it.

The Palm and the Heel of Your Hand

On areas where you can spread the pressure a little more, use the heel of your hand. If the area is large enough, use the whole spread of your palm for broad sliding strokes.

Avoid Tensing Your Fingers or Bending Your Wrist

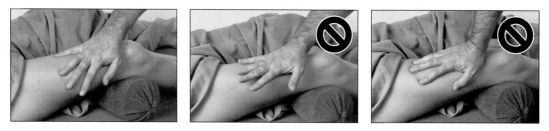

Figure 14.7: Using the heel/palm; a) using the heel/palm, b) tense fingers, c) bent wrist.

Keeping your thumb and fingers relaxed enables you to follow the contours of the client's body and to respond with your whole hand to the variations in muscle build and tensions. Take care not to bend your wrist too much.

Use One Hand on the Other to Increase the Pressure

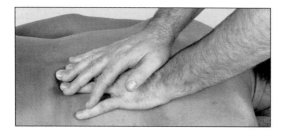

Figure 14.8: Hand-on-hand pressure.

If you need to increase the pressure, use one hand on the other. Lean your body for the pressure and keep both hands relaxed.

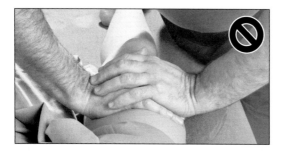

Fig 14.9: Sliding the hands sideways.

Make sure that you are not sliding your hands sideways with any great pressure as this puts pressure on your wrist.

Interlock Your Fingers to Use Both Heels Together

Wherever you can get your hands around the limbs, you can interlock your fingers. This enables you to clasp the muscles between the heels of your hands and squeeze and stretch them without needing to tense your shoulders or work your hands too hard. Once you've 'locked onto' the client's muscles, sway your body to move them. (If you are sitting on the table, sway your upper body, see figure 31.17). This works best on the leg muscles, particularly on the calf muscles when the client's leg is propped up or, if your hands are big enough, where the quadriceps muscles come together just above the knee. On a client with a large build, you might also find it useful on the arms.

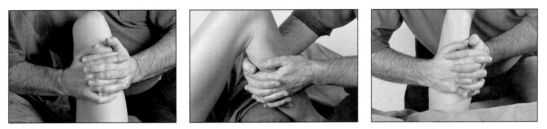

Figure 14.10: Interlocking the fingers to use the heels of the hands to squeeze muscles; a) squeezing the quadriceps, b), c) squeezing the calf muscles.

The Side of the Hand

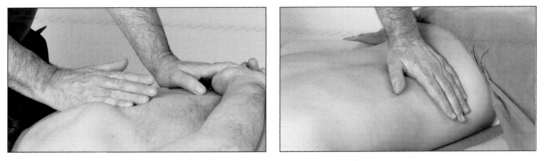

Figure 14.11: Using the outside edge of the hand for sliding strokes; a) sliding under the scapula, b) above the crest of the ilium.

Using the outside edge of your hand (the little finger side) will enable you to slide through narrow areas, for example between the scapula and the thoracic spine on a slender client. It is also useful for pressing into muscles next to bones such as the lumbar muscles that lie just above the crest of the ilium, particularly on slightly built clients. And it's a good tool for sliding under the medial edge of the scapula (if the client's scapula can be tilted up enough by bending the arm to take their hand behind their back).

Use the Other Hand for Guiding

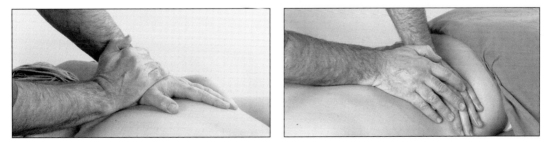

Figure 14.12: Guiding the working hand; a) under the scapula, b) above the crest of the ilium.

You cannot apply a lot of pressure directly *downwards* with the edge of your hand, even by pressing on it with your other hand. However, you can use the other hand to push it along more.

The Back of Your Hand

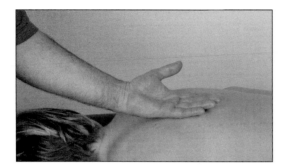

Figure 14.13: Back of the hand slide.

The back of the hand is an underrated tool for firm 'raking' strokes using the 'knuckles' at the base of the fingers (the metacarpophalangeal joints). Following general effleurage strokes on an area with your palm, this will enable you to dig in deeper. This is particularly useful on the client's back and hamstrings. Have your hand open and relaxed.

Which Hand to Use?

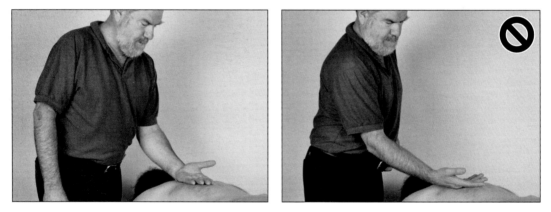

Figure 14.14: Which hand to use; a) the inside hand, b) the outside hand.

People are sometimes unsure about which hand to use for sliding strokes. Use your 'inside' hand (the one closest to the client) so that you can push it forward by swaying your body forward.

Use the Other Hand/Forearm to Increase the Pressure

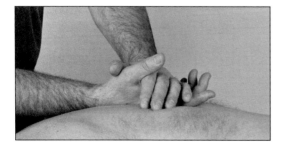

Figure 14.15: Increasing the pressure;
a) with the other hand (the 'frozen hand clap').

The depth and pressure can be regulated by pressing down on your upturned palm. For light pressure, lean your weight through your other hand to form a 'frozen hand clap'.

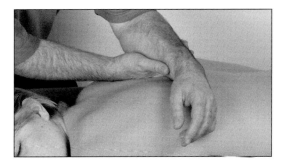

Figure 14.15 (cont.): b) with the other forearm.

For more pressure, lean your forearm across your working hand – across your palm and not across your fingers. Have the hand of your working forearm relaxed with your palm down so that the soft area of your forearm (the flexor muscles bellies – see figure 18.3) is across your working hand. Bend your knees and, if necessary, widen your stance (into the 'chimp' stance, see figure 18.24) so that you are not hunching over.

Avoid Bending Your Wrist

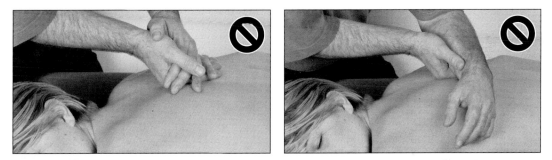

Figure 14.16: Bent wrist; a) using the frozen hand clap, b) using the forearm.

Whether you use your other hand or forearm to increase the pressure, take care not to let your working wrist bend.

The Medial Wrist Bone

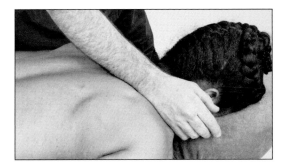

Figure 14.17: Using the medial wrist bone.

Use the small bulge of the medial 'wrist' bone (the distal end of the ulna) to focus the pressure more. You can apply pressure on a single point or deliver deeper sliding pressure than when you use the side of your hand.

Use the Other Hand to Increase the Pressure

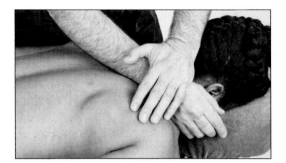

Figure 14.18: Using the other hand to increase the pressure.

Press on it with your other hand to increase the pressure and to guide your wrist bone. If you feel strain on your wrist bone as you do this or find that you need more pressure than you can easily apply, switch to using your knuckles (see Chapter 14), your fist (see Chapter 15) or your elbow (see Chapter 19).

The Lateral Wrist Bone

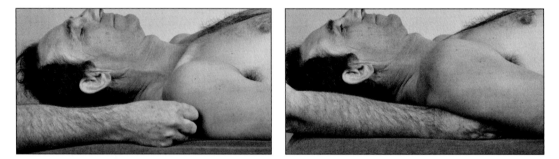

Figure 14.19: Using the lateral wrist bone; a) positioning the hand, b) 'pressing' up with the lateral wrist bone.

The lateral 'wrist' bone (the distal radius) can sometimes be useful for pressing up under the client's body by using the client's weight bearing down on it. Position your hand under the client's body to passively 'dig' up into the muscles, and wait for them to 'melt' onto it, *as long as you can comfortably take the pressure*. If possible, rest your arm on the table to keep it as relaxed as possible.

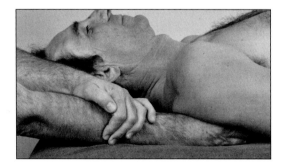

Figure 14.20: Dragging it back with the other hand.

If you want to slide it along under the client, use your other hand to drag it towards yourself. Do not just pull with your arm but sway your whole body to pull backwards.

Review

Many parts of your hands can be used to save your fingers and thumbs.

The base of the thumb can be used for applying general pressure.

Spread the pressure more by using the heel of your hand.

Use the whole spread of your palm for the broadest sliding strokes.

Interlock your fingers to use the heels of your hands to squeeze and stretch limb muscles.

Use the outside edge of your hand to slide through narrow areas or to slide in under the edge of bones.

Use the back of your hand for wide 'raking' strokes, using the other hand or forearm to increase the pressure.

Use your 'inside' hand (the one closest to the client), and avoid letting your wrist bend back.

Use the medial wrist bone (the distal ulna) to focus pressure on a single point or to slide along a narrow line. Press on it with the other hand to increase the pressure.

Use the lateral wrist bone (the distal radius) to dig up into the client's muscles, by placing your arm under the client's body to press up into it.

Vary the areas of your hands that you use in consecutive strokes.

With all of these techniques:

- Relax the non-working parts of your hand;
- Provide pressure by using the other hand whenever you can;
- Position and lean your body to provide the power, and;
- Sway forward to slide your hand forward, and sway back to pull it back.

CHAPTER 15

Using Your Knuckles

The skilled use of the knuckles for delivering concentrated, medium depth pressure can be a bridge between the comfortable limits of thumb and finger work and the firmer pressure that is possible with the fist. This chapter focuses on three aspects of using your knuckles:

1. Using them in order to conserve your fingers and thumbs;
2. Being effective without straining them, and;
3. Saving them by switching to larger tools such as your fist, forearm or elbow to deliver the massage.

Terminology – The 'Knuckles' and the 'Fist'

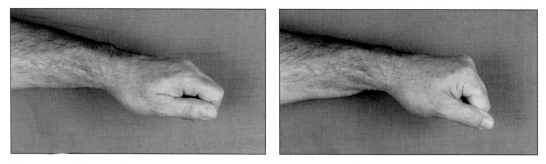

Figure 15.1: Terminology; a) the 'knuckles' – the IP joints, b) the 'fist' – the MP joints.

People most commonly use the term *knuckles* to refer to the first joints of the fingers (the proximal interphalangeal joints – the 'IP' joints). Knuckle techniques generally do not involve the little finger which is shorter than the others, and sometimes just use the knuckles of the index and middle fingers to concentrate the pressure.

The next chapter looks at using the *fist* for firm pressure on larger areas – the metacarpo-phalangeal joints of the fingers (the 'MP' joints) or the side of the fist. Although the MP joints are sometimes called 'knuckles', I'll refer to them as the 'fist' in this book for simplicity, and call them the MP joints whenever there could be any doubt. Many aspects of working with the knuckles that are covered in this chapter also apply to working with the fist.

A Few Cautions

Don't Overuse Your Knuckles

Although your knuckles are stronger than your fingertips, it is important *not to overuse* them, as they can be strained or even damaged by too much pressure. So use knuckle techniques sparingly. If you have small or slender fingers, and find that you can't use your knuckles without strain, DON'T include knuckle strokes in your repertoire.

Be Ambidextrous

As described below, you can reduce the pressure on your hands and wrists in knuckle kneading and friction strokes by using one hand at a time and supporting it with the other hand. When you do this, make sure that you regularly switch hands to avoid always working with the same hand.

Use Your Fist to Save Your Knuckles

And switch to using your fist whenever you can, especially when you want to increase the pressure, to sustain the pressure or to work over a large area. This too should not be used too much. So, for maximum pressure, learn to use your forearm and elbow (see Chapters 18 & 19).

Protective Exercises

Before and after using your knuckles, simple stretches will help to release tension from your hands. Useful exercises include curling and uncurling your fingers (see figure 11.46); shaking out your hands (see figure 11.47); and stretching your fingers (see figures 11.48 & 11.49).

Knuckle Percussion

You can use your knuckles in order to save your fingers for 'brushing' percussion across muscles. This enables you to 'shake' the muscles more forcefully than open finger brushing. It's most effective on the large muscles of the back and on well-developed thigh muscles. If it's appropriate, 'rapping' with your knuckles provides greater downward pressure on large muscle masses such as the gluteals.

Keep Your Wrists Loose

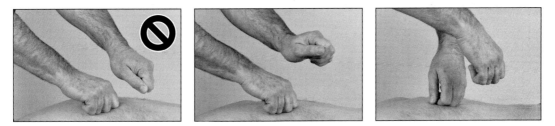

Figure 15.2: Knuckle percussion; a) 'rapping' with a stiff wrist, b) 'rapping' with a 'floppy' wrist, c) 'brushing' with a soft wrist.

In both of these strokes, let the movement come from the sweep of your whole forearm, rather than just using your hand. Keep your wrist soft so that your hand can move freely to avoid jarring either your hand or the client. And move around the table to keep your body behind your hands.

Knuckle Vibrations

The IP knuckles are also useful for saving your fingers in vibration strokes. You can rub them forward and back for a warming rub on muscles, one hand going forward as the other comes back.

Move Your Arms for the Stroke Not Just Your Hands

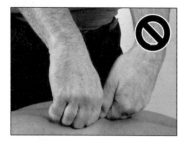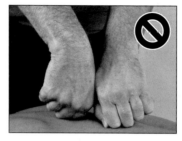

Figure 15.3: Knuckle vibration – hands moving in opposite directions; a), b) just moving the hands.

Keep your hands relaxed and do not just move them at the wrist, which is hard work and puts unnecessary pressure on your wrists.

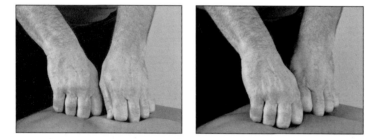

Figure 15.3 (cont.): c), d) moving the arms.

Move your whole arm to move each hand to save your wrists and deliver greater power and fluidity with less effort.

Knuckle Kneading

Wherever you can get your hands around muscles, you can knead them by 'grabbing' and squeezing them between your thumb and knuckles, using your knuckles as if they were strong, stubby fingers. This is most effective on clients' shoulders and limbs. You can knead with both hands simultaneously in 'classic' kneading fashion, one hand picking up the muscle tissue as your other hand releases it.

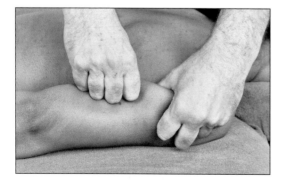

Figure 15.4: Knuckle kneading.

Support Your Wrist for Firm Strokes

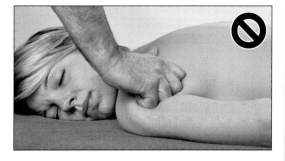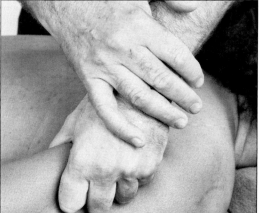

Figure 15.5: Looking after the wrist;
a) hyperextended wrist,
b) supporting your working hand.

However, if you are working on large, firm muscles or if you have small hands, knead with one hand only and support it with your other hand. This adds power to the stroke while reducing the pressure on your wrist. It also saves you from letting your wrist hyperextend.

Knuckle 'Friction'

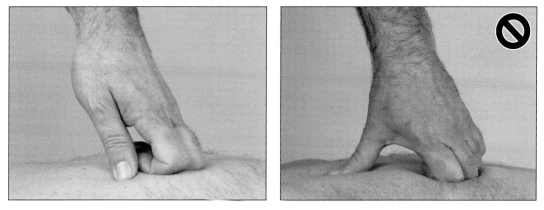

Figure 15.6: Knuckle 'friction'; a) the working 'tripod', b) thumb hyperextended.

You can also use your IP knuckles to work more deeply than your fingers in 'friction' strokes – small overlapping pressure circles, which gradually spiral along or across the muscles. This is especially effective on large well-muscled areas of the client's back or legs. (For deeper pressure, switch to your fist or learn to use your elbow).

Often, knuckle friction strokes just involve your index and middle finger knuckles, which project further than the others. Your thumb can form a 'tripod' with them to provide a stable base, acting as a pivot for this knuckle pressure, as long as you do not put too much pressure through it or let it bend back too far.

Move Your Hand as a Unit

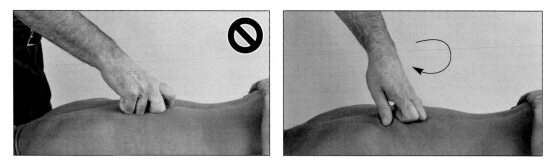

Figure 15.7: Moving over an area; a) just moving the fingers, b) moving the hand as a unit.

Knuckle friction soon becomes tiring for your fingers if you are moving them individually. Reduce their work by moving your whole hand as a unit for firm, concentrated pressure.

Keep Your Wrist Straight

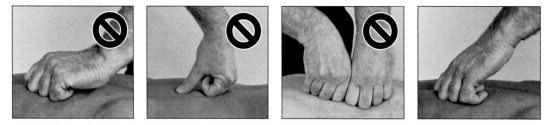

Figure 15.8: Keeping the wrist straight; a) overextended wrist, b) overflexed wrist, c) wrist bent to the side, d) straight wrist.

Avoid letting your wrist hyperextend, overflex, or bend sideways, each of which would put strain on it while reducing the effective transmission of force from your arm. Instead, keep it relatively straight but not rigid.

Support Your Working Hand

You can use both hands simultaneously for *light* knuckle friction. However, when you are applying pressure, it is quite an effort on each hand, and you are likely to be tensing your shoulders and hands to control the movements. Working with one hand while supporting it with the other reduces the pressure on your wrist and fingers. It enables you to relax your shoulders and use your bodyweight more for the pressure. It also gives you more control of the movement. This is particularly important when you need to focus the pressure precisely on small areas, for example when you are working on the muscles next to the client's spine.

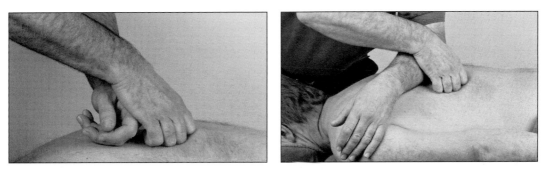

*Figure 15.9: Resting the working knuckles across the other arm; a) the other hand,
b) the other forearm.*

With practice, you will find a variety of ways of using your other hand to support, stabilise and guide your working knuckles. One way of doing this is to rest your working hand across the other hand or forearm, especially when you don't need such precise control.

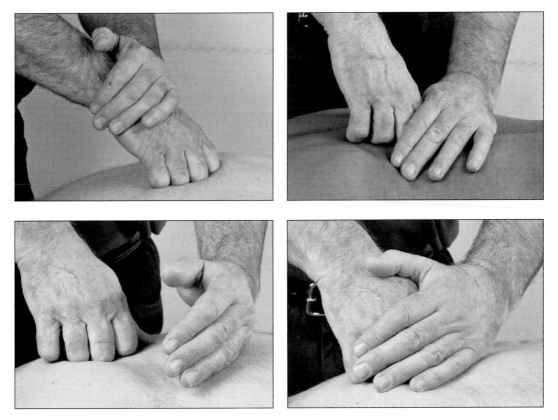

*Figure 15.10: Supporting the working hand; a) holding the working wrist,
b) holding the knuckles, c), d) 'wrapping' the other hand around the knuckles.*

Another way is to hold your working wrist, which will also remind you to keep it straight.

However, resting your working hand on the client's body will provide more stability for your working hand, making it easier to guide and enabling you to work with more precision. One way to do this is to hold your knuckles; another is to 'wrap' your supporting hand around your working hand. You can then use the supporting hand to help you to palpate the tissues that you are working on.

Mutual Hand Support

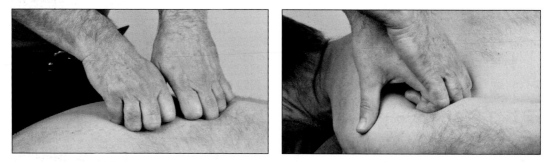

Figure 15.11: Mutual hand support; a) hands next to each other, b) one hand inside the other.

Another option is to use both sets of knuckles simultaneously, with each hand supporting the other. Because the pressure and 'steering' can then come primarily from leaning your bodyweight behind your hands, it requires less effort in your shoulders and arms for control. One way to do this is to have your hands next to each other; another is to have one hand inside the other.

Involving Your Body

Lean Forward for Pressure

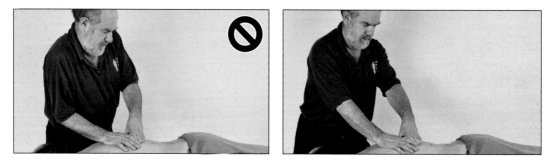

Figure 15.12: Delivering power; a) working stiffly, b) leaning bodyweight forward.

There are three important ways of involving your body in these strokes. Firstly, use your bodyweight to deliver power to your knuckles, rather than standing still, tensing your shoulders and trying to 'muscle through'. Lean forward for this. This also makes it easier to keep the pressure consistent. Be alert to the tendency to hold your body still (and to hold your breath) when focusing the pressure on small areas.

Change Position to Keep Your Body Behind Your Hands
Make sure that you do not have to twist as you apply force. Regularly reposition yourself so that you are directly behind your hands.

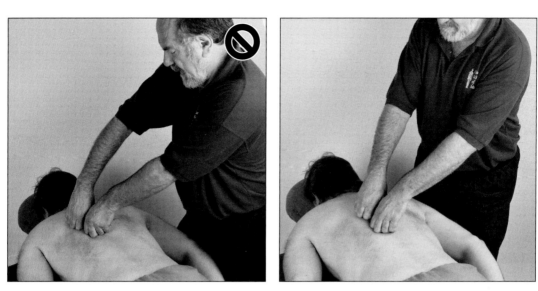

Figure 15.13: Aligning the body; a) not aligned, b) facing hands.

Don't Try to Reach Too Far

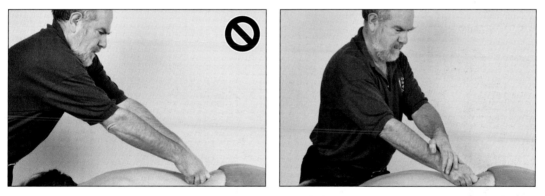

Figure 15.14: Reaching; a) Reaching too far from the head of the table, b) changing position.

And don't try to reach too far, which would put pressure on your lower back. For example, it is easy to apply knuckle pressure on the top of the client's back when you are standing at the head of the table. But do not try to continue this too far down the back, which would put strain on *your* lower back and lead to hyperextending your wrist. Instead, move to the side of the table.

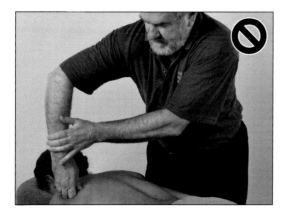

Similarly, there is no effective way of applying pressure on the far side of the client's back when you are standing at the side of the table. Instead cross to the other side of the table to work there.

Figure 15.15: Trying to apply pressure across the table.

Review

Use your knuckles in the middle range of pressure to save your fingers on large muscles, especially on the client's back and legs.

Switch to using your fist, forearm or elbow to avoid straining your knuckles when you want to apply more pressure.

When using your knuckles for percussion strokes, use your whole forearm and keep your wrist relaxed so that your hands can move freely.

When doing knuckle vibration strokes, keep your hand relaxed and make sure that your wrist doesn't bend too much when you are applying pressure.

Use your knuckles to save your fingers in kneading, taking care not to hyperextend your wrists.

For large muscles, use one hand for kneading and support it with your other hand.

For deeper pressure, use your knuckles to save your fingers in 'friction' strokes – small overlapping pressure circles.

Have your thumb and index and middle finger knuckles in a 'tripod' shape, and move your whole hand, taking care not to hyperextend your thumb.

For the deep knuckle pressure, use one hand and support it with the other.

Rest your working hand over your supporting hand or forearm, support your wrist to avoid hyperextending it, or wrap your supporting hand around your knuckles and rest it on the client's body for stability.

The power for working in depth with the knuckles comes from positioning and leaning your body behind your working hand(s).

Do not try to reach too far with knuckle strokes.

CHAPTER 16

Using Your Fist

The skilled use of the fist can be a bridge between the comfortable limits of knuckle work and the deeper pressure that is possible with the forearm and elbow. The fist is most often used for applying stationary pressure or for sliding pressure strokes, either along or across muscles. It is also used for some percussion techniques.

This chapter focuses on potential problems and effective practices when you are using your fist for applying pressure, which is when problems are most likely to arise. The main things to watch out for are:

• Clenching your fist;
• Letting your wrist bend;
• Applying pressure that is too much for your wrist, and;
• Standing still, rather than leaning and swaying your body for the pressure and movement.

Terminology – The 'Knuckles' and the 'Fist'

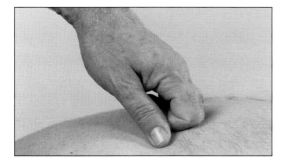

Figure 16.1: The 'knuckles': the IP joints.

The previous chapter covered the use of the IP joints (the proximal interphalangeal joints) of the fingers, which are commonly referred to as the *knuckles*.

When people talk about working with the *fist*, they are usually referring to either using the metacarpo-phalangeal joints of the fingers (the 'MP' joints) or the side of the fist (the medial / little finger side). Although the MP joints are sometimes called 'knuckles', I will refer to them as part of the 'fist', and call them the 'MP fist' when it's necessary to be absolutely clear.

Using the back of the hand is usually done with a relatively open hand rather than a closed fist, and primarily using the MP joints. It is covered in Chapter 14 (see figures 14.13–14.16).

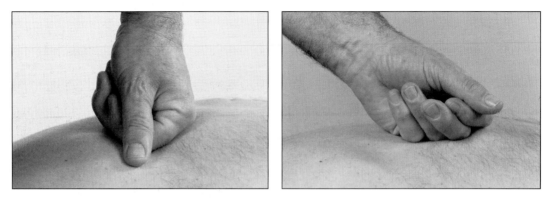

Figure 16.2: The 'fist'; a) the MP joints, b) the side of the fist.

Protective Exercises
Before and after using your fist, simple stretches of your fingers and wrist will help to release tension from your hands. Useful exercises include curling and uncurling your fingers (see figure 11.46), and mobilising the wrists (see figure 11.50).

A Few Notes of Caution

Don't Overuse Your Fist
Although the MP joints are bigger, stronger and less vulnerable than the IP joints, it is important *not to overuse* them, especially if you have small or slender hands. And there *are limits* to how much force your *wrist* can comfortably transmit (see Chapter 17). If you need to increase the pressure or to sustain it significantly, learn to use your forearm or elbow (see Chapters 18 & 19), particularly on the larger areas of the client's body.

Avoid Overusing Your Dominant Hand
Do not fall into the habit of constantly using your dominant hand when you are working with one fist and using the other hand to support it. Use whichever fist is most appropriate for the situation and mirror your technique on opposite sides of the massage table.

Monitor and Adapt to the Client's Responses
Monitor the client's responses carefully when you are first learning to use your fist as it is very easy to dig in too suddenly and/or too heavily. At the very least this will cause the client to tense against you because of the momentary pain. If you continue to apply pressure that is beyond the client's tolerable limits, you risk bruising their muscles. Instead of trying to force your way through the tissues, sustain a level of pressure that the client finds manageable. Wait to see if the muscles can soften ('melt') and release with this pressure. Ease the pressure off a little if there is a reaction against it.

Of course it takes time to master using your fist. However, as using it becomes familiar and easy, you may be applying more pressure than you realise, so it is important to continue monitoring your client's responses. Over time, with practice, you will develop greater sensitivity with the various parts of your fist.

Don't Try to Bulldoze Your Way Through Knots of Tension

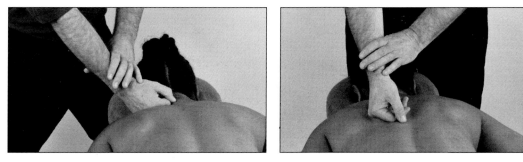

Figure 16.3: Approaching tension from different angles.

When you are sliding your fist along muscles, you'll encounter pockets of tension. Do not try to bulldoze your way through these 'stuck' areas, as this would increase the pressure on your fist and wrist, and is also likely to cause the client to tense against you. Instead, change the angle of your body and your fist. You will often find that these tensions will soften and let you through when you come at them from a different direction. This is like the side-to-side weavings of a water-skier to avoid hitting head-on into waves or the wake as s/he follows the boat.

Using the MP Fist

The MP fist is primarily used for applying stationary pressure or doing sliding pressure strokes. These are generally done by sliding the MP joints together in parallel shallow 'furrows', which is the focus of this part of the chapter. Sliding strokes are generally done along muscles ('stripping' the muscle) or across them (to encourage release by stretching the muscle sideways).

Avoid Clenching Your Fist

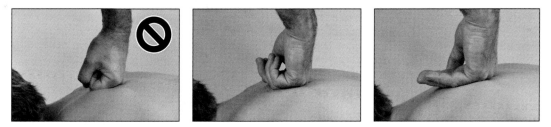

Figure 16.4: Using the MP fist; a) a clenched fist, b) a soft MP fist, c) open hand.

Whether you are applying stationary or sliding pressure, clenching your fist would take extra effort and cause you to stiffen your shoulders unnecessarily. It would also make it harder for you to feel the client's responses. Instead, loosely curl your fist or just have your fingers bent at the MP joints to keep your hand relaxed.

Don't Let Your Wrist Flex When Sliding Your MP Fist Forward

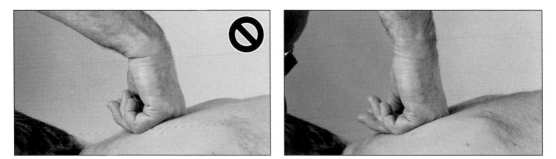

Figure 16.5: Sliding the MP fist too far; a) wrist flexing, b) keeping the wrist straight.

Be careful not to slide your fist so far that your wrist begins to bend into flexion, which puts pressure on it. Save it by dropping onto your IP knuckles (see figure 15.6) taking care not to let your wrist hyperextend (see figure 15.8), or turn over to use the back of your hand (see figure 14.13).

Support Your Wrist

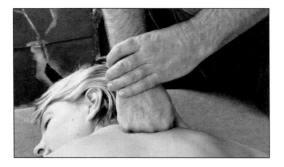

Figure 16.6: Holding the wrist to support the fist.

Rest Your Supporting Hand on the Client's Body for Stability and Precision

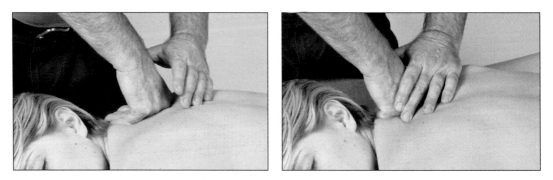

Figure 16.7: 'Wrapping' the other hand around the fist.

Holding your working fist with your other hand and resting this supporting hand on your client's body will provide more stability for your working fist and enable you to work with more precision than holding your wrist. One way to do this is by 'wrapping' your supporting hand around your working hand.

Use a Guiding Thumb Inside Your MP Fist

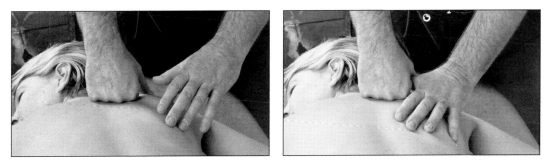

Figure 16.8: The thumb inside the fist; a) slipping the thumb inside the fist, b) guiding the fist.

Another option is to keep your guiding hand relatively relaxed by slipping your thumb inside your working fist. This gives you considerable control when a fist slide requires continuous, even pressure.

It also makes it easy to 'weave' your fist smoothly and easily as you slide it along (see figure 16.3). Be careful not to take it so far that you begin to twist your thumb, especially if you have a long, slender thumb and/or it is hypermobile.

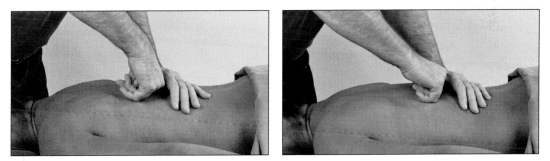

Figure 16.9: 'Cam and spindle' turning.

This way of guiding your fist is also frequently used for the 'cam and spindle' stroke in which the fist rotates around the thumb, twisting forward and back as it slides along. As you do this, be careful not to put too much pressure on your thumb or to twist it.

Use the Thumb Guide to Grip Areas

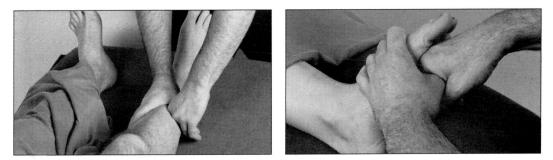

Figure 16.10: 'Gripping' MP fist slide; a) along the lateral shin muscles, b) on the client's sole.

As you slide your fist along the client's limbs, this way of guiding it enables you to 'grip' a little with your supporting hand for greater precision. Many people consider that this is the most effective way of using the fist to get into the compact, hardworking muscles on the lateral side of the shin (tibialis anterior, the toe extensors and the peroneals), both for sliding along them and for short zigzagging strokes across them. You can also use this grip to stabilise your fist when you are working on the client's sole.

Use Mutual Fist Support

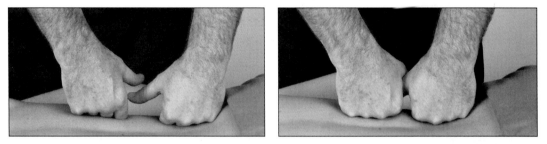

Figure 16.11: Side-by-side fists; a) slipping the thumb inside the other fist, b) mutual fist support.

If the working area is wide enough, you can use your MP fists side-by-side so that each hand provides support for the other. This is much easier than trying to control each fist separately. Slip one thumb inside the other fist for this mutual support. The steering and pressure can then come primarily from leaning and moving your body behind your hands, which reduces the work required of your shoulder and arm muscles.

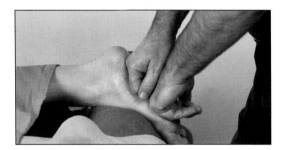

Figure 16.12: One fist following the other.

In narrower areas, have one hand follow the other, or have one inside the other. This is useful, for example, when you are sliding your MP fists towards yourself across the back of the client's armpit on the infraspinatus muscle. Curl your hands into loose fists which are touching, with one in front of the other. The front hand guides your working fist, which digs in as it slides down, and controls the speed of the movement, which is initiated by bending your knees.

You could also do this stroke with one fist inside the other, both facing the same way. Having your hands facing when one fist is inside the other is useful for applying stationary pressure or sliding your fists sideways.

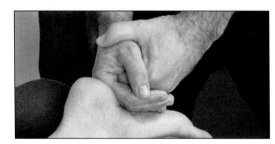
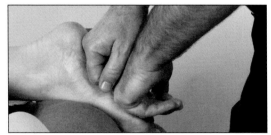

Figure 16.13: One fist inside the other.

Have Your Arms Relatively Straight to Transmit the Power

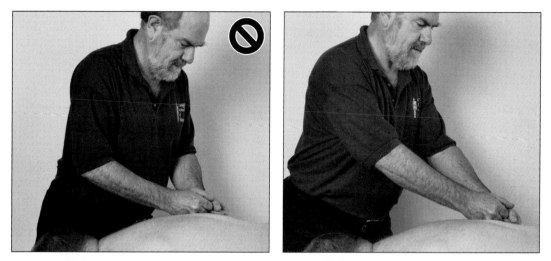

Figure 16.14: Effective transmission of power through your arms; a) bent arms, b) straight arms.

With all of these strokes, avoid bending your arms, which would reduce the effective transmission of power from your trunk. Have them relatively straight so that they can transmit the power with the least strain.

Avoid Overreaching

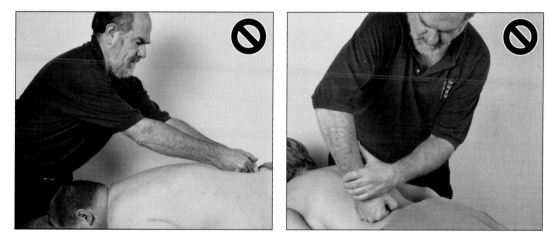

Figue 16.15: Trying to reach too far; a) from the head of the table, b) across the table.

Don't try to reach too far from the head of the table, which could put pressure on your back and reduce the effective power of your fist. Instead, move along the table. Similarly, do not try putting pressure on the far side of the client's back.

Position Your Bodyweight Above Your Fist to Slide it Towards Yourself

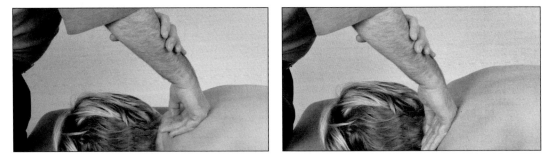

Figure 16.16: Sliding the MP fist towards oneself – lowering the body to slide the fist down.

To slide your fist towards yourself, rise up to get your bodyweight comfortably above your fist. Slide your fist down towards yourself by bending your knees to slowly lower your body, keeping your arms relatively straight (but not stiff) to transmit the power from your trunk.

Open Your Hand to Slide Smoothly Off an Area

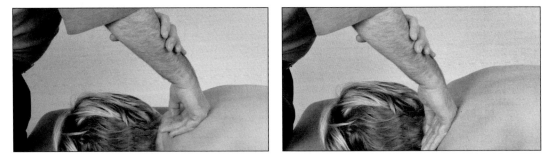

Figure 16.17: Sliding the MP fist towards yourself; a) sliding along,
b) opening the hand to slide off an area.

When you are sliding your MP fist towards yourself for example across the top of the shoulders or across the thigh, open your hand out as you slide it off the area. This enables you to come smoothly off without a jarring bump, which would be harder to control and more likely to produce a protective tensing in the client's tissues.

When You Cannot Use Your Other Hand, Guide the MP Fist With Your Thumb or Little Finger
Sometimes you will be using your other hand for another essential activity. For example, when the client is supine, you need to stabilise her forearm with one hand as you slide your fist down the flexor muscles. In this situation, make a 'horned' fist by extending your thumb and/or little finger, and use one or both 'horns' to channel the stroke along the client's arm.

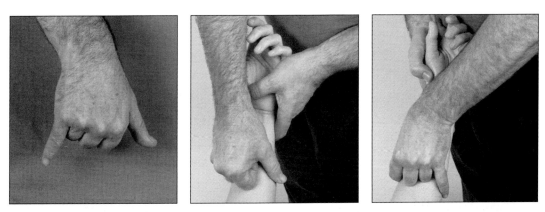

Figure 16.18: Guiding your hand; a) the guides, b) using the thumb guide,
c) using the little finger guide.

Sliding Your Fist Sideways

The MP fist strokes (above) enable you to dig into the tissue. Using the side of the fist (the medial / little finger side) for sliding strokes enables you to do longer strokes to stretch the tissue. These will have less pressure involved.

Don't Clench Your Fist

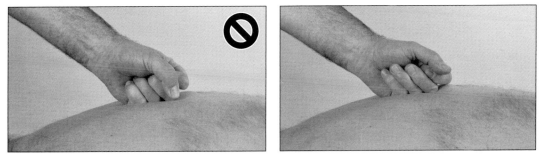

Figure 16.19: The sliding fist; a) tense fist, b) soft fist.

Have your fist open and relaxed as you use the side of it. Do not clench it, which is more awkward and harder work, and would lead to unnecessary tension in your shoulders as well.

Avoid Bending Your Wrist Sideways

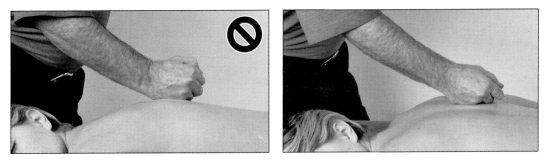

Figure 16.20: Looking after the wrist; a) letting the wrist bend sideways, b) keeping it straight.

Take care that your wrist does not sag into abduction (radial deviation), which could strain it and would reduce the force being transmitted to your fist.

Support Your Wrist

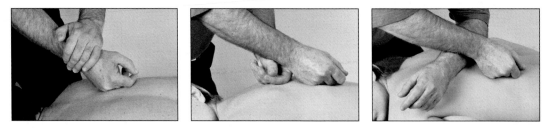

Figure 16.21: Supporting the wrist; a) holding it with the other hand,
b) resting it across the other hand, c) resting it across the other forearm.

Whenever you can, support your working fist with your other hand to reduce the pressure on it, and to work with more precision. Holding your wrist will help you to keep it straight. You can also rest it across your other hand to support it. However, resting it across your forearm will provide greater stability, and therefore help you to keep it more relaxed.

Use Mutual Hand Support
You can also use each hand to support the other when you are using both fists at the same time. You can then steer it and deliver consistent pressure by leaning and swaying your bodyweight behind your hands. This requires less effort in your shoulders and arms for control.

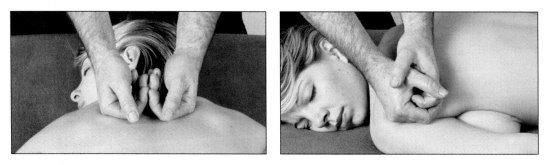

Figure 16.22: Mutual hand support; a) hands back-to-back, b) one inside the other.

If you are simultaneously sliding both fists sideways on a wide enough area, have them back-to-back, with the backs of your fingers touching for mutual stability. If you are sliding your fists down either side of the spine, make sure that you are not pressing on the spine itself.

Having one fist inside the other with your hands facing each other increases the power that you can apply and helps you to focus it on a small area.

Have Your Arms Straight to Transmit the Power

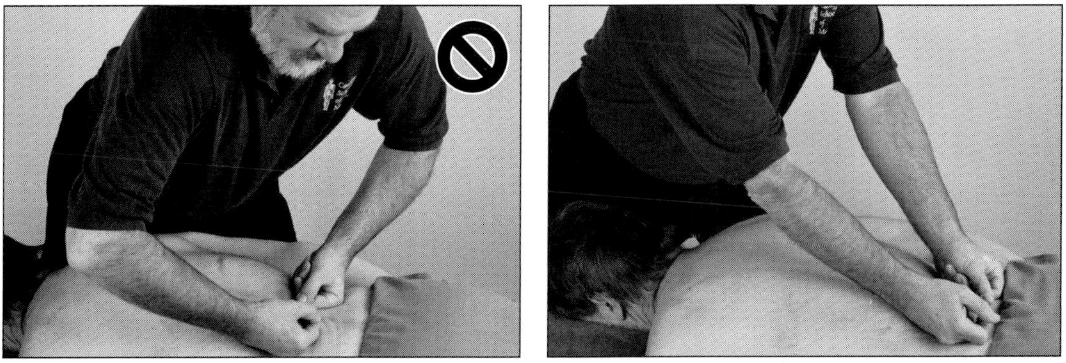

Figure 16.23: Transmission of power through the arms; a) bent arms, b) straight arms.

As with using the MP fist, having your arms bent would increase the effort needed in your shoulder muscles while reducing the transmission of power. So keep your arms relatively straight.

Backing Up Your Fist

Use Your Bodyweight for the Power
Do not try to force the client's tissues into submission, which is likely to cause the client to tense against you. In order to give the tissues time to 'trust' your pressure and to accommodate to it, you need to keep the pressure consistent. It is not easy to sustain even pressure for very long if you are standing still and just trying to 'muscle through' by tensing your shoulders and arms. This is hard work and would, in turn, cause you to tense your wrist and your hand. Instead, move your body with your fist. Using your bodyweight enables you to keep the pressure consistent without straining your upper body, and to move your fist slowly and evenly in sliding pressure strokes. (Of course, you can't effectively deliver fist pressure on the return stroke).

Get behind your fist and sway forward for applying stationary pressure or for sliding your fist forward. Step back to get behind your fist if your need to, and step forward, if necessary, to avoid overreaching. Rise up and get your bodyweight above your fist to slide it down towards yourself (see figure 16.16). Don't try to press down with the fist on the far side of the client's body when you are standing at the side of the table. Instead cross to the other side of the table (see figure 16.15).

Reposition Yourself to Change the Angle of Delivery

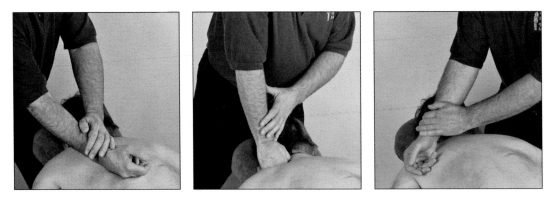

Figure 16.24: Angling oneself behind the fist.

Regularly reposition your body in order to keep your hips facing your fist(s), particularly as you work your way around bones, and approach muscles from different angles.

Balance Between Pressure and Sliding Forward

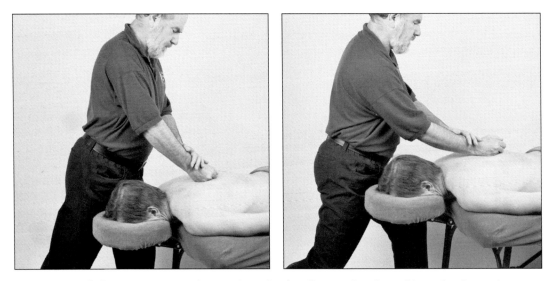

Figure 16.25: Balance pressure and movement; a) primarily pressing down, b) moving forward.

Rise up to apply more pressure with your fist and lower your body to move forward more.

Don't Hold Your Breath When Applying Force

There is a great temptation to breathe in forcefully or to hold your breath when you are applying pressure, which is likely to cause you to tense up. If it is difficult to break out of this habit, focus on breathing out (easily) as you apply the pressure.

Don't Hunch Over When You Are Working Seated

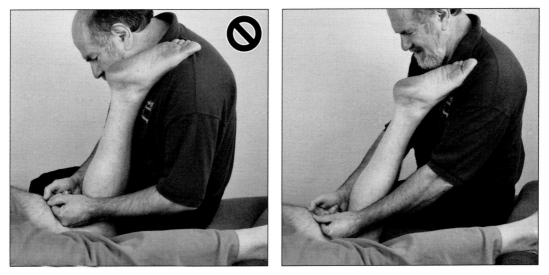

Figure 16.26: Sitting on the table; a) hunching over, b) leaning with the whole trunk.

Sitting on a seat or on the table may make it easier for you to comfortably sustain even pressure on a small area. Lean with your whole trunk to deliver pressure rather than hunching over and just using your shoulder muscles.

Review

Save your fingers, thumbs and knuckles by using your fist for applying pressure.

The two working areas of the fist are:

- The MP joints (the metacarpo-phalangeal joints) of the fingers, which are used for stationary pressure or to slide in parallel 'furrows';
- The side of the fist (the medial / little finger side) which is used for sliding strokes.

Before and after using your fist, simple stretches of your fingers and wrist will help to release tension from your hands.

The main things to watch out for when using your fist are:

- Clenching your fist;
- Letting your wrist bend, particularly when you are applying pressure;
- Applying pressure that is too much for your wrist, and;
- Standing still, rather than leaning and swaying your body for the pressure and movement.

In addition:

- Do not overuse it;
- Be careful how much you use it if you have small or slender hands;
- Support your wrist, whenever you can by holding it with your other hand or resting it over your other forearm;
- Avoid overusing your dominant hand, particularly when you are using one fist and supporting it with the other hand;
- Use whichever fist is most appropriate for the situation and mirror your technique on opposite sides of the massage table;
- Try approaching knots of tension from different directions, rather than trying to force your way through the tissues;
- Monitor and adapt to your client's responses, and;
- Switch to using your forearm or elbow for delivering more pressure.

Use your body to back up your fist by:

- Using your bodyweight for power to keep the pressure consistent without straining your upper body;
- Regularly repositioning yourself to change the angle of delivery;
- Not trying to press down with the fist on the far side of the client's body from the side of the table;
- Keeping your arms straight to transmit the power;
- Avoiding hunching over when you are seated, and;
- Not holding your breath when you are applying pressure.

When using your MP fist for applying stationary pressure or for sliding pressure strokes:

- Loosely curl your fist or just have your fingers bent at the MP joints to avoid clenching your fist;
- Open your hand out to slide smoothly off an area;
- Guide your fist with your thumb or little finger (in the 'horned fist' shape), when you are unable to use your other hand;
- Support your wrist whenever you can by holding it, by 'wrapping' your other hand around it, or using a guiding thumb inside it, or;
- Have your fists together so that they mutually support one another, either by having them side by side, one following the other, or one inside the other;
- Get your bodyweight above your fist and then bend your knees to slide your fist towards yourself;
- Position your body behind your fist to slide it away from yourself, and;
- If necessary, roll onto your IP knuckles or turn over to use the back of your hand to avoid letting your wrist bend into flexion by pushing too far.

When sliding your fist sideways:

- Avoid letting your wrist collapse into abduction (radial deviation);
- Do not clench your fist;
- Support your wrist by holding it or by resting it over your other forearm;
- Slide your fists together so that they can mutually support one another, either by having them with your fingers back to back, one behind the other, or one inside the other;
- Keep your arms straight to deliver the pressure and movement from your body, and;
- Step forward, if necessary, to avoid trying to reach too far with your fist(s).

CHAPTER 17

Looking After Your Wrists

The previous chapters in this section have touched on ways of looking after your wrists when you are using various parts of your hands for massage strokes. This chapter looks at the general principles of protecting your wrists.

Wrist Problems

It is primarily the cumulative effect of applying pressure with the wrist consistently bent that causes wrist problems in massage. Because pulling techniques put less pressure through the wrists, they are only likely to cause strain if they are done regularly with the wrist bent.

Straining the Wrists in Massage

The wrists are critical areas for massage practitioners to monitor, as they are one of the two most commonly strained areas of the body in massage (the other being the thumbs, see Chapter 13). Problems mainly arise from the *cumulative* effects of *applying pressure*, particularly with the *wrists hyperextended*. Because the application of pressure is such a major part of massage, this needs regular attention. Poor use of the wrists will not merely tire you; it can cause cumulative damage. This is a major cause of early retirement for practitioners. Don't ignore early warning signs of strain. Change your working practices to avoid long-term problems.

The main ways of reducing the pressure on your wrists and therefore the likelihood of straining them are:

- Keeping your wrists relatively straight when you are applying pressure;
- Using your other hand to support your working hand;
- Incorporating more passive stretches into your massage repertoire which open out your wrists rather than compressing them;
- Learning to use your forearm and elbow in order to save your hand and wrist entirely;
- Reducing the amount of hand-intensive activities in the rest of your life, and;
- Making sure that you are not doing those other activities, such as computer work, with your wrists bent.

Respect Your Limits

Bear in mind that there are limits to how much pressure a practitioner's wrist will take, even when it is used well. Those with small and/or slender wrists need to be particularly careful that they are not exceeding their comfortable limits. You also need to be very careful if your wrists are hypermobile as you are likely to be accustomed to bending them without noticing. The only way to *completely* rest your wrist is by learning to use your forearm and elbow, where appropriate (see Chapters 18 & 19).

Monitor Your Shoulder Tension

Note that, if you are straining or feeling pain in your wrists or hands, you are also likely to be instinctively tensing your shoulders. You may also be holding your breath and stiffening your back. In fact you could be unconsciously tensing throughout your body, which is likely to feed back into this cycle of strain and tensing. Therefore, if you are changing the way that you use your wrists, you need to consciously relax your whole body (particularly your upper body) to ensure that these associated tensions don't draw you back into old habits.

Wrist Problems in Other Activities

Wrist problems are not unique to massage practitioners of course. Any activity which involves the hands in *constant* or *repetitive* activity, especially with the wrists hyperextended, may lead to problems. Overuse injuries of the wrist are also occupational hazards for keyboard workers, musicians, hairdressers and factory workers.

Of course, if you are a massage practitioner and *also* doing other hand-intensive activities such as computer work (and, these days, who isn't?), gardening, DIY or playing musical instruments, you need to be especially careful of your wrists in your massage sessions *and also* in these other activities (see Chapter 47).

Wrist Strains

Work-related Upper Limb Disorders (WRULD) also called Repetitive Strain Injury (RSI), Repetitive Stress Injury or Occupational Overuse Syndrome) is a general term for cumulative strain in the upper limbs brought about by prolonged and repetitive use of the hands in restricted and/or repetitive activities, often in awkward positions. The wrist is the area most commonly affected.

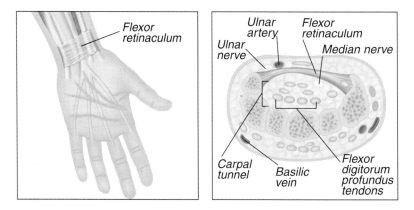

*Figure 17.1: Wrist; a) flexor retinaculum, palmar view,
b) cross-section of carpal tunnel at wrist.*

Muscles in the front of the forearm flex the wrist and the fingers, and control some thumb movements. As they pass over the wrist, each enclosed in its own sheath, the tendons of these muscles are held in place by the flexor retinaculum, a connective tissue band. The nerves and blood vessels which feed the hand pass with these tendons through the carpal tunnel, the space between the retinaculum and the carpal bones.

Tenosynovitis is the general term for inflammation of tendon sheaths, which is usually caused when the tendons in them swell up through overuse. The tendons can become swollen, tender and painful due to working awkwardly and/or repetitively. These swollen tendons may then press on the nerves and blood vessels in the restricted space under the flexor retinaculum, leading to carpal tunnel syndrome.

In *carpal tunnel syndrome*, pressure on the median nerve causes numbness, tingling or pain in the thumb, index and middle fingers. In the worst situation it can also lead to restricted movement and/or loss of control in the wrist and parts of the hand. This syndrome can also be caused by consistently having the wrists hyperextended when using the hand, which also restricts the area of the carpal tunnel (or by combinations of these causes). It can also have hormonal causes.

The Development of Wrist Strain

Although the pain and loss of function of full-blown WRULD in the wrist is quite unmistakable, there is usually a long, slow build up that precedes this, which is often ignored. However, if you regularly monitor your wrists, you will be able to adjust your massage techniques in response to discomforts that you notice. Bear in mind that strain does not usually develop evenly in both wrists. It generally develops much more in one wrist, although it can then develop in the second wrist if you begin to rely on that hand in order to save the strained one.

The First Stage – Discomfort When Working
In the first stage of problems developing, practitioners are only likely to notice discomfort in their wrists while they are actually working. Initially, these may be dull twinges or just a feeling that one is putting too much pressure through the wrist. If these small niggles are ignored, they are likely to develop into sharper pain when you are working.

The Second Stage – Persistent Pains or Aches, or Sudden Pains
If you continue to work in ways that put strain on your wrists, the next stage is aches or pain that persist when you are *not* working, initially intermittently and then more permanently. These can range from a sore or aching wrist to sharper, niggling pains or even throbbing pain. A further warning sign at this stage is sudden pain that comes on when you are relaxed, especially in the night.

The Third Stage – Persistent Pain Which is Aggravated by any Hand-intensive Activities
After a while, the persistent pains will often be aggravated in massage sessions, initially just by the type of massage strokes that sparked off the problems, and later by *any* strokes that put pressure on your wrist. These pains will also start to flare up in other activities in which you make extensive use of your hands, such as computer work. If it gets worse, pain will even be set off by everyday activities such as cleaning one's teeth, turning keys, opening doors, cooking, washing the dishes, and, in extreme cases, even dressing and feeding oneself. Obviously, this can be quite debilitating in one's life, and is a very frightening experience.

Responding to Wrist Strain

Reaching this stage has put paid to the careers of a significant number of massage practitioners who had not received information about the likelihood of this happening, about how it develops or how to monitor and avoid it. For some people, it has been the wake up call that spurred them into researching preventative / alternative ways of working and rehabilitation options (see, for example, the books of Laurianne Green and Gerry Pyves). For me, the warning signal came nearly twenty years ago when I had a few years break from doing regular massages. During the first months, I occasionally woke in the night with brief shooting pains through my wrists (a classic symptom of developing RSI). Although I had felt quite tired in my wrists when I was working, I had not experienced these pains until I had the break, which indicated that I had been straining my wrists without realising it. So, when I returned to doing massage, I knew that I needed to be more careful about how I positioned my wrists and the pressure that I put through them.

This all sounds quite alarming. *It is*. It is scary for the individual practitioner who is not only at risk of losing his/her livelihood but also of becoming debilitated in everyday life. It is also alarming for a profession whose aim is to *help others* to look after their bodies. It is an aspect of massage that needs to be highlighted much more than it currently is, because wrist problems are unfortunately prevalent in the profession, and they are largely *preventable* by using the guidelines in this chapter (and by learning the skilled use of the forearm and elbow).

Don't Continue Working in Ways That Strain Your Wrists
Therefore, treat discomforts or pains that you feel in your wrists as a warning sign. *Don't* continue doing strokes that strain your wrists. Use the information in this chapter to help you to work out what you are doing that is contributing and how to change it. Vary the massage techniques that you use, so that the pressure is not constant and not always on the same part of your wrists. Include pulling, lifting and stretching techniques, wherever possible, to lessen the compressive forces through your wrist. With many strokes, you can further reduce the pressure on your wrist by using your other hand to support and stabilise it (see figures 17.15 & 17.16).

Rest Your Wrists and Get Specialist Help to Prevent or Reverse Pain
Rest your wrists whenever you can. If you have persistent pain, especially if the pain persists when you are *not* working, seek specialist help. Regular massage can help as a preventative measure. It can also provide some relief from the pain/tensing cycle if there are already problems. Many people find that acupuncture, deep massage and osteopathy or chiropractic or physiotherapy, allied with changes in their way of working can reduce an established problem (see Chapter 45).

Learn to Use Your Forearm and Elbow
Bear in mind that using your hands for massage always involves your wrists. And using your body efficiently behind your hands, as advocated in this book, increases the power that is delivered through your wrists. So, even with the best positioning of your wrists, there is still quite a pressure passing through them. Therefore it is important to explore alternative ways of working, such as learning to use your forearm and elbows (see Chapters 18 & 19).

Reduce the Hand-intensive Activities in the Rest of Your Life
And look at how you use your wrist in hand-intensive activities in the rest of your life and the pressure that they put on your wrist. Think about how to change the way that you do them or consider stopping doing them entirely in order to reduce the pressure on your wrist.

At one point, for example, I realised that when playing acoustic guitar, one of my favourite 'winding-down' activities, I had (subconsciously) developed a technique which involved hyperextending my wrist. I had to retrain myself in a new technique, and also ration my guitar playing and find other ways of winding-down.

Wrist Exercises

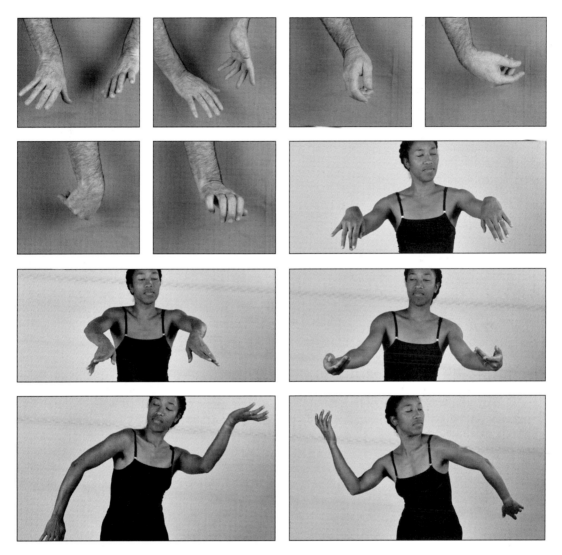

Figure 17.2: Wrist exercises; mobilising the wrist and involving the shoulders.

A reminder here – it is always useful to prepare for doing massages and to release any accumulated tensions afterwards by doing simple exercises that keep your wrists mobile. Begin by bending your hand forwards (flexion of the wrist), backwards (extension), and sideways (abduction and adduction). Then move your hand in a circular movement (circumduction), which incorporates pronation and supination of your forearm to make this movement more extensive and even. It is also important to exercise the closely related body areas – your shoulders and arms, and your thumbs and fingers (see figures 11.46–11.49).

In addition to mobility exercises, people with a small build may find it useful to do specific gym work or exercise routines under professional instruction to strengthen their wrists.

Avoid Working With Your Wrist Bent

Monitoring the angle of your wrists is crucial to avoid straining them. The ideal is to keep your wrist as straight as possible *without rigidifying* it when you are incorporating pressure in your massage strokes. Even when you are only applying light pressure, it is a good habit to cultivate. And when you are applying firm and/or sustained pressure, it is crucial to minimise the bending of your wrist.

Have a Supple Wrist for Percussion

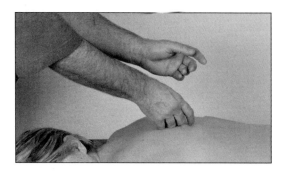

Figure 17.3: Having the wrist intermittently bent.

In many percussion strokes it is important that you keep your wrists supple and able to move. These are the only common techniques in which it is good to let your wrist bend.

Don't Apply Pressure With Your Wrist Hyperextended

However, *regularly applying pressure with your wrist bent will strain it.* If your wrist is bent, the transfer of power from your arm to your hand is inefficient, which often leads you to apply more force. In addition, part of your effort will go towards maintaining the stability of your wrist. These effects together put considerable pressure on the wrist, which is not adapted to working powerfully at an angle.

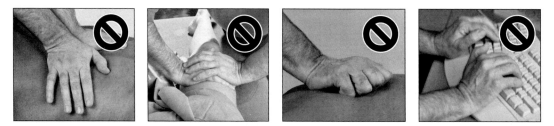

Figure 17.4: Working with the wrist hyperextended; a) applying pressure with the heels of the hands,
b) sliding the hands sideways up a limb with pressure, c) knuckle circling pressure,
d) poor wrist position for computer work.

Problems most commonly arise from having the wrist(s) hyperextended whilst applying pressure – with the heel of the hand, the fingers, the thumbs or the knuckles. Much of the power is then used just to stabilise the wrist. Doing strokes in this way is hard work on the arm muscles, inefficient and puts unnecessary strain on the wrist. (This is the same position that can cause such problems in computer work, both in typing and using the mouse).

If you are using a mechanical tool in order to save your thumbs or fingers when you are applying pressure, watch the angle of your wrist.

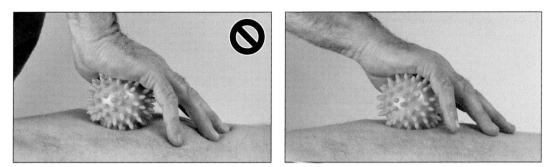

Figure 17.5: Using a spiky ball; a) with a bent wrist, b) with a straight wrist.

Don't Do Petrissage Strokes With Your Wrist Bent

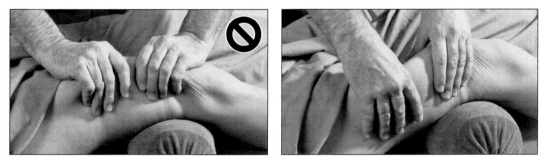

Figure 17.6: Squeezing muscles; a) with the wrist hyperextended, b) with the wrist straight.

Unfortunately, many people also knead and squeeze muscles with their wrists hyperextended, often without realising it.

Don't Hyperextend Your Wrist When Pulling

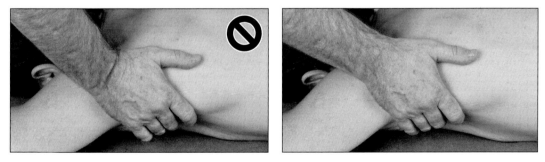

Figure 17.7: Pulling; a) with a hyperextended wrist, b) with a straight wrist.

And, when you are doing pulling strokes, it is also important to make sure that your wrists are relatively straight to minimise the pressure on them.

Monitor Your Wrist When You Are Working With it Bent

When you are using the palm or heel of your hand for the pressure, you can not keep your wrist straight of course. You can safely apply a certain amount of pressure through the heel of your hand with your wrist *somewhat* bent, as long as:

- The rest of your hand is relaxed;
- You generate the pressure by leaning your bodyweight rather than by tensing your shoulders and arms, which would produce more associated tension in your wrists;
- You don't do this too often or with too much pressure;
- You monitor your wrists carefully for any feelings of discomfort or strain, especially if you have small or slender or hypermobile wrists, and;
- You make sure that you are not also hyperextending your wrist regularly in other daily activities, such as typing or driving.

The Angle of Your Wrist When You Are Applying Pressure

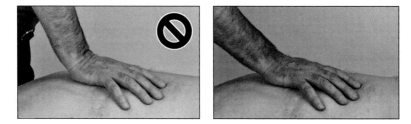

Fig 17.8: Wrist bent with relaxed hand when applying pressure; a) near 90˚, b) around 30˚.

Try the following experiment to discover the best working angles *for your own wrist*. Place your hand flat on your partner's back, and relax it so that it settles onto the contours of his/her body. Then bend your wrist towards 90°. Slowly increase the pressure that you apply through the heel of your hand by leaning your bodyweight forward, keeping your fingers relaxed. You are quite likely to feel a little niggle in the carpal tunnel area, even when your hand is very relaxed. This is a hint of the strain that you could cause by consistently working with your wrist bent to 90°.

Then, *keeping your hand relaxed* while still applying pressure through the heel, begin to straighten your wrist. Some people find that feelings of strain disappear from the wrist when it reaches an angle of around 45°. For many people, it needs to be less than this – often around 30°. Experiment with this a few times to find out what the comfortable *maximum* working angle is *for you* to have your wrist bent when applying pressure through your *relaxed* hand.

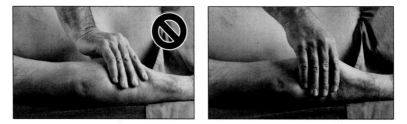

Fig 17.9: Squeezing a muscle; a) with the wrist bent, b) with a straight wrist.

Bear in mind that it is only a comfortable angle for applying pressure through the heel of your hand *when your hand is relaxed*. Notice that strain returns if you actively use your hand with your wrist at this angle. You will appreciate that this is *not* a good angle for your wrist, for example, when you are gripping, squeezing or kneading a muscle.

Instead, straighten your wrist more until you feel that you can do these strokes without any discomfort in your wrist. Most people find that they need to have their wrists virtually straight to be able to do this comfortably. Even in this position, if your wrists are *rigid*, you will probably feel little niggles of strain returning. So, even when you are applying pressure, make sure that your wrists are a little relaxed, and not stiff.

Avoid Overflexing the Wrist

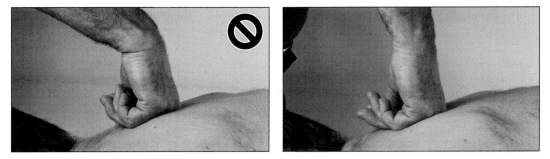

Figure 17.10: Fist pressure; a) have the wrist overflexed, b) having the wrist straighter.

Although having the wrist flexed is a less common problem, it can still affect the wrist if it is done too often.

Don't Let Your Wrist Bend Sideways

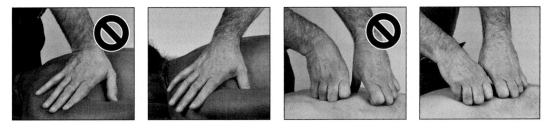

Figure 17.11: Having the wrist bent sideways or straight; a), b) hand pressure, c), d) knuckle kneading.

Applying pressure with your hand turned sideways will also place pressure on your wrist.

Reposition Your Body to Keep Your Wrist Straight

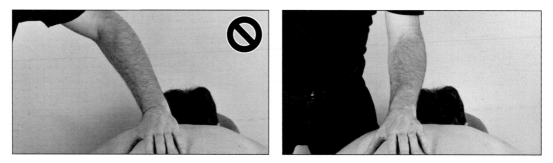

Figure 17.12: Positioning the body; a) in a position that causes the wrist to bend, b) repositioning to get the wrist straight.

Bear in mind that in order to keep your wrist straight, you will need to regularly reposition yourself to keep your body aligned behind your hands.

Supporting and Stabilising Your Wrist

Wearing wrist supports (see figure 8.5) will go a little way to supporting your wrists and remind you to keep them straight. However, supporting and stabilising your working hand with your other hand will help you to significantly reduce the workload on your wrist. This will also give you more control of your working hand, enabling you to work with more precision. This, in turn, reduces the need to tense your arm and shoulder muscles for control, both of which would put more pressure on your wrist. There are two ways of stabilising your wrist – either by holding it, or supporting it from underneath.

Hold Your Wrist to Support it

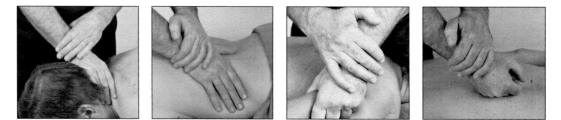

Figure 17.13: Holding your working wrist.

Holding your working wrist is one way of supporting and guiding it. This significantly reduces the workload on your wrist, and also gives you more control of your working hand, enabling you to apply and move the pressure more precisely. This in turn reduces the need to tense your arm and shoulder muscles for control, hence avoiding putting further pressure on your wrist.

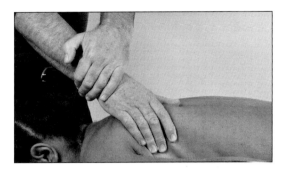

Figure 17.14: Holding your wrist for pulling.

Holding your wrist for pulling will also help you to guide your working hand and to reduce the pressure on your wrist.

Rest Your Wrist Over Your Other Hand or Forearm

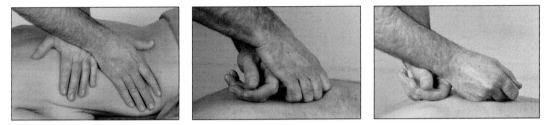

Figure 17.15: Resting the working wrist across the other hand.

You can use your other hand or fist to support your working wrist from underneath. The supporting hand acts as a platform, which derives its stability from resting on the client's body. Whenever possible move this support as a unit with your working hand for maintaining continuity in your strokes.

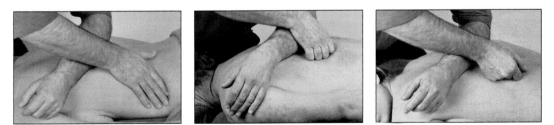

Figure 17.16: Resting the working wrist across the other forearm.

If, through practise, you can get comfortable with using your forearm for support, this will, of course, save your supporting hand completely.

Rest Your Wrist Over a Bolster or Your Own Thigh

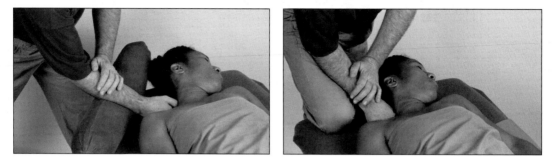

Figure 17.17: Supporting the working wrist; a) on a cushion, b) on practitioner's knee.

You can sometimes rest your working arm across a cushion or bolster, or across your own thigh by putting your knee on the table. This will provide more support, and will enable you to use your other hand primarily for precise guidance of your working hand.

Review

Wrist problems primarily arise from the cumulative effects of applying pressure and/or working with the wrists consistently bent, most commonly hyperextended.

Be careful if you are also regularly doing other hand-intensive activities such as keyboard work, gardening, DIY or playing musical instruments.

Practitioner's with small or slender wrists need to take special care of them, and may find it useful to do specific exercises or gym work under supervision to strengthen their wrists.

Watch out for the development of symptoms of wrist strain:

- Early warning signs such as dull twinges or niggles when doing massage strokes;
- Chronic aching or throbbing wrist pain;
- Numbness, tingling and/or pain in the thumb, index and middle fingers;
- Restricted movement and/or loss of control in the wrist and parts of the hand, and;
- Any pains that persist or regularly arise when you are not working.

Don't continue doing strokes that strain your wrists. Change your working practices, and, if necessary, the type of clients that you work with.

Rest your wrists when you can. Regular massage can help as a preventative measure.

Many people find acupuncture, deep massage and osteopathy / chiropractic / physiotherapy helpful for dealing with persistent pain.

If you are feeling strain in your wrists or hands, make sure that you are not also tensing your shoulders, which is likely to put extra pressure on your wrists.

Do mobilising exercises for your wrist to prepare for doing massages, and to release any accumulated tensions afterwards.

You may find it useful to wear wrist supports to help protect your wrists.

When you are *applying pressure*, try to keep your wrist relatively straight without rigidifying it.

Don't do sliding pressure strokes along a limb with your hands turned sideways.

You can apply a certain amount of pressure through the heel of your hand with your wrist *somewhat* bent, provided that your hand is relaxed and that you do not overdo it. For most people the best angle is about 30°.

Position yourself to keep your body aligned behind your hands and your wrist/s straight.

Holding your wrist will support it and give you more control of your working hand.

Reduce the pressure on the wrist of your working hand by resting it over your other hand or forearm.

Resting the forearm of your working hand on a cushion will provide stability for your working hand and wrist.

Conserve your wrists by learning to use your forearm and elbows.

Other Working Tools: 'Hands-free' Massage

The previous section of the book covers ways of reducing the strain on your hands in massage, particularly when you are applying pressure (see Chapters 11–16). This section looks at using other parts of your body in order to conserve your hands.

Although Swedish massage and its derivatives have relied fairly exclusively on the hands until recent decades, the use of other body parts is an integral part of most other massage traditions. For example, the feet are the main working tools in the Chavutti Thirumal massage of Southern India and some styles of shiatsu. In shiatsu and Thai yoga massage, other parts of the body are also used, especially when applying stretches.

Techniques from other traditions have filtered into Western massage in recent years. For example, the practice of using the forearms in Hawaii and both the forearm and elbow in Eastern Europe has influenced the development of many deep tissue massage techniques. And the use of the elbow as a penetrating tool for digging into small areas of tension, a common feature of many other massage traditions, is becoming widespread in Western massage. A number of massage approaches have recently been developed in the USA, based on Japanese barefoot shiatsu traditions. Recent British developments include the *No-hands Massage* style developed by Gerry Pyves, and my own *'Hands-free' Massage* approach.

This Section of the Book

The first two chapters in this section cover the use of the forearm and elbow, which are the commonly used substitutes for your vulnerable fingers, thumbs and knuckles for working on a massage table. You can use your forearm for light pressure strokes in order to give your hands a rest. Your forearm and elbow are *irreplaceable* when you are using firm pressure. This is especially important for practitioners with long, slender fingers and/or hypermobile digits, and those whose clientele require a firm massage.

The third chapter in this section covers the use of the knees and feet, which are common tools in floor massage, but can also be used a little when you are working on a massage table. The fourth chapter looks at ways of using your thigh, shoulder and hip to support the work of your hands in moving and stretching your client's limbs.

A Few Notes of Caution

This book presents *general* guidelines for using these massage tools. Experienced practitioners will, no doubt, be able to extract useful information from these chapters. However, for beginners, there is no substitute for a course of personal instruction with an experienced teacher as it is easy to strain yourself and/or bruise the client.

Using these tools in a massage session needs to be preceded by lighter strokes, and then gradually by firmer and deeper techniques in order to prepare the tissues. Rather than trying to *force* the tissues into submission (which generally causes the client to tense against you), apply pressure that is manageable for your client, and wait for the tissues to 'melt' and allow you through.

The transmission of force from the practitioner to the client is very direct when it is applied via the forearm, elbow, knees or feet, so it is easy to apply more pressure than you realise. Therefore it is crucial to *monitor and adapt to the client's responses* – both their verbal responses and also their bodily reactions such as holding the breath, or micro-flickers of reaction in the muscles that indicate that too much pressure is being applied. People often mistakenly assume that they will be unable to palpate with these massage tools. Of course they will never be as sensitive as your fingertips. However, with practise, it is possible to develop considerable sensitivity in palpating the client's tissues via your forearms, elbows, and feet.

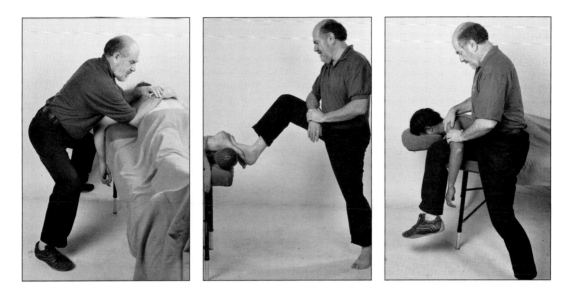

CHAPTER 18

Using the Forearm

Using your forearm enables you to save your hands in light to medium pressure massage strokes. It is irreplaceable for applying firm pressure, either stationary or sliding pressure, which is the main focus of this chapter. The last part of the chapter looks at using the forearm for passive stretches and to provide support for parts of the client's body as you move it.

The Main Working Areas – the 'Soft Forearm' and the 'Hard Forearm'

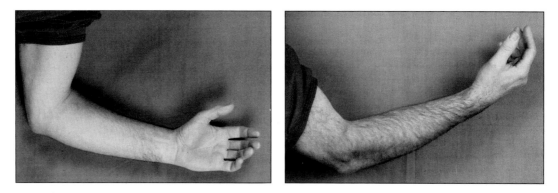

Figure 18.1: Main working areas of the forearm; a) the 'soft' forearm – the flexor muscle bellies, b) the 'hard' forearm – the edge of the ulna.

This chapter focuses on the two most commonly used parts of the forearm. Using the 'soft' forearm (the bellies of the flexor muscles) enables you to provide widespread general pressure, and the 'hard' forearm (the bony 'blade' of the ulna) will deliver harder, more focused pressure.

Although they are technically part of the forearm, the wrist bones are covered in Chapter 14 (see figures 14.17–14.20) because they can be used in similar ways to many other parts of the hand. The use of bony areas around the elbow, which can combine precision with more penetrating pressure, is the subject of the next chapter. Many of the principles of working with the forearm that are covered in this chapter also apply to working with the elbow.

Some Important Cautions

This chapter on using the forearm and the next on using the elbow are the ones that I am most hesitant about including in this book. I am concerned about people without prior experience bruising their clients and/or straining themselves in trying out the ideas presented here. If this is a new area for you, find an experienced teacher to help you to translate the ideas in this chapter into action.

Be Sensitive to the Client's Responses
Initially, you will need to focus on developing your ability to use your forearm. However, once you have gained some skill with it, it is important to focus on *feeling* (palpating) with it so that you can monitor the client's responses and adapt to them. Although your forearm will never be as sensitive as your fingertips, people are often surprised by how much that they can learn to feel with it through practice. Developing this skill can be greatly assisted in the early stages by feeling your way with your fingers in order to identify the landmarks and the 'texture' and tension of the muscles, prior to seeking to locate these with your forearm. You can also use the fingertips of your guiding hand (see figures 18.13–18.21) to help you to feel your way. Having your shoulders, arm and hand relaxed and aligning your body behind your forearm will all help this.

The transmission of force from the practitioner to the client is very direct when using the forearm. This is in contrast to the dissipation of the force when you use your hands because it is then spread through so many small joints. And, if you are using your body well (see figures 18.23–18.27), it will feel relatively effortless to apply pressure with your forearm. Therefore it is easy for you to be applying more pressure than you realise. So it is crucial to *be sensitive to your client's responses* – both verbal responses and also bodily reactions such as holding the breath, or micro-flickers of reaction in the muscles that indicate that the pressure is too much.

Monitor Your Breathing When Applying Pressure
When applying sustained pressure, practitioners also need to monitor *their own* breathing patterns. You may be subconsciously holding your breath or inhaling forcefully, either of which are likely to cause you to tense up. It is best to exhale gently as you apply the pressure (see figure 26.3).

Moving in Closer to the Client
Using the forearm involves moving in closer to the client. This should not be done too early in the massage or too abruptly, to allow the client to acclimatise to this closeness. Female practitioners with short arms and/or large breasts need to be particularly careful that you are not draping yourself over the client.

Using Your Body in an Unfamiliar Way
You may find that your legs feel sore at first as you accustom yourself to the lower stance (see figure 18.24) that is necessary to save your back. Practitioners with knee problems need to be especially careful about this. And some of your shoulder and arm muscles may initially feel sore as you use them in unfamiliar ways. As with any new activity, this will settle down when you become more familiar and skilled with using your forearm.

Don't Overuse Your Dominant Arm
As with using your hands, make sure that you don't overuse your dominant arm. This is particularly important for right-handers.

Respect Your Limits
Bear in mind that the way in which practitioners are able to use their forearms is affected by their build. Even with the most effective use of the body, there are *limits* to the capabilities of every practitioner.

Ease into Using Your Forearm
Using the forearm to apply pressure needs to be preceded by strokes that gradually work more firmly and deeply in order to prepare the tissues. So it is good to begin a massage with your hands to initially make contact and to palpate the area. Then, when using your forearm, gradually increase the pressure at a rate that is acceptable to your client.

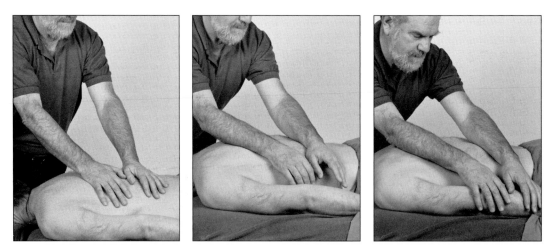

Figure 18.2: Moving from using the hands to using the forearms.

Practicing the execution of smooth transitions from using your hands in the familiar way into using your forearms (and back again) will aid this process. As you change the point of contact from the hand to the forearm, let your hand relax (see figure 18.4) and lower your bodyweight into the 'chimpanzee' stance by widening your stance and bending your knees in order to save your back (see figure 18.24).

Using the 'Soft' Forearm

The 'soft' forearm (the bellies of the flexor muscles) can be used for relatively light strokes in order to rest your hands. This area provides a large area to replace your palm and the heel of your hand for applying widespread pressure. On client's with soft muscles, the soft forearm is also effective on areas such as the shoulders when s/he is so 'wound up' that s/he would react against you digging in with thumb, knuckles or fist pressure.

Have Your Palm Turned Down

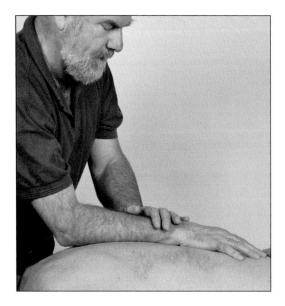

Figure 18.3: Using the 'soft' forearm – palm down.

Have the palm of your working forearm turned downwards to avoid rolling onto the edge of the ulna.

Relax the Hand of Your Working Forearm

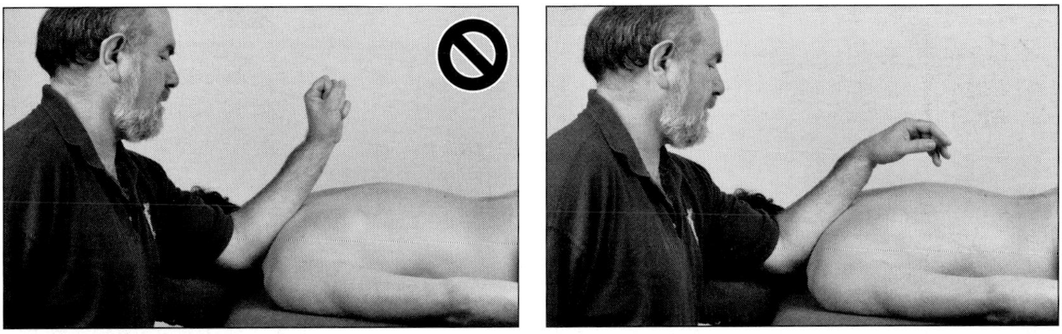

Figure 18.4: The hand of the working forearm; a) stiff hand, b) relaxing the hand – the 'swan neck' wrist.

Massage practitioners are so accustomed to using their hands, that most of us instinctively tighten them without realising it when we prepare to do a massage. Getting used to relaxing the hands is often one of the hardest aspects to master in using the forearm, so it takes continual monitoring for quite some time. Relaxing your hand enables you to give it a complete rest, while simultaneously giving yourself a massage on the normally hardworking flexor muscles (which, of course, are the muscles that you use to tighten your hand).

Unless you can relax the hand of your working arm, you will be using these flexor muscles unnecessarily. Because the bellies of your flexor muscles are the point of contact with your client, tightening them (to tense your hand) would produce the same instinctive wariness in the client as tensing your hands to do a massage, rather than encouraging him to relax. It would also make it harder for you to feel the responses in the area that you are massaging. So have the hand of your working forearm as relaxed as possible. Let it soften and hang loosely, so that it makes a 'swan neck' at your wrist when you are using your 'soft' forearm. This gives your hand a complete rest. Relaxing your hand like this is also crucial when you are using your elbow (see Chapter 19).

Use the Area of Your Forearm Close to Your Elbow for Pressure Strokes
In light sliding strokes, it doesn't matter which section of your forearm that you use. However, the best area through which to apply sustained pressure is close to the elbow. This enables the power to be most directly transmitted from your trunk to the client via your upper arm.

The Best Part of the Forearm for Applying Sustained Pressure

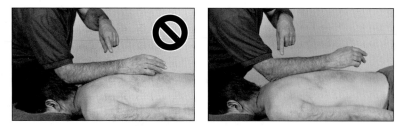

Figure 18.5: Applying pressure with the soft forearm;
a) using the forearm near the wrist, b) using the forearm near the elbow.

If you apply pressure close to the elbow, you will feel how the power is transferred fairly undiminished to the client, which enables you to remain relatively relaxed in your arm and shoulder muscles. Compare this with applying pressure through a more distal part of the forearm. As you move the point of delivery closer to your wrist, you will feel how you have to tense your upper arm and shoulder to control it, and that the proportion of the power reaching the client is reduced. This also applies to using the bony 'blade' of the ulna (see figure 18.7).

Use Your Soft Forearm Like a Snowplough for Sliding Pressure

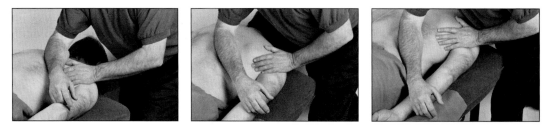

Figure 18.6: Sliding the forearm like a 'snowplough'.

As well as using your forearm to apply stationary pressure on one area, you can *slowly* push it forward across a wide muscle mass, using it like the blade of a road-grader or a snowplough. Moving slowly forward gives the tissues time to accommodate to your pressure, and to soften (to 'melt') and let you through. This is generally most effective on the thoracic and lumbar sections of the erector spinae muscles and on the hamstrings or quadriceps, especially for people with a medium to large build and/or with well-used muscles. On people with smaller builds, you'll need to angle it more side-on in order to avoid hitting bones, especially in the mid-thoracic 'channel' between the shoulder blade and the spine.

Using the 'Hard Forearm' / 'Bony Blade' of the Forearm

Have Your Palm Turned Up to Use the Ulna

Turning your palm upwards shifts the working area from the 'soft' to the 'hard' forearm (the edge of the ulna). When it is appropriate, this can provide you with a harder area for applying more focused pressure. This bony 'blade' can be quite a forceful tool so don't use it too suddenly or forcefully. Instead, make a series of light sweeps along or across the muscles, like spreading butter with a knife. This is different from the way that the point of the elbow is used to 'dig in' (see Chapter 19).

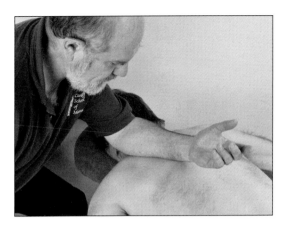

Figure 18.7: Using the bony 'blade' of the ulna – palm up.

Relax the Hand of Your Working Forearm

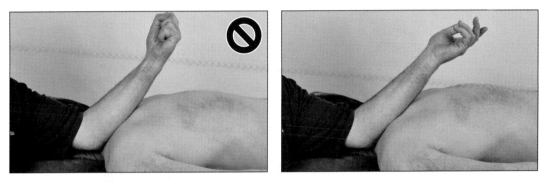

Figure 18.8: The hand of your working forearm; a) tense hand, b) relaxed hand.

As with using your soft forearm, keep the hand of your working forearm relaxed.

Vary the Width of the 'Blade' According to the Area That You're Working On

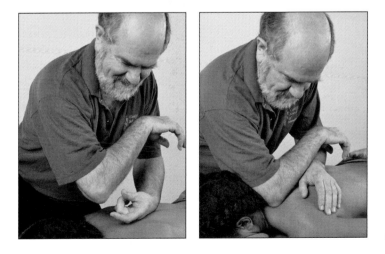

Figure 18.9: Narrow 'blade'.

The width of 'blade' that you are using can be varied, depending on the size and tension of the muscles that you're working on. A short section of 2–3 cm (about 1 inch) would be appropriate on the shoulders of a small-framed client.

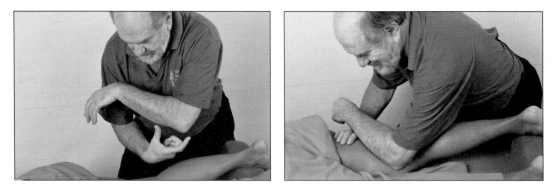

Figure 18.10: Wide 'blade'.

A wider 'blade' of 7–8 cm (3 inches) is better on the lower back or lower thoracic muscles of a larger person's back, or on a runner's hamstring muscles. Make sure that you are not unknowingly digging into muscles with the point of your elbow or scraping bones with it as you use this blade. As with the 'soft' forearm (see figure 18.5), the section closest to the elbow is the most effective to use for applying pressure.

Use the Hard Forearm Across Muscles to Stretch Them Sideways

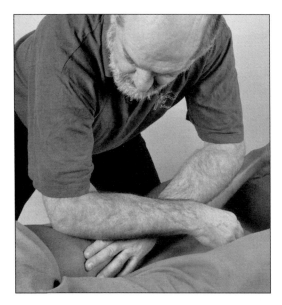

Figure 18.11: Working across the hamstrings.

This blade is quite useful for working across muscles to stretch them sideways. This is a cross between wringing and doing a cross-fibre stroke. It is most effective on the legs, especially on large and/or well-used hamstring and quadriceps muscles and across the calves.

Applying Pressure

Maintain Consistent Pressure

The massage practitioner who has mastered the use of the forearm and elbow can work quite firmly and deeply. The deeper that the pressure is, the more carefully it needs to be applied and monitored. Increase the pressure slowly and then keep it *consistent* in order to give the client's body time to 'trust' and accommodate to it. Similarly, move *slowly* forward with sliding strokes, waiting for the tissues to 'melt' and let you through. (Bear in mind that it is only easy to apply pressure as you push your forearm forward. Trying to apply pressure when you are pulling your forearm towards yourself requires you to tighten your shoulder muscles considerably and is neither easy nor very effective).

Trying to force too much with each slide is likely to cause the client to tense against you. Instead, make a series of sweeps in order to 'skim' off successive thin 'layers' of tension with each sweep. This is akin to using a carpentry plane effectively. Pressing too deeply with a plane gets you stuck, and often damages both the wood and the blade. If you press too deeply in massage, you may bruise the client, while overworking and perhaps even straining yourself. So it is best to cover the same area a number of times, 'shaving off' a little more tension with each sweep.

Follow the Contours of the Client's Body

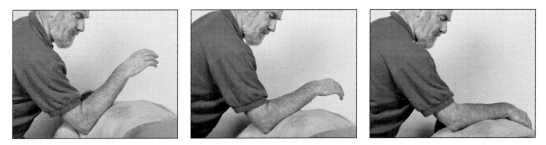

Figure 18.12: Tilting the forearm to follow the contours of the client's body.

It is easy to 'mould' your hands to the contours of the client's body because they have so many internal joints. However the forearm can't change shape in this way (although the flexor muscle bellies can be squashed or stretched a little as you use your forearm). Therefore, to cover an area, you need to tilt your forearm through a range of angles in order to follow the contours of the client's body. And you need to move your body behind your forearm in order to do this (see figure 18.26).

Reduce the Pressure and Tilt Your Forearm to Pass Over or Around Bones

Some years ago, a friend of mine bought an electrical vibrating massager for her back. She enjoyed me using it on her back because I steered around the bones, eased the pressure on thin muscles and increased it on the larger, tighter ones. However the first time that she used it on me, it was excruciating. She had no knowledge of anatomy, so she maintained the same pressure as she passed it over my bones (including my spine). Using the forearm in a similar indiscriminate way has given it an undeserved bad reputation.

Moving smoothly over the edge of bones, such as sliding from the midback muscles onto the back of the scapula, requires you to soften your pressure and tilt your forearm considerably. This is particularly important with clients who have prominent bones.

Practitioners with fleshy forearms can readily reduce the pressure and tilt over the edge of the client's bones to pass from one muscle mass to another. In fact, with practice they will find that they can even cross the client's spine in this way, provided that the vertebrae aren't too prominent. However, those with thinner forearm muscles will need to be much more careful about crossing bones. They may need to lift off entirely or return to using their hands to do this.

Guiding Your Working Forearm

Whenever your other hand is not involved in some other essential action, such as supporting a client's limb, use it to guide and stabilise your working forearm / elbow. Until you are well practiced at applying consistent, firm pressure without this support, you are likely to tense your arm and shoulders unnecessarily to control the movement. This reduces the power, precision and fluidity that you can deliver.

You can support your forearm either with your supporting hand on top of it to increase the pressure, or guiding it from underneath for more precision. You can easily change from one to the other of these supports as the situation demands. This support is most effective when it is applied *close to the working area* of the forearm.

Guide Your Forearm From Above to Increase the Pressure

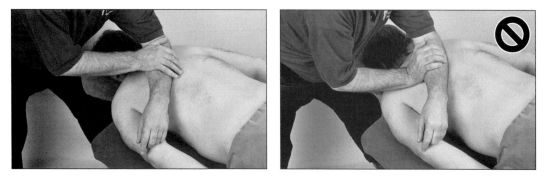

Figure 18.13: Supporting the working forearm from above; a) the guiding hand, b) bending the wrist.

Having your guiding hand on top enables you to increase the pressure by leaning your bodyweight forward. Guiding and adding weight works best when the pressure from your supporting hand is applied directly above the point of contact between your forearm and the client's body. Be alert to the tendency to tighten this guiding hand unnecessarily to control the forearm, and avoid bending your wrist too much.

Finding the Best Place for Supporting Your Working Forearm

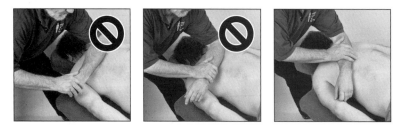

Figure 18.14: Poor support for the working forearm;
a) least support, b) poor support, c) best support.

The further away that your guiding hand is from the contact point between your forearm and the client's body, the harder that you have to work with it and the less fine-tuning control that it provides.

Try holding different parts of your working forearm to clarify this. If your try guiding your forearm by holding the hand of the working forearm, you will appreciate that this is *not* a very effective way of controlling your forearm. You have to tighten your wrist (and probably your fist too) for the technique to work at all. Even then, it only provides very general control. Holding your working forearm near the wrist gives a little more specific control and stability. However, because the support is so distant from the point of action in both of these situations, you have much less control than with your guiding hand close to the working area. And only a percentage of your extra pressure is delivered through your forearm to the client.

Use the Weight of Your Other Arm to Provide Pressure Whenever Possible

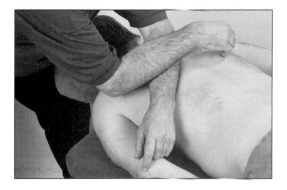

Figure 18.15: Guiding forearm.

Whenever possible, relax your guiding hand and provide the pressure with the weight of your other arm by resting your wrist or other forearm across your working forearm. With practice, you can learn to use your other forearm on top in order to conserve your hand while delivering more pressure with less effort.

Women with large breasts may want to have both forearms regularly crossed in front to create a barrier between you and the client as you move in close. This will save you from the tendency to hunch over in order to keep yourself back from the client.

Guide Your Working Forearm From Underneath for Precision

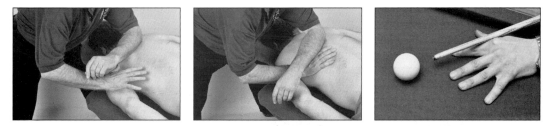

Figure 18.16: Guiding the working arm from underneath; a) the guiding hand shape, b) the guiding hand under the forearm, c) guiding a pool cue with the hand.

Guiding your working forearm from underneath enables you to use it with great precision by making use of the stability provided by resting it on the client's body. You can also palpate the tissues that you are working on with your guiding hand. This is particularly useful when you are working on sensitive areas or places that need a very precise application of pressure. (It is crucial for visually impaired/blind practitioners so that they can identify where they are working). However, the guiding hand does not supply pressure in this position, so you must rely on positioning and leaning your body for that.

Create a guide between your thumb and fingers so that you can use it in a similar way to a billiard player guiding his cue (although in the opposite direction).

Move Your Guiding Hand and Your Working Forearm as a Unit for Sliding Strokes

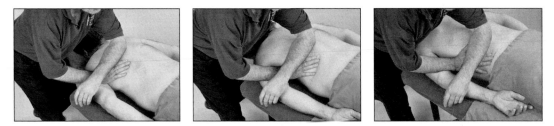

Figure 18.17: Moving the guiding hand and working forearm as a unit.

As you push your forearm over your client's body, slide your guiding hand (or forearm, see figure 18.15) with it as a unit. Sway your body to generate the power and fluidity of this movement, rather than standing still and just working with your shoulder and arm muscles.

Guiding Your Forearm From Underneath Enables You to Change the Amount and Direction of the Forearm That You're Using

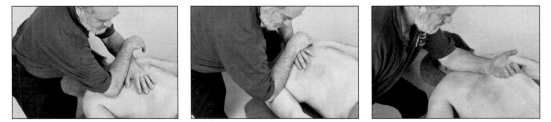

Figure 18.18: Moving the forearm in relation to the guiding hand;
a), b) shortening and lengthening the working forearm, c) rolling onto the 'hard' forearm.

This guide enables you to fluidly change the area of your forearm that you are using in mid stroke, for example:

- Shortening and lengthening the working surface of your forearm;
- Rolling from your 'soft forearm' onto your ulna, or;
- Moving from your forearm to your elbow.

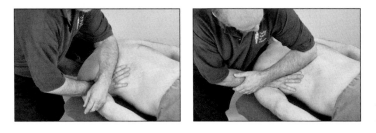

Figure 18.19: 'Rowing' the forearm; a) sweeping the forearm forward, b) sweeping the forearm backwards.

You can also sweep your forearm forward and back from this pivot point. This is like 'rowing' with your forearm, with the support acting like the oarlocks of a boat.

Guide From Underneath With Your Other Hand or Forearm to Save Your Hand

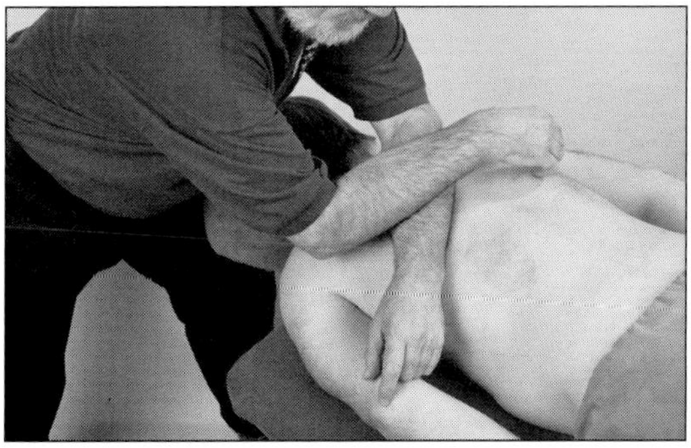

Figure 18.20: Guiding from underneath with the other forearm.

When you feel practiced enough at using your forearms, try providing a similar level of precision support with your other *forearm*, thus saving your supporting hand too. For example, you can 'wrap' your supporting forearm around the working forearm.

Use Your Thumb, Hand or Other Forearm to Protect the Client's Bones

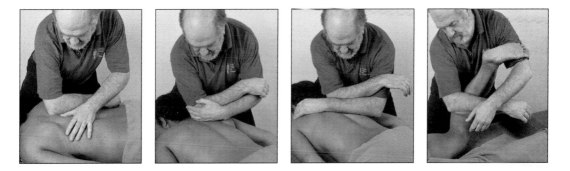

Figure 18.21: Protecting the client's bones; a) using the thumb to protect the client's spine, b) 'wrapping' the supporting hand around the working forearm, c), d) using the other forearm.

When you are working next to the client's spine, you can use the thumb of your supporting hand to protect the spine as well as guiding your forearm. This can be especially important when you are using the ulna. With practise, you will find that you can use your guiding hand in other areas in a more relaxed way without sacrificing precision control. For example you can 'wrap' it around your elbow.

Keep Your Shoulders Relaxed and Use Your Bodyweight When Working Without a Guiding Hand

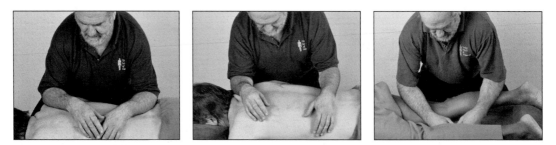

Figure 18.22: Working without the guiding hand – double forearm stretch; a), b) on the back, c) on the legs.

With practice, you can learn to apply *general* sliding strokes easily and fluidly without a guiding hand or forearm, *without stiffening your shoulders* or upper arm muscles, provided that you control the movement by positioning and moving your body behind your forearm (see figure 18.26). When you are pushing your forearms apart, for example, don't do it merely by using your arm and shoulder muscles. Instead lean your trunk forward as if you were going to fall onto your client, and use the momentum of this movement to spread your arms apart.

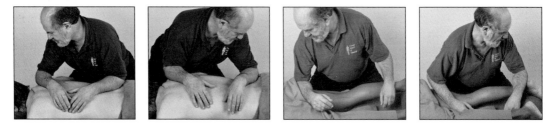

Figure 18.23: Swaying from side-to-side to push the forearm.

Practitioners with short arms and/or large breasts will need to adapt this movement. Instead of spreading your arms simultaneously, push one arm in one direction by turning a little and swaying to that side. Then, as you release this pressure, turn to push the other arm in the opposite direction.

Using Your Body With Your Forearm

Use the 'Chimp' Stance to Save Your Back – Widening Your Stance and Bending Your Knees

Hawaiian kahuna massage, which primarily uses the forearms, is often done on a high table. When you are working on a massage table which is set at the usual height, it is very easy to strain your back by hunching over the table when you add in forearm (and elbow) work. In contrast to massaging with your hands, you have to drop your body lower because you are only involving half of your arm length.

Widen your stance and bend your knees in order to lower your trunk. This saves your back and gives you greater control of the pressure that you're applying. You can then sway with your lower body to create the impulse for your arm movements, rather like the way that a chimpanzee moves. This enables you to work without straining your back. With practice you can get used to moving easily from using your hands to using your forearms by dropping into this 'chimp' stance.

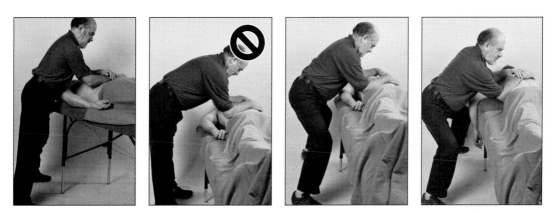

Figure 18.24: Body posture for using the forearms; a) high table,
b) hunching over on an ordinary height table, c), d) working like a 'chimp'.

At first the low working position may feel awkward. Don't be discouraged if your legs initially become a little sore, as it makes demands on muscles that may be unaccustomed to this sort of activity. If you persevere with it, you will find that your leg muscles will adapt. And, bear in mind that you are saving the smaller and much more vulnerable muscles of your hands by doing this.

Many Eastern martial arts involve these types of stances, so studying them can be good preparation for working in this way. Many of them, such as judo, Aikido and Tai Chi, also teach you to move from your centre (the 'hara' or 'tan tien' – the energy centre of the body, located in the lower abdomen – see figure 27.15). This will help you learn how to 'steer' your forearm strokes from your hips.

However, this low stance may not be comfortable if you have knee problems. In this situation, if you are going to make forearm work a major feature of your massages, you will need to consider getting a table that is electrically/hydraulically adjustable during a massage.

Kneel When Necessary to Avoid Hunching Over

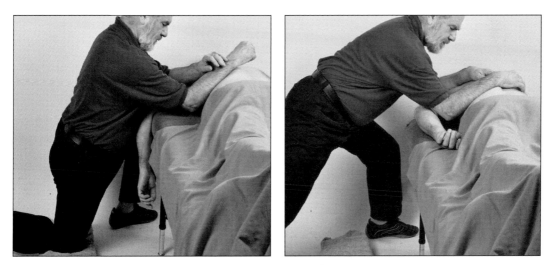

Figure 18.25: Working low down on the table; a) kneeling, b) low squat.

At times, you may need to kneel (ideally in the 'proposal' position – see figure 32.3) or take up a very low squat (by widening your stance further) to be able to work with your forearm on areas that are close to the table, for example along the top of a prone client's shoulders or the side of the hips (on the gluteus medius).

Sway Forward to Move Your Forearm Forward

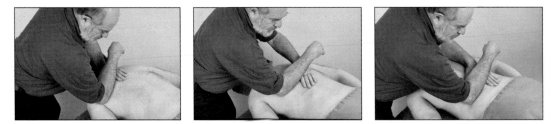

Figure 18.26: Lunging forward behind the forearm.

The fluidity and evenness of your forearm work and the power for maintaining pressure needs to come from using your bodyweight, rather than by tensing your shoulders and/or hunching over. Leaning your bodyweight provides the pressure. Aligning your body behind your forearm (having your forearm centered within your 'hip spotlight' – see figure 27.11) enables you to sway forward from your lower body in order to push your forearm smoothly forward with sustained, consistent pressure. Even when you are maintaining stationary pressure on one area, lean your bodyweight forward to apply the pressure, rather than hunching over and/or tensing your shoulders.

Position Your Body to Balance Between Pressing Downwards and Pushing Forward

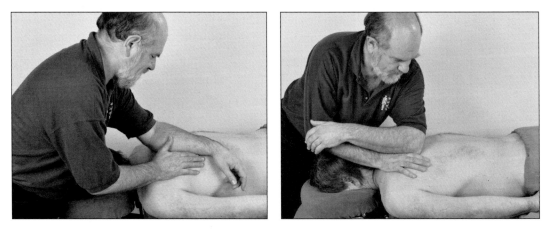

Figure 18.27: Balancing pressure and movement; a) moving forward, b) increasing the pressure.

As with using your hands, use your body position to regulate the balance between the pressure that you are applying and the movement of the stroke. You can increase the pressure by bringing your weight more directly above your working forearm. You can push forward more by lowering your body behind your forearm/elbow and swaying forward.

Using the Forearm for Lifting, Support and Stretches

You can often conserve your hands by using your forearms for stretches and for supporting the client's body. In these strokes too, you need to relax the hand of your working forearm.

Use Your Forearm for Support in Lifting Parts of the Client's Body

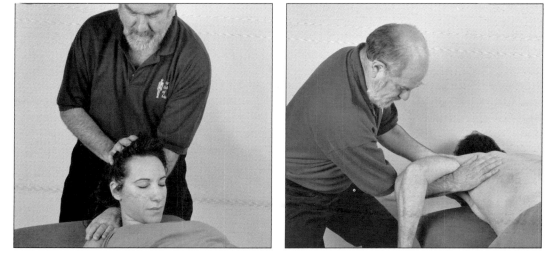

Figure 18.28: Forearms supporting client's body; a) lifting the head, b) supporting the arm.

You can use your forearm to support the client's head or their limbs when you are lifting these parts, for example to stretch the neck, shoulders or hip joints, or bending their knees.

Use Your Forearm for Stretches

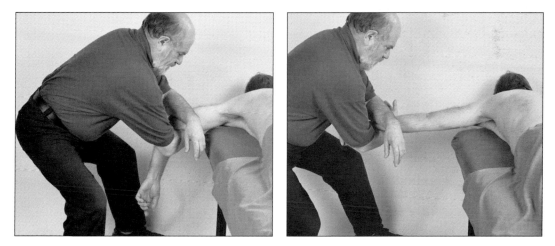

Figure 18.29: Using the forearm to stretch the client's arm.

Bend your arm a little to 'hook' the client's limb loosely in the crook of your elbow for stretches. You can also 'catch' the client's limb between both of your forearms to obtain sufficient 'grip' for a stretch.

'Sit' Back to Pull With Your Forearm

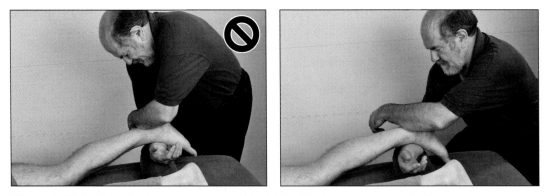

Figure 18.30: Pulling; a) with the arms only, b) by 'sitting' back with the whole body.

When the stretch involves pulling, do it by 'sitting' back from your hips, not by trying to use arm power only.

Review

Two areas of the forearm can substitute for your hands for applying stationary pressure or for sliding pressure strokes:

- The 'soft' forearm (the bellies of the flexor muscles) substituting for the palm or the heel of your hand, and;
- The 'hard' forearm (the edge of the ulna) for firmer, more specific pressure.

You can also use your forearm for stretching the client's limbs.

Prepare the client's tissues for using forearm pressure by applying strokes that gradually work more firmly and deeply.

Use your forearm carefully, monitoring and adapting to your client's responses so that you don't bruise them by using it too suddenly or too forcefully.

Don't overuse your dominant arm.

Recognise your limits. Don't strain yourself by trying to achieve force through your forearm that your body is not built for.

The area of the forearm close to the elbow is the best area to use for delivering pressure.

Keep the hand of your working forearm relaxed.

Use your other hand or forearm to guide your working forearm. Guiding your forearm from on top increases your ability to apply pressure, while guiding from underneath gives you greater precision.

Align your body behind your forearm and lean your bodyweight forward to deliver power, fluidity and evenness.

Control the pressure by how much you lean your bodyweight.

Sway forward with your whole body in sliding strokes, rather than standing still and tensing your shoulders.

To save your back, work 'like a chimp' by bending your knees and widening your stance to drop your body lower.

Lean more over the client to increase the pressure that you are applying, and drop lower and sway forward to push your forearm forward.

Follow the shape of the client's body by tilting your whole body behind your forearm.

To apply stationary pressure on an area, gradually lean your bodyweight forward to increase the pressure, and maintain it at an acceptable level to give the client's tissues time to 'trust' and accommodate to the pressure.

Proceed slowly in sliding strokes, waiting for the tissues to 'melt' and allow you through. Don't make the application of pressure at the beginning of each sweep or the release at the end too abrupt.

CHAPTER 19

Using the Elbow

Using the elbow can combine power and precision, while saving your fingers and thumbs. This chapter looks at the main areas around the elbow, which can be used for applying pressure on specific areas and for applying sliding pressure along a narrow area.

Many aspects of working with the elbow are similar to the ways of using the forearm, which were covered in the previous chapter. The working areas of the elbow need to be used with the same care as using the edge of the ulna (see figure 18.7). And, as with forearm strokes, position your body behind your working elbow to apply pressure and, if possible, guide the stroke with your other hand or forearm.

The Working Areas of the Elbow

This chapter focuses on four parts of the elbow. Unless one of these is specifically mentioned, references in this book to using the 'elbow' apply generally to all of them.

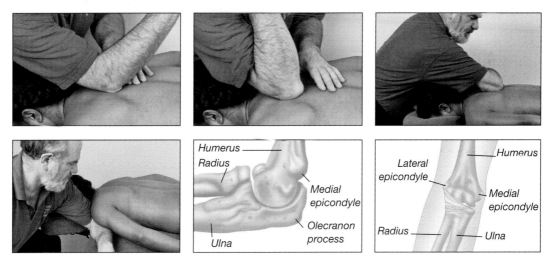

Figure 19.1: The common working areas of the elbow; a) the point of the elbow (the olecranon process of the ulna), b) the back of the elbow (the posterior olecranon), c) the inside of the elbow (the medial epicondyle of the humerus), d), e) the right elbow, medial view, f) anterior view.

The *point of the elbow* (the olecranon of the ulna) is the most commonly used area of the elbow. It can replace the thumb for digging into small areas of tension. This can be done with great precision and sensitivity when guided by the other hand. It can also save your fingers when you are doing sliding strokes that require sustained pressure concentrated along a narrow track.

The *back of the elbow* (the posterior surface of the olecranon) can be used to deliver similar pressure, which is spread over a wider area for sliding strokes.

The *inside of the elbow* (the medial epicondyle of the humerus) can also be used for wider-spread sliding pressure or for pulling. The *lateral epicondyle* can be used to apply pressure upwards by putting your arm under the client's body so that the client's weight presses on it.

Some Important Cautions

Don't Be Too Forceful

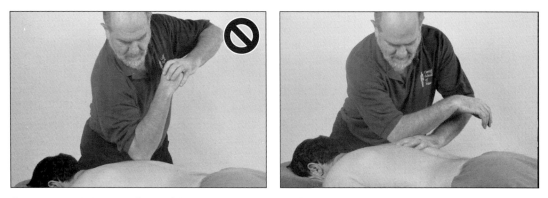

Figure 19.2: Using the elbow; a) in a gung-ho manner, b) with sensitive precision.

Using the elbow is the most extreme way of applying concentrated pressure with the arm. Unfortunately it has gained a bad reputation because of its over zealous use, which can cause pain and bruise the client. Instead of respecting its power and focusing on the precision that is possible with it, some people use the elbow too readily – too suddenly, too forcefully, and too early in massage sessions – and in a very 'gung-ho' way, like using a sledgehammer to crack open a nut.

Because the elbow is such a powerful tool, it needs to be used *carefully* and *sensitively*. The elbow, particularly the point of the elbow, should *only* be used when the tissues have been prepared for the appropriate level of pressure, and *not* as the first tool of choice. If using the elbow is new to you, find an experienced teacher to help you to translate the ideas in this chapter into action.

Use Your Elbow Sensitively
Your elbow will never be as sensitive as your fingertips for palpating the tissues and feeling the client's responses. However massage practitioners are often surprised at how much they *can* learn to palpate with the elbow when they take the time to 'tune-in' to what they can perceive with it. You can help yourself to develop the sensitivity of your elbow by initially feeling the area with your hands in order to identify the landmarks and the 'texture' and tension of the muscles, and then trying to locate these same elements with your elbow. You can also use the fingers of your supporting hand (see figure 19.9) to help you to feel your way.

As with using the forearm, it is very easy for practitioners to apply more pressure than they realise, so it is crucial to be *sensitive to the client's responses* and to be guided by them – both their verbal responses and also their bodily reactions. These can include holding the breath or micro-flickers of reaction in their muscles.

Maintain Even Pressure and Don't Try to *Force* Release
The massage practitioner who has mastered the use of the elbow can work quite firmly and deeply. The deeper that the pressure goes, the more carefully it needs to be applied. This pressure needs to be kept *consistent* in order to give the client's tissues time to 'trust' and accommodate to it, and sliding strokes need to move *slowly*.

Don't try to force the tissues into submission, which is likely to cause the client to tense against you. Apply sustained, static pressure by increasing the pressure gradually, maintaining it for a time and then taking time to slowly release it. For the same reason, when doing sliding pressure strokes, don't make the application of pressure at the beginning of each sweep or the release at the end too abrupt. Gradually push into the tissues and then wait for them to 'melt' and allow you to move through – in the way that a hot knife will gradually cut through frozen butter.

Guide Your Elbow
Whenever possible, control your elbow, especially the point or the back of your elbow, by guiding it with your other hand. If you are using your other hand for something else, rest the hand of your working elbow against your body. This takes the pressure off your working shoulder and arm, which you would otherwise tighten for this control. It enables you to use the working areas of your elbow as finely-tuned instruments. Even for skilled practitioners, it is difficult to use the *unsupported* elbow for sustained pressure with any great precision and without some tensing.

Moving in Closer to the Client
Using the elbow involves moving in closer to the client. This should not be done too early in the massage or too abruptly, to enable the client to acclimatise to this closeness. Female practitioners with short arms and/or large breasts need to be particularly careful that they are not draping themselves over the client.

Monitor Your Own Breathing
When applying sustained pressure, practitioners need to monitor *their own* breathing patterns. You may be unconsciously holding your breath or inhaling forcefully, either of which is likely to cause you to tense up and work too hard. It is best to exhale gently when applying pressure (see Chapter 26).

Don't Overuse Your Dominant Arm
As with using your hands, make sure that you don't overuse your dominant arm. This is particularly important for right-handers.

Respect Your Limits
Bear in mind that, even with such a powerful tool, there are limits to anyone's ability to apply pressure. Remain alert to your own limits, and don't strain yourself by trying to achieve force that your body is not built for.

Take Care of the Ulnar Nerve

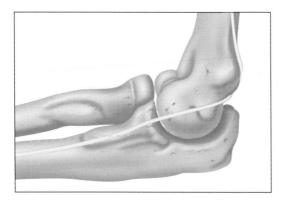

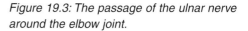

Figure 19.3: The passage of the ulnar nerve around the elbow joint.

When using your elbow, take care not to put pressure on your ulnar nerve (the 'funny bone' nerve) where it passes around the back of the elbow joint on the medial side of the ulna (between the olecranon and the medial epicondyle of the humerus). Regularly putting pressure on it can irritate the nerve and may even damage it.

Using the Point of the Elbow

The point of the elbow (the olecranon) is used for applying sustained pressure on one area or for sliding pressure forward along a narrow line. You can be quite precise about the depth and precision of using your olecranon by using the controls described below.

Control Your Depth of Working By How Much You Bend Your Elbow

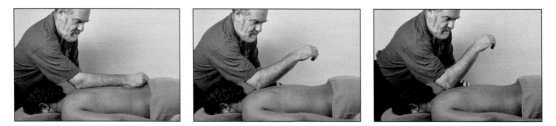

Figure 19.4: Bending the elbow more for the greater depth of 'cut'.

The depth to which you are pressing with your elbow is determined by how much you lean your weight and how much you bend your elbow. Having your arm almost straight gives a shallow 'cut'. Bending and straightening your arm enables you to increase and decrease the depth of working, like raising and lowering the blade of a circular saw to vary the depth of the cut. So it is best to begin with your arm relatively straight and only bend it when you are sure that greater penetration is appropriate. The more that you bend your elbow, the deeper the 'cut' that it gives.

Control the Pressure By How Much You Lean Forward

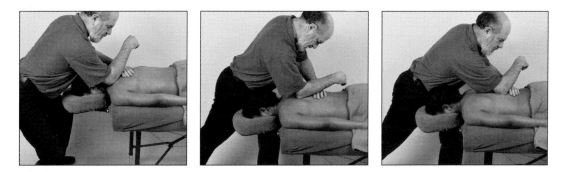

Figure 19.5: Controlling the pressure; a) leaning a little for light pressure,
b) leaning forward for more pressure, c) dropping down to move forward.

Whether you are applying stationary or moving pressure, control the pressure by how much you lean forward. Work lightly by just leaning a little. Lean more directly over your elbow to increase the power. Bear in mind that the point of the elbow is a very effective tool when your bodyweight is positioned behind it. It is easy to apply more pressure than you realise, so monitor the client's responses carefully.

Increase the push forward by lowering your body behind your elbow and swaying to slide it forward.

Slide Your Elbow Straight Forward for the Narrowest Sliding 'Cut'

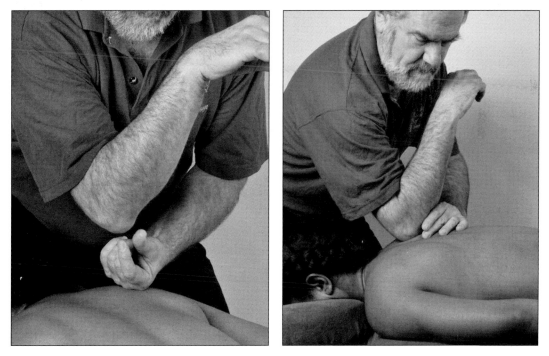

Figure 19.6: Using the olecranon for a narrow 'cut'; a) facing it forward, b) sliding it forward.

The olecranon is a strong, penetrating tool for sliding along a groove of tension in a muscle, and can 'cut' along a very narrow path.

Turn It Side-on for a Wider Sliding 'Cut'

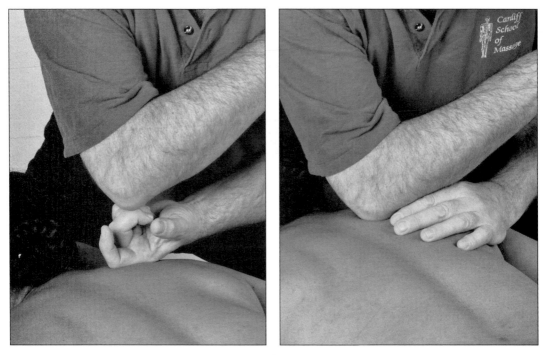

Figure 19.7: Using the olecranon for a wider 'cut'; a) turning the elbow side-on, b) sliding it side on.

Or it can be turned side-on to 'cut' a wider groove.

Relax Your Hand

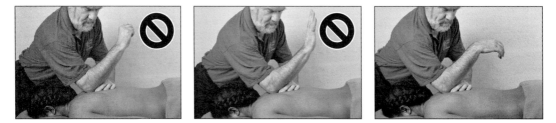

Figure 19.8: The hand of the working elbow; a) clenched hand, b) tense hand, c) letting the hand relax.

As with using the forearm, massage practitioners are so accustomed to using their hands, that most of us instinctively tighten them without realising it. However, unless you relax the hand of your working elbow, you will be unnecessarily tensing your arm (and shoulder). This would produce the same instinctive wariness in the client as tensing your hands to massage. It would also divert your attention away from your elbow and make it harder to feel what you're doing with it. So let your hand soften and hang loosely back, so that you can keep your arm and shoulders relaxed.

For the Greatest Precision, Guide Your Elbow With a 'Pincers' Grip

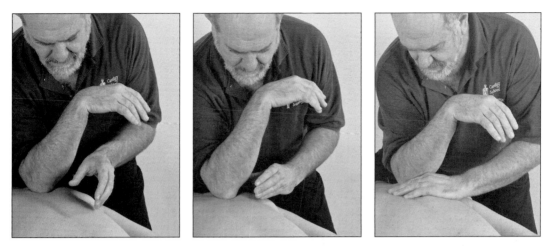

Figure 19.9: The guiding hand; a) a 'pincers' grip; b), c) controlling the elbow with the 'pincers'.

Guide your elbow by holding it in a gentle 'pincers' grip between your thumb and fingers to use it with the greatest precision. You can then pinpoint a specific area for the careful application of firm pressure. With practise, you can learn to 'wrap' your hand around your elbow or use the other forearm as a guide.

Protect the Spine With Your Thumb

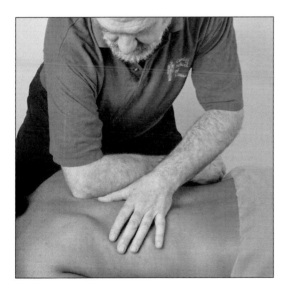

Figure 19.10: Protect the spine with your thumb.

When you are working next to the vulnerable bony prominences, you may feel that you need to be more precise about your control. As with using the forearm, placing your thumb against the spinous processes of the vertebrae will enable you to push towards them without fear of hitting them with your olecranon.

Rest Your Guiding Hand on the Client's Body

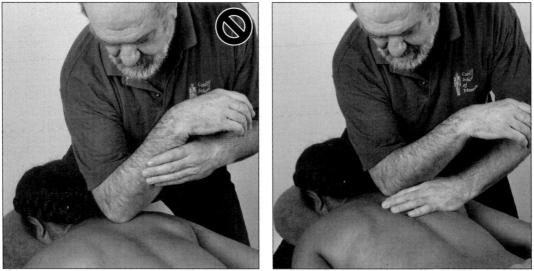

Figure 19.11: The guiding hand in relation to the client's body;
a) not in contact with client's body – less stability, b) resting on client's body for maximum stability.

Whenever you can, rest your guiding hand on the client's body for the greatest stability for your elbow.

Learn to Guide Your Elbow With Your Other Hand or Forearm

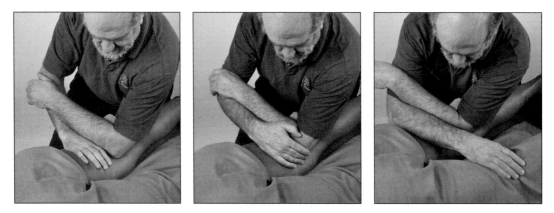

Figure 19.12: Guiding the elbow; a) 'pincer's' grip, b) 'wrapping' the supporting hand around the elbow,
c) guiding with the other forearm.

With practise, you can learn to control the elbow by 'wrapping' your guiding hand more loosely around it, or even using your other forearm to guide it.

Rest the Hand of Your Working Elbow Against Your Body When Your Other Hand is Occupied

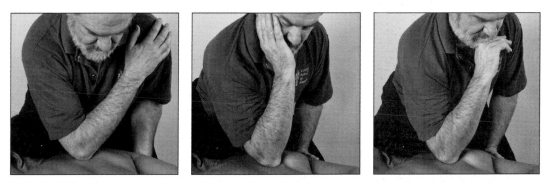

Figure 19.13: Working with one arm only by resting the hand against the body; a) against the shoulder, b), c) against the face.

If your other hand is unavailable for supporting your elbow, rest the hand of your working elbow against some part of your own body, such as your opposite shoulder, the side of your head, or your other arm. This enables you to 'steer' your elbow from two places (by using your body) with more ease and precision than by just tensing the muscles of your working arm and shoulder.

Involve Your Body

Whichever part of your elbow that you're using, there are three important aspects of using your body to support the power and evenness of your strokes:

1. Lowering your body by bending your knees and widening your stance to avoid straining your back by hunching over;
2. Leaning your bodyweight for the pressure, and;
3. Swaying forward or back to push your elbow forward or pull it back.

Use the 'Chimp' Stance to Save Your Back – Widening Your Stance and Bending Your Knees

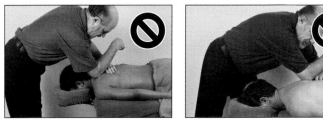
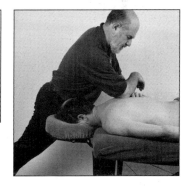

Figure 19.14: Body posture for using the elbow;
a) standing stiffly and hunching over,
b) leaning too far over the couch, c) working like a 'chimp'.

As with using your forearm, bend your knees and widen your stance in order to lower your body and position it behind your working elbow. This 'chimpanzee' position enables you to sway with your lower body to create the impulse for your arm movements, rather than standing stiffly, overusing your shoulder and arm muscles and/or hunching over, which would strain your back.

You may find that your legs get a little sore at first as they adjust to this stance. If you find that it remains awkward for you, consider studying an Eastern martial art such as judo, Aikido and Tai Chi, which involve this type of stances.

Sway Forward to Push Your Elbow Forward and Back to Pull It

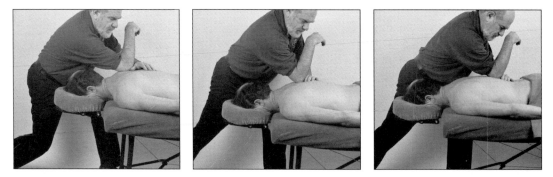

Figure 19.15: Lunging forward behind your elbow.

In a sliding stroke, sway smoothly forward with your whole body to push your arm forward, rather than standing still and tensing your shoulders.

Using the Back of the Elbow

The back of the elbow (the posterior surface of the olecranon) provides a solid pressure surface that is wider and not as sharp as the point for sliding pressure strokes. It is easier to apply pressure through the back of the elbow in pushing strokes, but it is also used for pulling strokes.

Use the Back of the Elbow on Sinewy or Wide, Flat Muscle Areas

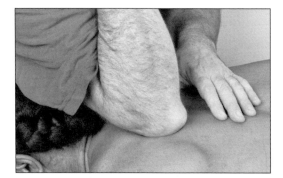

Figure 19.16: Using the back of the elbow.

The back of the elbow works well when you want to press as firmly as with the point without digging in so sharply. For example, it can be used on the thoracic section of sinewy erector spinae muscles.

Guide the Back of Your Elbow With Your Other Hand or Forearm
Whether you are pushing or pulling, use your other hand to guide the direction and control the rate of the movement. This will enable you to work with precision whilst saving you from unnecessarily tensing your shoulder and arm muscles. As for using the point of the elbow, rest your supporting hand on the client's body for the greatest control.

With practise, to save your guiding hand you can learn to use your other forearm for this instead.

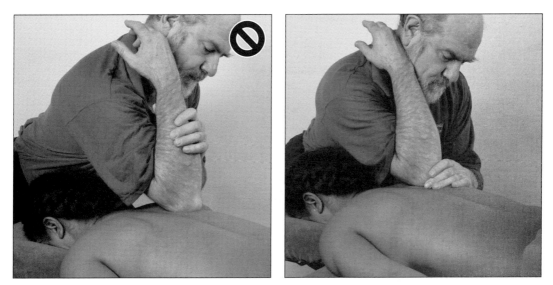

Figure 19.17: Guiding the back of the elbow with the other hand;
a) not in contact with client's body – less stability, b) resting on client's body for maximum stability.

Rest Your Hand Against Your Body When Your Other Hand/Arm Is Unavailable for Support

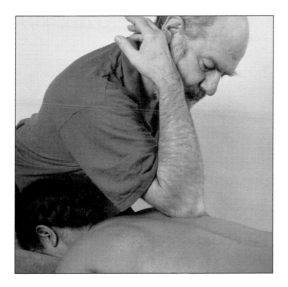

Figure 19.18: Resting the hand against the head.

As with using the point of your elbow (see figure 19.13), rest the hand of your working elbow against your body when your other hand is otherwise occupied, for example with supporting the client's limb. You can then move your body to guide your elbow from two points of 'steering', which will give you more control and enable you to keep your shoulders and arms relatively relaxed.

Avoid Standing Up Too High

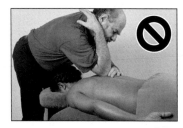

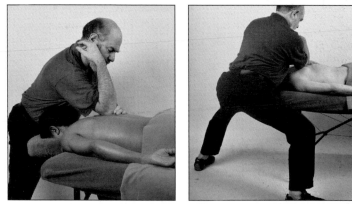

Figure 19.19: Stance to control the back of the elbow;
a) hunching over with stiff legs,
b) bending the knees,
c) the 'chimp' stance.

You need to keep your body low when you are using the back of your elbow. Don't stand up too much or you will find yourself rolling from the back of your elbow onto the point, as well as putting strain on your back. Instead, bend your knees and, if necessary, widen your stance.

Sway Your Body to Move the Back of Your Elbow

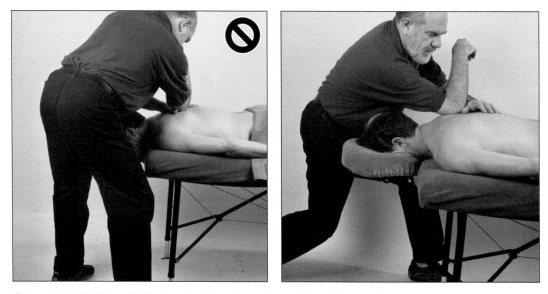

Figure 19.20: Pulling with the back of the elbow; a) standing stiffly to pull,
b) pulling by swaying backwards.

Swaying backwards with your body ('sitting' back) to pull your arm is easier and more effective than standing still and just doing the movement with your arm.

Using the Inner Side of the Elbow

The inner side of the elbow (the medial epicondyle of the humerus) also provides a small, 'blunt' working surface. It is most effective for pulling strokes, for example dragging it across the client's hamstrings. Guide it with your other hand and pull back with your body for the movement.

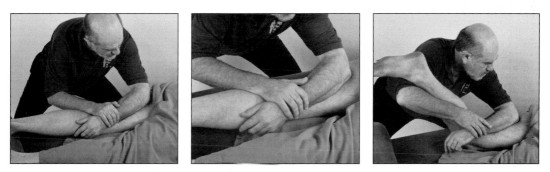

Figure 19.21: Pulling across the hamstrings with the inner elbow; a) pulling; b), c) moving with the stroke.

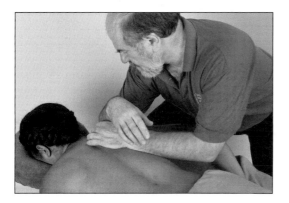

Figure 19.22: Stretching out along the client's shoulder with the inner elbow.

You can also 'catch' an area of the client's body to apply a stretch. For example, you can pull out along the top of the shoulder to stretch the trapezius, taking care to ease off the pressure before you hit the outer clavicle or the top of the scapula.

Using the Lateral Side of the Elbow

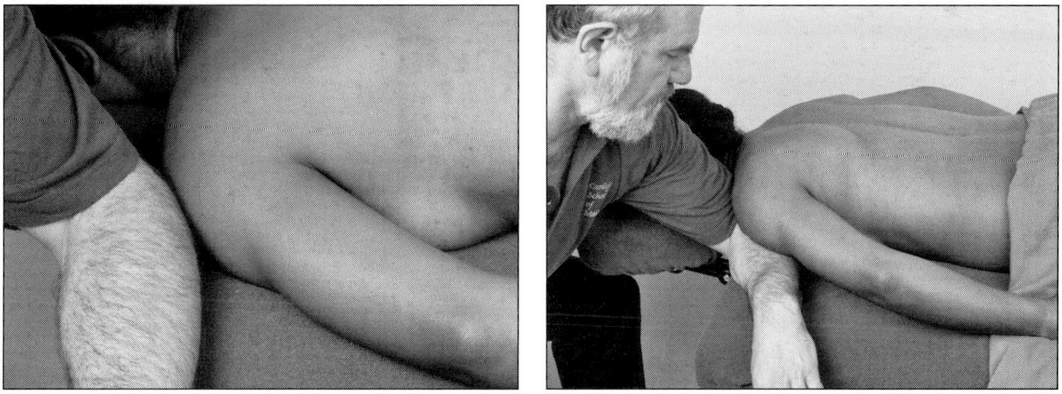

Figure 19.23: Using the lateral side of the elbow; a) the lateral side of the elbow,
b) sliding it under the client's shoulder.

The lateral epicondyle can be used to apply pressure upwards by putting your arm under the client's body so that the client's weight presses on it. You can focus this pressure under one point, or drag it under the client by swaying back to pull your arm towards yourself.

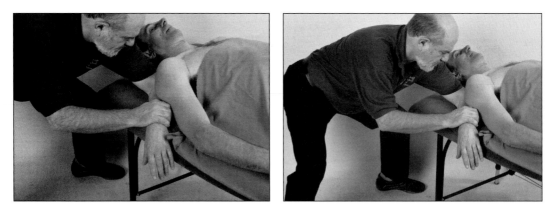

Figure 19.24: Pulling the lateral side of the elbow; a) using the other hand to help pull, b) swaying backwards.

Holding your forearm with your other hand will help you to reduce the pressure on your pulling shoulder and to keep the movement fluid and even.

Review

Save your thumbs and knuckles by using your elbow for applying pressure.

The useful areas around the elbow for massage are:

- The point of the elbow (the olecranon process of the ulna) for digging into small areas of tension, or for sliding strokes that require sustained pressure concentrated along a narrow channel;
- The back of the elbow (the posterior surface of the olecranon), which delivers firm but less single-pointed pressure;
- The inside of the elbow (the medial epicondyle of the humerus) for 'blunter' sliding pressure, and sometimes;
- The outer side of the elbow (the lateral epicondyle of the humerus) to apply pressure upwards from under the client's body.

Recognise your limits. Don't strain yourself by trying to achieve force through your elbow that your body is not built for.

Don't overuse your dominant arm.

Before using your elbow, prepare the tissues by applying strokes that gradually work more firmly and deeply.

Use your elbow carefully, monitoring and adapting to your client's responses so that you don't bruise them.

Use your other hand or forearm to guide your elbow with precision and sensitivity, and keep the hand of your working elbow relaxed.

Align your body behind your elbow and lean your bodyweight forward to deliver power, fluidity and evenness.

To save your back, work like a 'chimp' by bending your knees and widening your stance to drop your body lower.

Lean more over the client to increase the pressure that you are applying, and drop lower and sway forward to push your elbow forward.

When you are using the point of your elbow:

- Vary the depth of the 'cutting blade' by bending your elbow for more depth, and straightening it for a shallow 'cut';
- Vary the pressure that you are applying by how much you lean your bodyweight behind your elbow;
- Slide your bent elbow directly forward to use the narrowest cutting 'blade', and turn it side-on to widen it.

To apply stationary pressure on an area, gradually lean your bodyweight forward to increase the pressure, and maintain it at an acceptable level to give the client's tissues time to 'trust' and accommodate to the pressure.

Proceed slowly in sliding strokes, waiting for the tissues to 'melt' and allow you through. Don't make the application of pressure at the beginning of each sweep or the release at the end too abrupt.

CHAPTER 20

Using Your Knees and Feet

Historically, practitioners of Swedish massage have only been taught to use their hands for massage. However, the use of other body parts, which is integral to most other massage traditions, has filtered into Western massage in recent years. The forearm and elbow, which are covered in the two preceding chapters, are the most common tools in general use in Western massage to save the practitioner's hands.

Using the knees and feet for applying pressure (and, to a small extent, for stretching techniques) is a feature of many Asian massage traditions. It is much easier to do this in floor massage because you can get your bodyweight above the client. However, they also have some application in table massage for applying pressure, which is the main focus of this chapter.

The central knee, the upper shin and the foot can be used for applying 'pure' sustained pressure, for moving pressure or for maintaining pressure in an 'anchor and stretch' technique. In this situation, your weight is more *behind* your knee/foot, so it works best for pressing into the *side* of large muscles, such as gluteus medius or across the hamstrings or the sole of a prone client. This chapter also looks briefly at using your feet for applying pressure when you are working on a low table, which enables you to get your weight more *above* the client and therefore to press down more.

When you are working on an ordinary height table, you can only use your knees and feet in this way for occasional strokes, but it will enable you to rest your hands and arms for brief periods. However, working on a low table will make it more viable for a larger part of a massage session. You can get more of your bodyweight above the client and it is less demanding on your hip joint and your standing knee. If you have a table which is hydraulically / electrically adjustable during a massage, you can change the height to work in this way during the session without major disruption for the client. Note that the low table in these photos is 50 cm (20 inches) high; a lower table, set at 30 cm (12 inches), will make this easier. If you are working on the floor (see Chapter 42), you can incorporate many elements of using your feet that are covered here.

A Few Cautions

Use Them Sensitively
Both the knees and feet are primarily used for applying firm pressure, so take care not to use them too early or too suddenly in a massage. Apply the pressure and increase it slowly, monitoring the client's responses. Practise using these tools with colleagues who can give you helpful feedback before you try using them on clients. If this is a new area to you, find an experienced teacher to help you to translate the ideas in this chapter into action.

Monitor the Client's Responses

If you position yourself well, you can use your bodyweight to deliver considerable pressure through these tools without much effort. It is therefore very easy to apply more pressure than you realise. Your knee is not particularly sensitive, so it is important to ask for verbal feedback and to monitor the client's non-verbal responses. Although you can learn to feel more directly with your foot, it is also important to get feedback when using it.

Respect Your Limits

Using your knees and feet can be a powerful way of working. Bear in mind, however, that there are limits to what you can do, depending on your build and therefore the weight that you can put behind them. The mobility of your hip joint (see figures 20.19–20.22) will also affect your ability. Remain alert to your own limits, and don't strain yourself by trying to achieve force that your body is not built for.

Protect Yourself From Spreading Oil

Most of the knee and feet techniques covered below can be done with or without oil. However the focus of this chapter is on applying them without oil – on the skin before oil is applied, or through drapes or clothing – which is the usual way of incorporating them into Western massage. This avoids getting oil on your clothing when using your knees, or the need for special floor coverings and care in wiping your feet to avoid walking oil throughout your clinic when using your feet.

Using Your Knee to Apply Pressure

When practitioners talk about using the 'knee' to apply pressure into large muscle masses, they are usually referring to two areas – the centre of the knee (the knee cap (patella)) or the front of upper shin (the tibia). The way of using your body behind your knee (and feet) strokes is covered later in this Chapter (see figures 20.12–20.17).

Pressing Sideways With the Central Knee

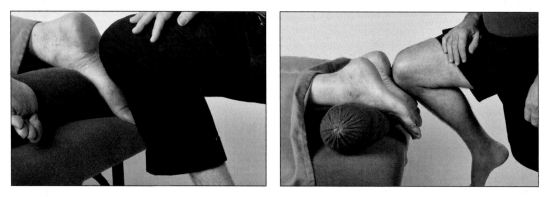

Figure 20.1: Using the central knee for applying pressure into the sole.

The centre of the knee provides a wide, fairly flat area with which to apply pressure. You can push it into the side of the gluteus medius. This is best done when the client is prone, because you then have leeway for pushing some way across the gluteus maximus as well. You can also press onto the prone client's sole with it.

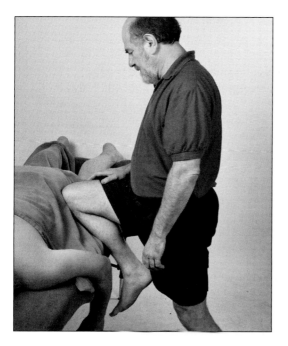

Figure 20.2: Pressing into the side of the buttock.

Pressing Across Muscles With the Upper Shin

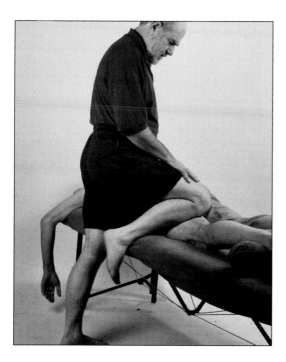

Figure 20.3: Using the upper shin for applying pressure across the hamstrings.

When you can't get the centre of your knee into a muscle mass, you may be able to get your upper shin across it. It is effective across the hamstrings for example. Because it focuses the pressure along a narrower line, practitioners with slender legs usually have a sharp front edge to their shins, so they need to be quite careful about how they use the upper shin.

Using Your Foot for Applying Pressure

Massage Styles That Use the Feet

The use of the feet (along with other parts of the body) is common in many non-oil massage traditions of Asia, which are done on the floor, such as Thai massage and many styles of shiatsu. The feet are also the main working tools in the Chavutti Thirumal massage of Southern India, in which a spice-laden coconut oil is used. This massage needs a warm climate or a very warm room (preferably with underfloor heating) as the client takes off all of his clothing (and just has a small covering over the genital area) to enable the practitioner to do strokes that cover the length of his body in a single sweep.

Many Western non-oil floor massages which use the feet combine aspects of Western style work on muscle tensions with pressure point techniques that are the mainstay of acupressure/shiatsu-based approaches. In the USA, where there are decades of experience of shiatsu, these include Compressive Deep Tissue Massage developed by John Harris and Fred Kenyon. If you want to work extensively with your feet, it is worth training in a floor massage such as barefoot shiatsu for non-oil work or in Chavutti Thiramul massage for using oil.

Working On an Ordinary Height Table Vs Working On a Low Table

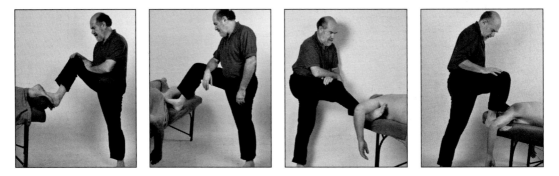

Figure 20.4: Using the feet; a) applying pressure on an ordinary height table,
b) applying pressure on a low table, c) applying a stretch on an ordinary height table,
d) applying a stretch on a low table.

The feet can be used on an ordinary height massage table for applying pressure. They are also occasionally used for stretches. These strokes are easier on a low table because it is easier to get your bodyweight above your feet to deliver pressure or to sway backwards for a stretch, and there's less strain on the hip joint.

Using Your Foot Skilfully

Applying pressure with your foot is most effective on well toned or tense muscle areas on clients with a medium to large build. It can also be useful on smaller people with a sinewy build or concentrated areas of tension. It works best on the back, buttocks and legs. Using the foot effectively requires you to learn to channel the skill and sensitivity through them that you've already developed with your hands. Therefore it is good for practitioners to spend time training each foot to locate the structures and tensions that you've previously identified by hand and then to practice working on them with the foot in equivalent ways.

The Working Areas of the Foot

Obviously the structure of the foot is similar to that of the hand. Therefore, because it has so many internal joints, your foot can adapt to the shape of the client's body much more than your forearm, elbow or knee. Three parts of the foot can easily be used for delivering pressure:

1. The heel can substitute for the heel of your hand for applying firm pressure;
2. The arch of your foot can contour around your client's limbs or around large shoulders for widespread pressure;
3. The balls of the toes can be used to concentrate pressure into a small area.

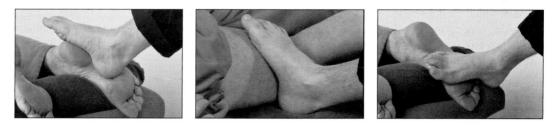

Figure 20.5: The working areas of the foot for applying pressure; a) using the heel for firm pressure, b), c), using the arch for widespread pressure.

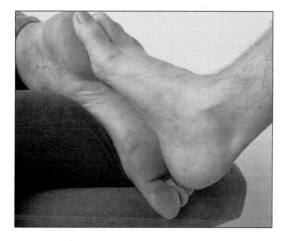

The best areas for applying *firm sustained pressure* are your heel and arch. Using them enables you to deliver the power from your leg directly through your ankle with the least need to tense your foot or ankle.

Figure 20.6: Using the whole foot.

You can also use your whole foot on an area such as the client's foot.

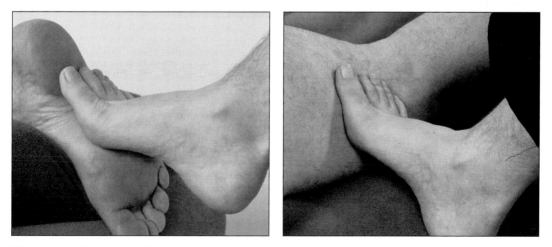

Figure 20.7: Using the balls of the toes for concentrated pressure.

Although using the balls of your toes can give you more precision, it requires muscular effort throughout your whole lower leg and foot to stabilise your foot at the necessary angle to deliver the pressure, so don't overuse them.

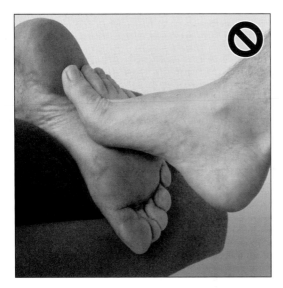

Figure 20.7 (cont.): c) using the ends of the toes.

Although, in theory, you could use the tips of your toes for applying pressure on small areas, it's hard work on them so it's best to avoid using them for this.

Keep Your Foot Relaxed

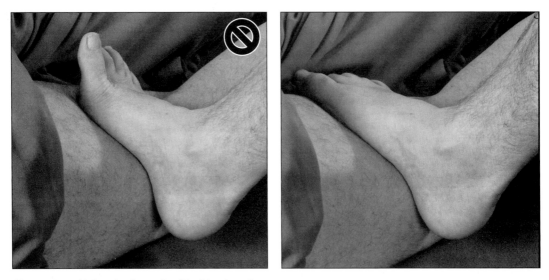

Figure 20.8: Using the foot; a) stiffly, b) relaxed.

Try not to stiffen your foot as you press with it. This would affect the massage in the same way as tensing your hand. It uses unnecessary energy, makes it harder for you to sense through your foot and tends to produce an instinctive wariness in clients rather than inviting them to relax.

Press Forward into the Side of the Client's Body

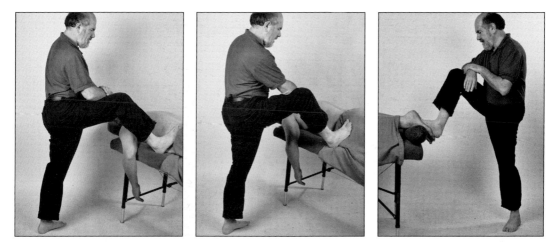

Figure 20.9: Using the foot to apply pressure to the side of the body; a) the waist, b) the buttock, c) the sole.

As with using the knee, you will find that it is easiest to apply pressure into the *side* of the prone client's body, for example into the side of the waist, buttocks, leg muscles, the sole of the foot and the top of the shoulders.

If you can't get your foot high enough to press down on an area such as the hamstrings, use your upper shin (see figure 20.3).

'Anchor and Stretch'/Pin and Stretch' Technique
In the 'anchor and stretch' technique ('pin and stretch'), you maintain pressure on a muscle while moving a distal part of the client's body in order to stretch the muscle under this anchoring pressure. You can either move the client's limb or ask the client to move it himself.

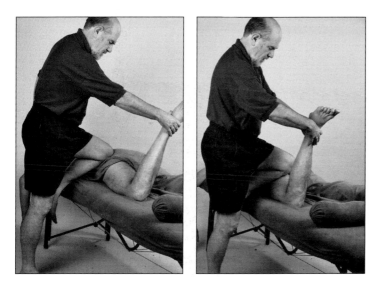

Figure 20.10: 'Anchor and stretch' technique; a) central knee pressure on the buttocks, b) shin pressure across the hamstrings.

Position yourself so that you can maintain pressure, for example on the client's buttocks or hamstrings. Then bend the client's lower leg up and move it until you feel the muscles being stretched under your pressing knee or shin. Side to side movement of the client's lower leg moves the gluteal muscles; you will find that you need a different range of movement for gluteus medius than for gluteus maximus. Bending and straightening the lower leg moves the hamstrings.

Use Your Foot for Stretches and for Rocking the Body

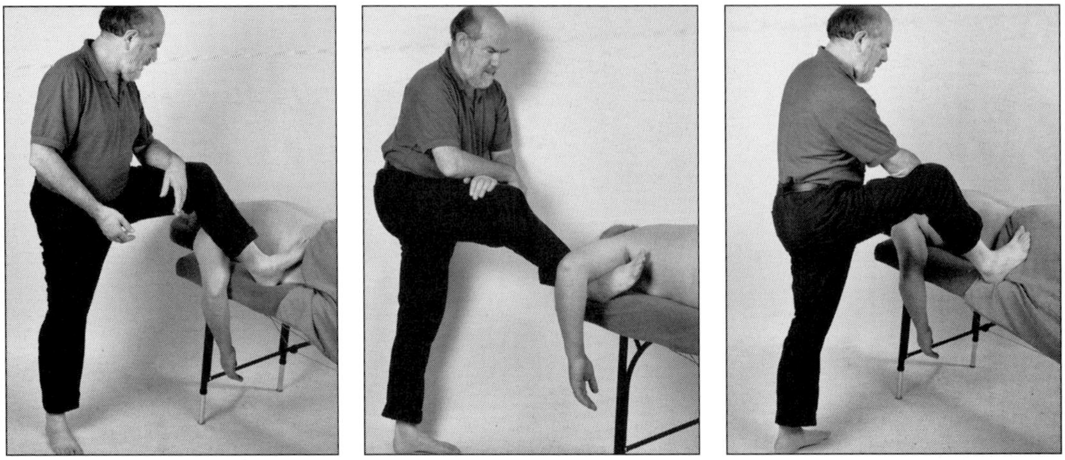

Figure 20.11: Stretches and body rocking; a) stretching the lower back, b) lifting the shoulder, c) body rocking.

On an ordinary height table, you can use your foot to push on the ilium to stretch the lower back. You could also 'hook' your foot under the client's shoulder to lift and stretch the shoulder in order to open the chest and stretch the pectoralis. You can also use your foot for rocking the client's body or rolling a limb. When you are pushing from the side, focus the thrust through the part of your sole that is appropriate to the size and power of your push. Don't stand stock-still and just push with your leg, which would quickly become tiring, but sway your body a little with the push.

These are all easier to do and you can take them further when you're working on a low table.

Involving Your Body to Apply Pressure With Your Knee/Foot

Use your body, rather than standing stiffly and just pushing with your leg.

Align Your Body Behind Your Knee/Foot
Whether you are using your knee or foot for applying the pressure, align your body behind it as much as possible. Being turned away would put strain on your hip joint while reducing your effectiveness. Change your position when necessary to change the direction of the pressure.

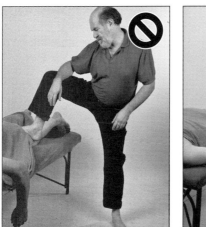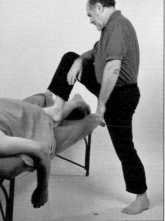

Figure 20.12: Aligning the body behind the working tool; a) turned away from the foot, b) aligned behind it.

Sway Your Body for Power

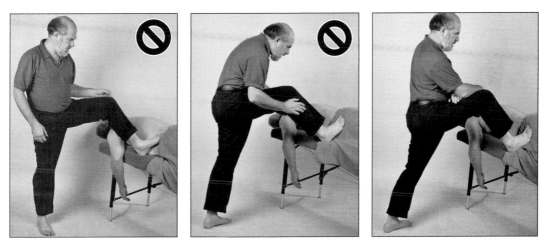

Figure 20.13: Delivering power; a) standing still and just pushing with the leg, b) tensing down to push hard, c) swaying forward.

Apply the pressure by swaying forward with your whole body. Lean forward to increase the pressure within the client's comfortable range and then slowly release it.

Monitor Your Breathing

When applying sustained pressure, practitioners need to monitor *their own* breathing patterns. You may be unconsciously holding your breath or inhaling forcefully, either of which are likely to cause you to tense up. It's best to exhale gently when applying the pressure (see figure 26.3).

Vary Your Working and Standing Legs

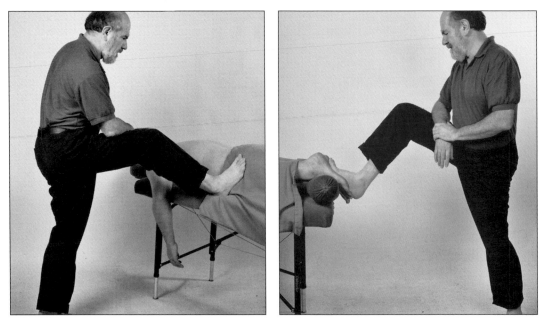

Figure 20.14: Varying the standing and working legs to fit the situation.

As with using your hands, there's a temptation to constantly use the same knee/foot for the massage. Learn to be 'ambidextrous', so that you use whichever foot/knee is most appropriate. And mirror strokes on the opposite side of the table to spread the workload, rather than constantly standing on the same leg.

Rest Your Arms or Use Them to Guide Your Leg

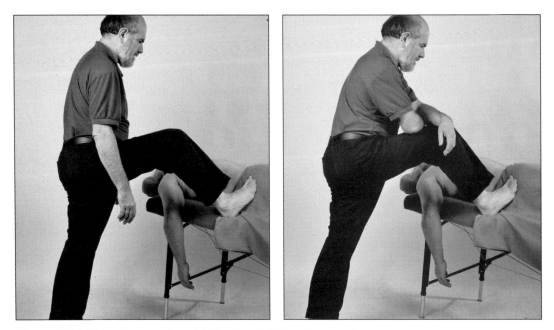

*Figure 20.15: Using the arms to guide the leg; a) letting the arms hang,
b) resting the arms across the working leg.*

As you lean and sway forward to deliver the pressure with your foot, you can let your arms hang down by your sides to give them a complete rest. Or you can rest one or both arms across your working leg to help guide your pressure.

Give Yourself Support

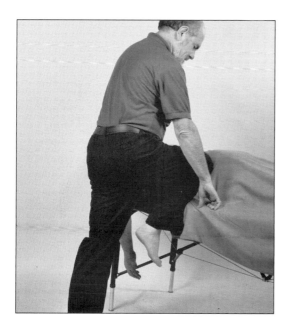

Figure 20.16: Hands on the table for support.

When using your knee, you might rest your hands on the table for stability.

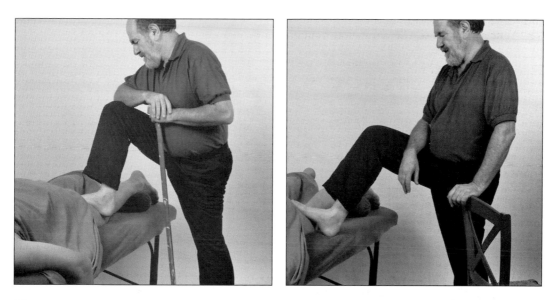

Figure 20.17: Using a support; a) a pole, b) a chair.

Or, when you are using your foot, you could use a pole or a chair back for support. (An Australian colleague of mine used to use his didgeridoo for balance when doing barefoot shiatsu; he also used to give clients a 'vibrational massage' by playing the didj over every part of their body – it was the '70s).

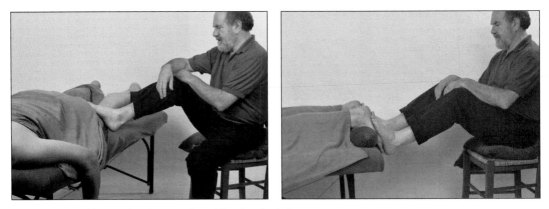

Figure 20.18: Sitting; a) using one foot, b) using both feet.

When you are using a low table, you can also sit down to use one foot at a time or both feet simultaneously. (The low table in these photos is 50 cm high/20 inches; sitting and using your leg/s is easier on a lower table – 30 cm high/12 inches).

Mobilising Your Hip Joints and Stretching Your Leg Muscles

Initially, your leg muscles may ache a little from spending time standing on one leg and from the stretch at your hip joint, so don't overdo it. You may find it helpful to do some of the following stretches before and after massages to ease these muscles. If you feel that opening up your hip joint and stretching the surrounding muscles feels like it needs more thorough attention, consider attending a yoga class or studying a martial art that involves high kicks.

Mobilising Your Hips

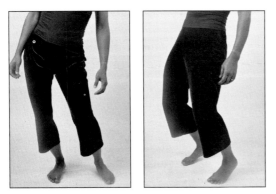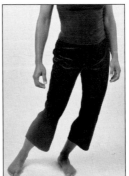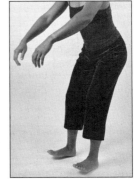

Figure 20.19: Swaying the hips in a circle.

Swaying your hips in a circle will help mobilise them.

Stretching the Muscles of the Hip Joint

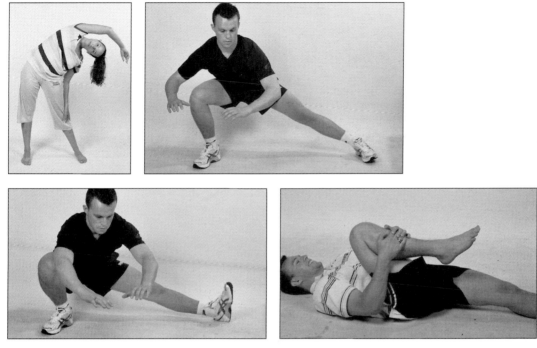

Figure 20.20: Stretching the hip and leg muscles.

These are some of the many stretches that you can do to stretch the muscles that cross the hip joint.

Stretch the Muscles of the Back of Your Leg

Having suppleness in the muscles of the back of your legs (particularly the hamstrings and the gastrocnemius) is crucial for being able to lift your leg up to the table for applying pressure.

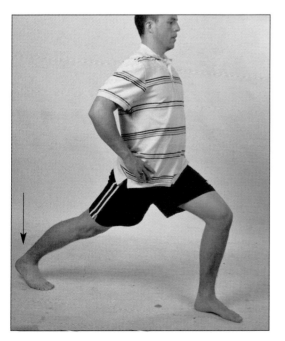

You can do this by stretching your leg back and lowering your heel towards the floor.

Figure 20.21: Stretching the leg back and lowering the heel to the floor.

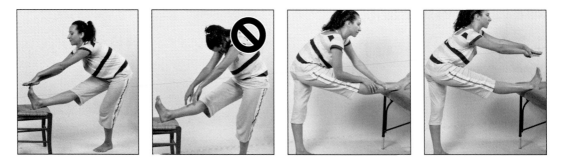

Figure 20.22: Stretches for the back of the legs; a) stretching with the foot on a chair,
b) crumpling the lower back, c) stretching with the foot on a high table, d) dorsiflexing the foot.

To stretch these muscles further, rest your foot on the seat of a chair. Lean your trunk forward, taking care to bend from your hips rather than hunching over, which would strain your back without affecting the hamstrings. This stretches your buttocks as well as your hamstrings and calf muscles.

Do this stretch on a high table to take it even further. Dorsiflexing your foot at the same time will make the stretch even more powerful.

Review

Using the knees and feet for applying pressure can have some application in table massage.

Use your foot also for applying stretches, or for rocking the client's body or for rolling their limbs.

Use your knee and foot carefully and sensitively, and monitor the client's responses.

Don't strain yourself by trying to achieve force that your body is not built for.

Protect yourself from spreading oil by using your knees or feet prior to applying oil to the area or by working through a drape.

Use the central knee (the patella) to press sideways into muscles such as the gluteus medius.

Place your shin across muscles, such as the hamstrings, to press down on them.

The heel of the foot can substitute for the heel of the hand for applying pressure.

The arch of the foot can contour around the client's limbs for applying pressure.

The balls of the toes can be used to concentrate pressure onto a small area.

When using your foot, keep it relaxed.

Align your body behind your working knee/foot, and sway your body to deliver pressure and movement.

Avoid constantly standing on the same leg, and mirror your techniques on the opposite side of the table.

Rest your arms, use them to guide and support your working leg, or use them on the table to support yourself.

Use a support, such as a pole or the back of a chair for balance, or, when you're working on a low table, sit in a chair to use your foot or both feet simultaneously.

Use exercises to mobilise your hips and to stretch your leg muscles, and/or attend yoga, martial arts or similar classes.

CHAPTER 21

Using Your Thigh, Shoulder or Hip as a 'Third Hand'

In floor massages such as Thai massage and shiatsu, the practitioner commonly uses his/her own body to support parts of the (clothed) client's body and to apply stretches. This chapter looks at ways of doing this at the massage table.

Many practitioners will be familiar with resting the prone client's ankle across your thigh or shoulder to support the lower leg. And, it is often useful to have cushions under the client's leg or shoulder so that you are freed up to massage with both hands from a range of angles (see figure 11.35). This chapter focuses on extending this by using your thigh and your shoulder as a 'third hand' – to simultaneously support *and mobilise* the client's limbs while you are also using your hands. It briefly looks at using your hip in this way too.

It takes practise to coordinate the 'third hand' with your hands, but it is a useful addition to your massage repertoire. It gives you more versatility while conserving your hands. This chapter gives a few examples of this concept in action; with practise, you will no doubt think of other ways of applying it. If you like this way of working, receiving treatments and/or studying with practitioners of Thai massage, shiatsu or similar modalities will give you more inspiration.

A Few Notes of Caution

If the ideas presented in this chapter are new to you, it is useful to get coaching from an experienced colleague and to practise with colleagues before trying them with clients.

Monitoring the Client's Responses
Monitor your client's comfort. Don't try to stretch them too far or in ways that put undue pressure on their bodies. And it is often helpful to explain to your clients what you're about to do, so that they are less likely to react against it, especially if you are applying a strong or unusual stretch.

Maintaining Professionalism
Because this way of working puts you closer to the client and in more intimate physical contact, it is important to maintain a professional attitude. This includes:

- Telling the client what you're doing (and maybe also why);
- Not exposing them in an oil massage;
- Not brushing against them inappropriately, or;
- Moving parts of their body inappropriately against your body (for example, when you are supporting and moving the client's arm, make sure that the dangling hand isn't brushing against your crutch).

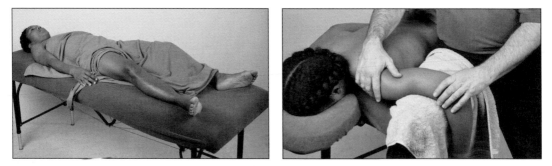

Figure 21.1: Using drapes; a) tucking in well around the client's upper leg,
b) towel to protect the practitioner's clothing and to maintain a professional distance.

When you are stretching the client's leg, make sure that the drapes are well tucked in around her hips. When you are resting the client's limbs on your own body, a small towel will protect your clothing from being stained by the massage oil. Even in a non-oil massage, you may sometimes want to use a towel to help you to maintain a professional distance.

Respect Your Limits
As with any technique, the possibilities are partly determined by your build. When trying out ideas from this chapter, be alert to your own comfort. Don't strain yourself by trying to lift the client's limbs if they're too heavy for you, or by attempting to achieve stretches that are beyond your comfortable capabilities.

And don't try to support parts of the client's body for longer than is comfortable. If you need them to be supported for long periods, use bolsters or cushions in order to free you up to move around the massage table.

Supporting and Moving the Client's Leg

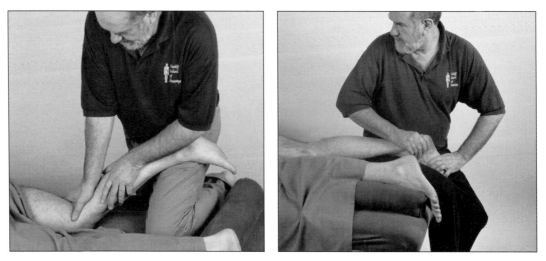

Figure 21.2: Supporting the prone client's ankle; a) kneeling on the table, b) sitting on the table.

Kneeling one leg on the table is a common way of supporting the client's ankle. This encourages him to relax his gastrocnemius and hamstrings for you to work on them. It is also common to sit on the table to work on his feet (although it is not good to stay in this position for too long because you need to regularly look back over your shoulder to monitor the client's responses).

Using Your Shoulder as a 'Third Hand'

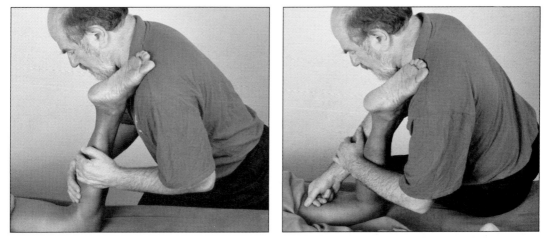

Figure 21.3: Supporting the ankle on the shoulder; a) standing, b) sitting on the table.

It is also common to rest his ankle on your shoulder (with a towel on your shoulder to keep oil off your clothing – and out of one's beard too!) in order to free up both hands for massaging. You can stand for this, or sit on the table (taking care not to hunch over). This enables you to dig deeply into the hamstrings and the gastrocnemius. Both of these working positions enable you to move the client's lower leg by swaying your body in order to stretch and mobilise the muscles as you apply pressure on them.

Using Your Forearm as a 'Third Hand'

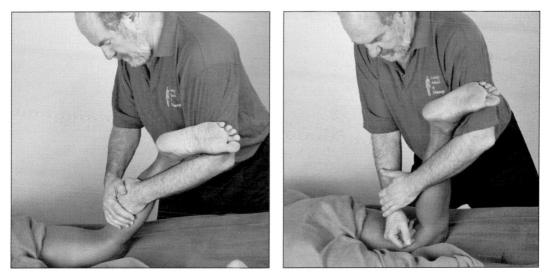

Figure 21.4: Supporting the lower leg over the forearm.

If the client's leg is not too heavy, you can also support it over your forearm, which will enable you to move it around even more. You can move her leg by swaying your body. When doing this, use both hands together in some way so that you're not tensing your shoulders and arm muscles to support the leg. For example you can work hand on hand to press into the gastrocnemius as you move the lower leg to stretch the muscle. Or you can support your working hand with your other hand as you apply pressure and move the leg to stretch the hamstrings.

Supporting the Client's Ankle Over Your Thigh

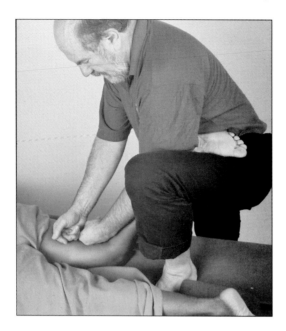

Figure 21.5: Supporting the client's ankle on the thigh.

Another option, if you're working in socks or bare feet, is to stand one foot on the table. You can then rest her ankle on your thigh and sway your body to move her leg as you massage it.

Supporting and Stretching the Side-lying Client's Leg

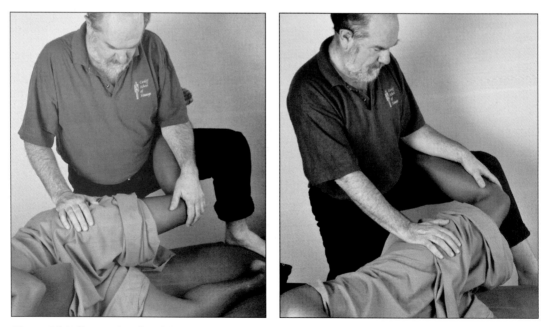

Figure 21.6: Supporting the side-lying client's leg; a), b) supporting and moving the client's leg.

When the client is lying on her side, standing with one foot on the table enables you to support her leg across your thigh and to bend it back by swaying and turning your body. You may need to stabilise it in this position with one hand. This can be a quite powerful stretch so monitor her responses.

Strain in the Hip Joint When Using the Thigh

If you feel strain in your hip joint in any of these positions, there are three things to consider.

Firstly, if you find that getting your leg up to the table height is strainful for your hip, try some hip joint stretches (see figures 20.20–20.22). If you still can't get your hip joint comfortable, especially when standing one foot on the table, don't do it.

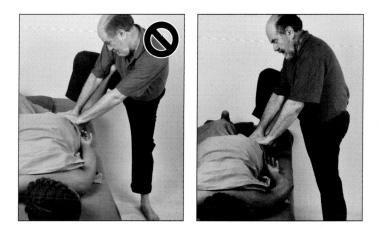

Figure 21.7: The angle of the standing foot; a) turned away from the table, b) so that the practitioner faces their work.

Then look at the way that you're working. Check that your standing foot is not turned too far away from the table which would put strain on your standing knee, and/or that hip joint, and possibly on your ankle too. Ideally, your foot should be turned so that your lower body (your hips) can face your working hands.

Bear in mind that when you stand with one foot on the table, you may not be able to turn your standing foot towards your working tools as much as when you sit or kneel on the table. However, make sure that your hips are behind your working tools as much as possible, and monitor that your hip joints are comfortable.

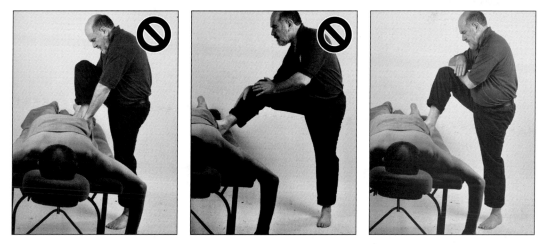

Figure 21.8: The distance from the table of the standing foot;
a) too close to the table, b) too far away from the table, c) a comfortable distance from the table.

Check to see if your standing foot is at the best distance from the table for comfortably supporting your body. Try moving it closer to the table and further away until you find the best position.

Supporting and Moving the Client's Shoulder

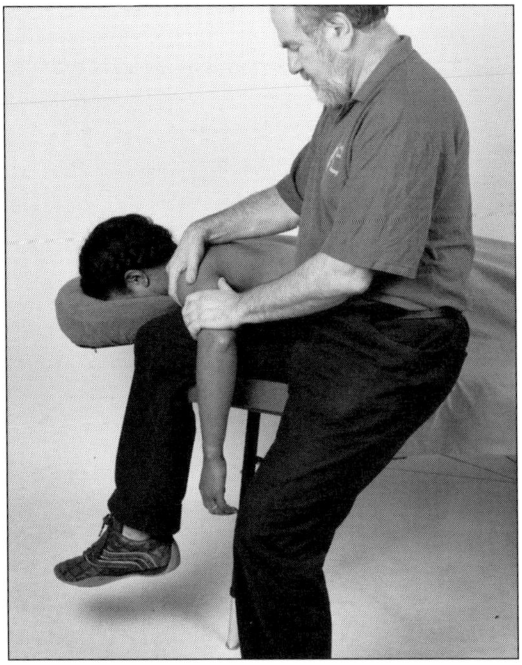

Figure 21.9 Sitting on the table to support the prone client's shoulder.

Sitting on the table with your thigh under a prone client's shoulder enables you to open the chest by stretching the pectoral muscle as you work on the shoulder muscles. This sitting position is easiest when the client's head is resting in a face cradle. Use a towel under the client's arm to protect your clothes from oil. Male practitioners might also consider placing a small cushion next to a female client's trunk to avoid brushing against her breast.

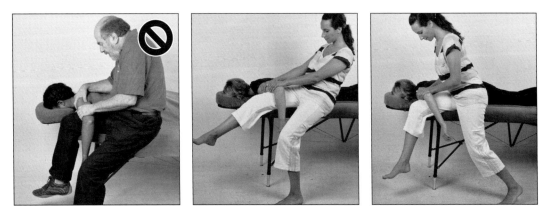

Figure 21.10: Pushing the shoulder back and forward; a) slumping down to pull, b) putting the standing foot forward to pull, c) putting the standing foot back to push.

Make sure that you're not cramped in or hunched over. If you lean forward to apply pressure, or lean back to stretch the upper trapezius, don't slump over.

Instead, sway from your hips to take pressure off your back. Moving your standing leg will help you balance and provide impetus for these strokes. Move your foot back a little to enable you to lean your body forward when you are applying pressure or pushing forward. Put your foot forward for pulling back.

As you sway forward and back, you could push the whole shoulder forward (towards the head of the table) and back (towards the foot of the table). You can extend this 'rowing' movement, by using your thigh like a 'third hand' to raise and lower your client's shoulder as well. Make sure that you're not tensing your body to lift and lower your thigh, especially if the client has a large, heavy arm. Swaying your body can be helpful for this; sway backwards a little for lifting your thigh and sway forward to lower it.

Supporting and Moving the Client's Arm

If it's comfortable, supporting a client's limb on your shoulder or hip will enable you to mobilise the joint by moving the limb through a range of angles, while simultaneously using your hands for massage techniques. (Don't do this if the limb is too heavy of course).

Use a small towel, when necessary, to protect your clothing from massage oil. And, when moving the limb in an oil massage, make sure that the drapes are well tucked in so that she doesn't feel exposed.

Resting the Client's Arm on Your Hip

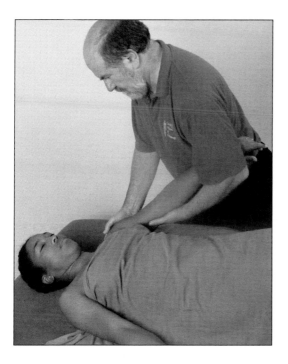

Figure 21.11: Supporting the client's arm on the hip.

If the client's arm is heavy, you can rest it on your hip, and if necessary, stabilise it with one hand. This saves you from holding the full weight with both hands, especially if it's heavy, as you mobilise her shoulder. It also enables you to sway your body to move her arm, while using both hands to massage around her shoulder or stretch her scapula.

Supporting the Client's Arm on Your Shoulder

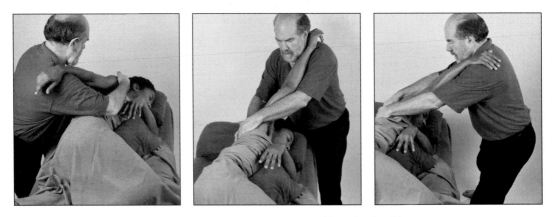

Figure 21.12: The side-lying client's arm resting on the practitioner's shoulder.

When your client is lying on her side, you can rest her arm on your own shoulder while you are massaging around her shoulder and mobilising it.

Review

You can use your thigh, shoulder or hip as a 'third hand' – for supporting and mobilising the client's limbs while you are simultaneously using your hands for massage techniques.

Don't strain yourself by trying to lift the client's limbs if they're too heavy for you.

Maintain professionalism by:

- Telling the client what you're doing and why;
- Not brushing against them inappropriately;
- Not trying to stretch the client beyond their limits;
- Protecting their modesty when doing stretches in an oil massage;
- Use a towel to protect your clothing from oil and, if necessary, to maintain a professional distance.

You can rest the prone client's bent up lower leg on your shoulder (either by sitting on the table or standing next to it), or on your thigh (by standing your foot on the table). This enables you to move it by swaying your body when you are massaging their calf muscles or hamstrings.

You can also rest the client's lower leg over your forearm to move it when you are using both hands together.

You can also stand one foot on the table to rest the side-lying client's leg on your thigh and sway your body to move her leg as you massage it.

If you feel strain in your hip joint as you use your thigh in this way, do some hip joint stretches, and check that:

- Your standing foot is facing towards your working hands, and;
- That you're not too close or far away from the table.

When sitting on the table and supporting the client's shoulder over your thigh, you can move it by swaying your body to move the shoulder forward and back and to raise and lower it with your thigh.

When you are working around a client's shoulder, it can be useful to rest her arm on your shoulder when she is lying on her side, or on your hip when the client is supine.

Using Your Body to Support Your Working Tools

This section focuses on how to use the rest of your body most effectively and with the least strain and effort to support the working tools described in the previous two sections. It also highlights unhelpful practices that could lead to cumulative problems over time. The next section (see Chapters 29–32) looks at how to integrate this in standing, sitting and kneeling.

Each chapter in this section covers one part of the body to look at the role that it plays in the overall way that you use your body. The ideal is to generate power and movement in your lower body, rather than standing still and only using your upper body which would make the massage stiffer and less fluid and would be harder work. Positioning your body well, leaning your bodyweight behind your hands, and swaying your body initiates movements which are translated up through your trunk. Keeping your shoulders relaxed enables the power to be transmitted through your arms to your hands, forearms or elbows, which you can then use with both strength and sensitivity.

A Dynamic Balance of Power and Ease

This way of working provides the massage practitioner with a balance between power (when appropriate) and ease by using natural body strength in a *dynamic* way that is neither hard nor rigid. Getting your body aligned behind your working tools and moving powerfully and fluidly enables you to stay relaxed and sensitive in your hands (or forearm, etc.) and therefore to be adaptable and creative with them.

As this becomes more familiar and comfortable, you will appreciate that this way of working is simultaneously relaxing and energising, enabling you to work with ease while still applying firm pressure. It takes the pressure off the commonest areas of strain for massage practitioners – the hands, shoulders and back. This is crucial if you are working with clients who require a firm massage. Even when you are using light pressure, it adds the essential qualities of fluidity and evenness to the massage. Once you build up your general stamina, this will enable you to do a number of massages in a day without exhaustion or straining your body.

Monitor the Client's Responses

Bear in mind that the transmission of force from your trunk to the client in this way is more powerful than standing still and just working with your shoulders and arms. So monitor your client's responses to be sure that you're not unknowingly applying more pressure than is appropriate.

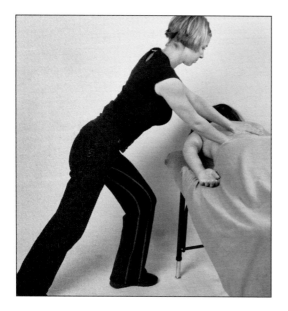

CHAPTER 22

Relaxing Your Shoulders

No matter how well we use our bodies, as massage practitioners, we have to use our shoulder muscles to some extent. However the ideal is to use minimal appropriate effort so that your shoulders are not tensed up around your ears or hunched forward around your chest. Their primary job in massage is to *transmit* the power that is generated by leaning and swaying your body to your arms, while remaining as relaxed as possible.

If your shoulders are tense as you massage, you will be working harder than necessary in your shoulder and arm muscles for your power, and the massage is less likely to be fluid. This chapter looks at common causes of tension in the shoulders, some simple exercises for relaxing them, and ideas on monitoring your shoulders so as to keep them relaxed while doing massages.

Anatomy of the Upper Back and Shoulders

A brief look at the musculature of the upper trunk is useful to review how much of it can be tied up in shoulder tension and therefore why relaxing the shoulders can make such a difference.

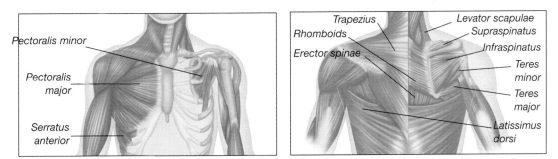

Fig 22.1: Main muscles of the upper back; a) anterior view, b) posterior view.

Underlying Postural Muscles
The only major muscles of the back that are not involved in arm movements are the postural muscles (the 'para-vertebrals') which consist of the erector spinae group, which extend from the sacrum to the base of the skull, and the transversospinalis network of small muscles between the vertebrae.

The Shoulder Muscles
All of the main muscles that overlay them in the back, chest and shoulders are involved in movements of the shoulder girdle (the clavicle and the scapula) and the arm. Some of those in the shoulder area, such as the trapezius and levator scapulae, also play a part in moving and stabilising the neck. Movements of the shoulder girdle and arm involve a complex interplay between the three groups of muscles – the prime movers of the arm, the muscles of scapular stabilisation, and the 'rotator cuff' muscles.

The shoulder muscles stabilise your shoulders for arm and hand movements. This can range from bracing your shoulders for large forceful movements, such as lifting a heavy case, to the small continuous 'fixator' role required for small hand and finger movements, such as typing. Thus tension in the shoulders can incorporate a large part of the musculature of the upper trunk and tie up a lot of energy.

The Prime Movers of the Arm

There are three prime movers of the arm. *Pectoralis major*, which forms the front of the chest and the armpit, moves the arm across the front of the chest. Because so much everyday activity (including massage) requires us to have our arms in this position, one can become accustomed to having the shoulders forward and the pectoralis shortened and tight. *Latissimus dorsi* covers the lower and mid back and forms the back of the armpit. It pulls the arm down in front of the body, for example in swimming or chopping wood, or moves the trunk in relation to the arm in climbing. The *deltoid* lifts the arm.

Scapular Stabilisation

The muscles of scapular stabilisation cover the shoulders and the side and back of the upper trunk and neck. Collectively they move the shoulder girdle around over the back and side of the ribs and then stabilise it in position for arm movements. *Trapezius* is the most significant muscle for massage practitioners, particularly the upper trapezius, which lifts the shoulders. It is assisted in this by *levator scapulae*, which lies under it. The *rhomboids* lie underneath the middle section of trapezius, and they work together with it in drawing the scapula back towards the spine. The lowest section of trapezius draws the shoulder blade back and downwards. The *serratus anterior* at the side of the chest draws the scapula forward towards the side of the ribs, for example in pushing movements. *Pectoralis minor* at the front of the chest (under pectoralis major) tilts the shoulder blade forward, or stabilises it for pushing downwards. It can become quite tight in people who habitually hunch their shoulders.

The 'Rotator Cuff'

A third group of muscles run between the scapula and the head of the humerus, forming the 'rotator cuff'. The main collective job of these four 'SITS' muscles – *supraspinatus, infraspinatus, teres minor* and *subscapularis* – is to keep the head of the humerus in place against the glenoid fossa (the shallow socket) of the scapula as the large prime movers move the arm. Infraspinatus and teres minor can also take the arm backwards and laterally/externally rotate it. (Teres major, which also runs between the scapula and humerus, assists latissimus dorsi).

Shoulder Tension

Shoulder tension has two components – tension that develops from the activities of our hands; and general stress that causes us to tense our shoulders up 'around our ears'. These often go together – doing physical activities under stress, such as typing up a document against a deadline.

Because we use our arms and hands so much in daily life, tension can slowly accumulate over time in the shoulders without one realising it. As massage practitioners know, this is the 'classic' area for everyday tension to build up, the area in which clients most often want a massage to relieve accumulated tension. And when there is shoulder tension, there will generally be related tension in the arms and hands.

Everyday Shoulder Tension

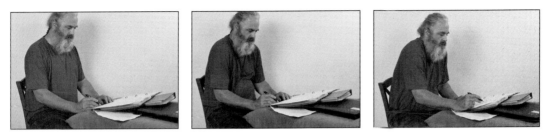

*Figure 22.2: Shoulder tension; a) sitting upright with relaxed shoulders,
b) hunched forward with rounded shoulders, c) tense shoulders 'around the ears'.*

Most activities in daily life, such as working at a desk or bench, using a keyboard, and driving require us to use our hands in front of our bodies, usually around the level of the lower chest or abdomen. So do most massage strokes. Over time, this can lead to the shoulders being held rounded towards the front of the chest and some hunching over in the upper back. Pectoralis major becomes shortened and stiff. There is often tension between the shoulder blades because the rhomboids and the thoracic section of the erectors are working hard in a stretched position to counterbalance the pull forward. And stress can cause the shoulders to rise 'around the ears' (upper trapezius tension).

Shoulder Tension in Massage

Of course the shoulders are often a major area of tension for massage practitioners. A common problem is that many of us have become habituated to having our shoulders in these positions. After a while we 'forget' that we can relax our shoulders and that we can move our shoulder blades back around our ribs to stretch pectoralis and open out the front of the chest. And, because shoulder tension is so common in daily life, many people who enter the field of massage already carry this tension, having unknowingly tightened their shoulders over the years.

Whatever the cause of shoulder tension, it will impede the transmission of power from your body to your arms as you massage, causing you to tighten your shoulders further in order to work harder. So, once established, this can develop into a vicious cycle. Because holding tension in the shoulders is such a common and unconscious habit, every practitioner needs to pay attention to their shoulders. Whenever you find yourself tightening your shoulders during a massage, relax them, and also make sure that you're using your whole body to initiate the massage movements.

Shoulder tension in massage can arise from a variety of factors, including:

- Habitual tension already held in the shoulders;
- The common unconscious habit of tensing the shoulders to do any physical activity;
- Trying too hard;
- Working on a table that is too high;
- Not using your body to support the work of your hands, and/or;
- As a reaction to straining your hands or wrist, or to attempting to apply more pressure than you can comfortably deliver.

The Height of the Table

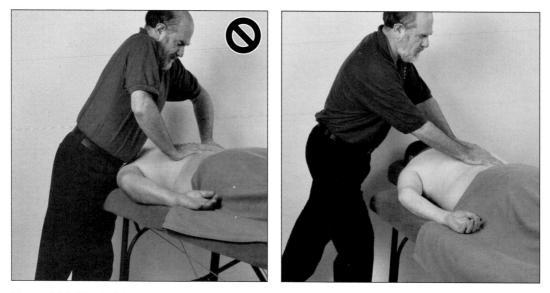

Figure 22.3: The height of the table; a) working on a table that's too high, b) working on a comfortable height.

Working on a table that is too high will prevent you from being able to get your bodyweight behind your hands. This will automatically force you to tense your shoulders in order to generate power.

Poor Bodyuse – Standing Stiffly or Hunching Over

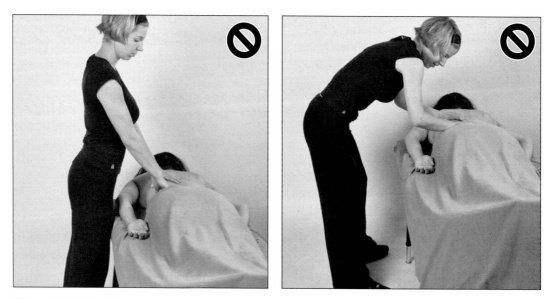

Figure 22.4: The effect on the shoulders of common postures; a) standing stiffly, b) hunched over.

If you are using your body poorly or awkwardly as you massage, you will find yourself tensing your shoulders in order to *generate* the power that they should ideally be *transmitting* from the trunk. If you are standing stiffly while massaging, for example, or you are hunched over, you will inevitably be overusing your shoulder muscles, instead of leaning and swaying your body to generate power.

Standing Too Close to the Table

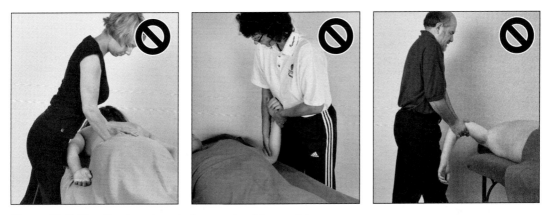

Figure 22.5: Standing too close to the couch; a) for applying pressure,
b) working on the bent forearm, c) applying a stretch.

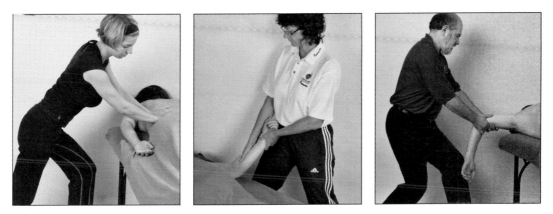

Fig 22.5 (cont.): Having enough space to lean forward; d) for applying pressure,
e) working on the bent forearm, f) applying a stretch.

Standing too close to the table when you're applying pressure often leads to tensing the shoulders. Stepping back so that you're not so cramped will enable you to lean your bodyweight more and thus save your shoulders. This will also apply for sliding strokes, for example when you're working on the client's bent up forearm. If you find that you're tensing your shoulders, lower the forearm and step back so that you can work on it at a better angle. Similarly, when you're doing stretches, give yourself space to sway back for the stretch, so that you avoid tensing your shoulders and just using your arms.

Focusing on Small Areas, Trying Too Hard
When people are first learning to massage, they often unconsciously tense their shoulders and arms and consequently use their hands unnecessarily stiffly. Even after learning to massage 'with the whole body', many of us revert to tensing our shoulders without realising it when we are using our fingers and/or thumbs to focus on a small area, when doing percussion strokes or when applying sustained pressure techniques. And, we are also quite likely to tense our shoulders whenever we are trying too hard to deliver pressure.

The Connection Between the Hands and Shoulders

Bear in mind that there is a strong connection between how we use our hands and how we hold our shoulders. If you are stiffening your hands or straining them, you will probably be tensing your shoulders as well. Conversely, being tense in your shoulders, which is an unconscious habit for many of us, is likely to result in unnecessary tension in your hands. So, whenever you notice tension in either your shoulders or your hands as you massage, check the other area as well.

The Connection Between the Hands and Shoulders

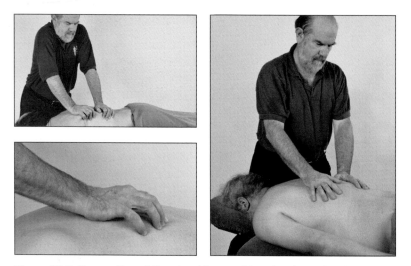

Figure 22.6: Connection of the shoulders and hands; a) tensing the shoulders, b) tensing the hand, c) relaxed shoulders and hands.

Check this connection for yourself. Rest your relaxed hand on your partner. Tense your shoulders and note how difficult it is not to tense your hand as well.

Then relax your shoulders and hand again. Tense your hand and notice the instinctive tightening of your shoulders.

Exercises to Relax and Mobilise the Shoulders

You will probably have familiar ways of relaxing and mobilising your shoulders gained from exercise and sports, so this section just covers some basic ideas. The Alexander Technique, yoga, and the Feldenkrais Method® also offer ways of helping you to learn to keep your shoulders and trunk relaxed in action. You can use these or similar exercises as part of your preparation at the beginning of the day, between clients, and to relax at the end of the working day.

Arm Stretches to Open the Chest

This first stretch is a good way to rebalance your upper body posture after you've had your arms and shoulders in front of your chest for long periods. It can be done either standing or seated.

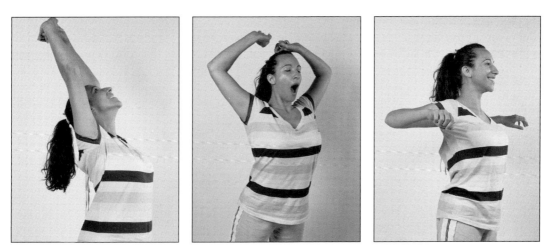

Figure 22.7: Arm stretches to open the chest.

Stretch your arms up and back, so that your shoulders are stretched back and the front of your chest opened and widened. It can be done with your arms separate or with your fingers interlocked. This stretch is what people instinctively do when they have been hunched over a desk for some time, often simultaneously yawning to gather more air into the expanded chest.

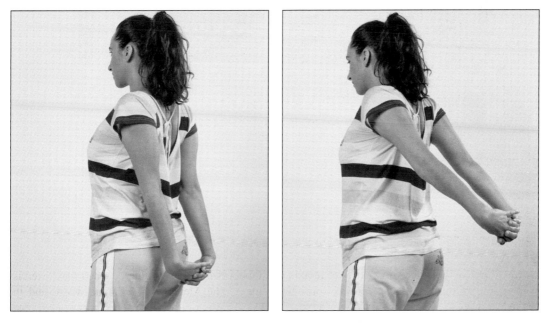

Figure 22.8: Stretching the arms back with interlocked fingers to open out the chest.

Another way of opening the chest is to stretch your arms behind your back with your fingers interlocked and your palms facing each other. To increase the stretch, straighten your arms. If it is not a strain, lift them a little to take the stretch even further.

Releasing the Shoulders

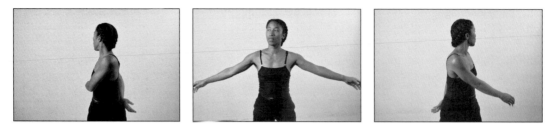

Figure 22.9: Turning with sweeping arms; a) one way, b) central position, c) the other way.

A simple way of releasing your shoulders is by turning your body from side to side and letting your arms sweep across your trunk. Begin by standing with your arms hanging at your sides. Then turn to one side with one arm sweeping across the front of your body and the other behind you. Turn your head in the same direction as part of the movement. Then as your arms 'uncurl', turn the other way to sweep your arms and turn your head in the opposite direction. As you turn to each side, you may find it helpful to lift the opposite heel from the floor, to reduce any potential strain in your lower back.

Mobilising the Shoulders

The following exercises will help you to regain mobility in your shoulders. They can be done either sitting or standing. Have your arms relaxed and hanging down by your sides, and try to keep them relaxed and dangling throughout the exercises.

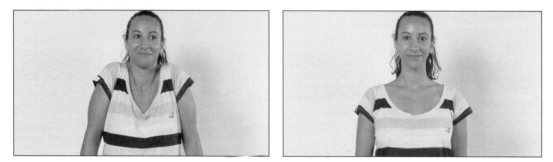

Figure 22.10: Tensing and relaxing the shoulders; a) Lifting the shoulders, b) releasing the shoulders.

Raise your shoulders up towards your ears while breathing in fully. Hold your breath for a few moments with your shoulders up in this position. Then let your shoulders drop gently down onto the top of your ribs as you simultaneously let your breath out in an easy exhalation.

To fine-tune this release, raise your shoulders and then release them and your breath in two stages, letting your shoulders drop halfway down and partly releasing your breath in the first stage, and then letting your shoulders and breath go the rest of the way in the second stage. Then do this in three stages and then four. The clearer you can make each stage of this movement and therefore the more finely-tuned that your sensing of your shoulders becomes, the more you will be able to notice any tension creeping into your shoulders as you massage and the sooner you can release it.

Next, bring your shoulders forward towards the front of the chest, without holding your breath. Then move them backwards so that your shoulder blades slide back around your ribs towards your spine. For many people taking the shoulder blades back is the least familiar of these movements and will therefore require the most concentration and practice to master.

Now move your shoulders through a circle that encompasses these four directions – up, backwards, down and forward. You may find it easiest to do it first with one shoulder and then the other before doing both together. Do these circular movements a few times in one direction, and then a few times in the opposite direction.

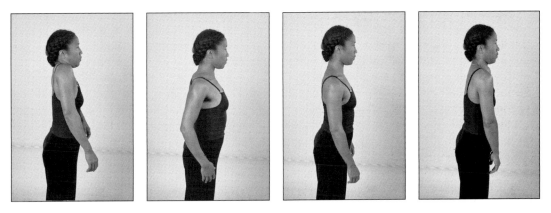

Figure 22.11: Moving the shoulders; a) taking the shoulders up, b) taking the shoulders backwards, c) taking the shoulders down, d) taking the shoulders forward.

Gaining Width in Your Shoulders

Even after doing the previous exercises, you may find that, through familiarity, your shoulders come to rest towards the front of your chest. This is very common because this is the shoulder position of so many daily activities (see figure 22.2). If so, take your shoulders backwards again, so that your shoulder blades move towards your spine. Then let them come a little way forward until they are positioned centrally between being pulled forwards and pulled backwards.

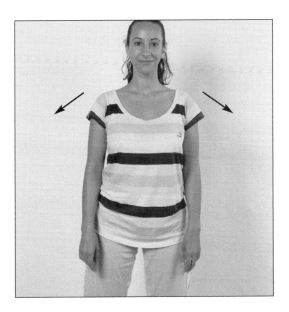

Figure 22.12: Widening the shoulders in the central position.

Once you have settled them in this central position, let them drop and widen out along this central line to retain maximum openness in your chest. Even if this is only a small movement, it is worth doing. See if you can let them move a little further outwards and downwards on each out breath.

Don't expect that your shoulders will automatically stay relaxed and in this position. You will need to continually monitor that you are not unconsciously tensing them or letting them move further forward than necessary. You may find it useful to regularly remind yourself of this feeling of 'relaxed width' in your morning warm-up and during your working day. You only need to take a few minutes to do the shoulder circling exercise and then let them settle into this position. Once this process is familiar, it only takes 15–20 seconds to focus on your shoulders and mentally 'nudge' them towards maximum relaxed width.

Then see if you can keep some width in your shoulders while you are doing massage treatments, instead of unconsciously letting them slip forward and get stuck in front of your chest. This will, of course, be hardest when your arms are stretched forward.

Monitoring Your Shoulders

All of these exercises have two purposes in relation to massage. Firstly, they help you to relax your shoulders. Secondly, by doing these or similar exercises regularly, you will become familiar with the *feeling* of relaxation and width in your shoulders. This will help you to monitor your shoulders *during* the massage. Then, whenever you notice yourself tensing up, you can relax them, rather than needing a shoulder massage yourself at the end of each massage that you do. And take a few moments at the end of a session to re-establish the sense of relaxed width.

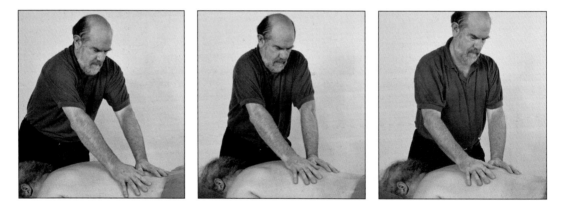

Figure 22.13: Shoulder position in massage strokes; a) shoulders forward, b) shoulders raised, c) shoulders relaxed and more retracted.

So, as you are massaging, regularly check the position of your shoulders. For most of us, it's useful to regularly give ourselves a little mental reminder to gently relax our shoulders and to take them slightly backwards for the feeling of 'relaxed width'. And make sure that you are also involving your whole body and breathing easily to support this release in your shoulders, rather than standing still and holding your breath (which would work against it).

Keeping Your Shoulders Relaxed When Pressing and Pulling

People with habitual shoulder tension may find that they need a great deal of practice to get used to monitoring their shoulders as they massage. The following experiment will develop your ability to monitor your shoulders as you do some simple pressure and pulling movements. If this seems helpful, you could then apply the same approach while you are doing other massage techniques. Try this initially without a client on the couch, so that you can just focus on your own body. Be aware that if you are tensing your shoulders, you are also quite likely to be holding your breath, which reinforces tensing up. So, as you observe your shoulders, also pay attention to your breathing.

In the accompanying photos, the difference between tense and relaxed shoulders is exaggerated to make them clearly distinguishable. With practice, you can learn to fine-tune your sensibilities so that you can catch the build up of tension earlier, and make the small adjustments necessary to nip it in the bud.

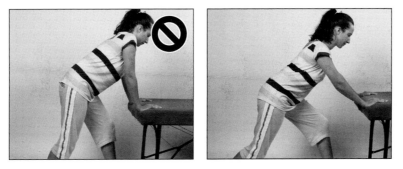

Figure 22.14: Pressing; a) with tense shoulders, b) with relaxed shoulders.

Stand facing the side of the massage couch, with your hands resting on it. Firstly, stand still and apply pressure by tensing your shoulders in order to gain a clear sense of how restricted it feels to work in this way, and the strains that are likely to arise. Then contrast it with good practice by relaxing your shoulders (and keeping them as relaxed as possible) as you press by gradually swaying your body forward.

Notice, as you do this, whether you are keeping your shoulders relatively relaxed and pushing from your body, or whether your shoulders automatically rise towards your ears. If the latter is happening, practice relaxing your shoulders, so that your shoulder muscles are still involved in the action but not overused, and coordinate this with swaying your body forward to increase the power of your push. If necessary, return to the shoulder circle exercise (see figure 22.11) to ensure that you start with relaxed shoulders.

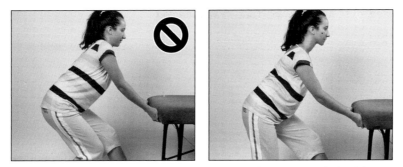

Figure 22.15: Pulling; a) with tense shoulders, b) with relaxed shoulders.

318 Dynamic Bodyuse for Effective Strain-free Massage

Now monitor and adjust the work of your shoulders in a similar way as you pull the couch by swaying backwards.

Once you are familiar with monitoring your shoulders, try these movements with a colleague on the table who can give you constructive feedback. Then get them to do this on you. Many people are surprised to discover the difference that tension or relaxation in the practitioner's shoulders can also make to the receiver. When the practitioner tenses his/her shoulders, it often invokes an instinctive wariness in the recipient or even tensing against the massage.

Integrating Shoulder Use With the Rest of the Body

Tensing the shoulders is often part of a bigger pattern of body tension or poor bodyuse. So learning to relax your shoulders isn't effective in isolation. It needs to be supported and integrated with the way that you use the rest of your body. As much as possible, initiate the power and fluidity for pushing, pulling and sustained pressure techniques from positioning and leaning your bodyweight behind your hands. If you are not positioning your body well and/or you are standing stiffly, your shoulders will inevitably tighten up again.

So, in addition to focusing on keeping your shoulders relaxed, do stretches to open your chest and to hyperextend your back (see figure 22.7). Or you could take up activities in which the chest is opened and the arms are stretched back, such swimming, yoga, or forms of martial arts or dance that incorporate this. And, of course, get regular massages yourself to release your shoulders, open your chest and to relax midback tension. And, as you work though this book and focus on other areas of your body, pay regular attention to your shoulders and how they contribute to or are affected by how you are using the rest of your body.

Review

The role of the shoulders in massage is to transmit power from the trunk to the arms, while remaining as relaxed as possible.

Shoulder tension accumulates through everyday use of one's hands and in response to stress.

In addition, shoulder tension can arise in massage due to:

- Standing still instead of moving your body to generate power;
- Hunching over;
- Working on a table that is too high;
- Not positioning your body behind your working hands;
- Straining your hands or wrists as you massage, or;
- Attempting to apply more pressure than you can comfortably deliver.

Because shoulder tension interferes with the easy transmission of power from your lower body, it can lead you into a vicious cycle of tensing your shoulders further in order to generate the power.

Release accumulated shoulder tension and mobilise your shoulders with regular exercises.

Monitor and adjust what you are doing with your shoulders as you massage, especially in pushing or pulling strokes.

CHAPTER 23

Transmitting Power Through Your Arms

You will inevitably build up the strength of your arm muscles through doing massage. However, just using your arms to apply pressure doesn't provide you with as much power as using your whole body. Strokes in which you rely on arm power to 'muscle through' will be stiffer, less powerful and less fluidly executed, and will ultimately become tiring to deliver. So this chapter looks at the role of your arms in delivering the *power* and *fluidity* to your hands that comes from positioning, leaning and swaying your body to support how you use your arms.

Different Builds

As you read through this chapter, bear in mind that practitioners with different length arms will need to vary their massage accordingly.

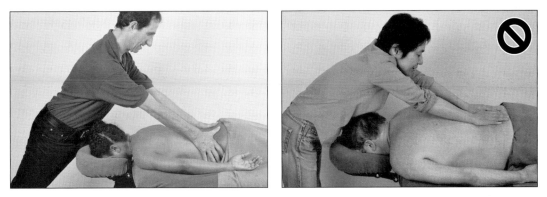

Figure 23.1: Reaching down the client's back; a) tall practitioner, b) short practitioner trying to reach too far.

For example, those with longer arms can reach further down the client's back without strain from the head of the table.

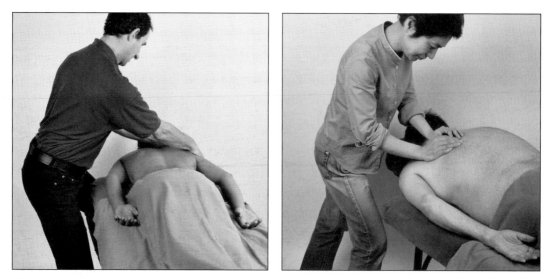

*Figure 23.2: Doing equivalent strokes; a) tall practitioner pulling the far shoulder,
b) short practitioner doing an equivalent pushing stroke on the close shoulder.*

When there is a choice, practitioners with short arms will generally find it easier to work on the close side of the client's back, while those with long arms will find the equivalent strokes more comfortable and effective to do on the further side. The short practitioner might just work on the close shoulder for example, while the tall practitioner could work on both shoulders at once, or just on the further shoulder.

Moving Your Arms With Massage Strokes

Of course, you need to keep your hands still for some massage strokes such as resting them on the client at the beginning of a relaxation massage ('holds' – see figure 33.17) or when you're applying stationary pressure. But, whenever you're moving your hands, try to move your arms as well to give strength and evenness to your strokes. It's obvious that you need to move your arms (by swaying your body – see figures 23.6 & 23.7) for large sliding strokes.

Avoid Clamping Your Arms By Your Side

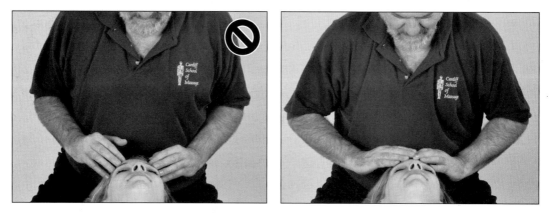

Figure 23.3: Small massage strokes with the fingers; a) with the elbows cramped by the side and the hands held still, b) spreading the elbows for stroking outwards.

Watch out for clamping your elbows stiffly by your sides, especially when you are working on small areas such as parts of the client's face. Even for these small strokes, holding your arms still would create unnecessarily hard work for your digits and put pressure on your wrists.

Move Your Arms With Strokes Whenever Possible

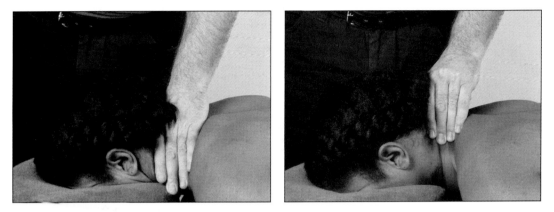

Figure 23.4: Moving the hand in a squeezing stroke; a) downwards to grip the tissues, b) upwards to stretch the tissues.

And moving your arms is important for strokes such as squeezing, even though you only need to move your hand a little forward as you take hold of the client's tissues and a little backwards to stretch them before releasing them. This will make the stroke much smoother and easier than if you were to hold your hand still.

Have Your Hands Echo Your Body Movements in Effleurage Strokes

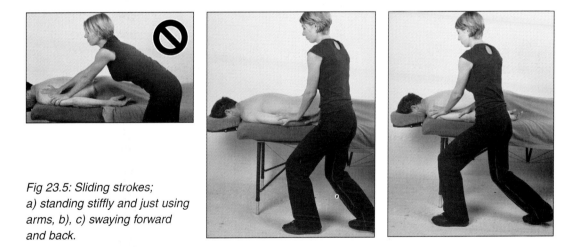

Fig 23.5: Sliding strokes; a) standing stiffly and just using arms, b), c) swaying forward and back.

In effleurage strokes, have your hands stay about the same distance from your hips. Initiate the movement of sliding them forward and back by swaying your body.

Images to Help Feel the Connection Between Your Hips and Arms

Many people have found the following images helpful in feeling how to transmit their body movements through their arms to their hands.

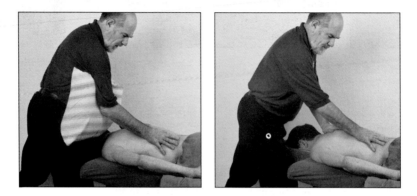

Figure 23.6: Feeling the hip and elbow connection in swaying forward; a) with a cushion, b) imagining the cushion.

When you are sliding your hands forward, imagine that you have a thick cushion between your respective hip and elbow as you sway forward. Some people find it useful to try this at first with a real cushion to help them to consolidate this feeling of how your body movement can propel your arms forward.

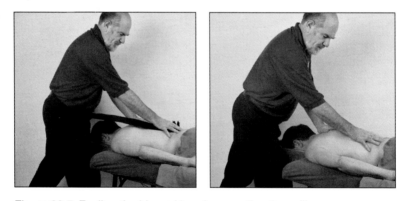

Figure 23.7: Feeling the hip and hand connection for pulling; a) with a ribbon, b) imagining the ribbon.

To feel the connection in pulling between the movement of your lower body and the consequent pull of your hands, imagine that you have a slightly elastic ribbon between your respective hip and hand so that, as you sway back, the movement of your hip pulls your hand.

These images may help you to clarify the feeling of initiating arm movements in the movements of your lower body. In effleurage strokes, you can alternate the images as you move between swaying forward and swaying back. As you twist your hips in a wringing stroke, you could imagine a cushion on the side that's moving forward and simultaneously a ribbon on the side that's pulling back.

Keep Your Arms Straight for Delivering Pressure

In lighter strokes, you might let your elbows bend. However, there is a temptation to stand still and overwork the arms for applying firm pressure, rather than straightening your arms to transmit the power of your body movement.

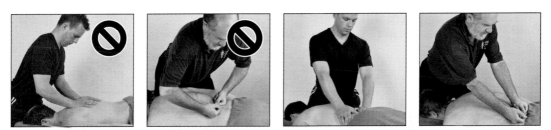

Figure 23.8: Transmitting the power through the arms; a) arms flexed, b) arms bent wide, c), d) arms relatively straight.

Whenever you are applying stationary pressure or incorporating pressure into a sliding stroke, bending your arms would dissipate your force away from the intended direction of application. This would force you to tense your arms to redirect the power back towards your hands. So straighten them to deliver the force directly. This applies whether you are using your hands separately or with one hand on the other.

Don't Try to Apply Pressure on the Far Side of the Client's Body

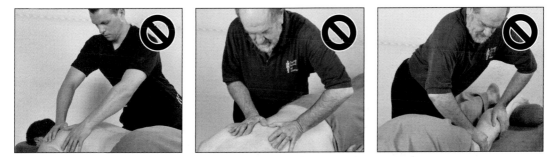

Figure 23.9: Attempting to apply pressure on the far side of client's body.

This is also the reason that you can't press down on the far side of the client's back or their further leg without strain. You would be bending your arm and/or leaning over too far, tensing your arm and shoulder muscles to direct your force, putting pressure on your back and still not delivering great power.

Keep Your Arms Relatively Straight for Strong Stretches

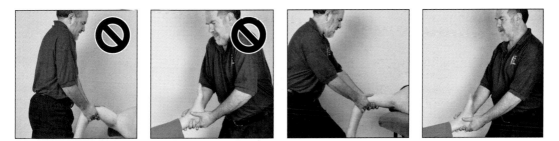

Figure 23.10: Applying stretches and lifting; a), b) with bent arms, c), d) swaying the body with straight arms.

There is quite a temptation to just pull with your arms for passive stretches and when you are lifting a client's heavy limb. Doing this would cause you to tense your arms and to work harder than necessary. For a stretch or lift, get your hands in position and then sway back to pull your arms straight to move the client's body part.

Bracing Your Arms

There are ways of bracing your arms to focus more power.

Brace Your Forearm on Your Thigh

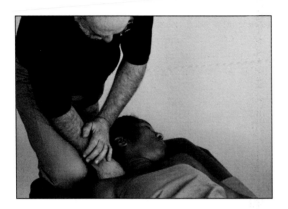

Figure 23.11: Bracing your forearm on your knee.

You can also use your own body for leverage. Put one knee on the table and rest your forearm across your thigh to use that as a pivot. This works well when you are sliding your fist along well-used shoulder muscles.

Push Your Elbow Directly With Your Body

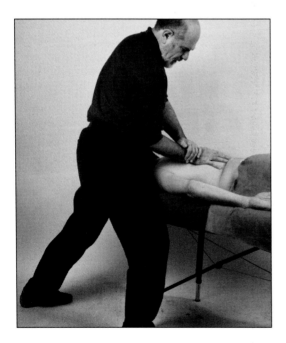

Figure 23.12: Pushing the arm from the hip.

Placing your elbow just inside your hip bone enables you to transmit the power of your bodyweight directly through your forearm to your fist as you sway forward. This will give you maximum power without working too hard with your shoulders or arm muscles. Be sure to monitor that this is not too much for your wrist. (If it is, switch to using your forearm or elbow for the massage).

Review

In massage, the power and fluidity for hand movements is conveyed through your arms from your trunk.

Reaching across the table is much easier for those with long arms, while those with short arms have a greater potential for pushing on the close side of the client.

Don't clamp your elbows stiffly by your sides when you are working on small areas.

In effleurage strokes, use your arms to deliver the movement of your body to your hands, so that your hands stay at roughly the same distance in front of your body.

In squeezing strokes, move your hand down and up a little as you take hold of the client's tissues and then release them.

When you are stroking outwards from the centre of the client's forehead or across the cheeks, initiate the movement by leading outwards with your elbows.

In strong massage strokes, bending your arms would dissipate your force so straighten your arms *without stiffening them* to transmit the power of your body movement.

Do not try to apply pressure on the far side of the client's body, because your arms will be bent as you reach over.

In stretches, take hold of the client's limb and stretch it by swaying backwards, letting your arms stretch out fully for the pull.

When you are applying pressure on one point, straighten and relax your arms and lean forward.

To help feel the connection between your body and your arm movements in sliding strokes, imagine that you have a thick cushion between your respective hip and elbow as you sway forward, and a ribbon between your hand and hip as you pull back.

Brace your forearm across your thigh with one knee on the table for sliding fist strokes.

When you are standing, placing your elbow just inside your hip bone enables you to transmit the power of your bodyweight directly to your forearm and hand as you sway forward.

Holding Your Head

The way that you hold your head can affect the way that you use the rest of your body. This chapter looks at three common habits which cause problems:

1. Dropping your head to watch your working hands, which often leads to hunching over;
2. Holding your head stiffly, which is often allied to shoulder tension and can cause you to stiffen the rest of your body, and;
3. Tensing your face, especially your jaw, which can be part of a pattern of tensing up to do massage strokes.

Watching Your Hands

When we are first learning to do massage, we need to look carefully at what we are doing with our hands.

Hunching Over

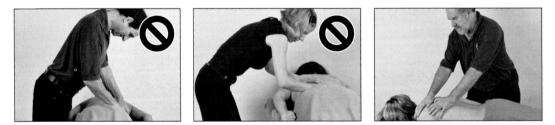

Figure 24.1: Watching the hands; a) dropping the head, b) hunching over, c) leaning with the trunk.

Initially, many of us do this by dropping our heads, which causes us to hunch over and impedes the transmission of power from the lower body. This can lead to overusing your shoulder and arm muscles. Unless this posture is addressed, it can become an unconscious fixed habit, leading to shoulder and neck tension and back problems. Tall practitioners need to be especially careful about this, because hunching over can already be such a habit for them. It is also a common problem for visually impaired massage practitioners, who are accustomed to hunching over to move their eyes close to objects for maximum visual input.

Dropping the head like this is also an occupational hazard for dentists and hairdressers. However massage practitioners have an advantage – as you become practiced at your profession, you can learn to bend your knees. This enables you to lean with your *whole trunk* so that your neck and head stay pretty much in line with your back (see figure 25.14). To bring your head down even closer to your work, bend your knees further, and, if necessary, also widen your stance.

If hunching over is an ingrained habit, you may need to receive deep tissue massage treatments and do some yoga, or Pilates, Feldenkrais or Alexander work to help change your posture.

Holding the Head Stiffly

There is another common habit associated with using your eyes. Sportspeople and dancers get used to focusing while they are moving. However, so much of modern life involves holding the head still while using the eyes, for example looking at computer screens or TVs while sitting in static positions, that many people come to massage sessions with the unconscious habit of stiffening the neck (and often the rest of the trunk) when using their eyes.

Shutting Your Eyes / Defocusing
A simple way of reducing this tendency is to regularly shut your eyes or to defocus them during a massage, or at least to look away from what you're doing every now and then. This gives you an opportunity to focus on moving your body with your massage strokes. It will also enable you to concentrate on your sense of touch with less distraction, more easily identifying the client's tensions and feeling the responses in their tissues as you massage.

Moving Fluidly Without Holding the Head Still
Bear in mind however that, even when we shut our eyes, many of us are still trying to 'look' through closed eyelids, which can lead back into the same problems of holding the head still and consequently also stiffening the rest of the body.

Moving Fluidly With the Eyes Shut or Open

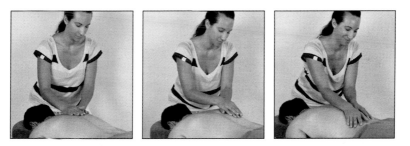

Figure 24.2: Moving fluidly with the eyes shut.

You can train yourself out of this. Stand at the side of the table and do a familiar effleurage stroke on your partner's leg or back by swaying your whole body forward and back. Shut your eyes and do the stroke a number of times until you've found a steady, relaxed rhythm for the movement. Sway smoothly to deliver fluidity and evenness to the movements of your hands. With practise, you will find that 'switching off' your eyes like this can also help you to tune into your hands during the massage.

Then open your eyes and bring them back into play. If this impedes the movement of your body and therefore the fluidity of the strokes that you're using or reduces your ability to palpate with your hands, shut your eyes again and re-establish the movement. Then try opening them again. Repeat this as many times as you need until you are able to move fluidly with your eyes open and focused.

Then practise the same process with less familiar strokes.

Don't Wear Loose Fitting Glasses

If you wear glasses, pay attention to the effect on how you hold your head. You may be unconsciously restricting the movement of your head (and therefore of your body) to ensure that your glasses do not fall off. In order to keep moving freely, take your glasses off to do massages, use contact lenses, or hold your glasses in place with a sports band.

There's something else to consider if you wear glasses. While we are able to focus on the whole picture at the centre of our vision, we register *movement* at the *edge* of our field of vision (see figure 24.7). In massage, this enables us to pick up the client's responses, which are expressed in other parts of their body than where we're focusing, such as changes in breathing patterns or facial expressions, or clenching the hands. Wide side levers on your glasses would impede this so wear glasses with *narrow* side levers.

Eye Exercises

If you feel the need for them, eye exercises can help you to break out of restricted visual patterns, relax your eyes and use them better. These exercises stretch and strengthen the eye muscles in the same way as stretching exercises do for the large muscles of the body. As you do these exercises, monitor that you're not holding your breath. (It's probably best to do them in private to avoid having to explain these unusual eyes activities).

A number of these eye exercises incorporate head movements as an essential part of the exercise. If you feel that mobilising your neck needs more specific attention, you will find some exercises which focus on this below (see figures 24.8 & 24.9). If you feel that this, in turn, needs to be supported by increasing the flexibility of your whole trunk, try the exercises for spinal suppleness in the next chapter (see figures 25.16–25.19).

If you find the following eye exercises useful, and want to go further with enhancing how you use your eyes and reducing eye strain and tension, try out Bates vision work or its derivatives.

Exercises for Softening Your Focus

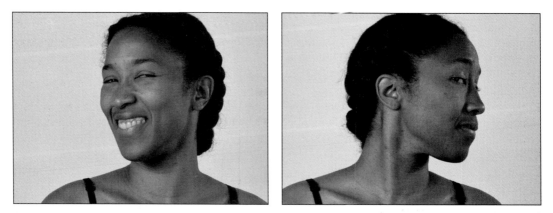

Figure 24.3: Eye focus exercise – turning the head while focusing on one spot.

A simple exercise is to focus on one spot while turning your head up and down and from side to side. Don't stare fixedly as this would tend to stiffen your neck. Instead let your focus be soft so that you can move your head easily; this will come with practise. This exercise enables you to feel how to soften and adjust your focus while also mobilising your neck.

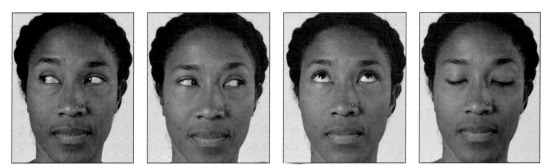

Figure 24.4: Moving the focus; a), b) looking from side to side, c), d) looking up and down.

Then do the opposite. Keep your head still, but not so that your neck is rigid. Move your gaze up and down and from side to side. Move your eyes slowly enough to be able to focus fully on each object that your gaze travels over. With practice you will gradually be able to move your eyes faster without losing the clarity of your focus. You could then move your gaze around in a continuous circle that encompasses the full range of your vision.

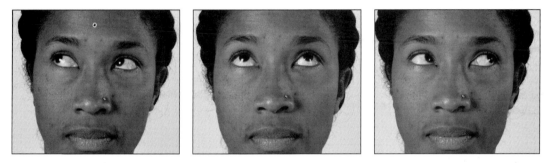

Figure 24.5: Expanding the upper field of vision; a) looking upper left, b) centrally upward, c) upper right.

Because we look downwards for most daily activities, including massage, looking upwards will be the least familiar and most challenging part of this exercise. You may find it productive, therefore, to spend more time working on the upper part of your visual range. Keeping your head still, focus centrally as high in your field of vision as you can, and then spend a few minutes moving your focus outwards to the upper left corner and to the upper right corner of your vision. This activates underused eye muscles and gives the others a rest.

Exercises for Shifting Focus
If you still find yourself staring, there is another simple exercise that will help you to get used to adjusting your focus. This is particularly helpful if you spend a lot of time focusing on a computer screen as well as looking at your clients, and not much time using your distance vision.

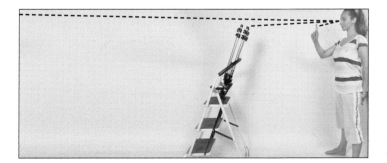

Figure 24.6: Eye exercise for distance accommodation.

Stand or sit for this exercise. Have an object at eye level about one metre (three feet) in front of you. Then position yourself so that you can also see a distant object such as a building or a tree directly behind this closer object. Then hold up one finger about 25–30 cm (10–12 inches) in front of your face at eye level in line with these other two points of focus.

Focus on your finger. Then move your attention to the object again one metre away and focus on it. Then focus on the distant object. Then focus on the middle object and then focus back on your finger. Continue to focus in turn on each one. In each position, take the time you need to focus clearly. Do not rush it, but, as you become more practiced, speed up the process of shifting focus at a rate that still enables you to focus clearly at each position.

Enhancing Peripheral Vision
There are also simple exercises that will enhance your ability to pick up movement at the edge of your field of vision. As noted above, your peripheral vision is helpful to pick up changes in breathing or facial expression or finger movements that indicate mini-reactions to the massage. The description of these exercises may sound strange, but, if you try them, you will find them effective.

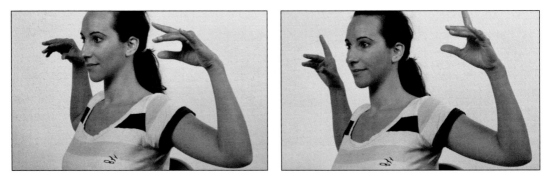

Figure 24.7: Enhancing peripheral vision of movement; a), b) solo exercise.

You can do the first exercise by yourself. Stand or sit at least 1.5–2 metres (5–6 feet) away from a wall that is bare or has very few distracting objects on it. Focus your gaze on the wall and keep your focus here throughout the exercise. Lift your hands so that each one is about 30 cm (one foot) to the side of your head. Move them forward and back at the side of your head so that they move just in and out of the edge of your vision. If you keep your focus directly ahead, you won't see the shapes of your hands clearly, but will get a sense of their movement. As you move your hands, also wiggle your fingers to enhance this sensing of movement.

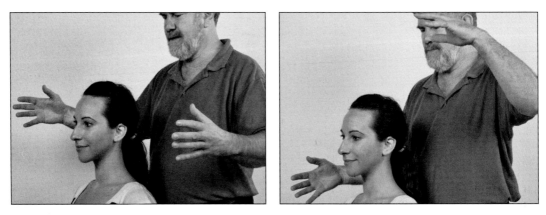

Figure 24.7 (cont.): c), d) paired exercise.

You can also try a variation of this exercise with a friend. Stand or sit facing the wall and focus on it. Your friend stands behind you, out of your field of vision. He then randomly sweeps his hands through the edge of your field of vision, fast enough so that you register the movement visually but without being able to actually focus on his hand. Your friend could use one hand at a time, or both simultaneously in different ways. To enhance the effect of movement, he could wriggle his fingers or twirl his hands around as he moves them.

Releasing the Neck

It is not only how you use your eyes that can lead to stiffness in your neck and restricted movement in your body. Irrespective of how they use their eyes, many people are habitually stiff in the neck, often due to general shoulder tension. The following exercises will help you to reduce neck tension. You could also do shoulder releasing exercises (see figures 24.12 & 24.13), so that you begin each massage with relaxed neck and shoulders.

Warming-up Neck Movements

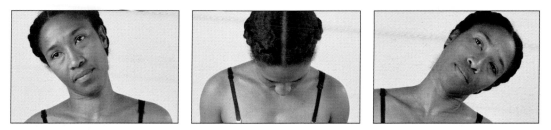

Figure 24.8: Head movements.

To focus on releasing neck tensions, include gentle head movements in your pre-massage warm-ups, drop your head to one side and then the other, keeping your face towards the front. Then drop your head forward. (These days, it is not recommended to drop your head backwards, as people can have undiagnosed cervical spine problems which this can aggravate).

Head Movements While Massaging

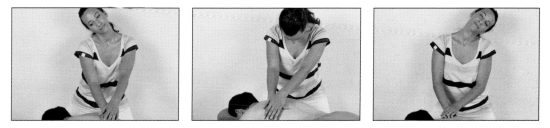

Figure 24.9: Small head movements while massaging.

The preceding head movements would probably be disruptive during a massage, but you can incorporate smaller movements, especially if you tend to get tight in your neck. During a slow sliding stroke or when you are applying sustained pressure on one area, for example, you could gently turn your head a little from side to side or gently tilt it up and down a little. It takes practise to incorporate these releases into your massage sessions without disruption, but it will pay off in the long term. If you find these movements too difficult to do when you are massaging, just regularly look away from your work for a few moments, to take pressure off your neck.

Massaging Your Neck

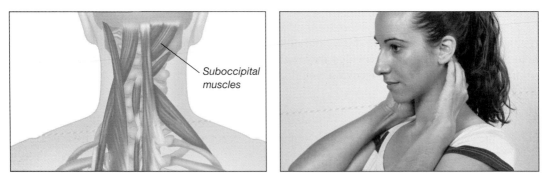

Figure 24.10: The suboccipital muscles; a) the muscles, b) massaging the muscles.

Massaging your neck regularly (or receiving massages) can also be helpful in releasing neck tension in the muscles, which balance your head. Pay particular attention to the suboccipital muscles under the base of the skull. These muscles are involved in fine-tuning the stability of your head on your neck, and can get very tight if you stare fixedly with your eyes, clench your jaw, or tense your shoulders.

Holding the Head to One Side
It is worth noting here, that many people habitually hold the head to one side, usually without knowing it. This can affect the ability to transfer a stroke symmetrically from one side of the massage table to the other. If you think that this may be a problem for you, get a skilled bodyworker to watch you in action and to coach you.

Determination

There is another cause of tension in the head that can relate to tension and stiffness throughout your body as you work. Some students and practitioners will approach any task by tensing up the jaw as part of their determination to 'do a good job'. Of course this is counterproductive. Tensing up will reduce your effectiveness, which is likely to lead you into a vicious cycle of tensing up more.

Tensing Your Face

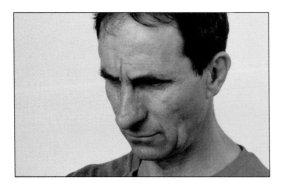

Figure 24.11: Tense facial expressions.

As a teacher I regularly see students frowning, gritting their teeth, clenching their jaws, pursing their lips, and/or sticking out their jaw when they are massaging. Tensing the face like this is generally quite subconscious. It's not a problem if these expressions are momentary. However if they are sustained, they often indicate an attitude of determination to 'do a good job' irrespective of the potential strain on one's own body. Monitor these facial tensions because they are likely to be accompanied by tensing the shoulders and probably tightening up many other areas of the body.

This grim determination can also be a reaction when the practitioner feels daunted by the build of a particular client and the pressure that they want. If you can't find *comfortable* ways of doing an effective job, it is important to recognise your limits and refer the client on to a colleague.

Relaxing Your Face
If you notice yourself regularly clenching your jaw, try to relax your face, neck and shoulders. To address the associated parts of this pattern, monitor and relax the rest of your body too and make sure that you are not holding your breath as you work.

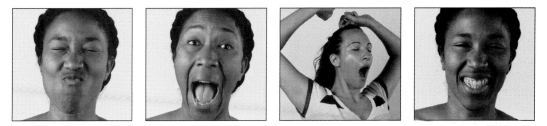

Figure 24.12: Exercises to mobilise the face; a) screwing up the face, b) stretching the face, c) yawning, d) laughing.

There are many exercises that practitioners can use to relax the jaw muscles and release tension from the face. Screwing up or stretching the face are easy ways of mobilising it. Yawning and laughing are good too. Self-massage of the face is also helpful.

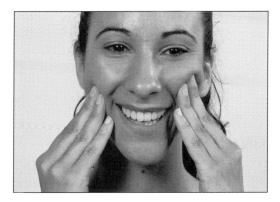

Figure 24.13: Self-massage of the face.

Review

Lean forward with your whole trunk to watch your working hands / forearm, rather than hunching over, or dropping your head.

Don't hold your head stiffly, which stiffens your neck.

Work without glasses, wear contacts or use a sports band to hold your glasses in place if they are loose.

Defocus your eyes or shut them regularly to focus on feeling with your hands, and to reduce the tendency to hold your body stiffly.

Regularly gritting your jaw, or tensing your face can be part of a pattern of determination about 'doing a good job' in which you ignore your own comfort.

Neck movements are a useful warm-up exercise to release neck tension.

During a massage, small head movements can help to relax your neck.

Yawning, screwing up and stretching your face and laughing will help mobilise it. So will self-massage of your face.

CHAPTER 25

Transmitting Power Through Your Trunk

As is emphasised throughout this book, you need to massage 'with your whole body'. The power and fluidity of your massage strokes comes from positioning your body, leaning forward to use your bodyweight and swaying for the movement. The role of your trunk in this is to transmit the power generated in your lower body to your arms. Poor postural habits can impede this transmission of power, reducing the ease and fluidity of delivery. This is likely to lead to overusing your shoulder and arm muscles and your hands. Over time, it may also lead to strain in your back.

This chapter focuses on how the way that you hold your trunk can affect your massage work. It firstly looks at practices that can put pressure on your back as you do massage, and ways of avoiding these. The following section looks at the effect of poor postural habits and then presents ideas on 'good' (dynamic) posture for your back. The last section looks at ways of maintaining the suppleness of your trunk.

Straining Your Back

The main causes of back strain in massage are:

- Standing still, rather than swaying your body to deliver strokes with power and fluidity;
- Trying to reach too far;
- Twisting your trunk, instead of aligning your body behind your hands;
- Lifting awkwardly;
- Lifting parts of the client's body that are too heavy for you;
- Hunching over or standing stiffly upright, rather than leaning your whole body forward.

Anything that puts pressure on your lower back is likely to cause you to stiffen up there, cutting off the transmission of power from your lower body and forcing you to rely on 'muscling through' with your upper body. This will lead to overusing your shoulder muscles. Your massage will consequently be harder work and more stilted.

Standing Still

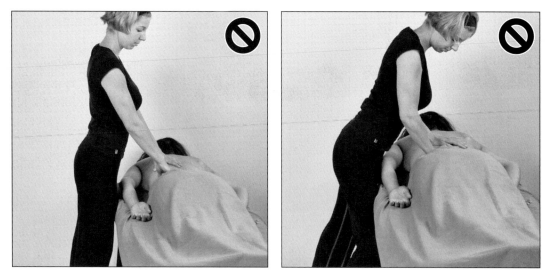

Figure 25.1: Standing still; a) standing still, b) leaning against the table.

Standing still cuts off the delivery of power and fluidity from your lower body and puts pressure on your lower back. Therefore you will have to tense your shoulders for power. It is also likely to make your massage stilted.

Leaning against the table compounds the problem. This also puts pressure on your lower back and can lead to backaches, particularly when your massage strokes involve pressure.

Overreaching

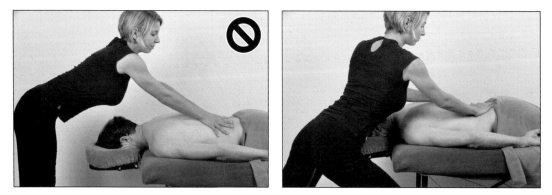

*Figure 25.2: Reaching down the client's back; a) from the head of the table,
b) moving more to the side of the table.*

Reaching further than is comfortable, for example trying to reach too far from the end of the table, also puts pressure on your lower back. To save your back, step to the side of the table so that you can sway your body to move your hands.

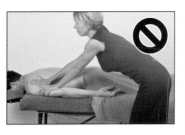

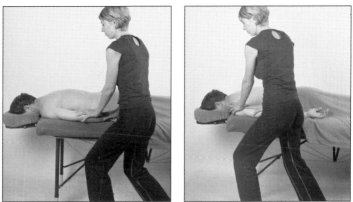

Figure 25.3: Doing long strokes; a) overreaching at the end of a long stroke, b), c), stepping forward for long sweeps.

Even when you are swaying your body with massage strokes, you can strain at the end of a long sliding stroke. So it is important to change position whenever you need to save your back. For example, step forward along the side of the table (see figure 28.9) to cover the whole of the client's back in one sweep, especially if you have short arms and/or you are massaging a tall client.

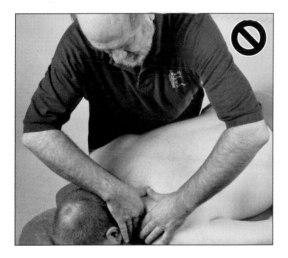

The same thing applies when you are reaching across the table. Only do wringing, kneading or pulling strokes on the far side of the client's body if you can comfortably reach without any strain in your lower back. Short practitioners need to be especially careful about this.

Figure 25.4: Reaching too far across the table.

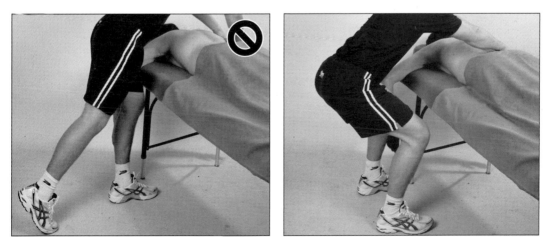

Figure 25.4 (cont.): b) rising onto tiptoes, c) dropping down to reach across.

People sometimes try rising up onto tiptoes to increase their reach but this puts pressure on the lower back. Instead, bend your knees to lower your trunk. If you can't reach comfortably across, move to the other side of the table.

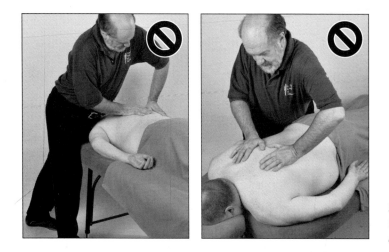

Figure 25.4 (cont.): d), e) trying to press down on the far side of the client's body.

And don't try to press down on the far side of the client's body, which is awkward and relatively ineffective. Instead, cross to the other side of the table to do this.

Twisting Your Trunk

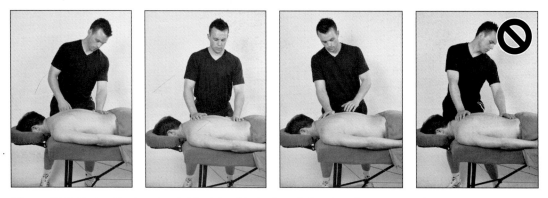

Figure 25.5: Facing the hands; a), b), c) turning body to follow hands, d) not turning lower body behind hands.

Reposition yourself regularly so that you can face your working hands. This enables you to work most effectively with the least strain in your trunk. Unfortunately, people sometimes twist the upper body towards their hands without moving their feet. This puts pressure on the lower back, reduces the effective transmission of force from your lower body and, over time, can lead to lumbar problems or reinforce existing ones. So always move your feet as part of aligning yourself behind your hands.

Poor Lifting
There are two things to watch out for when you are lifting:

1. Lifting a client's limb that is too heavy for you, and;
2. Lifting awkwardly.

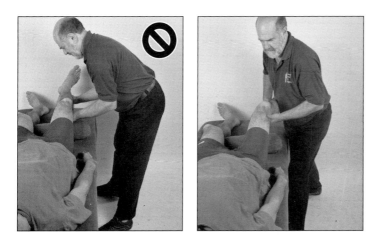

Figure 25.6: Lifting; a) holding the limb too far away from one's body, b) holding it closer.

Most of us have some idea of good lifting practice – that you hold the weight close to your body and lift with your legs and not your back. So when lifting the client's leg or arm, don't hold it too far away from your body, especially if it's heavy.

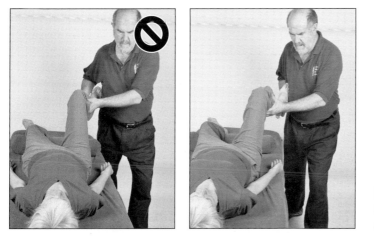

Figure 25.6 (cont.): c) not facing the part being lifted, d) facing the lift.

Face the part that you are lifting, so that your trunk is not twisted.

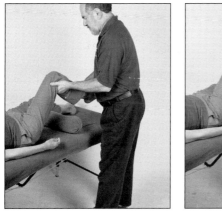
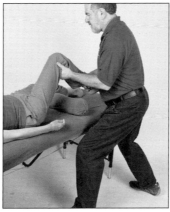

Fig 25.6 (cont.): e) just lifting with the arms, f) lifting with the legs.

And don't just lift with your arms, which puts unnecessary pressure on your lower back. Start low and *lift with your knees*, not your back. If it's too heavy, don't lift it.

Moving Your Whole Body to Save Your Back

In addition to looking after your back in the ways described above, keep the following principles in mind as you move around the massage table.

Align Your Lower and Upper Body Behind Your Working Hands

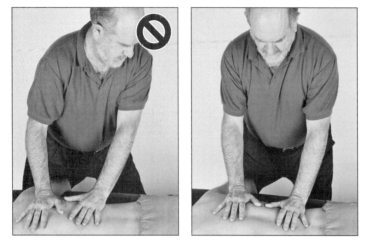

Figure 25.7: Alignment between upper and lower body and hands; a) trunk twisted, b) aligned.

Try to keep your lower and upper body aligned when you are applying force. This means having your shoulders, hips and feet facing in the same direction so that your body isn't twisted. When you are using both hands to apply pressure, keep them in front of your hips (within the 'hip spotlight', see figure 27.11), except when you are sliding your hands apart in a long stretch (see figure 28.37).

Bend Your Knees for Swaying

It is crucial to bend your knees to save your back. Don't drop into such a low squat that you strain them, but just soften them enough to have some 'give' in them.

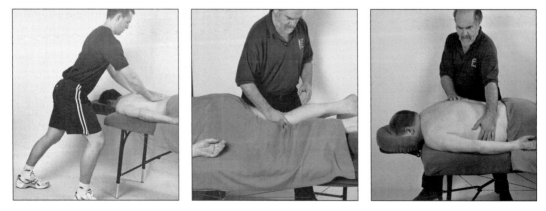

Figure 25.8: Bending the knees; a) bending the front knee to sway forward, b) in side to side swaying, c) twisting in a wringing stroke.

When you sway forward in the lunge stance, let your front knee bend. In the horse stance, bend both knees a little for swaying from side to side. In wringing strokes, let each knee bend in turn to alternately twist each hip forward behind each hand.

How Bending Your Knees Saves Your Back

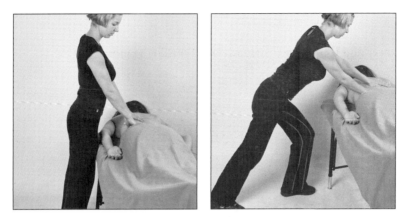

Figure 25.9: The effect on the back; a) with the knees straight,
b) when the knees can bend.

To clarify why bending your knees is essential, try standing with your knees locked back so that your legs are straight. You will notice that this stance puts great pressure on your lower back when you try to lean forward, because any bending can only happen here.

Contrast this with the way that letting your knees soften and bend eases the pressure on your lower back by enabling you to lean your whole trunk as a unit.

Rise Up or Lower Your Body to Control the Balance Between Pressure and Movement

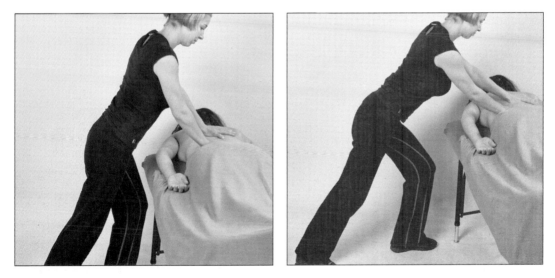

Figure 25.10: Balancing movement and pressure; a) applying more pressure, b) sliding more.

When you are applying sliding pressure, coordinate the balance between the pressure and the movement by how you position and lean your whole body, rather than just working harder in your upper body. You can increase the *pressure* by leaning forward to bring your weight more directly over the client (rather than just working harder with your upper body). Emphasise the *movement* forward by bending your knees to lower your body and then push forward from your legs.

Use Your Bodyweight for Stretches to Save Your Back

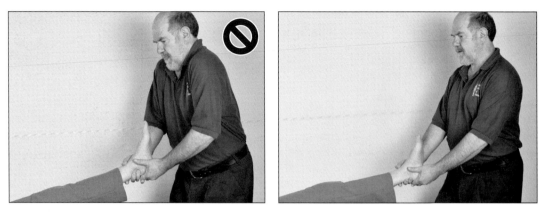

Figure 25.11: Pulling movements; a) pulling back with upper body only, b) 'sitting' back.

Similarly, when you are pulling a limb to stretch it, don't just pull back with your upper body. Instead, pull by 'sitting' back with your lower body, which is easier and more effective and reduces the pressure on your lower back.

Posture

Three common postural habits which many people have in everyday life will restrict them when they come to the massage table/chair – hunching over, standing stiffly upright, or leaning with stiff knees.

Hunching Over

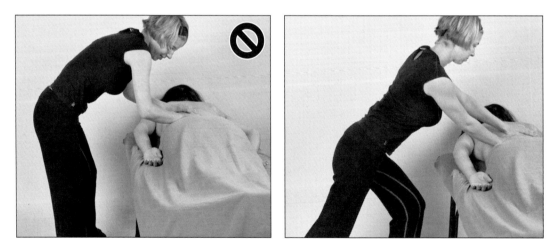

Figure 25.12: Hunching; a) hunching over, b) leaning with the whole trunk.

Hunching over is the most common postural problem in the trunk. This posture is often adapted by tall people, desk workers and many visually impaired people. In fact, most of us need to be careful not to slip into the habit of hunching over to look down when we are concentrating on the client's responses, learning new techniques, or working in very precise ways (see figure 24.1). This puts pressure on the back. Instead, when you need to lean forward, save your back by bending your knees to tilt your whole trunk as a unit. Bending your knees also enables you to drop your body when you need to work lower.

Standing Stiffly Upright

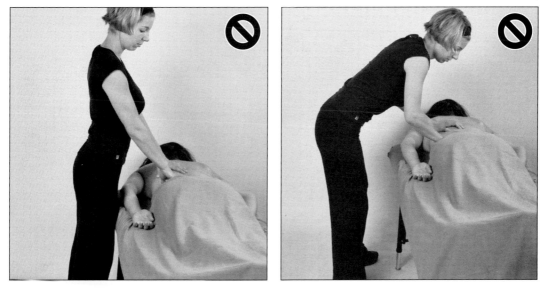

Figure 25.13: Standing stiffly; a) standing stiffly upright, b) having stiff knees.

Standing stiffly upright, which is less common, also cuts off the power from the lower body from being transmitted to the arms. A more common posture is to bend the trunk while keeping the knees stiff. Both of these put pressure on the back, especially the lower back in the latter posture. These postures also lead to overusing the shoulder and arm muscles, with a greater likelihood of shoulder stiffness and maybe also neck and back aches.

'Good Posture' for Massage

Dynamic Posture
So, what is the best 'posture' as you massage? I have reservations about using the word 'posture' as it often implies a stiffly held position. A more helpful idea of 'posture' is demonstrated in the *dynamic posture* of a tennis player preparing to return a serve. While s/he has a relatively straight back, it is not stiff but full of the potential to move into action. This is not easy to convey via the printed word and photos, but the intention of this book is to encourage you to develop a dynamic combination of strength and suppleness as part of your moving 'dance' around the massage table. Your breathing also plays a part in this dynamic posture; use your breathing to energise yourself without tensing up (see Chapter 26).

A Strong, Supple Back

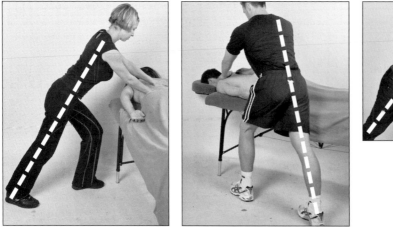
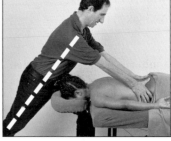

Figure 25.14: Good 'posture' when massaging; a), b), c) leaning with a long, supple back.

The ideal is to keep your back relatively 'straight' but not stiff, which enables you to keep your trunk both strong and supple. When leaning towards the table, you therefore need to do so with your *whole trunk* as a unit, rather than hunching over in the upper back or bending in your lower back. When you are seated, roll your hips forward on the seat to lean your whole spine as a unit, rather than crumpling your back.

Having a Wide Stance in the Lunge Stance

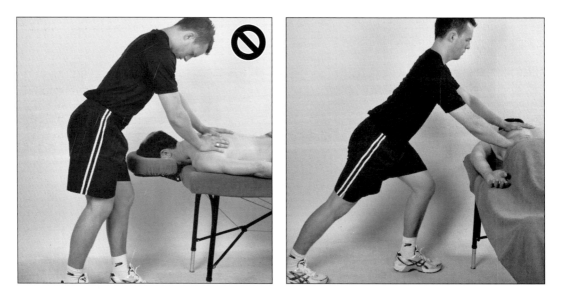

Figure 25.15: Leaning forward in lunge stance; a) with a narrow stance, b) with a wide stance.

In the lunge stance, this requires a wide enough stance that you can bend your front knee and straighten your back leg as you lean or sway forward, even if this lifts your back heel from the floor. Having your back foot too close dilutes the push coming from your back foot.

Monitoring Your Breathing

It is also important to monitor your breathing. If your back is strong, supple and well supported by your pelvis, this will also encourage easy, deep breathing. However, if you find yourself consistently breathing in forcefully or holding your breath with a particular stroke, you are likely to be tensing your body and working too hard to deliver the stroke. Try *exhaling* instead as you push into a strong stroke.

Monitoring Yourself in Action

Of course, when you first focus on all of this, you are quite likely to tense your back and to hold your breath as you concentrate on 'getting it right'. With practice you will discover how to lean without having a 'ramrod' straight back or holding your breath. As well as monitoring yourself as you massage, you can gain insights into your postural habits by getting coaching from a colleague or by having yourself videoed.

Maintaining Suppleness and Strength in Your Trunk

As described above (see figure 25.14), the ideal is to keep your trunk strong and supple. Obviously, receiving regular massages yourself will help to reduce the build-up of tension in your back. And deep tissue massage such as Rolfing® will help release and lengthen back muscles in a more systematic way. Activities such as walking, running, swimming, skipping and dancing will keep your back mobile. If you have a stiff back, it's worth doing regular exercises to help keep it supple. Disciplines such as yoga, the Feldenkrais Method®, the Alexander Technique, and Pilates can help you to develop a combination of strength and mobility in your trunk.

The following exercises will also help you to do this. Try them with an attentive but relaxed attitude. Don't go to your limits and then try to force your body further. Instead, focus on gaining ease and evenness *throughout* your comfortable range of movement. Respect your body's comfortable limits and perhaps nudge them a little.

The exercises are grouped in pairs – flexion/extension, side-bending to each side, and spinal twists to each side. When exercising, do each pair of movements enough times to get comfortable with your full range. Gradually reduce the movement in each direction until you find the central position, and then staying in this position for a short time, relaxed and breathing easily and deeply will get you familiar and comfortable with this position. This will give you the experience of having your trunk 'straight' (at its maximum length) *without rigidity.*

Curling Forward and Bending Back

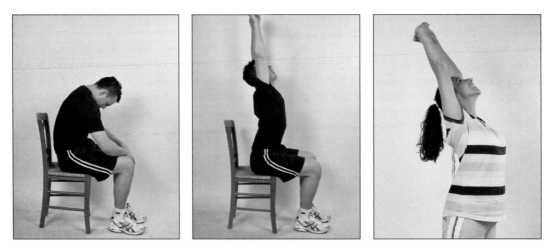

Figure 25.16: Flexion and extension; a) curling forward, b), c) back-bending.

Try this exercise seated at first in order to ensure that your whole trunk is involved. Slowly 'curl up' and then 'uncurl' your whole trunk (flexion and extension of the spine). Keep your head and shoulders balanced over your hips; otherwise the muscles that you are attempting to relax and stretch will tense up to stop you falling forward or backwards.

Don't move your head too far in this exercise – don't press your chin to your chest, and especially don't take your head too far back – but keep the movement of your head coordinated with the movement of your trunk.

Have good cushioning on the seat for your sitting bones. Make sure that your pelvis rolls on the seat – backwards (as you curl) and forwards (as you bend back). This ensures that the movement is not cut off in your lower back.

Then try the same movements standing.

Side-bending

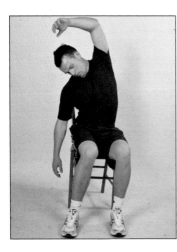 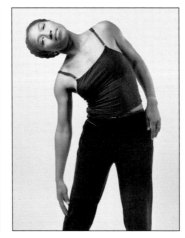

Figure 25.17: Side-bending.

Begin the side-bending exercise in standing. Slowly slide your hand down the side seam of your trousers to bend your trunk to that side. Then come up to the central position and bend to the other side. This gets your upper body bending a lot and will enable you to gradually also involve your hips. You are effectively shortening and lengthening each side of your trunk in turn.

To involve your lower body more, try the movement sitting. Rather than just bending down to each side, drop your shoulder and simultaneously lift your hip *on the same side*. This may feel a little awkward initially, but it's worth persevering as it will give you the maximum shortening and lengthening of each side of your trunk – between each respective shoulder and hip.

Rotating Your Spine

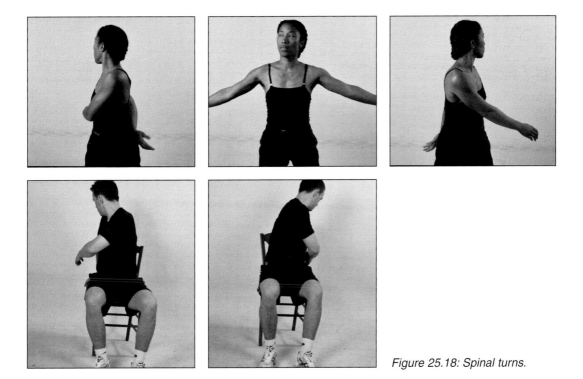

Figure 25.18: Spinal turns.

This can be done standing or seated by sweeping your arms across the front of your body as you turn to look behind yourself. Do it standing, or seated. When you are sitting, sit comfortably upright towards the front of a seat. Slowly twist to one side as if to look back over your shoulder, reaching one hand across the front of your body and the other behind yourself to help coordinate this rotation. Let the knee that you're turning away from slide forward, if it wants to, so that you don't put pressure on your lower back. Then do the equivalent twist to the other side. Spinal twists are a feature of many yoga postures.

Combining These Movements

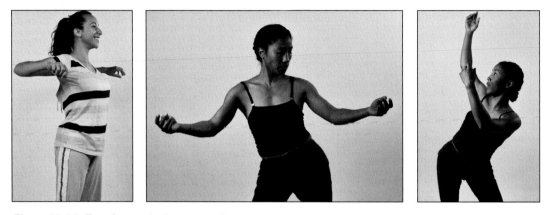

Figure 25.19: Free form spinal movements.

You can combine these movements in various ways, both structured and in a more 'free form' way to play with the inherent suppleness of your whole spine.

Strengthen the 'Core' Muscles of the Lower Trunk

It can be useful to follow these with Pilates, yoga or similar exercises to strengthen the 'core' muscles of the lower trunk, particularly if you have a tendency to hunch or bend in the lower back.

Review

The role of the trunk in massage is to transmit the power generated in your lower body to your arms.

Don't stand still as you massage, as this would cut you off from the power of your lower body and lead to overusing your upper back and shoulders.

Only reach along or across the table as far as you comfortably can without putting pressure on your lower back. Change position to avoid trying to reach too far.

Reposition yourself when necessary to keep your whole body facing your working hands so that you avoid twisting your trunk.

Bend your knees for swaying in order to take pressure off your lower back.

Bend your front knee when swaying forward in the lunge stance. Have a wide enough stance that you can bend your knee and straighten your back leg as you sway forward.

In the horse stance, soften both knees for swaying from side to side.

Increase the pressure by leaning your weight forward. Bend your knees and push from your legs to move forward more easily.

When lifting the client's leg or arm, use your legs to lift it and not your back.

When you are pulling a limb to stretch it, 'sit' back rather than just pulling with your upper body.

Be careful not to hunch over when focusing on your massage, or to stand stiffly upright rather than leaning your whole trunk forward.

The ideal is to keep your back relatively 'straight' but not stiff, which enables you to keep your trunk strong and supple.

Get regular massages and do activities that keep your back moving, and/or do stretching exercises to keep your back supple.

Simple exercises for maintaining trunk suppleness include flexion and extension, side-bending movements, spinal twists and combinations of these.

CHAPTER 26

Monitoring Your Breathing

Massage practitioners often instruct *clients* to focus on their breathing in order to help the process of letting go of tension. But we can forget to pay attention to *our own breathing* as we massage, and how it relates to the mood, rhythm and pacing of our work.

How do you, the practitioner, breathe as you massage? Do you find yourself holding your breath when you are applying pressure? Are you hunched over as you work and therefore unable to take in all the air that you need? Does your breathing 'wind you up' so that you end each massage exhausted? Or does it help you to remain calm and to pace yourself evenly?

Like many other aspects of bodyuse, our breathing patterns are usually unconscious until they cause us difficulties. This chapter highlights common breathing restrictions and offers suggestions for regaining the natural capacity of your breathing. It also focuses on how to coordinate your breathing with your massage strokes and how to use it to calm and pace yourself in massage sessions.

Breathing and Activity

The human body can build up reserves of many of the substances that it needs, but is unable to store more than a few minutes worth of oxygen, so we need to breathe constantly. Oxygen is used in the cells to help break down sugars, which releases energy to fuel the functioning of each cell and to maintain the body temperature. It is also the basis of the energy required for muscular activity, so we need to breathe more fully when we're involved in any physical activity – including massage.

Breathing plays an interesting role in the physiology of the body, because it can be consciously controlled but is also regulated by involuntary mechanisms. The autonomic nervous system regulates changes in our breathing patterns in response to the demands of the physical activities that we undertake, and our state of stress or relaxation. If you are involved in strenuous activity, for example, your breathing will speed up to get more air into your lungs (and your heart rate will increase to circulate the absorbed oxygen faster to your muscles). However we can also consciously control our breathing to some extent, for example by holding the breath, taking deep breaths to calm ourselves, or when we fit our breathing to the rhythms of physical activity.

The physiological needs of an activity is one factor in determining one's breathing. But breathing is also linked to one's habits and to one's frame of mind, whether this is conscious or not. Breathing is subject to unconscious control via our ingrained habits and the subconscious ways that we operate in our lives. This can be seen, for example, in the fulsome breathing developed through a lifetime of swimming, the tendency to restricted breathing due to a habitual hunched posture, the tense breathing pattern of someone with asthma (even when the asthma is not presently active), and the fast, shallow breathing that helps keep a 'born worrier' wound up. Breathing is thus a bridge between involuntary responses, conscious control and subconscious habits.

Restricted Breathing

How we hold our bodies can place physical restrictions on our capacity to breathe fully. Poor posture, being tense and holding the breath are common problems.

Hunching Over

If your back is strong and supple (see Chapter 25) and well supported by your pelvis (see Chapter 27), this will encourage easy, deep breathing.

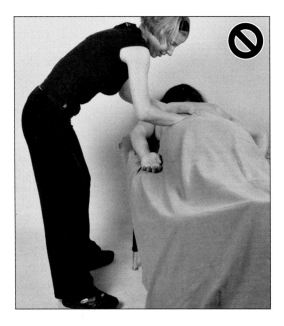

Figure 26.1: Hunching over, which restricts breathing.

However, if you are hunched over as you massage, this not only reduces your ability to transfer the power generated in your lower body (see Chapter 28) through your trunk (see Chapter 25) to your arms (see Chapter 23). It also impedes your ability to breathe fully, which of course reduces your ability to sustain your energy and stamina in massage sessions.

Many of us hunch over when we are focusing intently, for example when learning a new stroke or watching carefully for the client's reactions. In this case, you may just need to remind yourself to straighten up (and probably also to relax your shoulders, see Chapter 22), to bend forward with your whole trunk rather than hunching over, and to deepen your breathing.

However, if hunching over is a long-term habit, you will need to give it more attention. Receiving deep massage can be very helpful to release the muscular tensions that maintain this posture. Yoga, the Alexander Technique, the Feldenkrais Method® and Pilates also have valuable exercises that you can use to establish and maintain length in your trunk without rigidity. And you can also use the exercises in the previous chapter (see figures 25.16–25.18).

Stress

When we are stressed for any length of time and consequently tensing our bodies, there's a related tendency to hold the breath (which often feeds back into the cycle of tensing up). One way to break out of this impasse is to consciously take some deep breaths. Another is to undertake physical activity that requires fuller breathing to meet the demands of the body for oxygen to support the activity. These practices will get your breathing kick-started again. (Obviously, it is also important to address the situations that are causing you stress).

Tensing Up When Focusing on a Task

Many of us have the habit of tensing up (and holding the breath) when we focus on a physical task. If you notice this, take a few moments to consciously relax your body and let your breathing soften with as little disruption to the massage as you can manage. This is easiest when you are doing a slow sliding stroke or when you are applying static pressure. With practise it becomes possible to do this with any stroke without stopping or disrupting the massage.

Tension Due to Lack of Activity

And tension can build up from a lack of physical activity and a sedentary lifestyle. The slow accumulation of tension in the back muscles, which is very common, will reduce your capacity to breathe as fully as you otherwise could. Therefore simple exercises for trunk flexibility (see figures 25.16–25.18) will enhance your ability to breath more fully. (Conversely, breathing more fully will help you to keep your spine supple).

Holding Your Breath

When first learning a new stroke, many people often hold their breath (and also tense their shoulders) as they focus on 'getting it right'. So it's important to practise new strokes until they become familiar enough that you can relax as you do them. In the process, regularly remind yourself to breathe easily and to relax your shoulders until this becomes an automatic part of doing the stroke.

If you are regularly holding your breath as you massage, this will interfere with the evenness of your bodyuse and therefore of your massage strokes, even when you are otherwise using your body well. It will reduce your stamina and your ability to pace yourself in massage sessions. It is also likely that you will be tensing your body unnecessarily and working harder than is comfortable. It is especially common to hold the breath when applying firm pressure in massage. This is generally quite unconscious, but you can learn to change this habit once you begin paying attention to it. Try *exhaling* instead as you press or push (below).

Bear in mind that you may also be unconsciously tensing up and holding your breath at times in reaction to a client. This may happen, for example, when you are dealing with difficult, demanding or critical clients, or uncommunicative clients whose responses are therefore hard to read. Remind yourself to relax your breathing and your shoulders to avoid getting into the vicious cycle of becoming more and more 'wound up' which would make it harder for you to deal with the situation.

Using Your Breathing in Massage Sessions

Having focused on avoiding restricted breathing habits, it is also important to think about using your breathing in a more pro-active way. What can be applied to massage from the breathing protocols of exercise systems and sporting activities?

Building your physical stamina for doing massage includes the development of your breathing in a similar way to an athlete. Athletes generally have two main concerns with breathing – developing their overall breathing stamina (which is looked at below, see figures 26.5–26.8), and developing breathing patterns that fit their activity.

Breathing With the Rhythm of Massage Strokes

When they are first learning massage, people often work fast and jerkily in their desire to fit as many strokes as possible into each session. However, this is tiring for the practitioner and can be unsettling for the client. Many rhythmical activities, such as swimming and running, involve the conscious use of the breath to work with the rhythms of the activity. Using your breathing in a similar way in massage strokes will help you to establish an even working rhythm. This enables you to deliver your massage with ease, power and fluidity and to pace yourself in each massage session.

Establishing a Breathing Rhythm With Effleurage Strokes

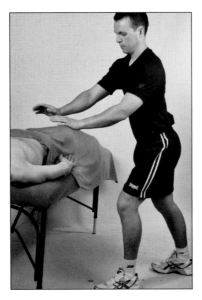

Figure 26.2: 'Miming' massage strokes to explore breathing patterns.

A simple way of connecting your breathing with massage strokes to pace yourself is to begin away from the table. Sway forward and back as you would for doing an effleurage stroke to establish a rhythm with it. Then incorporate a breathing pattern of breathing out as you push forward and breathing in as you pull back. When you have settled into this, do it with a partner on the massage table.

Exhaling When Applying Pressure

Another common problem is forcefully inhaling or holding your breath when you're applying pressure. This is likely to lead to stiffening up, instead of using your body in a powerful *and* relaxed way.

Therefore, if this is a habit, it's worth taking time to focus on this. When you are about to apply pressure, pause for a moment, relax your shoulders and trunk and then gently breathe out as you do the technique. This will enable you to combine ease with power and to maintain the evenness of the stroke.

Practice doing this at each stage of the massage at which you would usually tense up, until it becomes second nature to breathe out when you are applying pressure. Of course, you can also do this with any other strokes in which you tend to hold your breath or breathe in forcefully. The other types of strokes that most commonly need this attention are percussion strokes, pushing away from yourself in sliding strokes, and when you are lifting and/or stretching the client's limbs.

Breathing Patterns for Applying Pressure

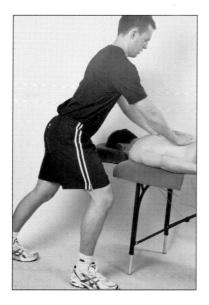

Fig 26.3: Leaning forward to apply pressure.

Try the following experiment to feel the effects of your breathing on firm massage strokes. Try it on a partner and then have them do it to you, so that you can feel the effects from both sides. Apply firm pressure on one place on your partner's body. Firstly, hold your breath as you apply and maintain the pressure. People generally notice a tendency to tense up as they do this. Then apply pressure again, this time breathing in strongly as you do so. Most people find that this produces a similar response. Finally, breathe out *evenly but not forcefully* as you apply the pressure. Then let your breathing remain as even as possible as you maintain the pressure. This generally enables the practitioner to remain more relaxed without losing power.

Then try doing a firm sliding stroke with each of these breathing patterns. Here too, people generally find that breathing out as they push forward enables them to remain more relaxed and to maintain an even pressure.

Then have your partner do the same to you. When she holds her breath as she delivers a powerful stroke, you're quite likely to notice the instinctive reactions to this in your own body. It commonly triggers an instinctive wariness in recipients, which may include holding *their* breath and tensing up.

If your partner then applies the same powerful stroke on you while breathing out easily, your body is less likely to react against it (unless the pressure is too much). Although your breathing may speed up a little as you 'meet the challenge' of the pressure and accustom yourself to it (and practitioners sometimes encourage the client to consciously deepen their breathing to 'go with it' more), your body is more likely to soften and let the pressure in (as long as it is manageable).

Sustaining Stamina

We often observe clients' breathing as an indication of their present state of stress and coping, and also of their character and approach to life, for example anxious, calm, excitable, high energy, or ponderous. We also use it as a monitor of the process of relaxation during the massage. Slowing and softening of the breathing is generally a sign of relaxation, a deep sigh often indicates a significant point of letting go, while a sharp intake of breath or a sudden holding of the breath indicate disruption to this process of relaxing. We can also watch for these same cues in our own breathing.

For example, stress and anxiety can lead to shallow breathing. If you are going through a stressful time in your life, you may find it helpful to start a massage session slowly while you focus on engaging your breathing and deepening it. Then, gradually increase the rhythm of your strokes at a rate at which you can comfortably maintain full, even breathing. This will enable you to sustain your energy for the whole massage without exhausting yourself. (At the end of the massage, you may also find that, as with any sustained physical activity, working in this way has given you renewed energy to tackle life's problems or, at the very least, to be less weighed down by them).

You can use strong and slightly faster breathing to *energise* yourself, but don't make it too fast or jerky to avoid winding yourself up.

Pacing Yourself

In many sports, breathing patterns are designed not only to fit the rhythm of movement and the energy requirements of the activity, but also to develop and maintain stamina and to focus mental concentration. Runners, swimmers and cyclists sustain and pace themselves with even, rhythmical breathing. Breathing patterns will be different for short bursts of activity, such as a short hurdle race, compared to more sustained activities such as a long distance run, a sports match or delivering a massage treatment. Keeping your breathing even and steady will help you to pace yourself, like a long distance runner or swimmer. This is preferable to exhausting yourself by expending all of your energy in a few minutes, in the equivalent of a one hundred metre dash.

At the other end of the scale, pacing does not mean working with a lacklustre level of energy, of course. You can pace yourself while varying the power, focus and rhythm appropriately throughout the massage session.

Of course, your breathing needs to deepen because you are doing physical work, but match it to the rhythm of your work to pace yourself. This is especially important when you need to retain your energy for a full working day, not just one session. If you have a tendency to wind yourself up with your breathing in massage sessions, you may find it useful to pause and breathe out when you catch yourself doing this, and then start again with a relaxed breathing cycle.

Obviously, your breathing rhythms will need to change as you do different types of strokes and also as you vary the 'mood' of the massage (from fast percussion to slow, deep pressure strokes, and from relaxing strokes to invigorating techniques). However, take care not to get into a cycle of just breathing fast and shallowly when you're doing fast strokes such as energising percussion, as this can quickly become tiring.

Bear in mind that if you are able to *gradually* increase your massage workload, your breathing will probably develop strength and efficiency to cope with the increasing requirements. If, however, you suddenly take on a full massage job, breathing will be just one of the aspects that you will need to concentrate on developing.

Calming and Centering

You can calm and centre yourself before a massage session, by taking a few deep breaths instead of just rushing in headlong. This can be useful at the beginning of your working day, especially if you have had a stressful time getting to work or you have home/work problems that you find difficult to disengage from. You may also find it helpful to take a few calming breaths if you are nervous about meeting a new client. This will help you to greet clients with a calm 'bedside manner' that helps to establish a relaxed, professional atmosphere for the session.

If you are feeling 'wound up', take a few minutes to focus on calming down if you can. Sit comfortably, mentally 'switch off' from your surroundings, and defocus or shut your eyes to help you to focus on your breathing. When you are tense, the tendency is to breathe shallowly and either to hold your breath or to be breathing quite fast. Therefore, without forcing it, gradually deepen your breathing a little more on each breath. At the same time, slow your breathing down by gently extending the length of each inhalation and exhalation. When you're breathing fully and slowly, maintain this for a minute to settle into it. If you want to focus more on relaxed breathing, yoga and meditation teachers and many stress management consultants can give you further practical instruction.

Of course, your breathing will speed up to meet the physical demands of doing a massage. However, keeping your breathing even will help you to sustain this centered attitude during the session. It also keeps the massage smooth and relaxing for the recipient, even if you are working firmly and deeply or doing strong stretches.

Expanding Your Breathing

The rest of this chapter looks at ways of expanding your breathing potential. It firstly covers some activities and exercise systems that incorporate a focus on breathing and then describes some simple breathing exercises that you may find helpful.

Activities That Help Breathing

A number of sports activities that include a focus on developing one's breathing and the ability to coordinate it with movement have already been mentioned in this chapter, such as swimming, running, and many martial arts. In addition, yoga, the Alexander Technique, and the Feldenkrais Method® all focus directly on relaxing and expanding the breathing, and many meditation systems focus on calming one's breathing.

Singing is helpful for expanding the energy and capacity of your breathing. (If you get singing coaching, make sure that your teacher is *not* of the old school approach, that demands great *tension* for singing). Learning to play a wind instrument will also help you to deepen and control your breathing. I have a friend who keeps his asthma under control by playing dijeridu.

Softening the Back Muscles

Bear in mind that tight back and chest muscles restrict one's ability to breathe. They can be softened via direct massage work, especially deep tissue massage, and also through stretches and body rocking movements applied by the practitioner. Many exercises systems include warm-up stretches that you can use to increase the suppleness of your trunk. You can also use the suppleness exercises in the previous chapter for this (see figures 25.16–25.18). Yoga, the Alexander Technique and the Feldenkrais Method® can all help to release back tension.

Images of the Lungs and Breathing

Before beginning the exercises below, it may be useful to review the structure of the lungs and the muscles that move them, and to look at images which some people find can help them to visualise and understand the working of the lungs.

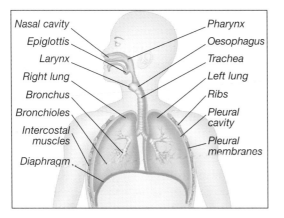
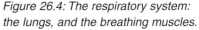

Figure 26.4: The respiratory system: the lungs, and the breathing muscles.

The lungs are soft spongy material, primarily made up of the air sacs (alveoli), the air tubes (bronchioles) that lead to them and the blood vessels which surround them. The lungs are surrounded by membranes (the pleural sacs), which attach them to the inside of the ribs and the top of the diaphragm. The expansion of the lungs in inhalation is due to muscles stretching them. The major breathing muscle is the diaphragm, which stretches the lungs downwards to expand their volume for inhalation. It is assisted by the external intercostal muscles, which run between consecutive ribs. They lift the ribs and thereby widen the chest cavity. When these muscles relax, it allows exhalation as the lungs reduce in size. In forceful inhalation and exhalation, other muscles in the chest, back and neck can come into play to increase the action of the ribs.

Imagining the Lungs as a Balloon

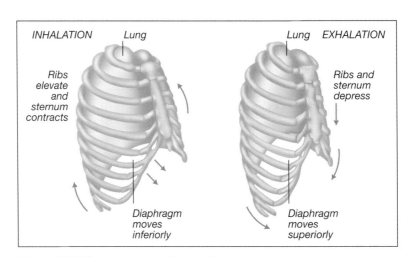

Figure 26.5: The mechanics of respiration.

Many people find it useful to imagine the lungs as a balloon (or as two balloons joined together – one for each lung) to help their understanding of breathing. In inhalation the balloon expands; and it deflates somewhat as we exhale. This balloon image makes it easier to picture the three-dimensional process of breathing. As we breathe in, the lungs have the potential for expansion downwards (the action of the diaphragm), and also forwards, backwards and sideways (via the action of the intercostal muscles in moving the ribs).

Exercises for Expanding Your Breathing Potential

The exercises below are designed to help you to reawaken your capacity to use your lungs in each of these dimensions. When doing them, bear in mind that different activities (including different massage strokes) require different breathing patterns. Therefore the exercises are only intended to expand your *general* breathing capacity; they don't offer a formula for 'correct' breathing. I emphasise this, because people sometimes have the idea that there is one single 'correct' way to breathe. However the best breathing practice utilises the capability of your lungs *according to the activity that you are doing,* depending on whether it's highly active such as playing sports or sitting quietly and reading or watching television.

The focus of the exercises is mostly on inhalation, as that is the active part of the breathing cycle when we are standing or sitting upright. Exhalation is more passive, unless we are controlling the rate of breathing out (as in singing, public speaking or playing a wind instrument), breathing out forcefully (for example, blowing out a candle or the yell that is often used to accompany a karate blow), or hanging upside down.

If focusing on breathing is unfamiliar to you, don't be discouraged if at first you feel that you are not able to achieve much change in your breathing. This takes time and practise, so persevere. It will also take practise to retain this extra capacity when you are focusing on doing a massage.

When you are first working with these breathing exercises, it is helpful to practise them regularly. Once they are somewhat familiar, it will only take a few minutes each time to reacquaint yourself with your breathing potential. You could do this between clients for example or during breaks. (This will also help you to re-centre yourself during your working day). Once you have established a feel for breathing in each area without needing to put your hands on, you can practice it anywhere at any time that you have a few minutes.

When you have expanded the capacity of your lungs in this way, regularly remind yourself to not hold your breath in massage sessions.

Breathing With the Front

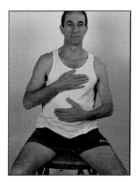

Figure 26.6: Breathing with the front of the trunk – hand positions.

Most people find it easiest to feel the front part of their breathing. Either sit, or lie on your back. Place one hand on your upper abdomen, just below the arch of your ribs, and the other across your upper chest. Your hands will help you to focus on the main areas that move as you breathe.

As you breathe in, focus firstly on breathing deeply 'into your belly'. It's not easy to sense the diaphragm directly, but this deep breathing which also involves the lower ribs (the lowest area of the actual lungs) will activate it. Don't deliberately push your belly out, but allow the action of your diaphragm to push down on your abdominal contents which in turn causes your belly to swell. Then continue breathing in, allowing your lower ribs to swell and then your upper chest to expand under your upper hand.

In breathing out, let these areas relax.

Breathing at the Side

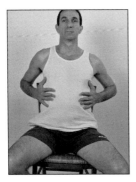

Figure 26.7: Side breathing – hand position.

Place your hands on the sides of your lower ribs to feel the sideways expansion and deflation, or, if you're trying this with a partner, have them place their hands on the side of your ribs. Do this breathing either sitting or standing.

It is easiest to feel the movement in this area, by firstly exhaling as completely as you can without strain. This produces a narrowing of your lower ribs. If you then hold your breath out for a few moments, so that you have to take in a full breath fairly quickly, you will feel the significant sideways expansion of your lower ribs with this reflex in-breath. Or you could yawn as you breathe in to maximise the extent of the in-breath. (You will probably also feel a swelling forward of your lower ribs and upper abdomen accompanying this).

Repeat this cycle a few times to establish a clear sense of the movement. As you become familiar with this sideways expansion and reduction and are able to exercise more control over it, you won't need to push your breath out so strongly to initiate the expansive movements of your ribs on the inhalation.

Breathing at the Back

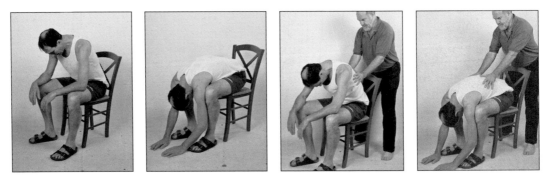

Figure 26.8: Sitting for back breathing exercises; a) sitting with forearms on the knees,
b) sitting with the chest on the knees, c), d) with partner's hands on the back of the lower ribs.

The backwards dimension of breathing is generally the least familiar. For many people, it's easiest to activate it by sitting in a chair and leaning forward. Rest your forearms on your knees or, if it is comfortable, drop your chest to your knees. By restricting your ability to use the front part of your breathing, this position will help you to focus on your back. It can be helpful to have a partner to help you to focus here too, by placing his hands on the back of your lower ribs.

With each in-breath, focus on a backwards expansion of the lower ribs. This will inevitably incorporate some sideways expansion as well. Let it relax on the out-breath.

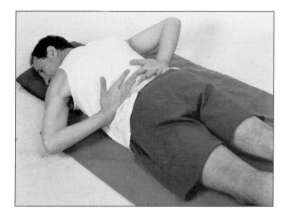

Figure 26.9: Back breathing while lying prone.

This can also be done lying on your front on a mat on the floor if it is comfortable for you, or on a massage table. Lie with your head turned to whichever side that you find most comfortable. Put the back of your hands on the back or side of your lower ribs, so that you are able to rest your elbows on the floor and relax your arms. This position will restrict your forward breathing, which invites you to focus even more on the breathing at the back. As you breathe in, let your hands be pushed a little backwards (up towards the ceiling) and a little sideways. They will settle back as you let your breath out.

Three-dimensional Breathing

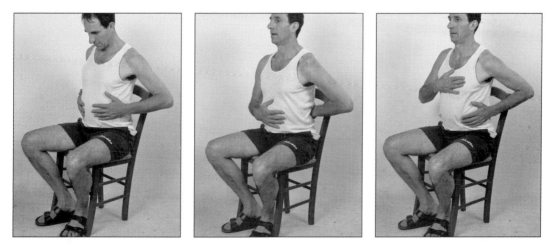

Figure 26.10: Placing the hands in different areas to help focus on breathing in three dimensions.

Then practice coordinating these three dimensions of breathing when you are sitting. Place your hands on each area in turn to focus there – on your lower ribs at the front, at the side, at the back, and simultaneously at the front and back. Do this initially with your hands on each area in turn for a full breath in to feel the expansion of that area as you inhale. When it becomes more familiar, moving your hands to each of these areas during each single in-breath will help you to focus on simultaneous, coordinated expansion of all of them.

Review

Paying attention to your breathing as you massage will help you to sustain your stamina, to maintain an even rhythm and to pace yourself.

If you need to calm and centre yourself in preparation for a massage session, take a few deep breaths.

If you are feeling quite 'wound up', take a few minutes to focus on calming down by gradually slowing and deepening your breathing.

Use strong and slightly faster breathing to *energise* yourself, but don't make it too fast or jerky to avoid winding yourself up.

Keeping your breathing even and steady will help you to pace yourself, like a long distance runner or swimmer, so that you don't end up exhausted after each massage that you do.

Avoid hunching over as you massage, which restricts your breathing.

Watch out for the tendency to hold your breath when you are learning new strokes, applying pressure, focusing intently on the client's responses, or dealing with a difficult client.

Take some deep breaths to relax your breathing whenever you notice yourself tensing up.

When doing strokes in which you habitually hold your breath, pause for a moment, relax your shoulders and then gently breathe out as you do the technique.

When you are applying pressure, try gently exhaling in order to avoid tensing up.

Tension in your back muscles will restrict your breathing, so keep your trunk supple through flexibility exercises and/or receiving massages.

Singing and playing wind instruments will help you to deepen and control your breathing.

When doing breathing exercises, focus on expanding your lungs for inhalation and allowing them to reduce on the exhalation. Placing your hands on various parts of your ribs will help you to feel this.

CHAPTER 27

The Central Role of the Pelvis

The primary role of the pelvis in massage is to transmit the power generated in your legs to your trunk, from where it can then be transmitted to your working hands or forearms. However the pelvis is not just the link between the legs and the trunk. It is also the area of the body around which movement can be centered for greatest power, fluidity and coordination.

The pelvis is also important in the alignment of your body. Your hips monitor whether your body is aligned behind your working hands, which enables the power of your lower body to be transmitted to your hands.

The Structure of the Pelvis

Before looking at the role of the pelvis in action, it's useful to briefly review relevant aspects of the bony structure and the associated musculature. It is also helpful to clarify some terminology. In this book, I am using the term *pelvis* in the anatomical sense for the combination of the innominate bones (the 'hip' bones) and the sacrum. I will use the term *hips* in the common language way to refer to the general area and *hip bones* to refer to the innominate bones, particularly the forward-projecting parts of the iliums (ilia). The *hip joint* is the junction between the head of the femur and the innominate bones at the acetabulum.

The Bones of the Pelvis

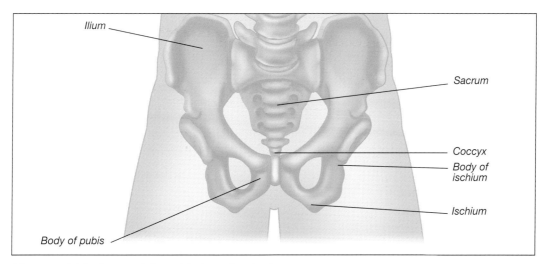

Figure 27.1: The bones of the pelvis (anterior view).

The pelvis is made up of the two innominate bones (the 'hip' bones, each comprised of an ilium, ischium and pubis) and the sacrum (the lowest weight bearing bone of the spine, which consists of five fused vertebrae) and the coccyx (the bottom fused bones of the spine).

The Muscles That Control the Pelvis

The strongest muscles of the body, coming from the legs and the trunk, attach to these central bones. The relationship between the legs and trunk is coordinated by these muscles, together with the iliopsoas muscles that cross the hip joint without directly attaching to the pelvis. Working together, all of these muscles control how you stand and walk, and how your trunk is balanced and supported on your legs. They enable us to control the movements of the pelvis and therefore to move around our centre of gravity in a powerful, coordinated way.

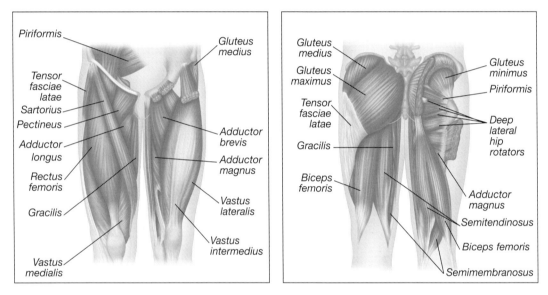

Figure 27.2i: The muscles of the pelvis; a) anterior view; b) posterior view.

The main muscles in this area are:

- Those of the buttocks, the gluteals and the deep lateral hip rotators, including piriformis, and;
- The thigh muscles which cross the hip joint; the hamstrings (biceps femoris, semitendinosus, semimembranosus) at the back of the thigh, the adductors, including gracilis, on the inner thigh, the tensor fasciae latae on the outside of the thigh, rectus femoris (part of quadriceps) at the front, and sartorius, which also crosses the front of the thigh.

Also the lower trunk muscles, which are involved in maintaining posture. The:

- Iliopsoas muscles, arising deep in the abdomen and attaching to the femur;
- Erector spinae muscle group, running from the sacrum up alongside the spine, and quadratus lumborum in the lower back, and;
- Abdominal muscles.

Via this last group of muscles, movement of the pelvis can initiate and support movement of the whole trunk. This is why developing the core strength of the lower trunk muscles (a particular focus of yoga and Pilates) will help this area to support upright posture.

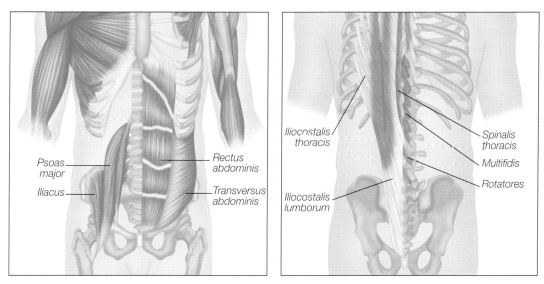

Figure 27.2ii: The muscles connecting the trunk and pelvis; a) anterior view, b) posterior view.

Movement Centered Around the Pelvis/Hips

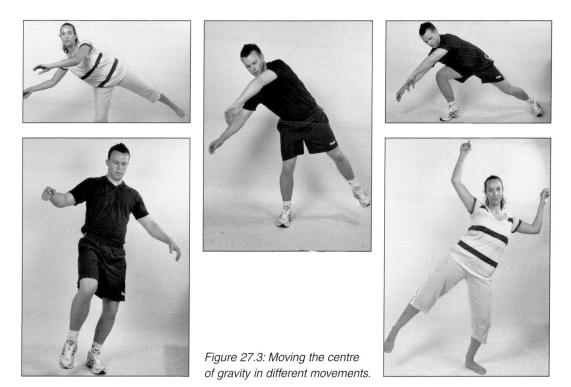

Figure 27.3: Moving the centre of gravity in different movements.

Functionally, in movement, the pelvis is at the centre of the body. The body's centre of gravity (the balance point of the body's weight) is within the lower abdomen. It is not located in a single point but moves around within a roughly spherical shape within this area, depending on our activities, for example leaning in one direction or stretching out our limbs. The bones of the pelvis surround this area. Movement which is centered around the pelvis is therefore also centered round the centre of gravity.

In Sport

Our increasingly sedentary lives tend to cut us off from our lower body and the potential power to be gained through the coordinated use of the legs and pelvis. However, when the power behind arm movements is centred around the pelvis (the hips), there is a combination of strength, evenness and precision in action. This can be seen in the gracefulness of a good golf swing or tennis stroke, in professional cricket and baseball games (both in batting and ball throwing), and in skilful judo or aikido throws. It can also be observed in Tai Chi, in which the movements are slower but still centered around the pelvis.

In Massage

Incorporating this quality of movement into massage enables us to work more strongly and fluidly and with less effort than if we stand stiffly and only use our shoulder and arm muscles. This takes pressure off the practitioner's back and shoulders while delivering power, where appropriate, and evenness to the massage strokes.

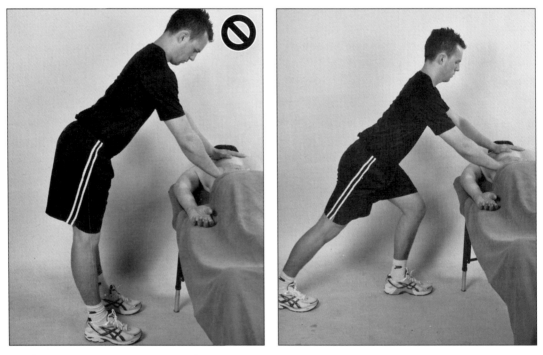

Figure 27.4: Stiff or moving pelvis; a) stiff legs leads to stiff pelvis and overusing the upper body, b) bending the knees when applying stationary pressure.

Many massage beginners stand with straight legs and only bend in the lower or midback as they initially focus on learning strokes. This stiffens the pelvis and stops the power from the legs being transmitted to the trunk. It puts pressure on the part of the back that is bending (usually the lower back) and leads to overusing the upper body. So the common instruction given to novices is to bend the knees (see figure 28.35) and sway the body. (This is usually combined with directions to relax the shoulders and breathing so that the power generated in the lower body can be transferred unimpeded to the arms and hands).

Even when you are applying stationary pressure, it is important to soften your knees and lean your body for the power.

Mobilising Your Hips

Exercises for Mobilising the Hips

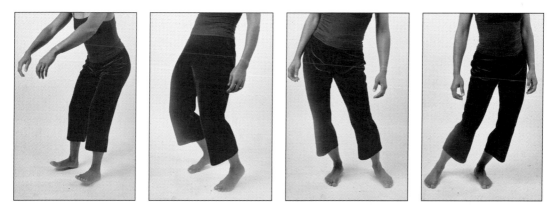

Figure 27.5: Mobilising the hips and lower back – swaying and circling the hips.

If you tend to stiffen your legs as you massage, simple warm-up exercises will help you to mobilise your hips. The easiest to do is a hip circle. Stand with your feet at least as far apart as the width of your hips. Sway your hips from side to side, and forward and back. Then take them in a circle as if you were keeping a hoop spinning. Of course, as you do these movements, you are simultaneously mobilising your lower back and also getting movement in your knees, your ankles and your feet. So this is a good way of getting movement throughout your lower body. As you do this, you will notice how moving your hips also gets your upper body moving.

Mobilising the Hips With Massage Movements

The following movements will help you to develop your sense of the relationship between the movement of your hips and your hands. Try them away from the table at first. When this 'air massage' feels comfortable and familiar, return to the massage table, and focus on creating the same feeling while working on a partner. Begin with the massage movements described below, and then try applying this principle to other strokes.

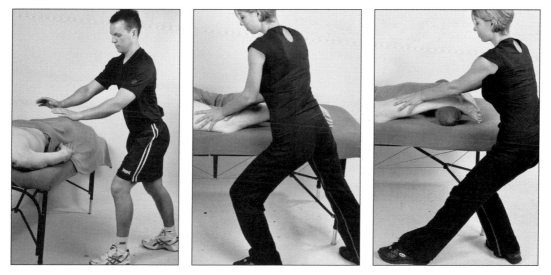

Figure 27.6: Mobilising the hips for effleurage movements; a) swaying forward and back, b), c), working on a partner.

Practise swaying your hips forward and back in the lunge stance, which is a common massage stance for effleurage strokes and travelling kneading and compression strokes. Stand with one foot forward from the other, and sway forward and backwards. These movements mobilise the whole of your lower body. It is useful to do them with your feet different distances apart to prepare for a range of massage situations. Then practice with your other foot forward. Reaching forward with your arms as you do this will help you to feel how this can deliver power and fluidity to effleurage strokes.

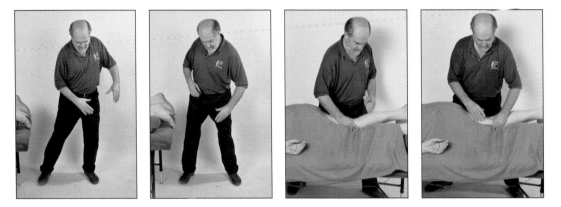

Figure 27.7: Swaying side to side for a hand-to-hand kneading movement; a), b) 'air' kneading, c), d) working on the adductors.

In the horse stance (with your feet alongside one another), you can sway side to side to move your hands as if you were doing a large hand to hand kneading stroke on the inner side of the client's thigh (on the adductors). Practise this as 'air massage' and then take it to the table.

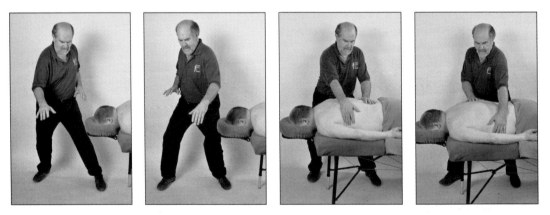

Figure 27.8: Twisting your hips in a wringing stroke; a), b) 'air' wringing, c), d) working on a partner.

It can also be useful to practise alternately twisting each hip forward, as in a wringing movement. Try this with your feet alongside one another (in a horse stance, see figure 28.32). Have your arms loosely reaching out in front of your body, so that you can feel how this movement can push one arm forward while simultaneously pulling the other back.

Aligning Your Body Behind Your Hands for Strokes That Involve Pressure

There is another way in which your hips are important in massage – as a monitor of whether your body is behind your working hands or forearm, etc. (The next chapter looks at the alignment between your feet, knees and hips, see figures 29.15–29.21).

Hands in Front of the Hips for Pressure Techniques

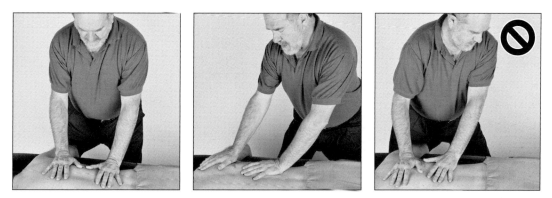

Figure 27.9: Working hands when applying pressure; a), b) in front of the hips, c) not in front of the hips.

When you are applying pressure, either stationary or sliding, have your hips facing towards your working hand(s). Otherwise, your upper body will be twisted, causing possible strain and reducing the effective transmission of force from your lower body. Having your hips aligned with your hands enables you to keep your hands relatively relaxed for the delivery of strong pressure, when appropriate.

Turning to Change the Direction of Applying Power

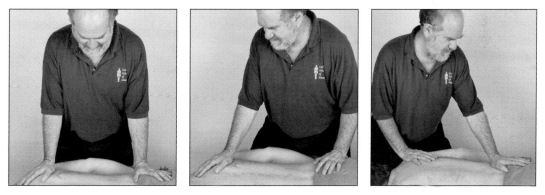

Figure 27.10: Hands safely in front of the hips; a) stretching equally along the length of the client's back, b), c) turning to lean more weight onto one hand.

When you are applying *equal pressure* with your hands (or forearms), it's only safe to move your hands out of this alignment when you are sliding them apart equally as you lean your weight forward, for example when you are doing a stretch which spreads up and down the client's back or limb.

If you want to deliver more weight to one hand, turn your hips so that they face more towards this hand. The other hand may then be out of the spotlight. This is not a problem unless you are trying to maintain the same pressure through it, in which case you will be overusing your shoulder muscles (and probably still not achieving equal pressure).

The 'Hip Spotlight'

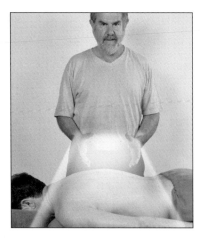

Figure 27.11: The 'hip spotlight'.

An image that helps many people maintain the alignment of their hips and working hands is to imagine that you have a spotlight shining forward from your hips. When you are using *both* hands at the same time to apply *equal pressure*, keeping your hands within the hip spotlight will help you to keep your hands and hips aligned. The following experiment will help you to work with the feeling of this hip spotlight.

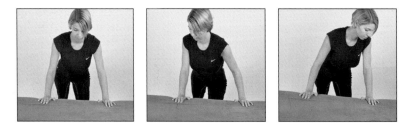

Figure 27.12: Feeling the 'hip spotlight' as the hips are turned;
a) weight centrally, b) weight more on one hand,
c) weight more on the other hand.

Stand facing across the massage couch in a lunge stance and put both hands on the surface of the couch. Lean forward a little so that some of your weight is on your hands. Then turn your hips slowly to the right and to the left. Notice that your weight is only delivered equally to both hands when they are both centrally within the spotlight. Your weight will be delivered much more to one hand when the 'spotlight' is focused primarily on that hand.

You may then find it useful to try this on a partner on the couch, to help you to get used to focusing in this way when you are working on a client.

When you are seated, it is important to regularly reposition yourself so that your hips face your working hands as much as possible for the same reasons.

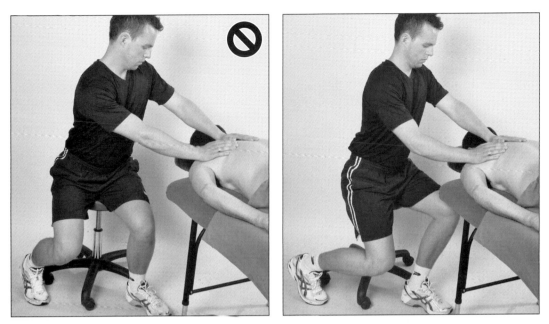

Figure 27.13: Seated massage; a) hips turned away from hands, b) hips towards hands.

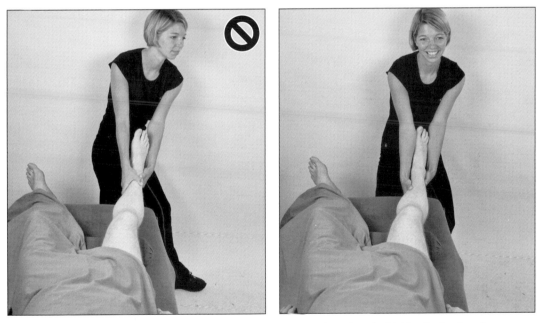

Figure 27.14: Stretching the client's leg, a) hips turned away from hands, b) hips facing hands.

When you are applying stretches, have your hips facing the client and the back of your pelvis towards the direction in which you will need to move for the stretch. If you want to sway from side to side while maintaining the stretch, for example when stretching a prone client's leg (see figure 39.19), keep the back of your pelvis facing away from the client.

The Energy Centre

In addition to these structural ways of thinking about the pelvis and using it, practitioners of shiatsu and many Eastern martial arts refer to centering yourself in the *hara* – the energy centre of the body in the lower abdomen – in order to work simultaneously with vitality and relaxation. This area is considered to be the centre of one's life force. The 'tan tien', the centre point of the hara, is described as being in the lower abdomen, three fingers width below the navel. In shiatsu practice, 'working from the hara' incorporates the idea of moving from the postural centre, but also includes the sense of paying attention to and working with the energy of this centre of vitality.

Tuning in to the 'Hara'

Here is an exercise to help you to 'tune in' to the hara. It's hard to do more than hint at this process in a book. So, if you want to follow this up, find a shiatsu or martial arts teacher who can give you personal instruction that suits your style of learning.

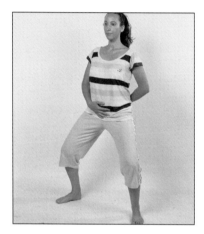

Figure 27.15: Tuning in to the hara.

Stand comfortably in the horse stance. Gently bend your knees a little and, if necessary, sway from side to side every little while to ensure that you don't stiffen in this position. (The exercise for mobilising your hips Is a useful preparation for tuning in to this area of your body, see figure 27.5).

Place one hand on the front of your lower abdomen and the other on your lower back directly behind it. Use your breathing to help you focus here. As you inhale, direct some of your breath into your lower abdomen, so that this area expands a little under your hands. As you are breathing in, imagine that you are also taking 'energy' into this area. Depending on what works for you, you might visualise this in the form of light or a particular colour, or feel it as a sense of expansiveness or filling up (for example with warmth), or as a vibration (such as an inner hum or 'buzz'). Let this area physically contract as you let your breath out, while you maintain the feeling of the 'energy' in your hara. Practise until you have consolidated the feeling of filling up your energy centre as you inhale and comfortably retaining this feeling of energy as you breathe out.

Then, each time that you exhale, imagine spreading this energy out into the rest of your body. Start with a small expansion, for example a little higher into your abdomen, and then, as you become more familiar with it, spread it further through your body with each breath. (Shiatsu practitioners often focus on two aspects – the energy connection to the ground, and the feeling that energy from the hara flows through the trunk and arms and to the hands).

When this process is familiar, combine it with movements of your hips. Begin to sway from side to side, forward and back, and then to turn from one side to the other. Start with small movements in each direction and keep them smooth while keeping your focus on the hara. Gradually make your movements more expansive as long as you are able to maintain this central focus. Then reach out with your arms as you sway. When all this is comfortable, try this at the massage table. With practise, you can learn to simultaneously focus on your hara to keep your movements centered and energised *and* on the client.

Review

The primary role of the pelvis in massage is to transmit the power generated in your legs to your trunk, from where it can then be transmitted to your working hands or forearms.

When the power behind arm movements is centered around the pelvis (the hips), there is a combination of strength, fluidity and evenness in action.

Centre yourself in your hara in order to work with a combination of vitality and relaxation.

Swaying forward and backwards, from side to side and moving your hips in a circle are simple exercises to mobilise your hips.

When you are applying pressure with both hands, align your hips with your working hands (or forearm) to ensure that the power of your lower body is being transmitted to your hands.

Use the image of keeping your hands in the hip spotlight to help you to maintain this alignment.

When using both hands to apply pressure, only let your hands move out of the spotlight when you are sliding them apart to do a long sliding stretch.

If you want to deliver more weight to one hand, turn your hips so that they face more towards this hand.

Sway forward and back to initiate the ebb and flow of effleurage movements.

Sway from side to side to initiate the movement of large kneading strokes, for example when kneading the adductors on the inner thigh.

Practise twisting each hip forward alternately in the horse stance to initiate wringing strokes.

When stretching parts of the client's body, have your hips facing the client and the back of your pelvis facing the direction in which you move to do the stretch (the opposite direction).

CHAPTER 28

Generating Power From Your Lower Body

For people who have been taught to focus only on their hands, it can come as a surprise that the lower body has an equally significant role in massage. In order to save the smaller muscles of your arms and hands, *power* for your massage strokes and *fluidity* of delivery needs to be initiated in the large muscles of your legs. So, rather than standing still and relying on your shoulder muscles, the ideal is to lean and sway your body for this. The massage then starts 'from the ground up' and is transferred through your body to your hands.

This chapter focuses on this essential role of your legs in generating and transmitting power and fluidity to your upper body, and how the positioning and alignment of your feet, knees and hips supports this. It firstly covers some general principles about using your legs. It then looks in detail at how this applies in the lunge stance (having one foot forward) and the horse stance (having your feet side by side). The last part of the chapter covers ways of maintaining suppleness in your hips, knees, and ankles.

Using Your Legs Dynamically

Using your legs dynamically can be unfamiliar because life has become so sedentary for many of us in recent decades, due to the prevalence of computers, television, and cars. Most people do less everyday activities that exercise the legs such as walking, running, or cycling. Many people have little or no experience of activities which are built around lower body movements such as skiing, skating, surfing, or skateboarding, or of activities in which movement initiated in the legs is directed through the arms such as tennis, basketball, dancing or martial arts such as judo. Without this background, people often stand stiffly when they first work at the massage table, or stand in other ways that don't support dynamic activity.

Consequently, it may take you some time to develop the combination of mobility and stamina in your legs. Don't overdo it when you are first learning massage, but persevere in order to take pressure off your upper body. You may even find it helpful to take up one of the activities mentioned above to help the process along. While you may initially feel some aches in your legs as you use unfamiliar muscles, these will pass as you become more practised. And bear in mind that the leg muscles that you are using are bigger and stronger than the muscles of your shoulders and arms, which you are conserving.

Footwear

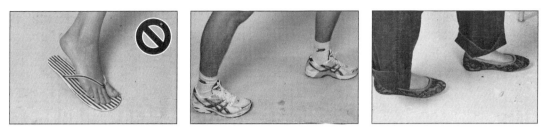

Figure 28.1: Working footwear; a) open-heeled footwear, b) trainers, c) flat-soled shoes.

As mentioned in Chapter 7, you need footwear that enables you to bend your knees and that will move with your feet. Open-heeled footwear would limit how freely you could move. If you are not accustomed to wearing flat-soled footwear, you may need to regularly stretch your calf muscles and quite possibly your hamstrings too (see figure 28.41).

Initiating Movement and Power From Your Lower Body

Align Your Feet and Hips Behind Your Hands
The position of your feet will determine the direction that your hips face.

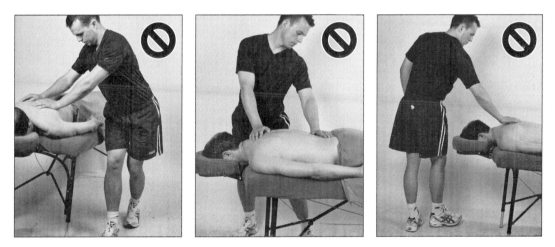

Figure 28.2: Not aligning the feet, hips and hands.

If your feet are turned away from your working hands, that will also turn your hips away from them (i.e. your hands will not be within the area of your hip spotlight, see figure 27.11). If your hips are not facing your hands when you are applying stationary or sliding pressure or pulling, your body will be twisted. This would diminish the force that is transmitted to your hands. It would also put pressure on your trunk, especially your lower back, and also on your hip joints, your knees and perhaps also your ankles.

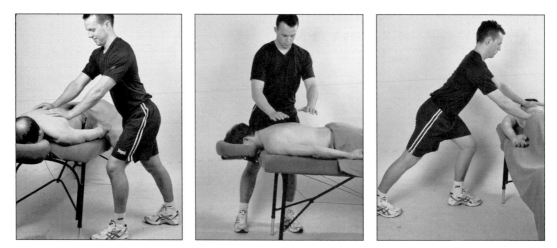

Figure 28.3: Aligning the feet, hips and hands.

The alignment of your feet, knees and hips is essential for the effective transfer of power from the ground up to your working tools (your hands/forearm, etc.). This, in turn, enables you to keep your shoulders and arms relatively relaxed, and to keep your hands free for the fine-tuning of the massage techniques.

Change Position to Keep Your Body Behind Your Hands

Two main stances are used in massage – the 'lunge' stance and the 'horse' stance (below). As you become skilled, you will no doubt discover ways of modifying and adapting them when you need to. After you are familiar with them, practise changing position so that you don't get stuck in any position for too long. And practise making the transitions smooth so that this doesn't interrupt the fluidity of the massage.

If you change the direction of your pressure and/or movement *without* reorienting yourself, you will be twisting your body and losing effectiveness. Initially, most people find it helpful to practise repositioning themselves for each new massage stroke, like a snooker player lining up for each successive shot (see figure 4.12). With experience, you will learn to move smoothly between strokes and, when appropriate, within strokes, and to coordinate this into a continuous, fluid '*dance*', like the moving 'dance' of a skilled tennis player (see figure 4.21).

Let Your Knees Bend

Standing stiff-legged prevents you from powering your massage strokes from your lower body. *Softening* your knees enough so that you have some 'give' in them is essential for being able to sway with your massage strokes. (However, don't bend them so much that you have to tense them to keep balance and end up in a stiff, awkward stance).

At first, your knees may be stiff and creaky as you bend them and sway your body, and you may be using leg muscles in unfamiliar ways. However, unless you have serious knee problems which are aggravated by bending and moving them, you will find that the joints will become more lubricated over time and your muscles will develop the stamina that you are asking of them. Many people find that this way of moving can also be applied to other activities in their lives, such as ironing, washing dishes at the sink, and sawing wood.

The Effect of Standing Stiff-legged

Stiffening your knees not only restricts your lower body movement and therefore the power of your massage strokes. It also puts pressure on your lower back, which is the first area that can then bend. If you want to clarify this for yourself, try the following exercise.

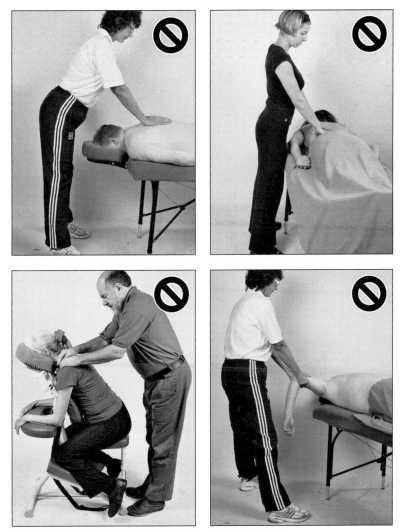

Figure 28.4: Standing stiff-legged;
a), b), c) sliding strokes and applying pressure, d) applying a stretch.

If you lock your knees back and then try doing a sliding stroke, you will feel how this cuts off the power of your lower body, making the stroke less powerful and more stilted, and forcing you to overuse your upper body. It puts all of the pressure for the movement on your lower back, which can be a strain if you regularly work in this way. You may also find that your breathing is restricted. You'll feel how this also happens if you stiffen your knees back when you're applying a stretch.

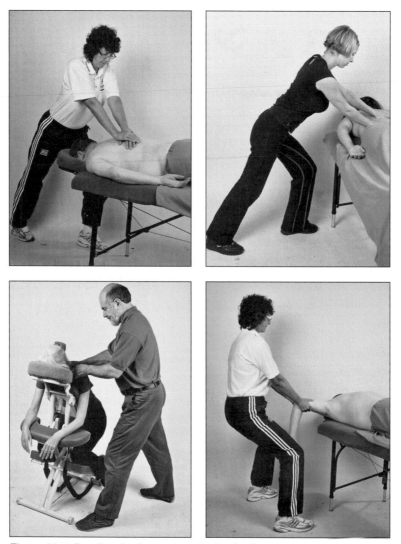

Figure 28.5: Bending the knees to save the back;
a), b), c) sliding strokes and applying pressure, d) applying a stretch.

Compare this with softening your knees so that there is some 'give' in them. This enables you to sway your body for massage strokes, making them more fluid and even, and taking the pressure off your lower back.

Avoid Standing Still or Jamming Yourself Against the Table
Standing still limits your ability to initiate the massage from your legs in the same way that standing just in one place would restrict your ability to play tennis. It puts all the work onto your upper body and reduces the power and ease that you can generate, and can put pressure on your lower back. Massage novices sometimes also lean against the table, which has the same effect.

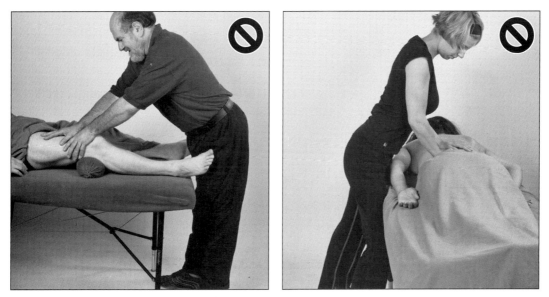

Figure 28.6: Restricted ways of standing; a) standing still and trying to reach too far, b) leaning against the table.

Have a Wide Stance

Having your feet far enough apart is essential for being able to bend your knees and sway your body. If this is unfamiliar to you, you could undertake training in martial arts such as judo, aikido or Tai Chi to accustom your leg muscles to moving when you're in this wide stance.

The Distance Between Your Feet

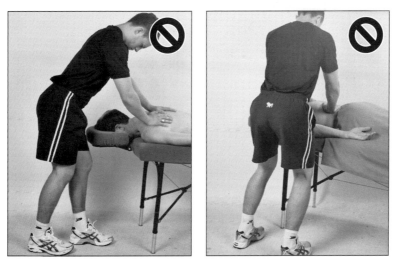

Figure 28.7: Feet too close together for comfortable swaying; a) in lunge stance, b) in horse stance.

If you stand with your feet close together and try swaying, you will feel how this restricts you and puts strain on your lower back when you are reaching. This applies in both the lunge stance and also the horse stance.

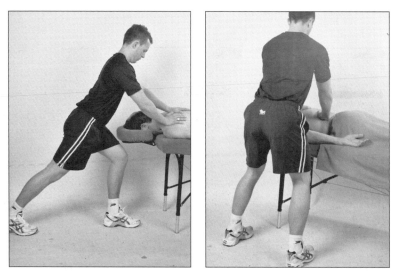

Figure 28.8: Feet far enough apart to sway; a) in the lunge stance, b) in the horse stance.

Widening your stance enables you to sway, i.e. to involve your lower body in your strokes. You will find that you need to widen your stance even further when you are massaging with your forearm or elbow (see figures 18.24 & 19.14).

Lean Forward to Deliver Pressure

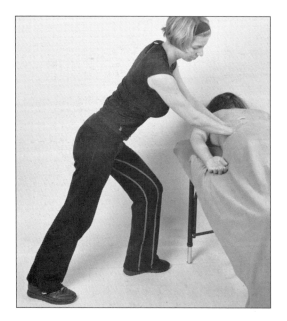

Figure 28.9: Leaning forward to deliver pressure.

Whether you are apply stationary or sliding pressure, lean forward with your whole body to deliver that pressure.

Move Your Body to Support Your Hands

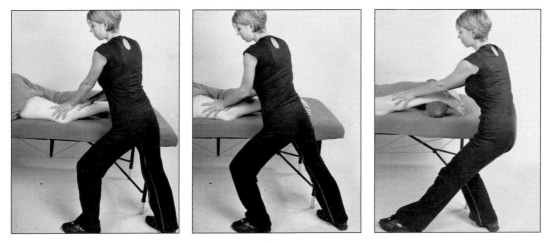

Figure 28.10: Swaying with hand movements; a), b) swaying forward, c) swaying back.

Fluid movement can only come from moving your body. So it is essential to sway your body for the fluidity and evenness of sliding massage strokes, whether it is the ebb and flow of light effleurage strokes or the concentrated pressure of deep tissue work. Your massage can then be strong, when it is appropriate, while your hands remain relatively relaxed for fine-tuning your massage delivery and also able to monitor the client's responses. This will also help you to pace yourself throughout a massage session.

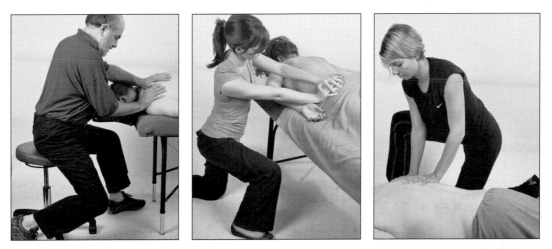

Figure 28.11: Swaying forward to deliver pressure and movement; a) when seated, b) when kneeling, c) in floor massage.

If you are seated (see Chapter 31), you can still sway your trunk provided that you can keep your feet comfortably planted on the floor so that your legs can support your movements. Even when you are kneeling at the massage table (see Chapter 32) or working on the floor (see Chapter 42), it is crucial to underpin the movements of your hands by swaying your body.

Sway Back for Pulling

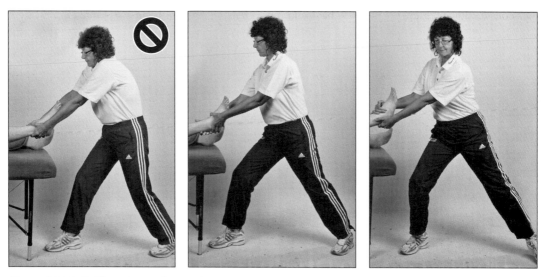

Figure 28.12: Pulling; a) standing and pulling only with the upper body, b) pulling by 'sitting' back, c) reaching back with the back leg.

Practitioners sometimes try to do pulling movements or stretches by standing still and merely using the upper body. However, the pull is much stronger and more even with considerably less effort when you use the weight of your lower body to pull your arms. Do this by swaying. If you need to increase the power of this movement, sink your weight lower by bending your knees more as you sway back and/or stretch or step back with your back leg.

Stay Grounded
Apart from when you're stepping around the table, try to keep as much of your soles on the ground as possible.

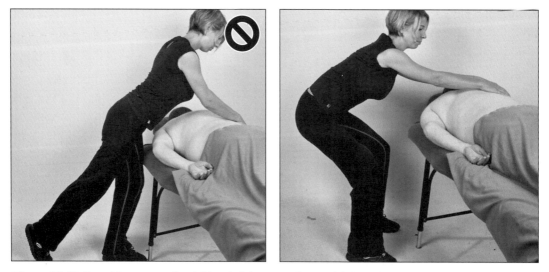

Figure 28.13: Reaching across the table; a) rising onto tiptoes, b) dropping down.

When reaching across the client's body, be careful not to rise up onto tiptoes for any length of time. It is not a stable position to hold and cuts off your lower body from delivering power to your hands. It puts considerable pressure on the lower back and causes tension in the calf muscles to maintain balance. Instead, as you reach, lower your body's centre of gravity by bending your knees. And don't try to reach too far. Instead, if your need to, cross to the other side of the table.

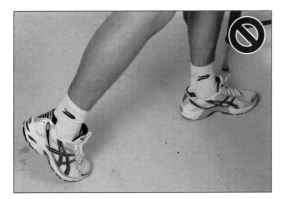

Figure 28.13 (cont.):
c) back heel lifted from the floor for long periods.

Of course you will sometimes need to lift the heel of your back foot from the floor. Try not to stay in this position for too long. It overworks your calf muscles, and doesn't give you as much push as when your foot is flat on the floor.

Keep a Spring in Your Step

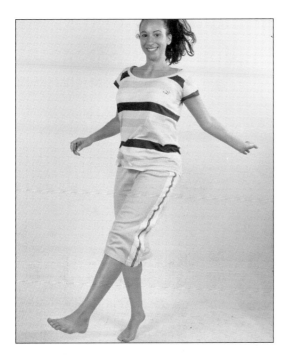

Figure 28.14: Energising the legs through skipping/jumping.

You may find that when you've used your legs in this grounded way for a full working day, you are left with a sense of heaviness and sluggishness in your legs. You can lighten and energise them by activities such as running, skipping, jumping or trampolining. Many forms of dance also promote nimbleness in the feet and a 'spring' in your step (see figure 10.13).

The Lunge Stance

The lunge stance, in which one foot is forward and the other back, is the most commonly used stance. The name comes from the starting position in fencing. This stance is sometimes called the 'archer' stance or the 'bow' stance.

When you are applying stationary pressure, this stance enables you to lean forward for the pressure and to remain forward to sustain it (see figure 28.9). This is also the basic stance for strokes in which you sway forwards and backwards, using the momentum of your body to give fluidity and evenness to your hand movements, and to add power when it is appropriate (see figure 28.10).

Therefore it is the primary stance for long effleurage strokes and for sliding deep tissue strokes with the fist or forearm. It also enables you to gradually sway forward to support travelling strokes such as kneading along the client's arm or leg.

Which Foot to Have in Front

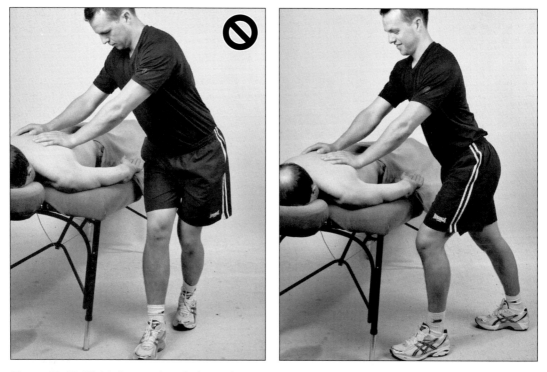

Figure 28.15: Which foot to place in front; a) the inside foot forward, b) the outside foot in front.

Practitioners sometimes get confused about which foot to place in front. Whenever you are standing alongside the table and facing towards either end of it, have your outside foot (the one furthest from the table) forward, and your inside foot (the one closest to the table) back. This keeps your lower body turned in towards your hands. If you were to have your legs the opposite way (the inside leg forward and the outside leg back), you would feel how this turns your hips away from the table and your hands.

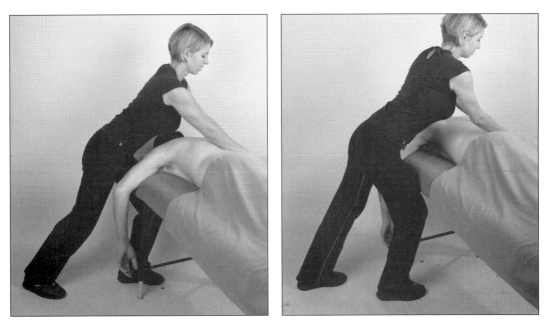

Figure 28.16: Facing across the table with either foot forward.

When you are standing in the lunge position at the side of the table and facing directly across it, for example for doing a double-handed sliding stroke across the client's back, it doesn't matter which foot that you have forward. However, make sure that you don't habitually always have the same foot in front, as this will use your body (and hands) very unevenly over time.

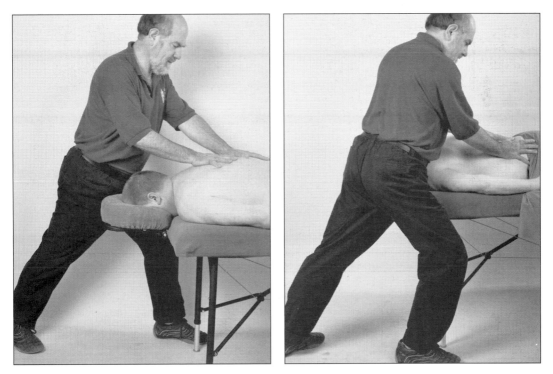

Figure 28.17: Stance for sliding the hands down the client's back.

When you are sliding both hands down the client's back from the head of the table, change the foot that you have in front in order to reach further down one or other side of the table.

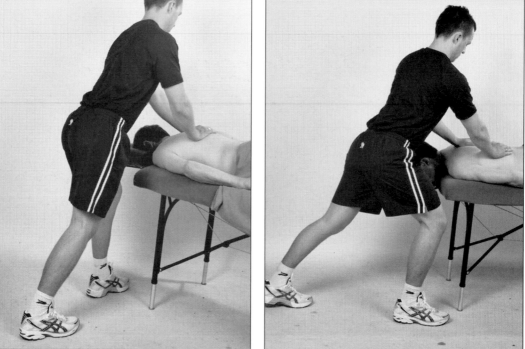

Figure 28.18: Standing at the corner of the table; a) facing across the table, b) facing along the table.

When you are standing at the corner of the table, the foot that you place in front will determine whether you are facing along the table or across it.

Mirror Your Posture on Opposite Sides of the Table

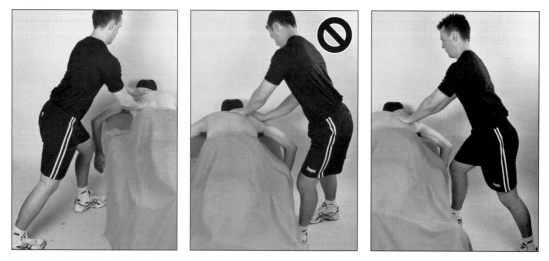

Figure 28.19: 'Mirroring' strokes on the opposite sides of the table;
a) doing the stroke on one side of the table, b) not mirroring the posture on the other side of the table,
c) mirroring the posture on the other side of the table.

When crossing from one side of the table to the other, there's a temptation to take up the same posture for the equivalent stroke on the opposite side of the table, i.e. to stand with the same foot forward, so that you can continue to use your dominant hand. Instead, mirror your posture and hand use.

Avoid Having the Back Foot Turned Away

Early in my career, I often finished massage sessions with a pain in one knee that hadn't been there before the massage. I also sometimes had a faint echo of niggling discomfort in the same side of my lower back. What had caused it? It was clearly due to something that I was doing as I massaged. With the help of a Tai Chi teacher, I looked at the alignment of my feet and hips as I worked, and discovered how I was putting pressure on my knee by turning my back foot outwards, away from the direction of the movement. In my years of teaching since, I've seen that this is a very common problem.

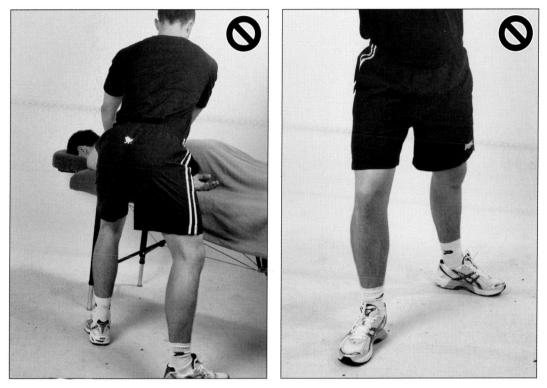

Figure 28.20: The back foot turned across the direction of movement.

Massage beginners often take up the lunge stance in the same way that caused my problems – standing alongside the massage table with the back foot turned at right angles to the direction of the massage stroke. This limits your ability to move your body in the direction of the massage stroke, which reduces your effectiveness. Because it turns your lower body away from the direction of your hands, you will be working in a twisted position. Because part of your body will be turned towards your hands and part towards your foot, the greatest pressure will generally be on the point of the greatest twist in your body. However there is also likely to be pressure and therefore the potential for cumulative strain throughout your lower body on the turned away side. This could show up in your lower back through your hip, knee and ankle joints and down into that foot.

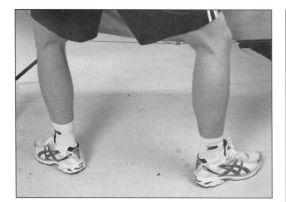

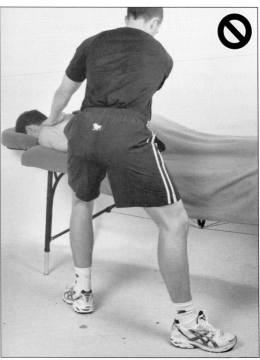

Figure 28.21: The back foot turned away from the direction of movement; a) the position of the feet, b) twisting the body to reach along the table.

Sometimes the back foot is turned even further away from the hands. This is often a habit for tall practitioners, who take up one position by the side of the table, and then depend on their long arms to reach the full length of the client's body. It can also be a legacy of dance training. As the practitioner turns to reach along the table, it twists the trunk and puts strain on the back and the joints of the leg, and reduces their effectiveness.

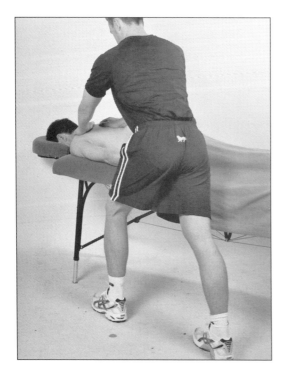

Figure 28.22: The back foot turned towards the hands.

Turning the back foot away is a subconscious habit for most people, which needs attention to change. The crucial thing is to turn your foot so that your hips are facing your hands whenever you are applying pressure and/or doing sliding strokes. If turning your back foot towards your hands is unfamiliar, it can feel awkward at first. Don't be discouraged if this initially makes unaccustomed demands on your leg muscles. You may need to regularly stretch your calf muscles to make it possible (see figure 28.41). With practice these muscles will adapt and you will feel how this helps align your lower body behind your hands.

Finding the Best Angle for Your Foot in the Lunge Stance

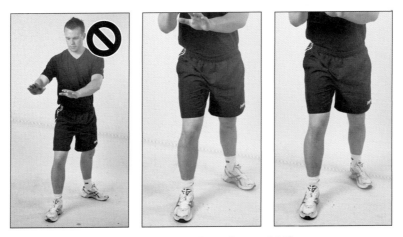

Figure 28.23: The angle of the back foot; a) turned 90˚ away,
b) turned 45˚ away, c) turned 30˚ away.

If turning your back foot away is a habit for you, it is worth taking time to find the best angle for your foot. Stand with your back foot at 90° to the direction of your hand movements to feel how this turns your lower body away from the movement. Then gradually turn your foot towards your hands, until you find the angle that enables you to have your hips facing in the direction of your hands without any discomfort in your hip joint (i.e. that your hands are within the 'hip spotlight', see figure 27.11). The most comfortable angle varies from person to person, but most people find that between 30° and 45° suits them best.

Have the Front Foot Facing Forward

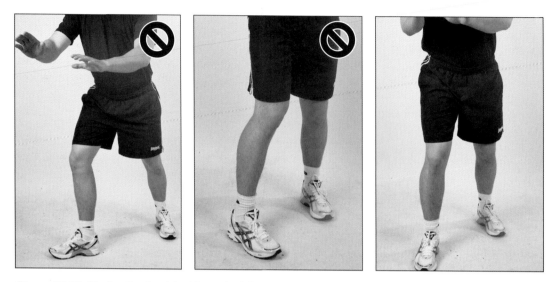

Figure 28.24: Having the front foot turned; a) foot turned out, b) foot turned in, c) front foot facing towards the hands.

Occasionally people turn the front foot too far out or, very occasionally, too far in. Turning the foot out can be a legacy of dance training, In dance, the turnout enables the dancer to stand tall and to spring *upwards*. However, in massage, it interferes with the ability to sway *forward* behind your hands. As you try to sway forward, it also puts pressure on your front knee, which can twist it.

Very occasionally, practitioners have the habit of turning the front foot too far in towards the table. This too will interfere with an easy swaying forward of your body without strain.

Bending the Front Knee

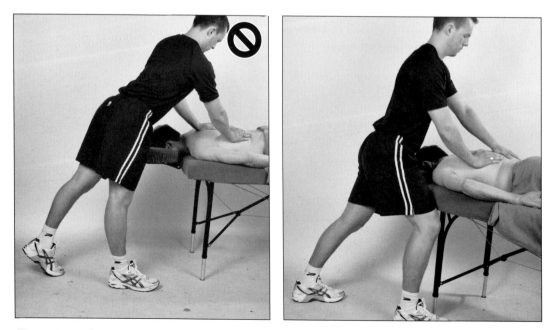

Figure 28.25: Swaying forward; a) keeping the front knee straight, b) bending the front knee.

If you were to keep your front knee straight as you sway forward in the lunge stance, this would put you in a very unstable stance, which would reduce the transfer of power to your hands and the fluidity of your massage movements.

Instead, as you sway forward, let your front knee bend so that your hips glide easily forward, staying on much the same level. Let your back leg straighten. This enables you to keep the power and movement of your lower body even, which then translates to your hands so that you can deliver the massage stroke smoothly.

Keep Your Front Knee Over Your Foot

As you sway forward in the lunge stance, your front knee takes a major part of your weight. It therefore comes under considerable strain if it is no longer over your foot as you bend it forward. There are two aspects to watch out for to maintain your stability and avoid straining your knee.

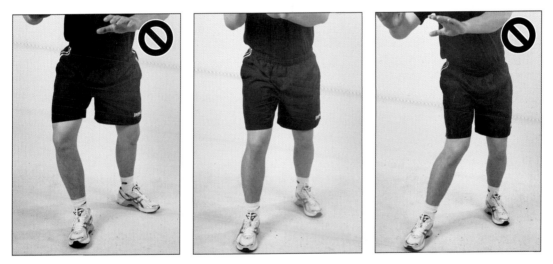

Figure 28.26: Bending the front knee forward; a) leaning to the outside,
b) safely above the foot, c) leaning to the inside.

Firstly, take care that your knee doesn't lean too far to the inside or the outside of your foot. (This is more likely to happen if your front foot is turned out or in, see figure 28.24).

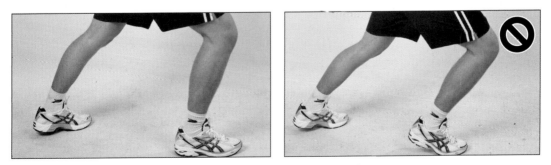

Figure 28.27: Bending the front knee forward; a) bent knee safely over the foot,
b) bent knee beyond the foot.

Secondly, take care that you don't slide your bent knee so far forward that it is beyond your foot. This is also an unstable position that will put pressure on your knee.

Step Forward Alongside the Table to Avoid Overreaching

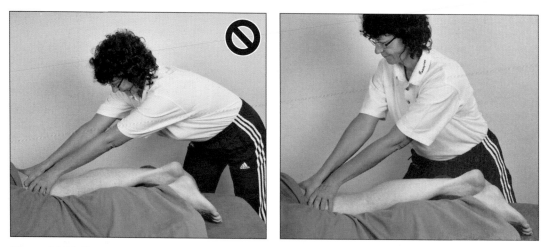

Figure 28.28: Reaching forward; a) overreaching from one position, b) moving forward.

Do not try to reach further than is comfortable from one position. Instead, change position.

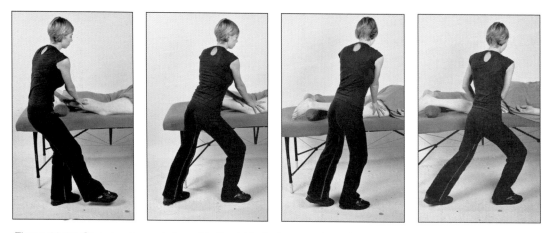

Figure 28.29: Stepping forward alongside the table for long strokes; a) stepping forward to begin the stroke,
b) swaying forward, c) stepping up with the back foot to move along,
d) stepping forward with the front foot to complete the stroke.

Step forward alongside the table to maintain the sweep of a long sliding stroke (and step back on the return stroke). To step forward, bring your back foot up behind your front one, and let your weight move onto your back foot as you step forward with the front one, somewhat like a waltz step. Then sway forward again.

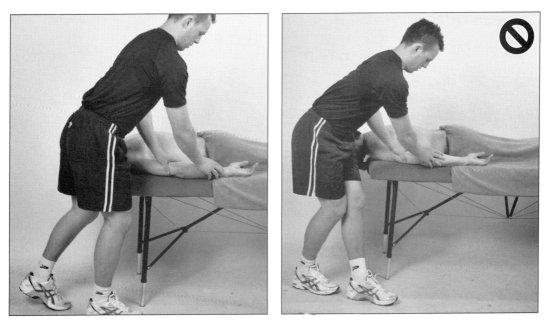

Figure 28.30: Crossing the legs when stepping up; a) preparing to step forward,
b) bringing the back leg past the front.

When stepping forward, don't bring your back leg past your front leg, as this would turn your hips away from the table, twisting your body and interfering with the continuity of the stroke.

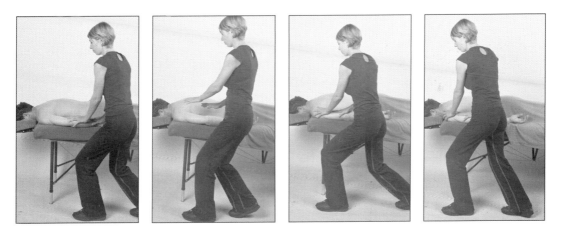

Figure 28.31: Stepping up alongside the table for short overlapping strokes; a) first stroke,
b) lifting the hands off and stepping up, c) starting the next stroke, d) finishing the stroke.

Another option is to do a series of shorter overlapping strokes instead of trying to maintain a single long one. As you finish each short stroke, lighten your hands and step up along the table so that you can start the next stroke a little further back from where you finished the previous one. Gradually move forward doing these overlapping strokes, making a smooth lift off and remaking contact smoothly to give the client a sense of continuity of progression. Reverse the process to work your way back.

The Horse Stance

When you want to use both hands *equally*, take up the 'horse' stance, in which your feet are side by side. The name comes from martial arts, where it refers to the horse rider's posture. This stance is most often used when you are standing at the side of the table and facing across it.

Don't Stand Stiff-legged

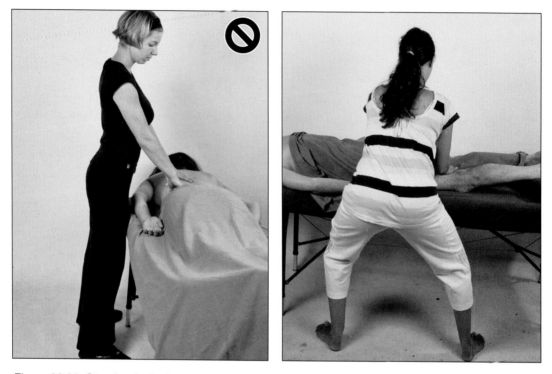

Figure 28.32: Standing in the horse stance; a) standing with stiff knees, b) bend the knees.

As in the lunge stance, don't stand stiff-legged. Bending your knees will enable you to move without putting pressure on your lower back. There are three main ways of moving in this stance; swaying from side to side, leaning forward for applying pressure, and twisting (rotating).

Have a Wide Enough Stance to Be Able to Sway Comfortably From Side to Side
Have your knees far enough apart so that you can comfortably sway without losing balance (see figures 28.7 & 28.8).

Look After Your Knees When Swaying

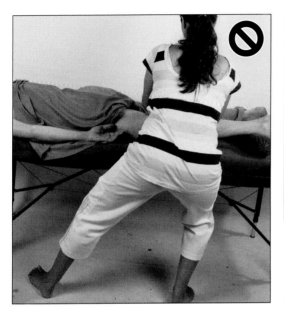
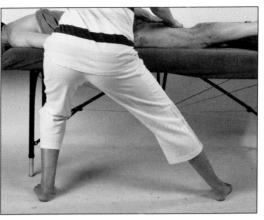

Figure 28.33: Swaying from side to side;
a) knee moving beyond the foot,
b) knee safely above the foot.

As you sway from side to side, take care that your knee doesn't move beyond your foot, as this would put great pressure on it.

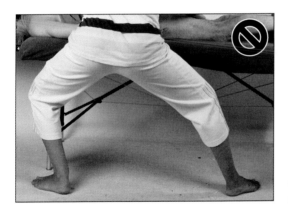

Figure 28.34: Foot turned out too far compromises the knee.

Bear in mind also that turning your foot out too far also has the potential to turn extra pressure on your knee as you sway sideways.

Sway From Side to Side With Each Hand in Large Kneading Strokes

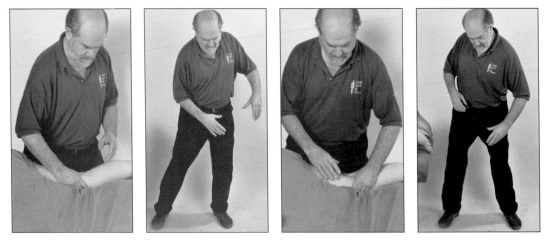

Figure 28.35: Moving for large hand kneading strokes.

When you are doing large hand kneading strokes, for example up and down the client's inner thigh, sway from side to side to echo and support the movements of your hands.

Twist Your Body for Wringing Strokes

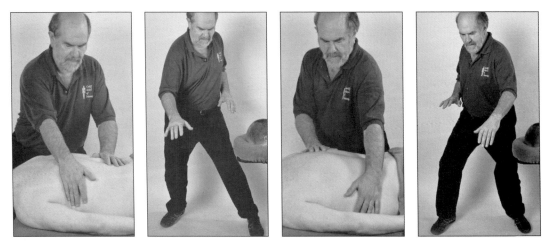

Figure 28.36: Moving for wringing strokes.

The horse stance is the best position for doing wringing strokes across the client's back or leg, because it enables you to twist your hips with the movements of your hands. Twist one hip forward to push the same hand forward, while you twist the other hip back to pull the respective hand back.

Lean Forward to Push Your Hands Apart for a Long Stretch

The horse stance is also a useful position for doing stretches in which you push your hands apart. Lean forward to push equally with each hand. To put more weight behind one hand, turn towards that hand by turning your feet to move into a lunge stance.

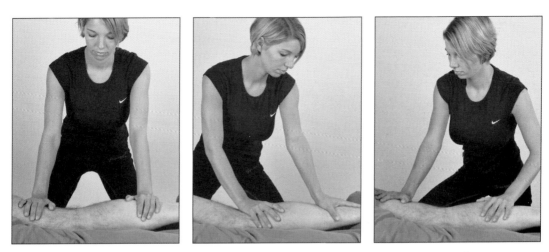

Figure 28.37: Pushing the hands apart; a) the horse stance for pushing the hands equally apart, b), c) turning towards each hand.

Don't Try to Reach Too Far in the Horse Stance

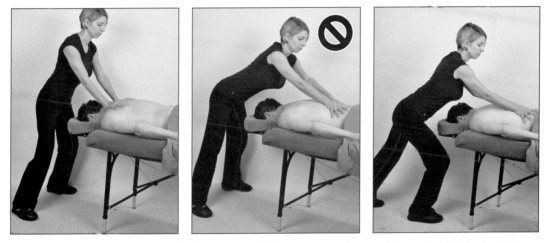

Figure 28.38: Working at the end of the table; a) the horse stance for pressing on the client's shoulders, b) trying to reach too far, c) switching to the lunge stance to reach further.

You can also use the horse stance when you are pressing equally on the client's shoulders from the head end of the table. Place your hands on the client's shoulders and increase the pressure by leaning forward. This stance will also enable you to apply pressure a short distance down the client's back. However, you will need to switch into a lunge stance to apply pressure further down the client's back.

Similarly, you can work in a horse stance at the foot of the table to work on a client's foot, but change to the lunge stance (and perhaps move more to the side of the table) for strokes that slide up the client's leg.

Poor Postural Habits in the Horse Stance

There are two postural habits to watch out for in the horse stance because of the pressure that they put on your legs; standing too much on one leg, and letting your knees sag inwards.

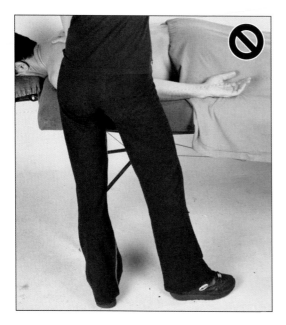

Figure 28.39: Standing with the weight on one leg.

Many of us have the unconscious habit of standing with our weight more on one leg much of the time, which puts extra pressure on the joints of that leg. It is important to monitor that you are not consistently standing in this way in the horse stance. This particularly applies when you are standing relatively still. If you are not sure of how you stand, get yourself videoed, or get coaching from a skilled bodywork colleague, a martial arts teacher or a sports trainer.

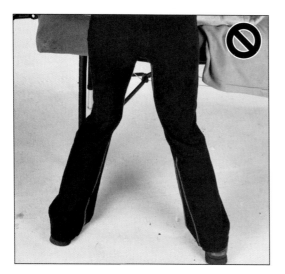

Figure 28.40: Letting the knees sag inwards.

Take care also not to let your knees sag or drop in towards one another. This cuts off the power arising from your lower body. Instead of your legs acting as a 'springboard' for massage strokes, you are likely to slump a little and to stiffen your upper body to compensate. This can cause lower back problems and sometimes strain in the upper back as well. Practitioners can become heavy-handed without realising it because of the lack of lower body support for their massage strokes.

Having the knees sag in towards one another can be a cause or consequence of having 'flat feet', i.e. low arches. If this is a problem for you, there are some simple ways to re-establish the arch, which will also lift your knees. You could wear trainers with raised arch supports. If you find yourself standing with your feet turned outwards, turn them in a little so that they are more parallel. This makes it easier to keep your knees above your feet and, for most people, will lift the arch a little. You could also do activities such as running, skipping, jumping, dancing or trampolining that involve pushing up from the legs to give a 'lift' to your arch and therefore also lift the inside of your knee.

Maintaining Flexible Hips, Knees, and Ankles

Leg Stretches
It is good to stretch your leg muscles before doing a massage. This is particularly important for people who sit a lot, because they can become used to having their knees flexed and their hamstrings and calf muscles shortened. Also, their lateral hip muscles don't get much exercise.

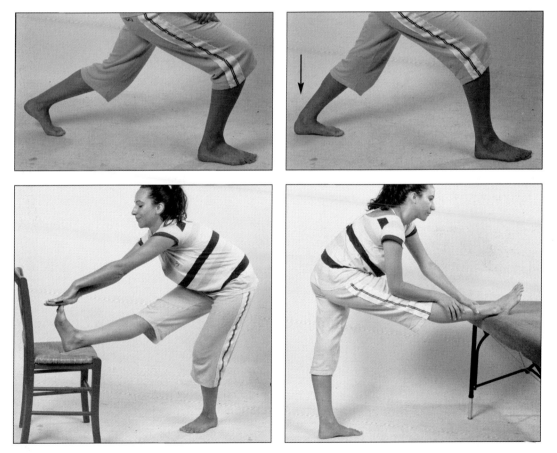

Figure 28.41: Back of leg stretches; a), b) lowering the heel to the floor,
c) resting the leg on a chair to stretch the muscles, d) resting the leg on a table to stretch the muscles.

To stretch the hamstrings and calf muscles, stand with one foot forward. Stretch out your back leg, straighten it, and slowly lower your heel towards the floor. Another way to stretch them is to put your foot up on a chair or table and slowly lower your knee to straighten your leg and/or lean forward from the hips, taking care not to just bend in your lower or midback. Dorsiflexing your foot in these positions will extend the stretch further.

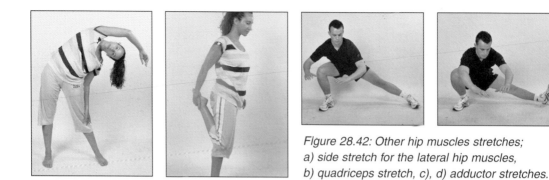

Figure 28.42: Other hip muscles stretches;
a) side stretch for the lateral hip muscles,
b) quadriceps stretch, c), d) adductor stretches.

A side stretch will stretch the muscles at the side of the hips, particularly gluteus medius and the tensor fasciae latae. Keep your body and head facing the front as you lean your trunk sideways to slide your hand down the side-seam of your trousers. Come up through the central position and slowly drop to the other side.

Bending your leg back will stretch your quadriceps. Stretching your leg sideways from a low squat will stretch your adductors, and turning your foot up will extend the stretch.

Developing Leg Suppleness in Activity
Being able to bend your knees and sway your body requires flexibility in your hips, knees, and ankles. Each of the following exercises focuses on one of these joints, while also mobilising the other. If, after doing these exercises, you feel the need to do more work on getting flexibility in your legs while you are involved in dynamic activity, try skiing, skating, surfing, skate-boarding, snow boarding, or martial arts such as judo, aikido and Tai Chi. These will be particularly effective for developing ankle flexibility in action.

Mobilising the Hips

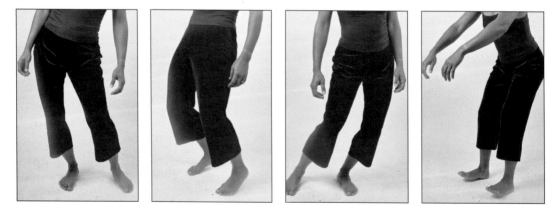

Figure 28.43: Hip circles.

For hip mobilisation, stand with your feet at least as far apart as the width of your hips. Sway your hips from side to side, and then forward and back. Then take them in a circle that encompasses these four directions. Rather than just mechanically doing each circular movement a set number of times, focus on the quality of the movement. Practice smoothing out the uneven, jerky parts of the movement. Do this by softening and relaxing your body, not by tensing up. If one part of the circle seems much stiffer than other parts, you could focus on moving back and forward through that area until it becomes easier.

When this becomes easy, give yourself a fresh challenge. Try moving from side to side in the shape of an infinity sign ∞ in one direction and then the other. This adds rotation to the movement. Similarly, once you've established this movement, focus on making it smoother.

Mobilising the Knees

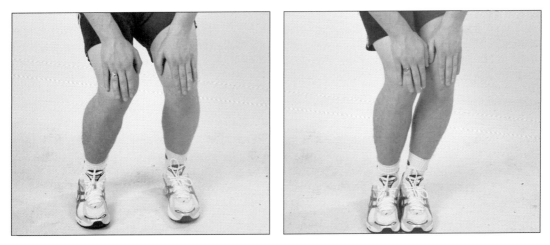

Figure 28.44: Knee circles; a) with the feet apart, b) with the feet together.

To focus on mobilising your knees, stand with your feet a short distance apart. Put your hands on your knees and sway them forward and back and sideways and then move them in a circle (and, if this is easy, in the shape of an infinity sign). This activates each part of your knees in turn, and also involves your ankles. If you feel ready to undertake a more challenging version of this exercise, try it with your feet right next to one another.

Ankle Movements

It is crucial to have supple ankles in order to avoid standing stiffly as you massage. Stretching your calf muscles (see figure 28.41) is good preparation for this. The hip circles (see figure 28.43) will mobilise your ankles to some extent.

However, keeping your sole flat on the floor as you circle your legs will stretch and mobilise your ankles more. It will also wake up each part of your foot in turn as it takes your weight. This accustoms your ankles to retaining flexibility whilst also supporting your weight. The knee circles (above) will therefore have more effect on your ankles.

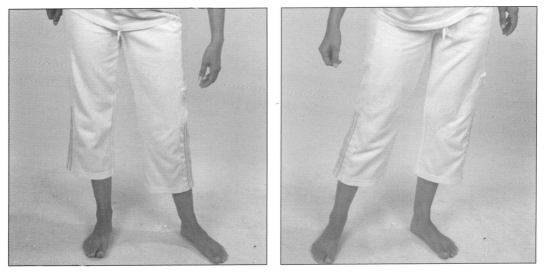

Figure 28.45: Swaying with the soles on the floor to mobilise the ankles.

To focus directly on your ankles, stand with your feet some distance apart, and rock forward and back and from side to side, keeping your feet flat on the floor and also bending and swaying your knees and hips and using your arms to avoid overbalancing. (Having your feet further apart will enable you to work your ankles more than in the knee circles). Then extend the movement into a circular movement, continuing to use your bodyweight as a counterbalance. Make sure in these movements that you don't strain your knees by bending them too far sideways. If you want more of a challenge, this movement could also be taken into the infinity shape.

Review

Your legs are essential to the power, movement, fluidity and evenness of massage strokes.

Standing still at the massage table restricts your ability to initiate the massage from your legs. So does leaning against the massage table.

Instead of standing stiff-legged, soften your knees a little so they can bend as you move.

Wear low-heeled shoes that will move with your feet.

Have a wide enough stance that enables you to sway easily without overbalancing.

Position your body so that the power of your bodyweight is directly behind your working hands / forearm and then move in the direction of the massage stroke.

Reorient yourself to change the direction of applying pressure or of movement.

Develop this into the continuous moving dance of massage.

Lean towards the massage table to sustain the force in sliding strokes or to apply pressure on one area of the client's body.

Regulate the amount of pressure that you are applying by how much you lean.

Be careful not to stay on tiptoes for any length of time.

Sway forward and back for sliding strokes.

When swaying, keep your bent knee above your foot.

Pull by 'sitting' back to use the weight of your lower body.

Use the lunge stance for swaying forward and back, to lean behind travelling strokes including deep sliding pressure strokes, for focusing sustained pressure on a single point and for pulling strokes.

At the side of the table, stand with your outside foot forward and your inside foot back.

Bend your front knee as you sway forward to keep the movement even.

When you are doing long sliding strokes, step up alongside the table (without crossing your legs) to avoid overreaching.

Don't turn your back foot away from your hands, as this will also turn your hips away. Find the angle that enables you to have your hips facing towards your hands.

Make sure that your front foot is not turned out.

Use the horse stance for using your hands equally. Sway from side to side for large hand kneading. Twist your hips for wringing strokes. Lean forward to apply pressure with both hands, or to push your hands apart in a long stretch.

Be careful not to stand with your weight on one leg for too long, or to let your knees sag inwards.

To lift your arches and the inner side of your knees, wear shoes with inbuilt arch supports, and turn your feet to be more parallel.

Warm up your legs by doing stretches for your calf muscles and hamstrings, and mobilising exercises for your hips, knees, and ankles.

If using your legs dynamically is unfamiliar, take up regular walking, running or cycling, or consider taking up sports, which are built around lower body movements.

SECTION 6
Integrated Bodyuse for Massage

As is emphasised throughout this book, doing massage is not just a matter of using your hands to deliver the massage. Equally, it involves positioning and moving your body to support the actions of your hands (or other working tools). This enables you to work with the least strain while being most effective, especially when you are applying pressure. This is particularly important for practitioners with a small build and/or short arms. It will also help those with larger builds to conserve their energy, and reduce the wear and tear on their bodies.

Even if you are working lightly, using your body in this way imparts a quality to the massage that is simultaneously dynamic *and* relaxed. Once you have built up your general stamina, it will also enable you to pace yourself comfortably during a working day without exhaustion or straining your body.

This section pulls together information from Section 3: *Using Your Hands* (see Chapters 11–17) and Section 5: *Using Your Body* (see Chapters 22–28), to focus on coordinating how you use your hands and your body for delivering massage techniques with power and fluidity. Chapter 29 focuses on how this applies when you are standing, and Chapters 31 & 32 look at sitting and kneeling. This section also looks at 'positional intelligence' – how your position in relation to the client determines the sort of techniques that will be effective and those that would be strainful to attempt. The principles covered here also apply when you are using your forearm or elbow, which are covered in detail in Chapters 18 & 19.

The next section of the book looks at the specific hand-body relationships in a range of common massage techniques, and the following section on working with the client in positions other than lying on a massage table.

Focusing simultaneously on your hands and your body (while also monitoring the client's responses) takes practice. Monitor yourself regularly as you work (see Chapter 5) to develop your ability to feel this connection between what you are doing with your body and your hands (or forearm or elbow), until effective bodyuse becomes an automatic and instinctive part of delivering each massage technique.

The Massage Dance

The guidelines in this section are presented in a fairly static way to highlight one principle at a time. However, bear in mind that the ideal is to blend them into a continuous, fluid 'dance' around the massage table or chair (see Chapter 4). Sometimes this will involve leaning and swaying in one position for a period of time. At other times, it will involve moving fluidly from position to position between and within strokes, like the graceful, fluid 'dance' of a champion skater or skilled sports player. You can develop this ability to 'dance' around the massage table or chair through practice, through watching and receiving massages from other people, and by getting coaching from skilled practitioners and teachers.

You may find yourself stiffening up again in the future, especially when you are stressed or learning new strokes. If you feel this happening, deliberately exaggerate the body movements and repositioning until you settle back again into the massage dance. Later, as this coordinated 'dance' becomes second nature, you can make it smaller and quieter.

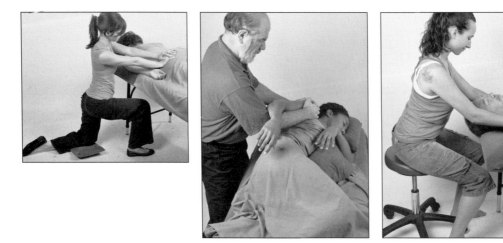

CHAPTER 29

Integrating Hand and Body Use

This chapter looks at coordinating how you use your body and your hands at the massage table or chair. It reviews and pulls together information from Section 3: *Using Your Hands* (see Chapters 11–17) and Section 5: *Using Your Body* (see Chapters 22–28).

The next chapter extends one aspect of this – how your position in relation to the client determines the sort of techniques that will be effective and those that would be strainful and/or ineffective. Many of the principles covered in this chapter also apply when you are seated or kneeling, which are covered in Chapters 31 & 32. Much of it is also relevant when you are using your forearm or elbow, which are covered in detail in Chapters 18 & 19.

Coordinated Bodyuse: a Brief Review
It is useful to begin with a review of the main principles of good bodyuse covered in this book. They are:

* *Conserving your hands* by using them skilfully;
* *Saving them* by using other body areas such as your forearms and elbows whenever possible;
* Getting *your body behind your working tools* to use your bodyweight;
* *Leaning and swaying your body* to generate the power and movement that supports your working tools;
* Continually *repositioning yourself* around the massage couch for best advantage.

The ideal is to work with the least strain while being most effective, so that you can pace yourself, conserve your energy, and reduce the wear and tear on your body.

Using Your Body to Support Your Hands

It is useful to briefly review the contribution of each part of the body, and how they can be blended together into the 'dance' of massage. (Look back at Chapters 22–28 for more detailed information). The ideal is to generate power for pushing, pulling and sustained pressure techniques from your lower body and to transmit this to your hands or other massage tools. This enables you to take the pressure off the common areas of strain for massage practitioners – the hands, shoulders and back.

Try to find a balance in these movements between strength (when necessary) and ease, so that you are working in a way that is simultaneously dynamic, flexible and relatively relaxed. Even when you are using light pressure, this will add the essential qualities of rhythm, fluidity and evenness to the massage. It is crucial when you are working firmly.

Power From Your Lower Body

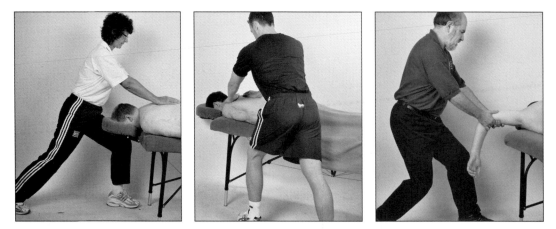

Figure 29.1: Power from the legs; a), b) swaying forward for pushing, c) swaying back for pulling.

The role of your legs in massage is to generate the power of your massage techniques and the rhythm and evenness with which you deliver them. Softening your knees so that they have a little 'give' in them is essential for swaying with your massage strokes. Having your feet far enough apart gives you a wide base to keep you stable as you sway.

Aligning Your Feet, Hips and Hands

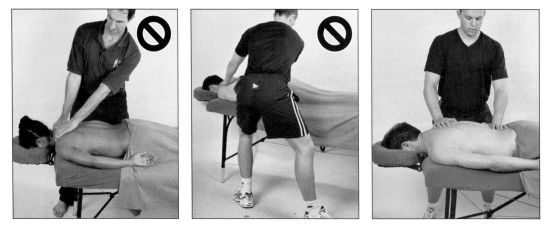

Figure 29.2: Aligning your feet, hips and hands; a), b) not aligned, c) aligned.

The position of your feet determines the direction that your hips face. If your feet are turned away from your working hands, that will also turn your hips away from them. If your hips are not facing your hands when you are applying pressure (either stationary or sliding) or pulling, your body will be twisted. This would diminish the force that is transmitted to your hands. It would also put pressure on your trunk, especially your lower back, and also on your hip joints, your knees and perhaps also your ankles.

Aligning your feet and hips behind your hands enables you to move easily and fluidly in the intended direction of your massage stroke. In the lunge position, you can lean forward to deliver pressure, sway forward and back for sliding strokes, and sway back for stretches. In the horse position, you can sway sideways or twist your hips behind strokes.

Transmitting the Power Up Through Your Trunk

Positioning your body well enables the power of your lower body to be transmitted through your trunk to your arms.

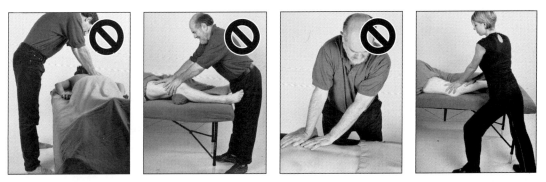

Figure 29.3: Trunk; a) hunched over, b) trying to reach too far, c) twisted, d) trunk long and supple.

Hunching over or twisting your trunk would impede this transmission of power. Therefore, it is important to keep your trunk strong and supple and to 'stand tall' (to maintain your length) without rigidity (see figure 25.14).

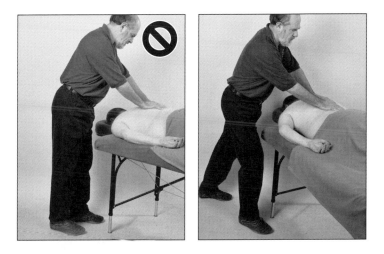

Figure 29.4: Leaning forward;
a) stiff knees,
b) bending the knees
to save the back.

When leaning forward, bend your knees to save your back. Bending your knees also enables you to drop your body when you need to work lower.

Centering Movement Around the Pelvis

Functionally, the pelvis, the lowest part of the trunk, is the centre of the body in movement (see figure 27.3). When the power for arm movements is centered around the pelvis, there is a combination of power and evenness in the follow-through. This can be seen in the simultaneous power, gracefulness and precision of a good golf swing or tennis stroke. In massage, as in those other sports, this reduces the demands on your lower back and shoulders.

Even Breathing

Having your back strong, supple and well supported by your pelvis will encourage easy, deep breathing. Your breathing needs to deepen as you massage to support the physical activity, but to remain even for pacing and stamina.

Monitor your breathing, particularly when you are applying pressure (see figure 26.3). Holding your breath or inhaling strongly when you are doing firm strokes is likely to lead you into tensing up and working too hard. Instead, try to breathe out easily as you push into the stroke.

Keeping Your Shoulders Relaxed

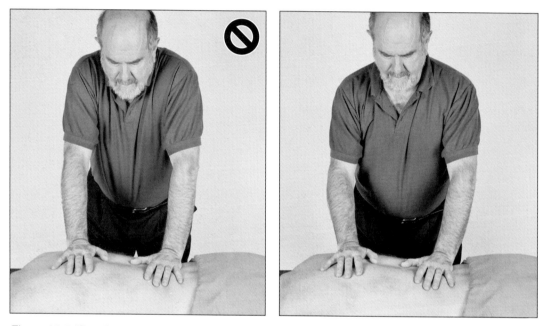

Figure 29.5: The shoulders; a) tensed, b) relaxed.

When the power comes from your lower body, it enables you to keep your shoulders relaxed so that you can transmit this power from your trunk to your arms. This reduces the effort needed in your shoulder and arm muscles, and leaves your hands free for the fine-tuning of your massage techniques.

Tensing the shoulders is such a common, unconscious habit that you need to regularly pay attention to keeping them relaxed. This is important, because having tense shoulders impedes the transmission of power. This is likely to lead into a cycle of tensing up and overusing your upper body in order to 'muscle through'. This process often includes holding the breath, which further reinforces this tension.

Working on a table that is too high or standing still/with stiff knees when you are massaging will lead to tensing the shoulders, so pay attention to these possible contributing factors.

Involving Your Arms

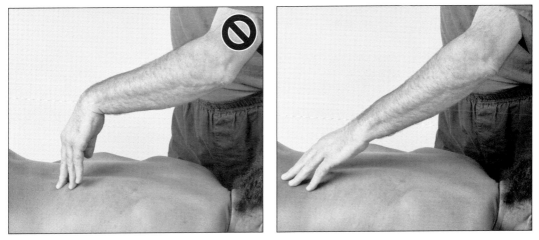

Figure 29.6: Moving with massage strokes; a) just moving the hand, b) moving the arm.

Don't just move your hands with massage strokes. Move your arms and your body with the strokes.

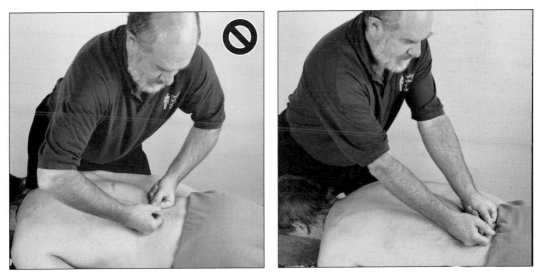

Figure 29.7: Applying pressure; a) bent arms dissipating the pressure,
b) straight arms directing the pressure.

Keep your arms straight when you are applying pressure, so that the power comes directly from your trunk to your hands without being dissipated.

Working Hands

All of this preparation enables you to channel the power from your body through your hands (or forearm or elbow, see Chapters 18 & 19) to deliver it to your client. Using your body well helps you to keep your hands relatively relaxed. This makes it easier to use them for the twin tasks of delivering the massage and simultaneously palpating the client's structure and their responses to guide your work.

Having Relaxed Hands

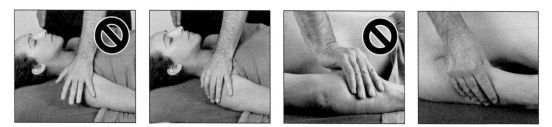

Figure 29.8: Relaxing the hands; a) stiff hand for effleurage, b) relaxed hand for effleurage, c) stiff hand for squeezing, d) relaxed hand for squeezing.

Relaxing your hands enables you to mould them to the surface contours of the client's body in the initial effleurage strokes, and to keep them relaxed and responsive as you then knead and squeeze the muscles and apply firmer pressure.

Relax the Non-working Parts of Your Hands

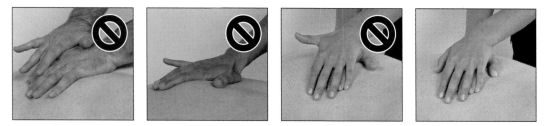

Fig 29.9: The non-working parts of your hand; a), b), c) tensing the non-working parts of the hand, d) relaxing the non-working areas.

Practitioners sometimes unconsciously stiffen their fingers or thumbs when using other parts of their hands. This uses unnecessary energy, tends to stiffen your whole hand and reduces your ability to palpate the client's responses.

Don't Overuse Your Thumbs or Fingers
The areas of the hands that are most at risk in massage are the thumbs (see Chapter 13) and the wrists (see Chapter 17), and, to a lesser extent, the fingers (see Chapter 12). Save your fingers or thumbs for the situations in which you can't use other parts of your hands, such as working around the client's head and neck.

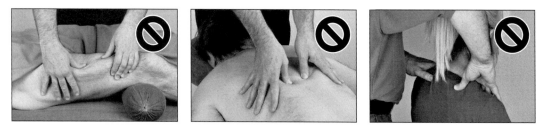

Figure 29.10: Straining the thumbs; a) in kneading, b), c) for applying pressure.

Be especially careful of your thumbs (see figure 13.1), which can easily be overused in strong kneading strokes, such as working on the thigh muscles, or for applying pressure.

Use the Largest Appropriate Part of Your Hand (or Forearm)

Whenever it's appropriate, save your fingers and thumbs by using larger 'tools' for the massage, such as the heel (see figure 14.7) or the back of your hand (see figure 14.13), your knuckles (see Chapter 15) or your fist (see Chapter 16). And find an experienced teacher who can train you in the use of your forearm and elbow to save your hands completely (see Chapters 18 & 19).

Use Both Hands Together Whenever You Can

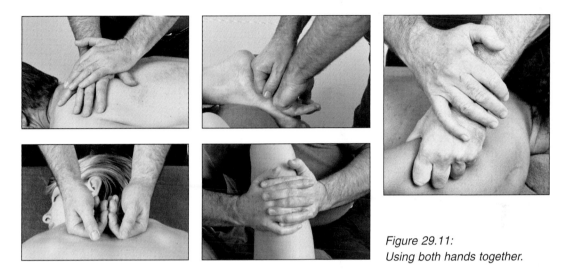

Figure 29.11:
Using both hands together.

Use your other hand to support and stabilise your working hand, and work 'double-handed' whenever possible.

Take Care of Your Wrists

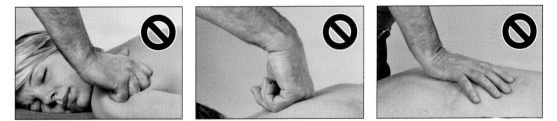

Figure 29.12: Bent wrist when using pressure.

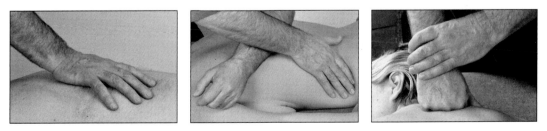

Figure 29.13: Looking after the wrist; a) straight wrist, b), c) supporting the wrist.

Whenever you are incorporating pressure into a massage technique, keep your wrist relatively straight but not stiff, and make sure that the pressure isn't too much for it. Support it with your other hand to reduce the pressure on it, and learn to use your forearm and elbow to take the pressure off it entirely.

Integrating Hands and Body

One aim of this book is to encourage you to develop your ability to focus on the connection between what you are doing with your body and what you are doing with your hands (or forearm). The long-term ideal is for effective bodyuse to become an automatic and instinctive part of delivering each massage technique. The rest of this chapter reviews some general guidelines for this. (The next two sections of the book, Chapters 33–42, look at how these principles apply in specific types of massage strokes and working situations).

Align Your Bodyweight Behind Your Working Tools

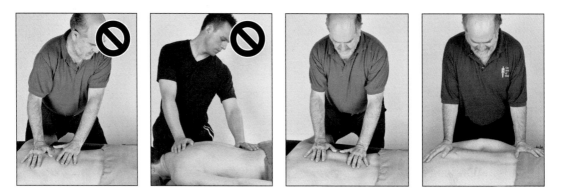

Figure 29.14: Applying pressure; a), b) body turned away from the hands,
c) body aligned behind the hands, d) body facing between the hands for a stretch.

When you are doing *light* sweeping strokes, it is not essential to keep your body directly behind your hands all the time, as long as your body is *not twisted*. However, when your massage strokes involve pressure, position your bodyweight directly behind your hands, so that you can lean or sway forward to deliver the power from your lower body to your hands. To be sure that your body is aligned with your working hands (or forearm), check that your hands are framed in the beam of your 'hip spotlight' (see figure 27.11). Otherwise you would be twisting your body, which would increase the likelihood of strain and reduce the power available to your hands. This usually leads to overusing your upper body.

Not only does this enable you to use your bodyweight to deliver the pressure. It also enables you to sway directly forward in the direction of the stroke, and therefore to maintain the pressure and to give fluidity and evenness to the movement.

Change Position to Remain Aligned With Your Hands

Reposition yourself to keep your body behind your working hands (or forearms), and to change the direction in which you are applying pressure. If you try to change the direction of pressure without reorienting your body, you will be twisting your body and losing effectiveness.

Lean Forward to Give Weight to Your Strokes

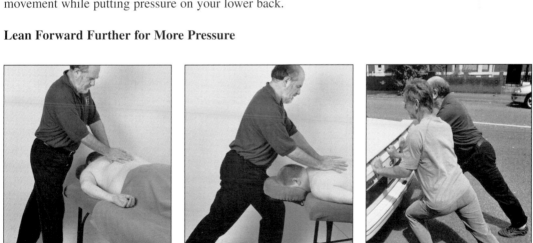

Figure 29.15: Applying pressure; a) tensing the shoulders for pressure, b) leaning forward for pressure.

Even when you are applying stationary pressure, lean forward for the pressure rather than standing stiff-legged and just using your upper body to generate it. Bend your knees so that you can lean with your whole trunk. Stay relaxed enough so that you would fall forward if the client was not there on the table for you to lean on. Don't tense your shoulders which would reduce the evenness and power of the movement while putting pressure on your lower back.

Lean Forward Further for More Pressure

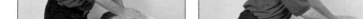

Figure 29.16: Regulating the pressure; a) leaning forward for light pressure,
b) leaning forward more to increase the force, c) pushing a car.

Regulate the amount of pressure that you are applying by how much you lean forward. Lean forward to deliver more pressure, as you would for pushing a car.

Move With Your Massage Strokes

Avoid standing still and just massaging with your arms. This would make your strokes stilted, and lead to overstretching as you reach forward.

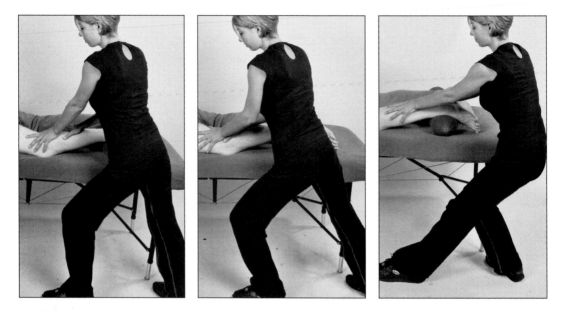

Figure 29.17: Swaying for sliding strokes; a), b) swaying forward, c) swaying back.

Instead, lean and sway forward and back with your whole body to deliver sliding strokes with ease, power and evenness, and to sustain the force throughout the stroke. Bend your knees in these movements to save your lower back. Even for light strokes, this provides fluidity and an evenness that you couldn't create by just using your upper body. And it is essential for supplying the power for firm strokes. Obviously, in sliding strokes, you can't apply the same pressure on the return stroke.

Swaying to Feel the Hand-body Connection

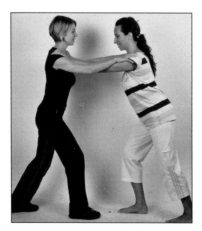

Figure 29.18: Swaying forward and back.

It can be useful to practice movements that help you to internalise the feeling of swaying your whole body to move your hands. One way of doing this is by working with a partner in the 'push me-pull you waltz' to practise lunge stance movements. Stand facing your partner in the lunge stance, both of you with the same foot forward (both right feet for example), and place your hands on each other's shoulders. Sway forward and back, one of you swaying forward as the other sways back. Let your front knee bend and your back leg straighten as you sway forward. Do this for a while to feel the connection between the movement of your hands and the rest of your body.

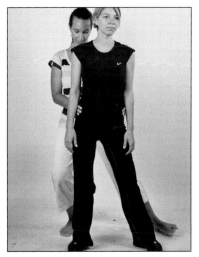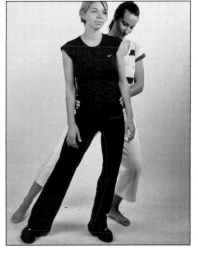

Figure 29.19: Swaying sideways.

To practice swaying sideways in the horse stance, have your partner stand in front of you with both of you in the horse stance. As you sway from side to side, push your partner's hips so that they sway from side to side with you. Then change places so that each of you gets both sides of this experience.

Rise Up or Sink Down to Balance Between Pressure and Movement

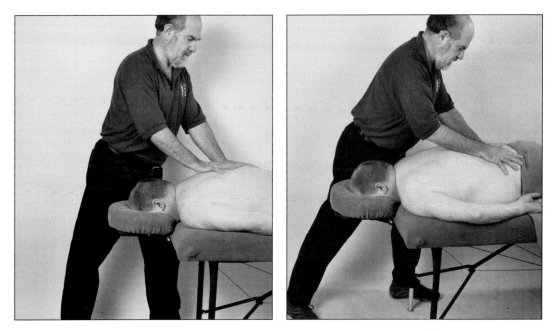

Figure 29.20: Incorporating pressure in a sliding stroke; a) rising up to increase the pressure, b) sinking lower to push forward.

When you are sliding forward there are two components to balance – the pressure and the movement of the stroke. Leaning your bodyweight provides the pressure for the stroke (see figure 29.16). You can increase the pressure by bringing your weight more directly above your hands (or forearm). Bear in mind that the deeper you are working, the slower that you need to move to give the client's body time to accommodate to the pressure. Stepping back a little and sinking lower makes it easier to push forward. Move between these two positions to regulate the balance between them.

Move Fluidly Around the Table – in the Massage 'Dance'

When you first focus on this, you may need to take a few seconds before each stroke to reposition yourself, like a snooker player lining up for each consecutive shot. With practise, you will develop the ability to move fluidly from stroke to stroke, like a musician joining up separately learnt musical phrases into a continuous stream of music. And you will need to practice changing position or direction *within* some strokes so that you can do this fluidly too.

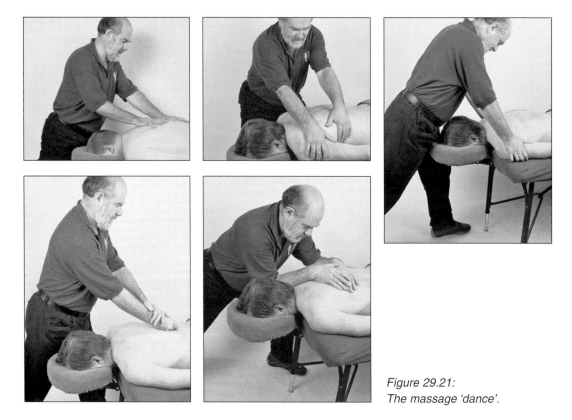

Figure 29.21:
The massage 'dance'.

The ideal is to develop this into a fluid, continuous 'dance', like the 'dance' of tennis players as they move around the court to position themselves for each stroke (see Chapter 4). Obviously, the words and illustrations in this book can only hint at this dance. You can develop this ability to 'dance' around the massage table or chair through practice, through watching and receiving massages from other people, and by getting coaching from skilled practitioners and teachers.

You may find yourself stiffening up again in the future, especially when you are stressed or learning new strokes. If you feel this happening, deliberately exaggerate the body movements and repositioning until you settle back again into the massage dance. Later, as this coordinated dance becomes second nature, you can make it smaller and quieter.

Review

Coordinate how you use your hands (or forearms, etc.) with how you position and move your body to support them.

Don't overuse your thumbs or fingers. Save them for the situations in which you can't use other parts of your hands or your forearms.

Use the largest appropriate part of your hand/forearm for massage techniques, and use both hands together whenever you can.

Keep the non-working parts of your hands relaxed as you use other parts.

When you are applying pressure, keep your wrists relatively straight but not stiff, and make sure that the pressure isn't too much for them.

Keep your shoulders relaxed so that you can transmit the power unimpeded from your trunk to your arms, and keep your arms straight when you are applying pressure to deliver the power to your hands.

Let your breathing deepen as you massage to support the physical activity, but keep it even for pacing and stamina.

Don't just move your hands with massage strokes, but move your arms, and sway your body too.

Generate the power and the fluidity of your massage techniques from your lower body.

Keep your trunk strong, supple and long without rigidity to transmit the power from your legs.

Lean forward to create the power for each stroke, rather than standing still and relying on the muscle power of your upper body.

Bend your knees to lean forward to take the pressure off your back, rather than hunching over.

Regulate the amount of pressure that you are applying by how much you lean forward.

In sliding strokes, position and lean your body, and then sway to move your hands forward and backwards.

Apply stretches by 'sitting' back, rather than just pulling with your upper body.

Align your feet, hips and hands for applying pressure, pushing or pulling.

Reposition yourself regularly in massage sessions to keep your body behind your working hands/forearms.

Rise and sink between or within strokes to change your angle of delivery.

Blend these ingredients into a continuous, fluid 'dance' around the massage table or chair.

CHAPTER 30

'Positional Intelligence'

The previous chapter included information about positioning your body to best support each stroke. However, the converse also applies – your position will determine the type of stroke and pressure that you are able to apply. So this chapter focuses on how to bring 'positional intelligence' to bear by:

- Recognising the possibilities and limitations of your position in relation to the client, and;
- Changing your techniques or your position, when necessary, to work effectively and avoid strain.

Applying Pressure

This is particularly crucial *when you are applying pressure*, because this is the aspect of massage that has the potential to put most strain on your body. The most common situations in which people get into problems are:

- Working across the table;
- Trying to cover the length of the client's back or legs;
- Being too close in or too far away from the table, and;
- Working on the prone client's shoulders.

As has been emphasised throughout this book, you need to get your body *behind* your hands to apply pressure so that you can use your bodyweight and avoid having to rely solely on the muscle power of your shoulders and arms. However, you also need to be able to get yourself *above* your hands in order to be able to deliver pressure (downwards) to them (through relatively straight arms, see figure 23.8).

Therefore, a major principle of this chapter is that you can only comfortably apply *pressure* when you can lean your body for the power, although you can reach further for pushing and pulling strokes (as long as you sway forward and backwards for these strokes). In practical terms this means that, if their arms are long enough, practitioners can do *pushing and pulling strokes* on the far side of the client's body or on the client's shoulders from the side of the table, or a certain distance down the client's back from the head of the table. However it is only possible to comfortably *apply pressure* onto the *close* side of the client's body or the close leg from the side of the table, and onto the client's shoulders from the head of the table.

The Client's Position
Of course, how *the client* is positioned will also affect how you are able to work. This chapter, like most of this book, mainly focuses on working with the client lying prone or supine on the massage table. The last part of the chapter looks briefly at working with the client lying on the side to illustrate this.

Working Across the Table

Facing across the massage table enables you to do some strokes comfortably on the far side of the client's back (or their further away leg), and makes others difficult and/or strainful to execute.

Push and Pull Across the Far Side of the Client's Back

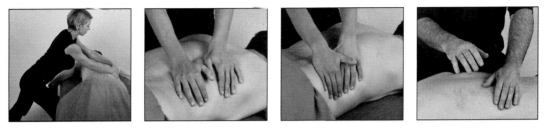

Figure 30.1: Working comfortably on the far side of the client's back; a) reaching across, b) pushing the erector spinae muscles, c) pulling the erectors, d) percussion.

For example, it is easy to push the erector spinae muscles away from the spine on the far side or pull them towards the spine. You can even reach to the far side of the client's back for kneading, wringing and percussion strokes, provided that your arms are long enough for you to comfortably reach across without straining your back.

Don't Try to Apply Pressure on the Far Side of the Client's Back

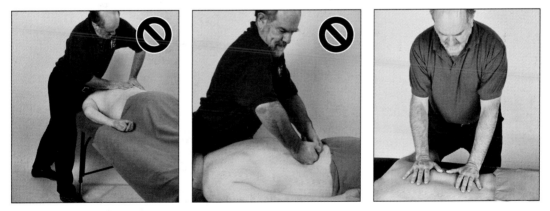

Figure 30.2: Straining to work on the far side of the client's back;
a), b) trying to apply pressure on the far side of client's back, c) working comfortably on the close side.

However, you can only position yourself comfortably to *apply pressure* without strain on the *close* side of the client's back. If you tried to apply firm pressure on the far side of the client's back, you would find yourself tensing your shoulder/s. It would also put pressure on your back, and it's not effective. So work firmly on the close side and then cross to the other side of the table to apply pressure there.

Don't Try to Apply Equal Pressure on Both Sides of the Client's Back

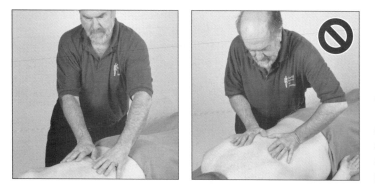

Figure 30.3:
Working equally on both sides
of the client's back;
a) light sliding strokes,
b) trying to apply equal pressure
from the side of the table.

When you are standing alongside the table, trying to apply pressure equally on both sides of the client's back creates the same problems. You can do *light* sliding strokes on both sides of the client's back, as long as you carefully monitor your own shoulders and back as you reach across. However, it would only be possible to simultaneously apply equal pressure by climbing up onto the table and straddling the client like a shiatsu practitioner.

Don't Try to Apply Pressure on the Client's Further Leg

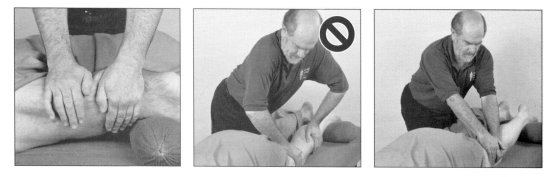

Figure 30.4: Working on the legs from the side of the table; a) wringing the far leg,
b) trying to press on the back of the far leg, c) pulling comfortably on the far leg.

This also applies on the client's legs. You can easily press on the close leg. You can also knead and wring on the far leg if your arms are long enough. You can even press onto the *inner side* of the far leg. However it's not possible to comfortably press on the back or the outer side of the far leg.

Trying to Reach Too Far

Trying to reach further than is comfortable makes strokes awkward and puts pressure on your lower back.

Avoid Overreaching From the End of the Table
This happens when practitioners try to slide their hands too far down the client's back from the head of the table, or too far up the leg from the foot of the table. (Obviously tall practitioners can comfortably reach further down the client's back than shorter practitioners). Instead, step to the side of the table, to cover the whole length of the client's back (one side at a time) or the full length of one leg.

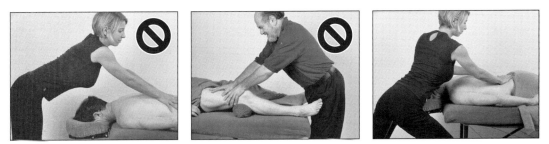

Figure 30.5: Reaching; a) overreaching from the head end of the table,
b) overreaching from the foot of the table, c) moving to the side of the table to avoid overreaching.

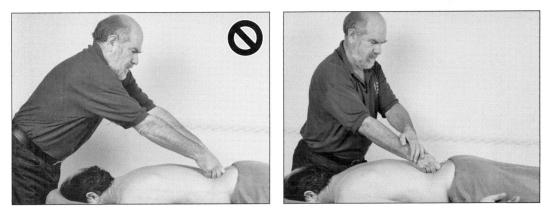

Figure 30.6: Applying pressure down the back; a) overreaching from the end of the table,
b) moving to the side of the table.

Similarly, when you are at the end of the table, don't try to *apply pressure* further down than the midback area, because you won't be able to get your weight above your hands. Instead move to the side of the table to press on the close side of the client's back.

Move to Avoid Overreaching When You're Alongside the Table

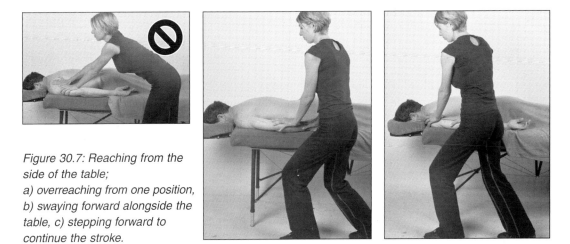

Figure 30.7: Reaching from the side of the table;
a) overreaching from one position,
b) swaying forward alongside the table, c) stepping forward to continue the stroke.

When you are standing alongside the table, don't stay in one position when you're doing long strokes, for example covering the length of the client's leg or back. Instead, maintain the pressure by stepping forward and stepping back on the return stroke.

Take Your Build into Account

Take your build into account as well, not only to determine how far to reach but also to decide what type of strokes to do. For example, tall practitioners will generally find it easier to reach across to do strokes on the far side of the client's body, such as working around the shoulder, that the short practitioner will only be able to comfortably execute on the close side. And the short practitioner's build will lend itself more to pushing strokes, that the tall practitioner will often find easier to replicate by pulling (from across the table).

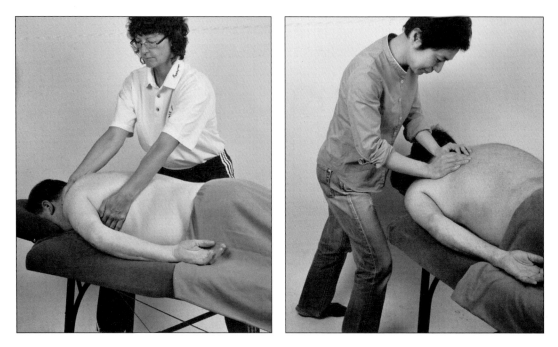

Figure 30.8: The length of the practitioner's arms; a) tall practitioner working across the table, b) short practitioner working on the close side of the table.

Moving In and Moving Away From the Table

Take care not to get in too close when you are applying pressure. Position yourself so that you can have your arms fairly straight (but not stiff) to deliver the pressure. If you are too close, your arms will be bent, which dissipates the power from your trunk.

Don't Cramp Yourself

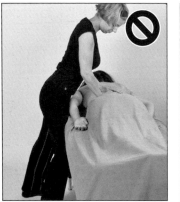
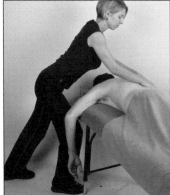
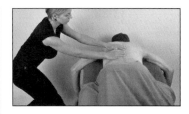

Figure 30.9: Distance from the table; a) jammed against table, b) close to the table for working comfortably across the client's body, c) further away from the table.

Standing against the table would restrict your ability to sway with your strokes and cause you to work with your upper body only, and could also put pressure on your back. Move in closer to the table or further away from it as your massage techniques demand so that you can use your bodyweight.

Working on the Prone Client's Shoulders

Working on the prone client's shoulders requires constant repositioning to avoid getting into awkward and potentially strainful positions.

Beware of Kneading the Client's Shoulders From the Side of the Table

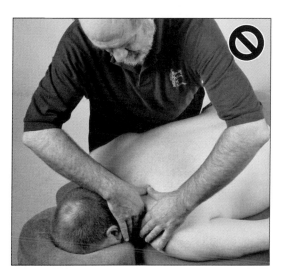

Figure 30.10: Kneading and wringing the client's shoulders; reaching over too far from the side of the table.

When you have been working at the side of the table, you can stay there to knead or wring the upper trapezius from this position. Work on the opposite shoulder if you can comfortably reach across, or the close one if you can't (see figure 30.8). Take care not to lean too far forward to work on the shoulder in this way.

Wring the Client's Shoulders if You Can Comfortably Reach Across

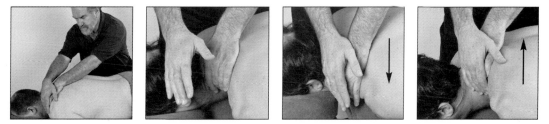

Figure 30.11: Double-handed wringing; a) using a two-handed stretch, b) the position of the hands, c) pushing with the heels, d) pulling back with the fingers.

If you can comfortably reach the opposite shoulder, use double-handed wringing instead.

Face the Shoulder That You're Working on at the Top of the Table

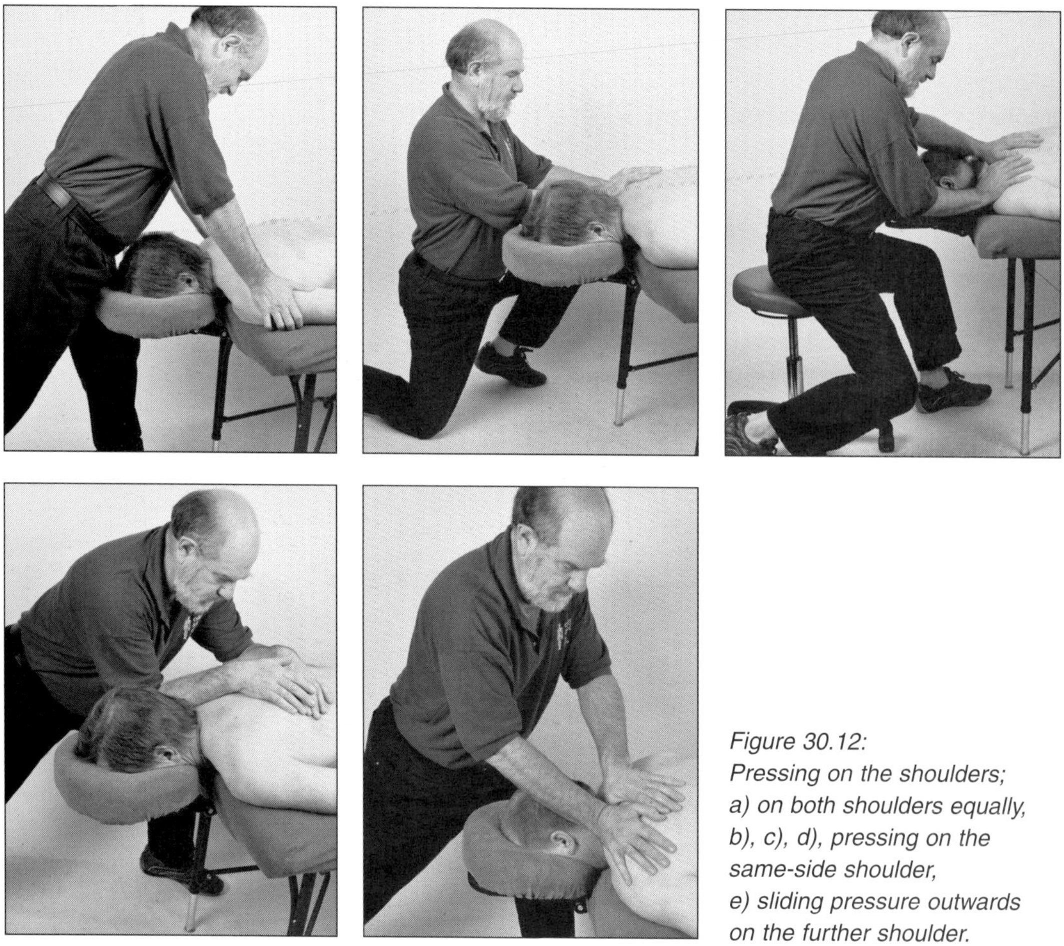

Figure 30.12:
Pressing on the shoulders;
a) on both shoulders equally,
b), c), d), pressing on the
same-side shoulder,
e) sliding pressure outwards
on the further shoulder.

It is impossible to comfortably press down on the top of the client's shoulders from the side of the table. Stand beyond the client's head to apply equal pressure on both shoulders simultaneously. Move a little to the side to press on the same-side shoulder. Or face diagonally across the table to slide the pressure out along the opposite shoulder.

The Advantages and Limitations of Each Client Position

Bear in mind that each position that your client takes up will have its advantages and limitations. You will find that you can work effectively on certain parts of the client's body or do particular stretches when s/he is in one position that are difficult or impossible in another position. This chapter finishes with a brief look at some of the special features of having the client lying on the side to illustrate this. Chapters 38 & 39 look at working with the client seated or lying on a futon on the floor.

Having the Client Lying on the Side

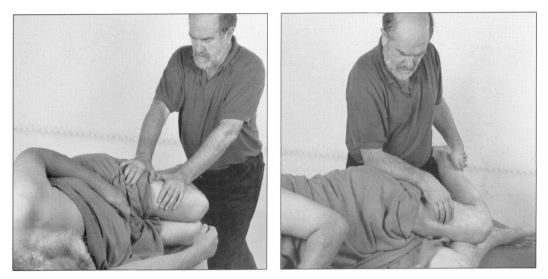

Figure 30.13: Working with the client lying on the side; a) working on the iliotibial band, b) working on the client's gluteus medius.

This position gives you easier and more extensive access to the outer side of the hip and thigh (gluteus medius and the iliotibial band) than you can get with the client either prone or supine. It also enables you to work on the adductors (on the inner thigh) of the client's other leg.

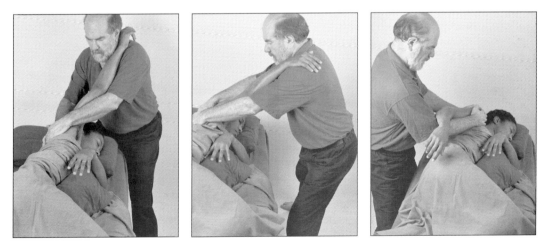

Figure 30.14: Working with the side-lying client's shoulder.

The same position gives you 360° access to the shoulder. This enables you to massage the client's shoulder from the front and the back, and from the top end of the table. You can also stretch her arm through its full range of movement without her needing to move.

Review

Your position around the massage table determines the type of stroke and pressure that will be effective and those that would be strainful to attempt.

Don't try to apply pressure on the far side of the client's back or their far leg.

Avoid trying to reach too far down the client's back from the head of the table or up the leg from the foot of the table.

Tall practitioner's can reach further without strain and often prefer to do pulling movements.

Short practitioners need to move more to prevent trying to reach too far, and have more potency in pushing and pressing techniques.

Don't cramp yourself by standing too close to the massage table.

Don't try to press on the client's shoulders from the side of the table.

Apply equal pressure on the shoulders from the top of the table.

Face each shoulder in turn to work on it from the head of the table.

Work in ways that suit the position that clients are in, or have them move into positions that give you easier access to particular areas of their body.

CHAPTER 31

Massaging While Seated

The previous chapters focused on standing at the massage table or massage chair. This chapter looks at bodyuse principles to keep in mind when you are seated on a chair or stool, or sitting on the massage couch.

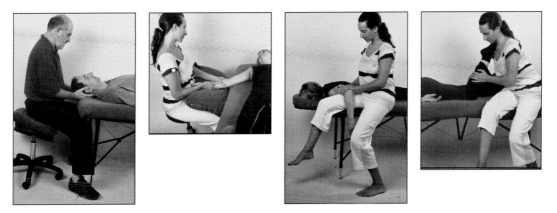

Figure 31.1: Seated practitioner; a) working on the client's head, b) nurturing stroking of the client's arm, c), d) sitting on the table.

Many practitioners sit down when working on small and/or sensitive areas of the client's body, particularly the head and neck, and sometimes areas such as the feet. This provides better stability than standing for this focused work. It's also useful for resting the client's arms/hands on your own body (on a towel, if you're using oil) to give them some nurturing stroking.

Many people also sit on the table, for example to support a client's limb, or to work deeply into the client's calves when the leg is propped up.

Sitting On a Stool or Chair

A Stool on Wheels

A stool on wheels with an easily adjustable height seat is the best seating. It moves with you as you change direction, which enables you to make small shifts in mid-massage with the least disruption. For example, you can gradually change the direction that you are facing as you slide your hand or your fist down the client's neck and out along the shoulder.

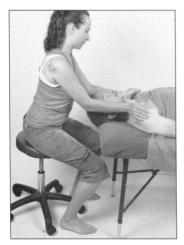 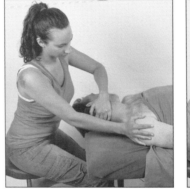 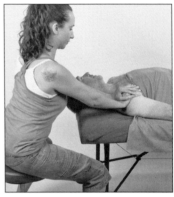

Figure 31.2: A stool on wheels; changing the angle of working.

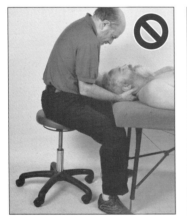 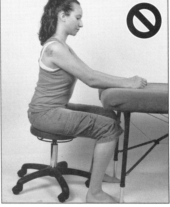 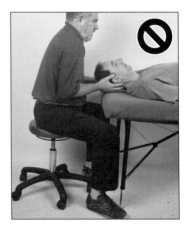

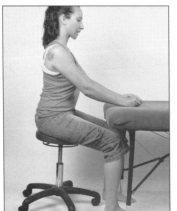 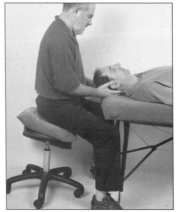

Figure 31.3:
Working at different heights;
a) hunching down,
b), c) seat too low for
comfortable working,
d) raising the seat for
comfortable working,
e) putting cushions on the seat.

If the seat height is readily adjustable, you can easily change the level that you are working on. This enables you to avoid hunching down if the seat is too high, or straining to get high enough for comfortable working. If the seat is too low for comfortable table work, build it up with cushions.

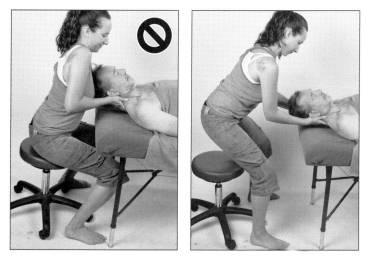

Figure 31.4:
Rising up from the stool;
a) trying to lift while seated,
b) rising to standing.

If necessary you can rise up smoothly to a low squat or to standing, and then sit back easily on the stool. If you need to stay standing, it's easy to push a stool on wheels out of your way with your foot, with minimal disruption to the massage. Or to retrieve it with your foot to sit again.

Using an Ordinary Stool
If neither of these are available, use an ordinary stool or chair. When you need to reposition your body, you can either slide across the seat or move the stool/chair. This is more difficult to do while sustaining the pressure than when you have a stool on wheels.

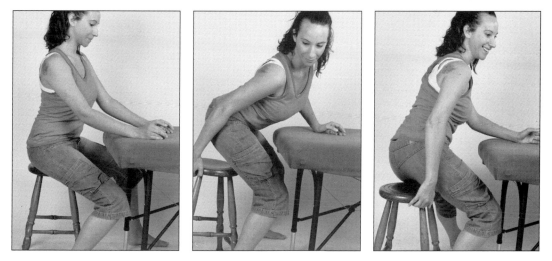

Figure 31.5: Repositioning yourself by shifting the stool.

It is obviously easier to move a stool in mid-massage than a chair, so they are preferable. You may find that you can rise up enough to shift the stool with one hand and then sit back on it in the new position.

Using a Chair

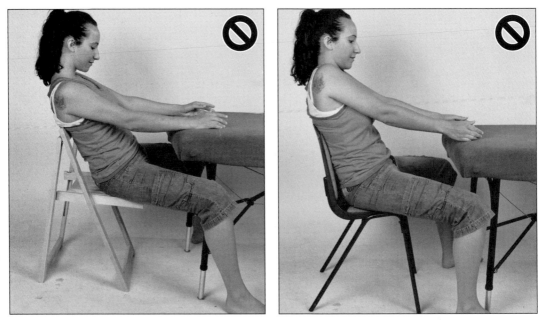

*Figure 31.6: Backward tilting chair back and sloping back seat; a) at the mercy of the chair,
b) consequent tensing and overusing the shoulders.*

If you are using a chair, try to avoid those which have a back that leans backwards or a seat that tilts
your hips backwards (as so many chairs do). They will push you into a slouch so that you'll have to
tense and overuse your shoulders to have any effect. Look for a chair with an upright back and a
horizontal seat.

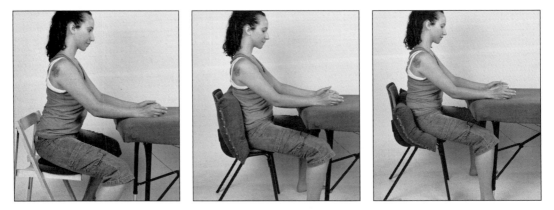

*Figure 31.7: Sitting up in the chair; a) sit forward, b) having a cushion behind the back to sit upright,
c) wedging a cushion under the butt to tilt the hips forward.*

If you find yourself slouching, try to sit towards the front of the chair so that you are able to sit upright,
plant your feet on the floor and lean or sway forward to engage your body in the massage. Putting a
cushion behind your back to keep you upright or under the back of your hips will help tilt you forward.

Relative Positions of the Seat and the Massage Table

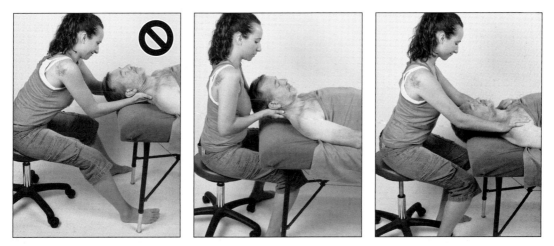

Figure 31.8: Sitting distance; a) too far away for comfortable lifting,
b) close enough to comfortably lift the client's head, c) further away for applying pressure by leaning.

You need to be able to move in close to the table, for example to comfortably lift the client's head without straining your back, and further away to apply pressure by leaning your trunk. Either move on your seat or move the stool/chair.

Involving Your Body When Seated

Align Your Trunk and Hands

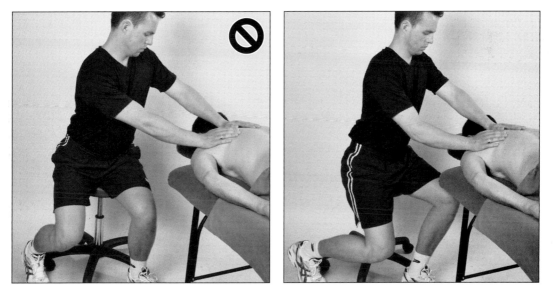

Figure 31.9: Aligning the trunk; a) body twisted away, b) lower body aligned behind the working hands.

Keep your trunk aligned behind your working hands/forearm to transmit the power of your bodyweight to them, rather than being twisted as you work.

Lean With Your Whole Trunk

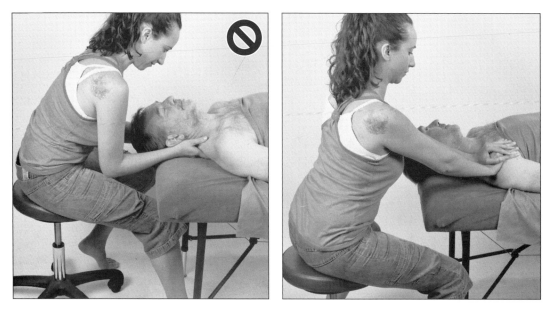

Figure 31.10: Leaning forward; a) crumpling the back, b) leaning forward with the whole trunk.

Use your bodyweight as much as possible to save your shoulders and hands. As you lean forward to apply pressure or do a sliding stroke, or lean back in a pulling stroke, maintain length in your trunk by rolling your hips on the seat, rather than hunching over or crumpling your back. This involves rolling your sitting bones (ischiums) on the chair, so make sure that the seat has adequate cushioning to make this comfortable.

The ideal is to keep your back like the dynamic posture of a good tennis player – long and *supple* (not stiff, see Chapter 25). There are many physically based disciplines such as yoga and Pilates that can help you to learn to lengthen and strengthen your back in action without rigidifying it in the process (see Chapter 44).

Avoid Overreaching

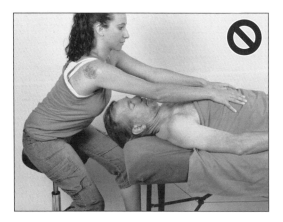

Figure 31.11: Overreaching while seated.

Don't try to reach further than is comfortable, which puts pressure on your back and will generally cause you to tense your shoulders and arms.

Involve Your Legs

If your legs don't provide adequate stability, you will tend to slouch and/or tighten your back (especially your lower back) in order to compensate. This, in turn, will force you to rely on your upper body only for your massage techniques.

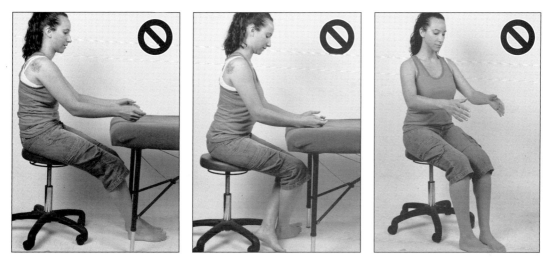

Figure 31.12: Lack of leg support when sitting; a) feet too far forward, b) legs crossed, c) feet too close together.

Having your legs stretched too far forward or crossed will not give good support for your trunk. Even having your feet too close together will restrict your ability to move and sway behind your hands, making your delivery more restricted and stilted.

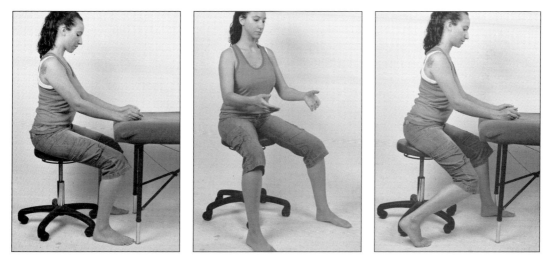

Figure 31.13: Leg support when sitting; a) feet planted, b) feet comfortably apart, c) one foot planted and the other leg bent.

Even for small movements of your hands, for example while massaging the client's head, make sure that you can sway and lean a little from your hips so that you don't become locked into a rigid position. Having your feet planted on the floor and your legs comfortably spread will steady your body for this.

You may find it easier at times to have only one foot in front and the other bent back, as long as you can still use them to comfortably stabilise and support your trunk.

Seated at the Head of the Couch

How you work at the head of a massage couch will be affected by the position of the table legs and the connection between them. Make sure that you aren't forced into positions that are uncomfortable for your back and/or force you to rely on just your upper body for your power by preventing you from swaying or leaning your lower body behind your strokes.

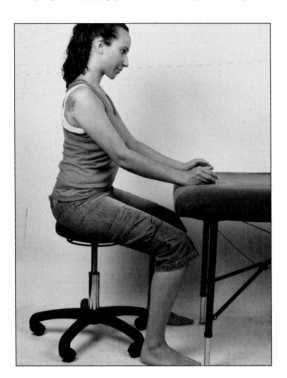

Figure 31.14: Sitting at a couch with recessed legs.

Some couches have recessed legs at the head end to make space for your legs when you are seated. The table pictured also has a high arch connecting the legs so that there's room for your knees to go straight forward under the table, which is a great advantage if you have long legs.

Other tables have the cross-stays between the couch legs low enough that you can position one or both legs relatively comfortably between the couch legs. This is more restrictive, as it takes time and attention to put your legs over the cross-stays and to take them out. Therefore you are more likely to work with one leg forward and the other back so that you can more easily change position. Take care that this doesn't compromise your back by forcing you into a twisted position.

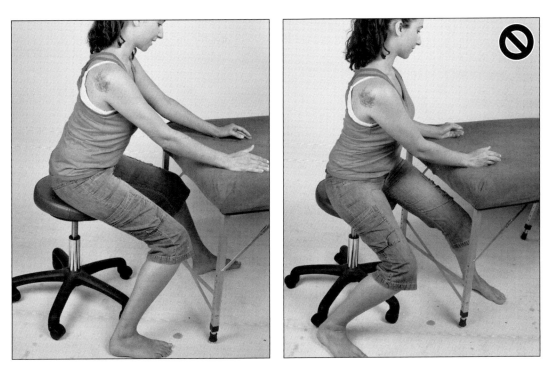

Figure 31.15: Sitting at a table with low cross-stays; a) one leg forward, b) working twisted.

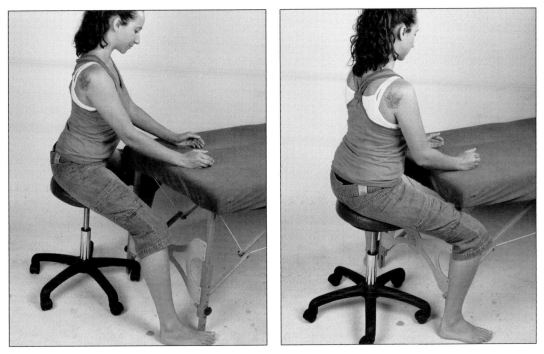

Figure 31.16: Spreading your legs wide; a) sitting at the corner of the table, b) sitting centrally.

However, with many couches, there's no room for your legs under the couch. On these tables, you need to spread your legs widely to get close enough to your client. Make sure that this spread of your legs doesn't put strain onto your lower back, particularly when you are sitting centrally.

Sitting on the Table

Many people also sit on the table to support a client's limb. When you are using oil, draping a towel over your clothing will protect it.

Don't Collapse into a Slouch

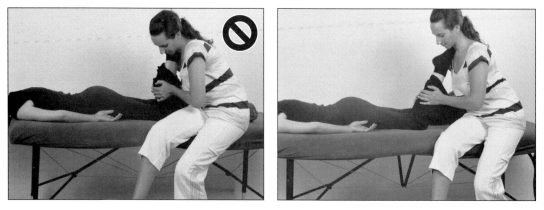

Figure 31.17: Sitting; a) slouching through sitting too close, b) further away to maintain length in the trunk.

Position yourself to avoid slouching, which can happen if you are too close to the area that you are working on.

Support From Your Leg

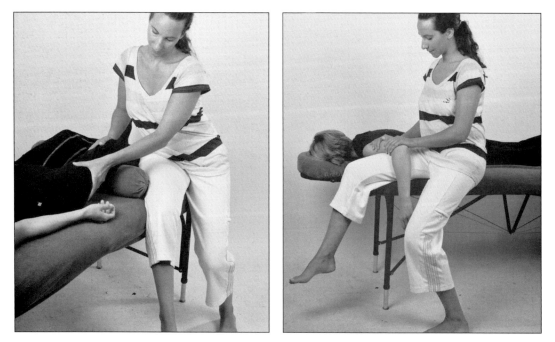

Figure 31.18: Sitting on the table with the supporting foot planted on the floor.

Try to keep one foot on the ground to stabilise your trunk and to generate the power that comes to your hands. Keep the other leg free to act as a helpful counterbalance when needed.

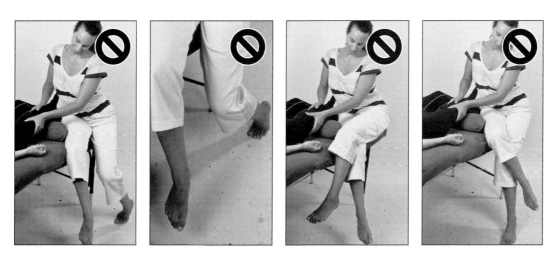

Figure 31.19: Unstable ways of sitting; a), b) with the supporting foot on tiptoes, c), d) crossing the legs.

Try not to be on tiptoe with this foot for any length of time, as that will reduce your stability and may lead to cramp in your calf. Don't cross your legs, which will also restrict you (even if you have one foot on the floor).

Lean Your Whole Body for Pushing and Pulling Movements

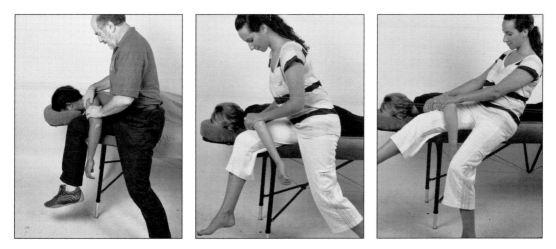

Figure 31.20: Leaning while seated on the table; a) using the free leg to counterbalance,
b) leaning forward to push, c) leaning back to pull.

To apply pressure or to push, push from the grounded leg as you lean forward with your whole trunk. Maintain the length in your trunk rather than hunching over.

To pull, lean back with your trunk. It can be helpful to bring your supporting leg forward to help this movement and to move your free leg forward as a counterbalance.

As you do these movements, you may find yourself momentarily flexing or turning your trunk. Don't keep your trunk in these postures for an extended period of time.

Don't Hold Your Breath

If you are using your body well, but still stiffening each time you push, apply pressure or pull, try to breathe out with the stroke rather than inhaling or holding your breath – both of which reinforce stiffening up when you're doing firm strokes.

Review

Sitting down gives you greater stability for working on small and/or sensitive areas of the client's body.

Make sure that your seat doesn't tilt your hips backwards. Use a wedge-shaped cushion or a rolled towel under the back of your pelvis to help tilt you forward if you find yourself slouching.

The best seating is an adjustable height stool on wheels.

Try to use a stool that puts your hips at roughly the same height as your knees. Build up the seat with cushions if necessary.

Lean forward with your whole trunk to apply pressure or do a sliding stroke, rather than hunching over or crumpling your back.

Have enough cushioning on the seat that you can comfortably roll on your sitting bones.

Sit towards the front of the seat so that you can plant your feet on the floor to give you stability as you sway with your strokes.

Keep your trunk aligned behind your working hands, rather than being twisted as you work.

Slide across the seat and/or move the stool or chair to reposition your body behind each stroke.

Move in close to the table for lifting and further away to apply pressure by leaning your trunk.

Don't try to reach further than is comfortable.

Plant your feet on the floor for stability. Don't have your feet too close together, or have your legs crossed and/or tucked under the stool.

Take care of your back when you are seated at the head of a massage couch.

If you have to slide one leg between the table legs and work slightly turned to the side, make sure that your body is not uncomfortably twisted.

Move between positions so that you don't stiffen into an awkward posture.

Sit on the table to support a client's limb, or to work deeply into the client's calves when their leg is propped up.

Don't sit so close to the area that you're working on that you have to hunch over.

When you are sitting on the table, try to keep one foot on the ground to stabilise your trunk.

Push from your foot to apply pressure or do a sliding stroke. Try not to be on tiptoe for any length of time.

To pull, lean back and bring your supporting leg forward.

CHAPTER 32

Kneeling While Massaging

This chapter focuses on kneeling on the floor when you are working at the massage table or massage chair to work lower than is comfortable in standing. It also looks briefly at kneeling one knee on the massage table to get your weight above the client. (Chapter 42 looks at kneeling and sitting for floor massage).

As in standing, the power for pushing, pulling, or sustained pressure techniques is ideally generated from your lower body. The strength of the massage then comes from positioning your bodyweight behind your hands and leaning forward or pulling back, rather than by tensing your shoulders and relying solely on upper body muscle power. This keeps your hands relatively relaxed for fine-tuning your massage techniques.

Kneeling on the Floor

There are two interrelated aspects of bodyuse to monitor:

- The comfort of your knees, and;
- Looking after your back.

Supporting Your Knees

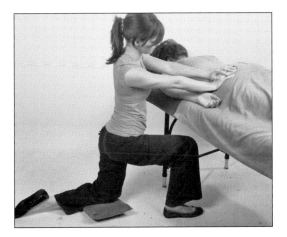

Figure 32.1: Supporting your knees with a cushion.

When you are kneeling on the floor, it is good to have padding under your knees to protect them. Have cushions at hand to slide under your knee/s.

Looking After Your Back

When you are kneeling (or sitting on the floor, see figure 42.3), it is important to monitor your back. Lean and sway your trunk to underpin the work of your hands. This need only be a small sway of your trunk, but it has a very different effect from just using your arms. The main principles are to:

- Keep your body aligned behind your hands;
- Avoid trying to reach too far;
- Lean with your whole trunk rather than hunching over, and;
- Only lift parts of the client's body if you can use your legs and not just your back.

Don't 'Kneel Up' on Both Knees

You might want to sit on one or both heels for short periods, if it is comfortable for you (see figure 42.5), for example to massage the client's arm when it is dangling off the side of the table. However, the main focus of doing massage when you are kneeling will be to work on the areas of the client's body that are close to the level of the tabletop, and too low for you to comfortably get to in standing.

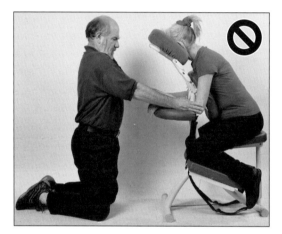

Figure 32.2: 'Standing up' on both knees.

Therefore, beware of 'standing up' on your knees to apply pressure. This will cause you to stiffen your lower back for balance and stability, putting pressure on it. This position is quite restricting, so move instead into the 'proposal position'.

The 'Proposal' Position

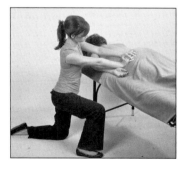 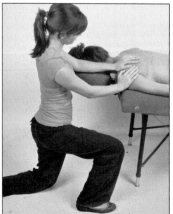 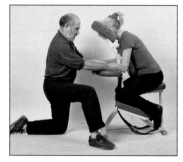

Figure 32.3: The 'proposal' position.

The 'proposal' position (having one knee and one foot on the floor) provides a more mobile and dynamic way of working. It enables you to work higher without tensing your back. You can range over a wider area without losing balance or power, and without having to reposition yourself.

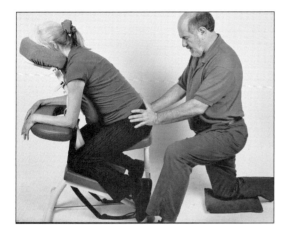

Figure 32.4: Cushion under the knee.

Have a cushion under your knee if necessary.

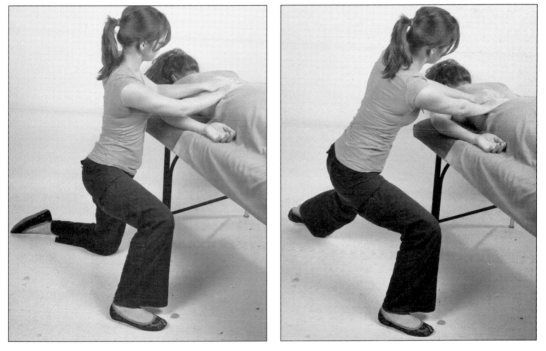

Figure 32.5: Rising; a) from the 'proposal' position, b) to standing.

And it is easy to rise up from the 'proposal' position into a low squat as the need arises, and then drop back into the proposal position without strain or disruption to the massage.

Aligning Your Feet, Knees and Hips

It is important to keep your hips facing in the direction of your massage tools and the direction of movement when you are applying sustained pressure or doing strokes that sway forward and back.

As for standing at the table, which foot you have standing in front will determine the way that you are able to face (see figure 28.18). For example, when you are kneeling at the head of the table to work on the client's shoulder, having one foot forward will face you across the table, while having the other foot forward will turn you to face along the side of the table.

Also, as for standing, don't let your front foot turn out too far (see figure 28.24), which could strain your knee, and don't let your knee fall to the inside or outside of your foot as you sway forward (see figure 28.26).

Kneeling One Knee on the Table

Sometimes it is useful to kneel one knee onto the massage table.

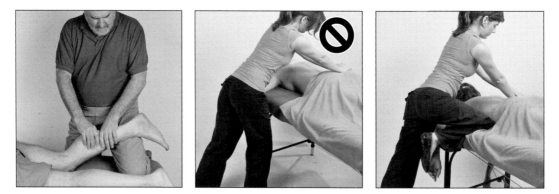

Figure 32.6: Kneeling one knee on the massage table; a) to support the client's ankle,
b) straining to reach across the table, c) getting closer to the client.

You might do it to support parts of the client's body, such as their ankle. It's also useful to save your back when you need to get closer to your client on a wide table, especially if you have short legs. Don't kneel up if the table is too high for you to comfortably reach.

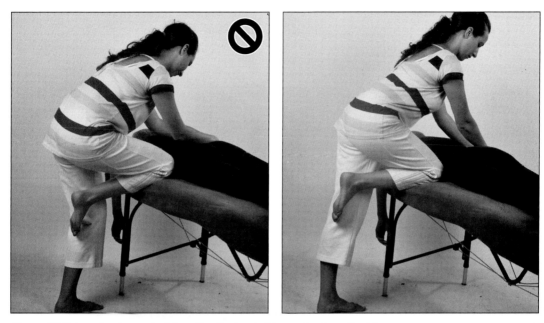

Figure 32.7: Leaning forward; a) bending the back, b) swaying from the hips.

When leaning forward for massage strokes, sway from your hips, rather than hunching over.

Review

When you're kneeling, have cushions under your knees to protect them if necessary.

Position your bodyweight behind your hands and lean forward or pull back with your trunk, rather than by tensing your shoulders.

Keep your hips aligned behind your working hands/forearm, and bend and sway from your hips, rather than hunching over.

Don't try to reach further than is easily comfortable.

Use the proposal position to get at areas of the client's body that are close to the surface of the massage table (rising into a slow squat if you need to), or to work on low parts of the client's back when s/he is in a massage chair.

In the 'proposal' position (being on one knee and one foot):

- Sway forward for sliding strokes;
- Change the direction that you are facing by changing the foot that you are standing on;
- Don't let your front foot turn out too far;
- Keep your knee balanced over your foot as you sway forward.

When you kneel one knee on the massage table, lean forward with your whole trunk, rather than hunching over.

Bodyuse for Common Massage Strokes

This section of the book looks at coordinating how you use your body and your hands for 'classic' Swedish massage strokes – effleurage, petrissage, compression strokes, and percussion and vibration techniques – and other commonly used techniques such as applied stretches and body rocking. These chapters synthesise information from Section 3 on hand use (Chapters 11–17) and Section 5 on bodyuse (Chapters 22–28). This section emphasises working *defensively* – looking after your hands, particularly conserving your fingers and thumbs, and using your body to support them.

The Terminology of Swedish Massage

Swedish Massage is the name given in Sweden and throughout the English-speaking world to the massage sequence that was put together by Per Henrik Ling in Stockholm in the early 1800s. The same style of massage is known as *Classical Massage* in other parts of Europe. The terminology coined by the Dutch physician, Georg Mezger, in the mid-1800s, is today used by massage practitioners, physiotherapists, osteopaths, and beauty therapists. In this book, I'm using the most commonly agreed categories, grouping types of strokes according to how they are applied and how they affect the soft tissue.

In the 'classic' Swedish massage sequence, each group of strokes is seen as belonging to a set stage of the massage. The general sequence of working is to begin lightly and gradually work more deeply, taking it at a pace and to a depth and pressure that is appropriate for the client. The practitioner then gradually lightens the pressure to finish the massage.

The Limits of the Terminology

Each chapter in this section looks at a different type of stroke, describing them as if massage consisted of a set of completely separate, distinctively different 'strokes'. Most massage teaching begins in this way because it makes it easier for description and learning. However, while this terminology can cover the underpinning 'building blocks' of massage, it has its limits.

For example, many common strokes don't fit neatly into the generally agreed groupings. Draining / 'milking' strokes are often seen as the crossover between effleurage and petrissage, and the heaviest effleurage (sliding) strokes blur into compression strokes. And elements of two types of strokes are sometimes deliberately blended for particular effects, such as using a sliding (effleurage) vibration along a limb, incorporating aspects of kneading into a sliding stroke, or including deep pressure in wringing movements. A further blurring has occurred with the influx of techniques from other traditions and the development of new types of techniques in recent decades.

The distinctions between strokes is also blurred by the need to join strokes together into a fluid, continuous sequence for a massage to be effective. In fact, the individual ways that practitioners develop of moving between strokes and between different parts of the body, which is part of the development of their own style, would often be hard to describe in terms of the 'classical' grouping of the strokes. In addition, many people find themselves developing the 'transition' strokes that they discover in this process into 'full' strokes in their own right.

Also, while it is customary to view each set of strokes in the classic massage sequence as a preparation for the next (and this can be very useful for the novice), the boundaries between these 'stages' are not clear-cut in practice. Experienced practitioners often combine strokes, incorporate other types of strokes and bend the 'rules' of the classical sequence.

And, of course, each massage needs to suit the individual client. You will need to modify or expand strokes or leave them out according to the needs and responses of your clients. For example, you would primarily use effleurage strokes for giving a nurturing massage to a baby or a frail senior citizen. In contrast, a sportsperson with well-used muscles would expect you to fairly quickly to get to a deep level of pressure and operate there for most of the massage.

CHAPTER 33

Effleurage Strokes

This chapter looks at the best ways of using and *saving* your hands in effleurage strokes and how to coordinate your bodyuse to support them. Most massage begins with light effleurage strokes, and then the pressure is increased as a prelude to other, deeper strokes. Sometimes effleurage is the main or only type of stroke used, especially with babies and frail older people where the focus is on nurturing massage, or when clients have conditions which preclude the use of deeper work, such as certain severe forms of multiple sclerosis. In relaxation massage, effleurage strokes are usually begun slowly and evenly to start relaxing the client. In sports massage they are done more briskly to warm up and energise the tissues in preparation for the deeper strokes.

Draining / 'milking' strokes are sometimes classed as effleurage strokes because of the way that they slide along the length of limb muscles. However they also involve squeezing the muscle, so they will be covered in the next chapter with other petrissage strokes.

'Holds' are not usually considered to be a part of the 'classic' Swedish massage sequence but are often used to begin massage treatments, especially in relaxation massages. They are done by resting your hands quietly for a time on the client's body. Because holds are used to prepare the way for effleurage strokes and are done in a similar way, there is a brief section on them at the end of this chapter.

Using Your Hands

Use as Much of Your Hands as You Can

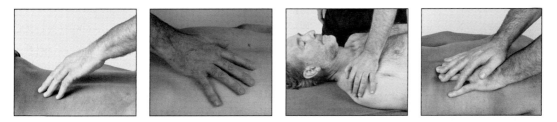

Figure 33.1: Using large areas of the hand; a) fingertips for 'feathering', b) front surface of fingers, c) whole hand stroking, d) hand on hand pressure.

There is a temptation to use just your fingers for stroking because of the sensitivity of the tips. Your fingertips work well when you're brushing lightly across the skin in a 'feathering' stroke. And you can use the front surface of your fingers for stroking small, delicate areas such as the face. However, it is important to save your fingers by using the whole front surface of your hand whenever you can, particularly when you're incorporating pressure into the strokes.

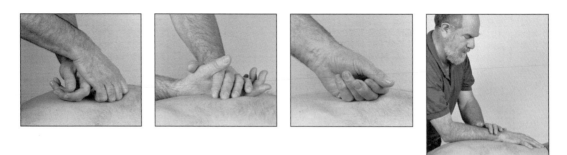

Figure 33.2: Saving the fingers; a) using the knuckles,
b) using the back of the hand, c) using the fist, d) using the forearm.

If you need to apply firm pressure, switch to using your knuckles, the back of your hand, your fist, or your forearm. If you need to, return briefly to using your fingers to palpate an area. But use the larger areas regularly so that you develop your ability to palpate with them.

Keep Your Hand Relaxed
Stiff and unresponsive hands use unnecessary energy and make sliding strokes stilted and uneven. They also tend to evoke an instinctive wariness in clients rather than inviting them to relax.

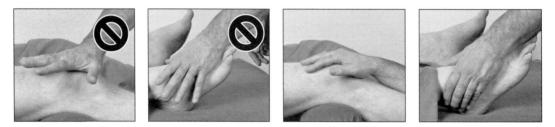

Figure 33.3: Stroking; a), b) with a stiff hand, c), d) a relaxed hand following body shapes.

Whether you're doing light 'feathering' strokes or firm stroking, it is important to keep your hands relaxed. This enables you to continuously mould them to the contours of the client's body as you slide them over the different shapes. It also makes it easier to sense the state of the client's muscles, and to feel the responses which help you to gauge how soon and how much pressure to apply. You can vary your pressure according to the 'terrain' and these responses. Lighten your pressure to slide over bones. Slide lightly over thin or soft muscles and press more deeply into areas of thick, sinewy and/or well-used muscles.

Use Your Other Hand to Increase the Pressure
When you're using your palm, increase the pressure by putting one hand on the other, while keeping both hands as relaxed as possible. Lean your body to deliver more weight via your top hand (see figure 33.9). You can also use your other hand across your fingers to increase the pressure that you deliver through the tips. Don't overdo this because of the pressure that it puts on your fingers.

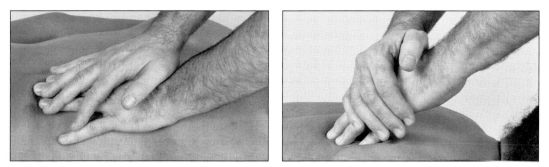

Figure 33.4: Using the other hand to increase the pressure; a) hand-on-hand pressure, b) pressing on the fingers.

Keep the Non-working Parts of Your Hands Relaxed

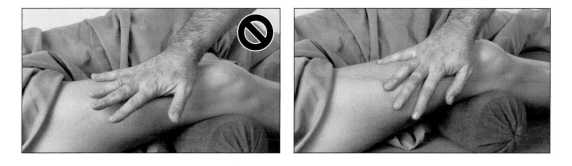

Figure 33.5: Focusing pressure through the heel of the hand; a) with stiff fingers, b) with relaxed hand.

At times, you will want to focus pressure through specific areas of your hand. As you direct the pressure through one part of your hand, such as your heel or palm, try to keep the other parts, such as your thumb or fingers, as relaxed as possible.

Moving the Focus of Pressure Through Different Parts of the Hand

Try this exercise to get used to changing the area of your hand through which you focus pressure while keeping the rest of your hand relaxed. Place your hand on your partner's back or thigh where you can rest it relatively flat. Relax your hand so that it can take up the shape of your partner's body.

Lean forward to apply general pressure through your hand. Then without moving your hand or tensing any part of it, sway your body to move the point of delivery of the pressure through different parts of your hand.

When you feel comfortable with this, give yourself the challenge of focusing pressure through different parts of your hand (and keeping it relaxed) while sliding it.

Take Care of Your Wrists

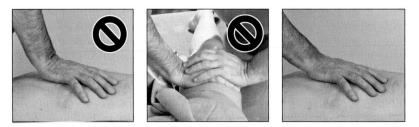

Figure 33.6:
The angle of the wrist;
a), b) bent,
c) straight.

When you increase the pressure that you are applying, make sure that your wrist is not significantly bent which would put pressure on it (see figures 17.4–17.8). Even when you are doing light stroking, take care that it is not bent for long periods.

Involving Your Body

Aligning Your Body Behind Your Hands

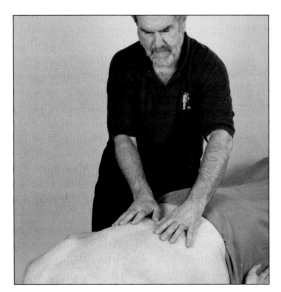

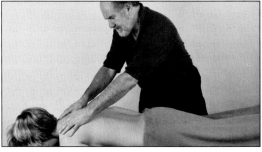

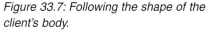

Figure 33.7: Following the shape of the client's body.

Keep your hips aligned directly behind your hands (see figure 27.9), so that your bodyweight is the powerhouse for your hand movements. Therefore, when you're following the broad contours of the body, you may need to sway a little from side to side and/or change position so that the movement of your hips echoes the weaving movements of your hands.

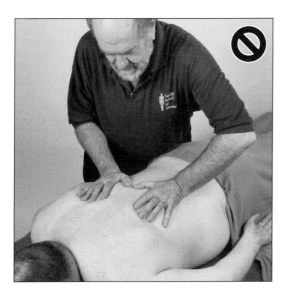

Figure 33.8: Trying to apply pressure on both sides.

When you're standing alongside the table, it's fine to do *light* stroking simultaneously on both sides of the client's back. However, it's not possible to apply firm pressure evenly. Trying to do this is awkward. You will find yourself tensing your shoulder and it puts pressure on your lower back. So, apply firm pressure on the close side only and then cross to the other side of the table.

Lean Forward to Increase the Power

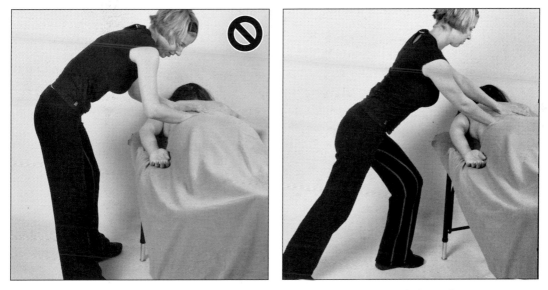

Figure 33.9: Increasing the pressure; a) hunching over, b) leaning with the whole trunk.

Lean forward with your whole trunk to increase the pressure, rather than hunching over.

Sway for Sliding Hand Movements

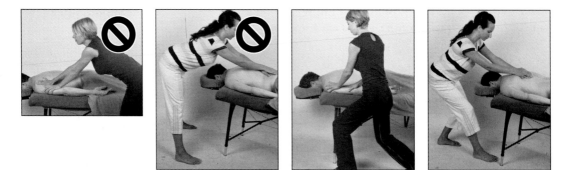

*Figure 33.10: Body movement with effleurage strokes; a), b) standing still,
c), d) swaying and stepping forward with the stroke.*

Standing still leads to stilted sliding strokes which are unnecessarily hard work. So, even for light sliding strokes, sway forward and back to support the movement of your hands (and step forward and back if you need to). This will give fluidity to the stroke, and deliver power when it's appropriate. It will also enable you to keep your hands relaxed. This makes it easy to vary the pressure within a stroke in response to the client's build and responses.

Bend Your Front Knee as You Sway Forward

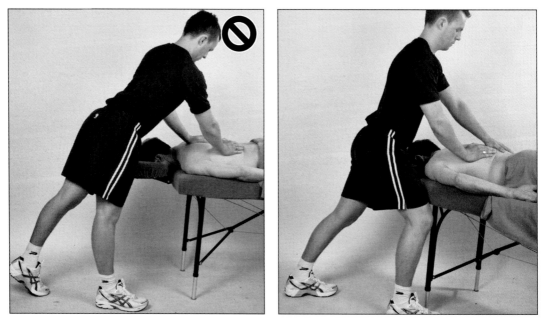

*Figure 33.11: Swaying forward for an effleurage stroke; a) stiffening the front knee,
b) bending the front knee.*

Sway forward and back in the lunge position (see figure 28.15) for long effleurage strokes along the length of the body. When you are swaying forward, let your front knee bend so that your body movement remains smooth. Keeping the front knee straight would cause you to rise up into a stiff, less balanced position, which would disrupt the continuity of your hand movements.

Use Your Breathing to Help Make Sliding Strokes More Fluid

When you are doing long, slow effleurage strokes, you can also use your breathing to help pace the strokes and keep them even. Breathe out as you push rather than breathing in or holding your breath, both of which are likely to cause you to tense up (see figure 27.3).

Avoid Overreaching

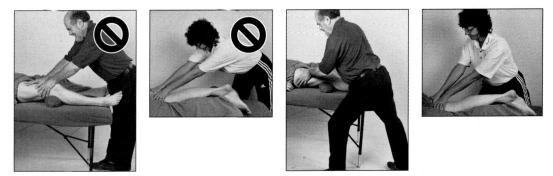

Figure 33.12: Position for full leg effleurage; a), b) reaching from the foot of the table, c), d) standing alongside the client's lower leg.

When you are doing long sliding strokes, don't try to reach too far, which puts strain on your back. This is especially important for short practitioners, particularly if the client is tall.

For example, don't stand at the foot of the table to slide your hands up the whole length of a client's leg. Instead stand by the lower leg. Similarly stand alongside the client's forearm when you are working on his/her arms.

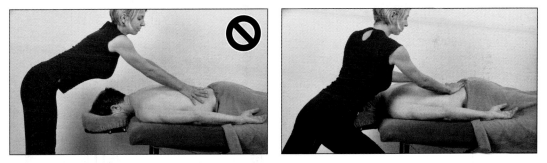

Figure 33.13: Reaching from the head of the table; a) trying to reach too far, b) moving to the side to reach further down the back.

Similarly there is a limit to how far you can comfortably reach down the client's back from the top of the table. Overreaching will put strain on your lower back, and will not be particularly effective. Instead, move to the side of the table to work on the client's lower back, one side at a time.

Step Forward Alongside the Table to Avoid Overreaching

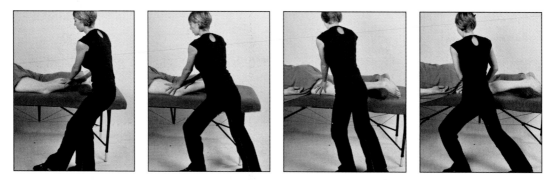

Figure 33.14: Stepping forward alongside the table for long strokes;
a) stepping forward to begin the stroke, b) swaying forward, c) stepping up with the back foot to move along,
d) stepping forward with the front foot to complete the stroke.

You may not be able to comfortably reach the whole length of a client's leg or back in one sweep without straining your own back. If this is the case, step forward along the side of the table in mid-stroke. Do it by bringing your back foot up behind the front one, and then taking your weight onto your back foot so that you can step out with the front one and sway forward again. Reverse the process when you are sliding back on the return.

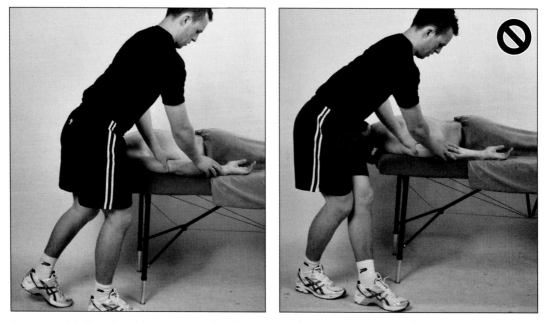

Figure 33.15: Crossing the legs when stepping up; a) preparing to step forward,
b) bringing the back leg past the front.

When stepping forward, don't bring your back leg past your front leg as this would turn your hips away from the table, twisting your body and interfering with the continuity of the stroke.

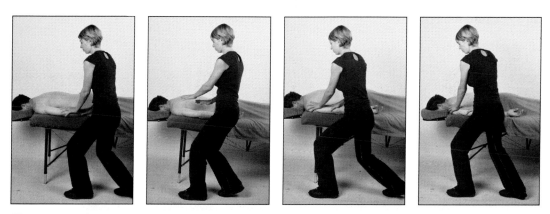

Figure 33.16: Stepping up alongside the table for short overlapping strokes; a) first stroke, b) lifting off the hands and stepping up, c) starting the next stroke, d) finishing the stroke.

Another option is to do a series of shorter overlapping strokes instead of trying to maintain a single long one. As you finish each short stroke, lighten your hands and step up along the table so that you can start the next stroke a little further back from where you finished the previous one. Gradually move forward doing these overlapping strokes, making a smooth lift off and remaking contact smoothly to give the client a sense of continuity of progression. Reverse the process to work your way back.

'Holds'

'Holds' are not usually considered to be a part of the 'classic' Swedish Massage sequence but are in widespread use. They are done by resting your hands quietly for a time on the client's body. Many massage practitioners begin and end the massage with them, and also use them intermittently throughout the massage, especially in relaxation massage.

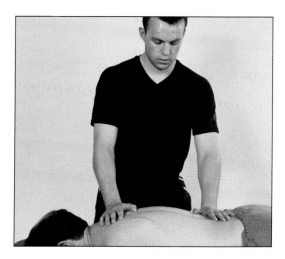

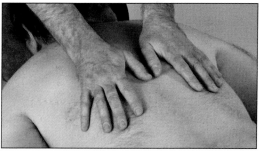

Figure 33.17: Holds; a) standing comfortably, b) relaxed 'melting' hand.

When doing them, it is important to keep your hands and your body relaxed. Stand in a position which you will be able to comfortably maintain for a period of time. Allow your hands to relax so that they mould to the contours of the client's body. And don't be heavy-handed. If your hands are resting on the client's back for example, keep them light enough so that they can gently rise and fall with the client's breathing cycle without impeding it.

Review

Use the largest appropriate area of your hands for doing effleurage strokes. Save your fingers by using your palm, knuckles or forearm.

Keep your hand relaxed so that it can continuously adapt to the contours of the client's body.

Where appropriate, focus pressure through specific areas of your hand, keeping the other parts as relaxed as possible.

Press on your working hand with your other hand to increase the pressure.

Take care not to let your wrists bend, especially when you're applying pressure.

Align your body behind your hands, and lean forward to increase the pressure (rather than hunching over).

Sway your body to deliver power and fluidity to sliding hand movements.

Bend your front knee as you sway forward.

Use your breathing to help make sliding strokes more fluid, focusing in particular on breathing out as you push forward.

Position yourself alongside the client's limbs or back to avoid overreaching as you cover the whole limb. Move to the side of the table to avoid trying to reach the whole of the client's back from the head of the table.

In long strokes, step forward in mid-stroke to avoid straining to reach too far, taking care not to cross your legs as you step, which would turn you away from the table.

When doing 'holds', position yourself so that you can stay comfortably in the same position for a period of time, and let your hands relax so that they mould to the contours of the client's body.

CHAPTER 34

Petrissage Strokes

Once the tissues have been warmed with effleurage, petrissage strokes focus on restoring pliability to tense, contracted muscles. This rejuvenation is helped by the 'pumping' action of alternately squeezing and releasing the muscles, which also stimulates blood circulation through them. Petrissage strokes are most effective on the long muscles of the limbs and the areas of the trunk where you can get your hands around the muscles. Heavy petrissage strokes, in which pressure is directed to the underlying tissue to help free adhesions, lead into and overlap with compression strokes (see Chapter 35).

Looking After Your Hands

Petrissage strokes make more demands of your thumbs and fingers than most other strokes, apart from applying pressure with your thumbs (see Chapter 35). So this chapter emphasises working *defensively*. Use petrissage strokes sparingly and appropriately. For example, kneading strokes that are fine on small, soft muscles can cause cumulative strain if you regularly use them on large, sinewy and/or well-used muscles (and they won't be very effective).

Use Other Tools to Achieve Similar Effects
Think about whether the particular stroke is absolutely essential to the massage. Try to save thumb and finger-intensive petrissage strokes, particularly kneading, for areas where you feel that you have no other options. Whenever possible, find other ways of achieving similar effects, for example by using larger areas of your hands, or your forearm, or elbow. You may still need to palpate the area initially with your sensitive fingertips. With practise, as you get accustomed to using these other massage tools, you will learn to pick up more information through them.

Take Into Account the Size of Your Hands
Petrissage strokes don't often cause problems for practitioners with large, strong hands. If this is your build, the information here will help you to avoid tiring your hands.

However, other practitioners, *especially* those with small hands, or long, slender or hypermobile digits, need to be very careful about doing petrissage strokes. The information in this chapter is particularly directed towards you, as you are more at risk of straining your thumbs, and perhaps your fingers too.

General Principles to Look After Your Hands

This chapter looks at the potential problems and how to avoid them for four main petrissage strokes – kneading, squeezing, wringing, and 'draining' strokes. General principles for using petrissage strokes are to:

- Try not to use your finger and thumb tips too often, but try to use as much of your fingers and thumbs as you can;
- Conserve your thumbs and fingers, for example by using kneading sparingly;
- Avoid having your thumbs hyperextended;
- Save your thumbs by using the base of your thumb or your knuckles instead, and by using the heels of your hands only for wringing;
- Reduce the pressure on your fingers by using them together rather than separately;
- Use both hands together whenever possible, either one hand supporting the other for example for squeezing, or using one hand on the other, for example for double-handed wringing;
- Move your hand for the strokes rather than holding it stiffly, and;
- Move your body to power the stroke rather than standing still.

The Terminology of Petrissage

There is more disagreement about the terminology of petrissage strokes than any other group of strokes – both about the types of strokes included in this grouping, and the specific names for each of these strokes. So, if you have learnt to group strokes in different ways or with different names, I hope you will bear with the way that I've categorised them in this chapter.

For example, some people class draining/'milking' strokes as effleurage strokes because they slide along muscles, and others as petrissage because of the 'muscle pumping' effect. I have included them in this chapter.

Because the deeper petrissage strokes 'blur' into compression strokes, some authorities put both into one collective grouping. Although there is quite an overlap, I find it useful to distinguish between strokes that primarily move and stretch the tissue (petrissage) and those that press or dig down into it (compression, see Chapter 35). Deep knuckle kneading, which operates at the crossover, is covered in this chapter.

Squeezing

Squeezing strokes can vary from pinching, to 'grabbing' with the whole hand or with both hands together.

Don't Overuse Your Finger or Thumb Tips

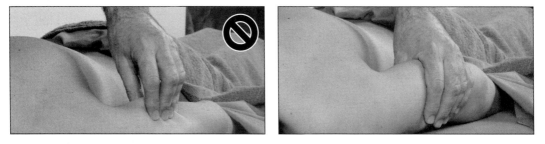

Figure 34.1: Squeezing; a) just using the tips of the finger and thumbs, b) using more of the digits.

Use as much of your thumb and fingers as you can for squeezing the muscles to avoid just using the tips.

Don't Let Your Wrist Hyperextend

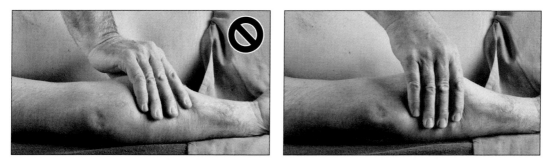

Figure 34.2: The angle of the wrist; a) hyperextended, b) relatively straight.

Don't let your wrist bend back as you take hold of the muscles.

Move Your Hand

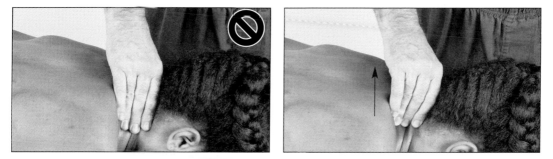

Figure 34.3: Squeezing; a) holding the hand still; b) moving the arm.

When you are squeezing muscles with your thumb and fingers, don't hold your hand still. Instead, move it forward to take hold of the tissue, and then move it back a little as you squeeze. This reduces the work of your fingers and thumbs, while giving more power and fluidity to the stroke.

Support Your Hand

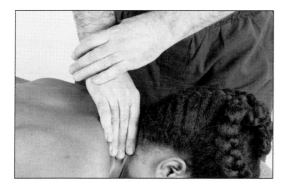

Figure 34.4: Supporting the squeezing hand.

Unless you are using your other hand for some other crucial action, use it to support your working hand. This reduces the work of your working hand. It is particularly important when you are working on large, well-used muscles.

Save Your Digits

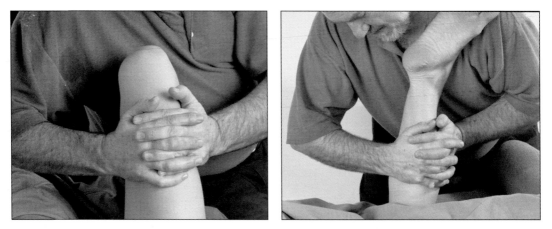

Figure 34.5: Using the heels with interlocked fingers; a) squeezing and stretching quadriceps, b) squeezing and stretching the calf muscles.

Where you can get your hands around the muscles of the limbs, you can interlock your fingers and squeeze with the heels of your hands to save your digits. For example, prop up the client's leg to work in this way on the quadriceps and the calf muscles.

Move Your Body for the 'Squeeze and Stretch' Technique

You can get more release in the muscles by stretching them while maintaining the squeeze on them – the 'squeeze and stretch' technique. Take hold of the muscles and lean or sway back while maintaining the grip, rather than just pulling with your arms.

'Draining'/'Milking' Strokes

'Draining' or 'milking' strokes, which combine sliding along muscles with squeezing them, are used to 'pump' the limb muscles, particularly in the forearm and lower leg.

Conserve Your Hands

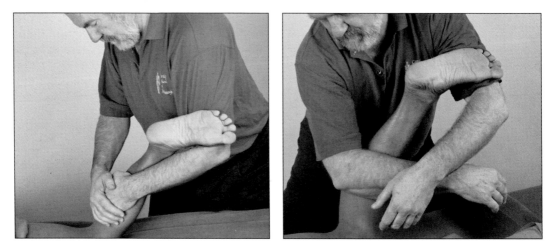

Figure 34.6: Saving the hands in draining strokes; a) using both hands together, b) using the forearm.

Take care not to hold your hands stiffly. On large, well-developed muscles, conserve your hands, especially if they are small, by using both hands together. Or switch to using your forearm for a sliding pressure stroke (see figure 18.6).

Move With the Stroke

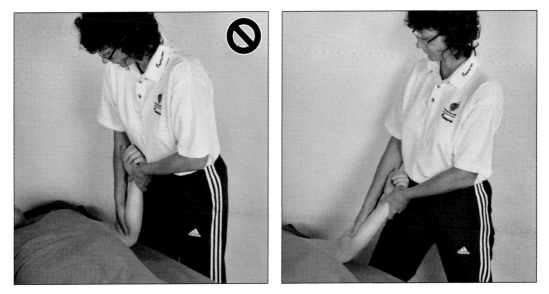

Figure 34.7: Moving your body for 'milking' strokes; a) standing too close to be able to move, b) leaning for 'milking' down a limb.

Give yourself enough space to be able to lean forward for the power, and sway forward for the draining movement. It will sometimes be easier to hold the distal section of the arm or leg upright to 'milk' down ('towards the heart'). In this position, slide your hand/s by bending your knees to slowly drop down. If necessary, widen your stance to make this easier.

Kneading

A range of strokes are classed as 'kneading', ranging from small, focused techniques in which you use your fingers and thumbs to squeeze the tissues to large hand movements in which you pick up and twist the tissues as you pass them from hand to hand. For the sake of clarity, I am calling these strokes respectively 'thumb kneading' and 'breadmaking'. 'Thumb kneading' can also include deeper kneading in which you dig into the tissues. These strokes, which overlap with wringing and compression strokes, all involve picking up the tissues with one hand as you release them with the other. In 'circular kneading', you have one hand supporting the other.

Use Thumb Kneading Sparingly
Although kneading is a classic massage technique because of its effectiveness in softening tissue, it is energy consuming to do. Practitioners with large, strong hands (and a strong build to support their hands) can generally do a reasonable amount of kneading without problems, although they need to avoid overusing their thumbs. However, practitioners with small hands or long slender digits and those with hypermobile thumbs need to use kneading strokes sparingly and with care, especially thumb kneading. And take care that you are not also using your thumbs extensively for pressure point work.

Don't Hyperextend Your Thumbs

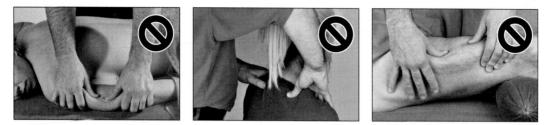

Figure 34.8: Kneading with hyperextended thumbs.

The greatest problem in thumb kneading strokes is the pressure that it puts on your thumbs, which is increased if you have them hyperextended.

Use the Reinforced Thumb Technique to Reduce the Pressure on Your Thumbs

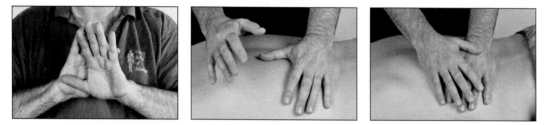

Figure 34.9: The reinforced thumb; a) hand positions, b), c) using the reinforced thumb.

If you feel the need to use your thumb to focus pressure on a small area, use the reinforced thumb. This enables you to reduce the pressure on your thumb when you're doing short thumb strokes. Have your working hand deliver pressure to your thumb. Push it forward for a short stroke, lift it and then push forward for the next overlapping stroke.

Conserve Your Thumbs by Using Other Tools for Kneading or Equivalent Strokes

However, there is a limit to the pressure that you can comfortably carry. So, monitor that you are not putting more power through them than they can comfortably handle.

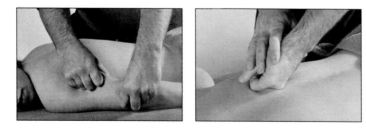

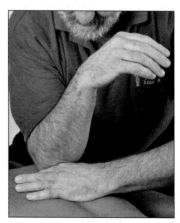

*Figure 34.10: Substitutes to save the thumbs in firm kneading;
a) the knuckles, b) the fist, c) the elbow.*

Save your thumbs for lighter work and, whenever possible, use other tools such as your knuckles for deeper kneading (see figure 15.4 – although be careful not to overuse them either). Or use your fist (see Chapter 16) or your guided elbow (see Chapter 19) for firmer 'digging' pressure.

Use Large Hand Kneading ('Breadmaking') Sparingly if You Have Small Hands

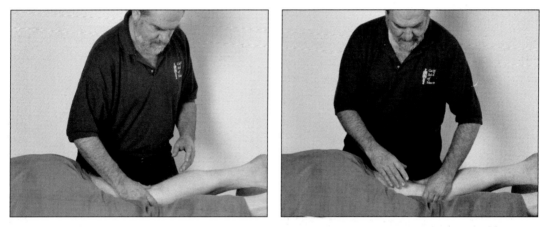

Figure 34.11: 'Breadmaking' – one hand picking up tissue as the other releases it.

Thumb kneading (above) is used to focus on small areas. 'Breadmaking', the full hand version, is used for large areas of muscle. In this stroke, the muscles are picked up and stretched or twisted as they are passed between the hands, each hand picking up the tissue that the other has just released.

If you have small or slender hands, you are likely to find this stroke tiring and ineffective on clients with a large build or well-used muscles. Even for those with larger hands, regularly gripping and letting go of the muscles is hard work on the hands.

Sway Your Body From Side to Side for Large Hand Kneading

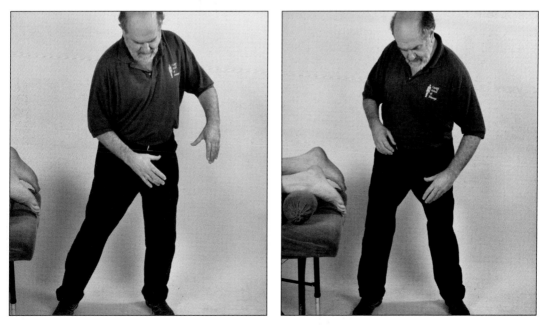

Figure 34.12: Swaying from side to side for large kneading strokes.

Don't just use you arms for this stroke, but sway from side to side (in the 'horse stance', see figure 28.32–28.40) when doing large kneading strokes, such as on the client's thigh.

Support One Hand With the Other to Reduce the Workload on Each Hand

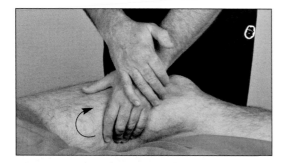

Figure 34.13: 'Circular kneading', one hand supporting the other.

If it becomes tiring to do this stroke with two hands, have one hand support the other in 'circular kneading' strokes. This will reduce the workload on each hand, and enable you to initiate the stroke from body movement even more easily.

Don't Try to Reach Too Far Across the Client's Body

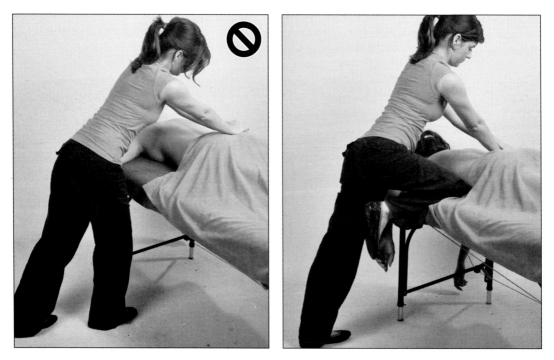

Figure 34.14: Reaching across the client; a) straining to reach too far,
b) kneeling one knee on the table to reach comfortably.

Take care of your back when reaching across the table to do large hand kneading on the far side of the client's back. Don't try to reach too far, especially when you are working on a broad client. If you have a small build, kneeling one knee on the table may make it possible for you to comfortably reach across without strain.

Wringing

Wringing is done across groups of muscles, across a limb or right across the back. One hand pushes forward as the other pulls back to wring the muscles between them.

Save Your Thumbs

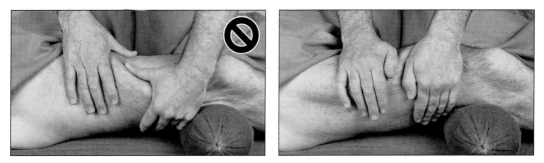

Figure 34.15: Saving the thumbs in wringing; a) with hyperextended thumbs, b) thumbs moving with the fingers.

Your thumbs are ineffective in all but the smallest wringing strokes. And if you try to use them, you are likely to hyperextend them, which puts pressure on them for little useful effect. Save them by keeping them next to your fingers and using the heels of your hands to push instead.

Relax the Non-working Parts of Your Hands

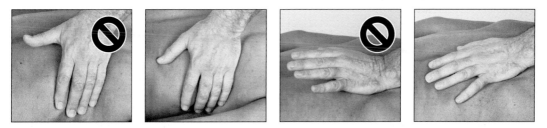

Figure 34.16: Relaxing the non-working parts of the hand; a) stiffening the thumb when pushing, b) relaxing the thumb, c) stiffening the fingers, d) relaxing the fingers.

Relax the non-working parts of your hands to conserve energy and to help keep the strokes even. Watch out for the common tendency to stiffen the fingers or the thumb when pushing forward with the heel of the hand.

Avoid Hyperextending Your Wrist

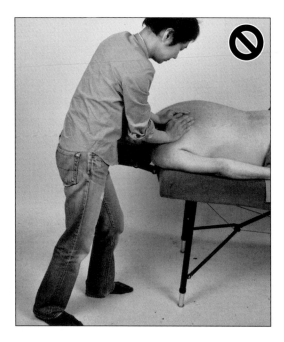

Figure 34.17: Monitoring the wrist; hyperextended wrist.

When you are pushing forward with the heel of the hand, take care not to hyperextend your wrist, particularly when you are pushing on the close side. If necessary, bend your knees to drop lower on the close side to avoid this.

Rotate Each Hip Forward in Turn to Propel Your Hand Movements

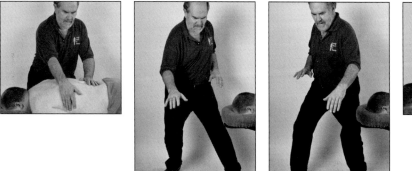

Figure 34.18: Twisting the body for wringing strokes.

As with the other petrissage strokes, standing still and just using your arms would make this harder work and less fluid than moving your body. Take up the horse stance, and twist each hip forward in turn to push its respective hand forward with power and fluidity. As you twist one hip forward to push your hand, you will be simultaneously twisting the other hip back to pull your other hand back towards yourself.

Move Sideways to Cover a Long Area

When you are gradually wringing up and down the length of the client's back or leg, sway or step sideways along the table to stay behind your hands.

Use Double-handed Wringing to Reduce the Workload on Each Hand

As with circular kneading, double-handed wringing enables you to work more effectively on large, well-used, tight muscles whilst conserving your hands.

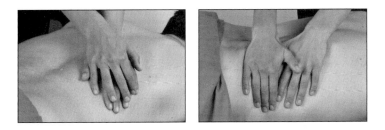

Figure 34.19: Double-handed wringing; a) hand-on-hand, b) hands next to one another.

Use one hand on top of the other, or have your hands next to one another, to push and pull them together across the muscles. This stretches the muscles sideways in a similar way to 'classical' wringing. Use your top hand to focus the push through the heel of your underhand, and then to help pull with the 'hooked' fingers of your underhand.

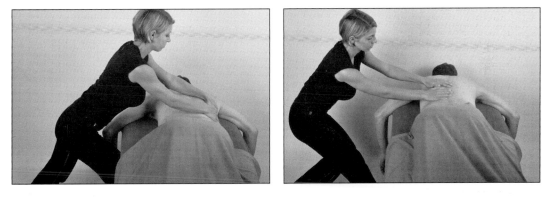

Figure 34.20: Swaying forward and back for double-handed wringing.

Take up the lunge stance so that you can sway forward and back with your whole body to initiate the movements of your hands. Bend your front knee as you sway forward for pushing to keep the movement forward fluid and even. Pull by 'sitting' back, rather than standing still and just moving your arms.

Use Forearm Wringing to Save Your Hands Entirely

When you are working on the client's legs, you can save your hands entirely by using your forearm to 'wring' the muscles in a similar way to double-handed wringing.

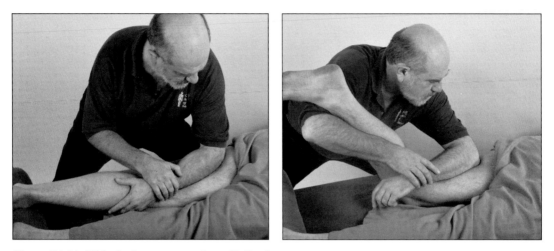

Figure 34.21: 'Wringing' across muscles with the forearm.

Widen your stance and bend your knees to avoid hunching over (see figure 18.24). It is generally easiest to do this in the horse stance because it enables you to twist your hips to deliver power to your forearm as you push and pull with it. Push forward across the muscle with the distal section of your ulna (the bony 'blade', see figure 18.9). Pull back with your inside elbow bone (the medial epicondyle of the humerus, see figure 19.21). Use your other hand as a support on which to pivot your forearm.

Review

Petrissage strokes make more demands of your thumbs and fingers than most other strokes, so use them carefully and sparingly.

Be particularly careful if you have small hands, or slender and/or hypermobile digits.

Whenever possible, use other larger tools to achieve the same effects.

In petrissage strokes, look after your hands by:

- Avoiding using your finger and thumb tips too often;
- Conserving your thumbs and fingers, for example by using kneading sparingly;
- Avoiding having your thumbs hyperextended;
- Reducing the pressure on your fingers by using them together rather than separately;
- Use both hands together whenever possible;
- Moving your hand for the strokes rather than holding it stiffly, and;
- Moving your body to power the stroke rather than standing still.

In squeezing strokes:

- Don't overuse your finger or thumb tips;
- Don't let your wrist hyperextend;
- Move your hand for the stroke rather than keeping it still;
- Use your other hand to support your working hand whenever possible;
- Save your digits by using the heel of your hands for squeezing with your fingers interlocked, and;
- Sway your body back for 'squeeze and stretch' techniques rather than just pulling with your arms.

In draining/'milking' strokes:

- Conserve your hands by using both hands together, and;
- Move your body with the stroke rather than just using your arms.

In kneading strokes:

- Use thumb kneading sparingly to save your thumbs;
- Don't hyperextend your thumbs;
- Use the reinforced thumb technique to reduce the pressure on your thumbs;
- Conserve your thumbs by using other tools for kneading or equivalent strokes;
- Use large hand kneading ('breadmaking') sparingly if you have small hands;
- Sway your body from side to side for large hand kneading;
- Support one hand with the other to reduce the workload on each hand;
- Don't try to reach too far across the client's body.

In wringing strokes:

- Save your thumbs by keeping them with your fingers;
- Relax the non-working parts of your hands to conserve energy and help keep the strokes even;
- Avoid hyperextending your wrist;
- Rotate your hips forward in turn to propel your hand movements;
- Step or sway sideways to cover the length of the client's back or leg;
- Use double-handed wringing to reduce the workload on each hand;
- Use forearm wringing to save your hands entirely.

CHAPTER 35

Pressure Strokes

The compression strokes used in Swedish massage include:

- Small, specific rubbing strokes (often called *friction* or *frictions*), such as circular friction and transverse / 'cross-fibre' friction, and;
- The general application of stationary or sliding pressure over an area (sometimes exclusively called *compression*).

These strokes overlap with other pressure strokes, which have come into common use in massage in recent decades such as pressure point techniques, deep tissue massage techniques, techniques from reflexology, and adaptations of shiatsu pressure techniques.

This chapter looks at the potential strains on your digits in these strokes and ways of reducing these, using other parts of your hands, forearm and elbow, and ways of using your body to support these working tools.

Caution – Fingers and Thumbs at Risk

These strokes are the firmest strokes in the general massage repertoire. Because of the pressure that you're delivering, you need to be careful about which parts of your hands that you use and how you use them.

Friction Strokes
This is particularly important in friction strokes because of the pressure that they put on your digits. People are usually taught to use either the fingers, the thumbs, the index knuckle or two or three knuckles together for the small movements of circular friction. Cross-fibre / transverse friction is generally done with one or two fingers, sometimes with the index finger on the middle finger, or with the thumbs.

If you have large, strong hands, friction strokes probably won't cause you problems, unless you use them too often, too forcefully, or with your digits hyperextended. However, if you have small, slender, or hypermobile fingers and thumbs, use friction strokes carefully and sparingly. If you feel discomfort developing in your digits, reduce how much you use these strokes or avoid using them altogether. Whenever you can, use larger tools such as your knuckles (Chapter 15), your fist (Chapter 16) or your elbow (Chapter 19) for concentrated pressure, or your forearm (Chapter 18) for widespread pressure.

To reduce the pressure on your fingers and thumbs in friction strokes, avoid:

- Having your digits or wrist hyperextended;
- Only using one or two fingers when you can use them all together;

- Just moving your fingers or thumb when you could move your whole hand;
- Consistently applying more pressure than is comfortable for them;
- Using your fingers or thumbs when you could use your knuckles or fist.

Pressure Point Techniques and Reflexology

Much of this also applies to using the thumbs for pressure point techniques such as trigger point work and for many reflexology techniques. Unless you have quite strong thumbs, you need to be careful about how much of this that you do. People with large, strong hands or those with strong, stocky digits are least likely to have problems. If you have small, slender and/or hypermobile thumbs, use these techniques sparingly, as they put considerable pressure through your thumbs. Be aware that, when you are applying pressure, there's a temptation to stand (or sit) still, and often to hunch over as well, and to tense your shoulders and rely on muscle power alone, which stiffens your hands.

Compression

In 'classic' Swedish massage, compression strokes are a group of broad strokes in which stationary or sliding pressure is applied over the large muscles of the trunk and limbs. In present-day massage, these strokes overlap with more specific pressure strokes such as pressure point techniques and deep tissue massage techniques, and are often used to lead into them.

Because of the pressure that you're delivering, you need to use the largest appropriate tools for these strokes – your palm (see figure 14.7), your fist (see Chapter 16), or your forearm (see Chapter 18). If you have small or slender hands, save them by learning to use your forearm whenever possible.

Deep Tissue Massage Techniques

In recent years, a range of deep tissue techniques has come into widespread use in massage. They put quite a lot of pressure on your working tools, so it's important to conserve them. Your fingers are the most vulnerable tools, so only use them when you feel that nothing else will do the job. Be especially careful about using them if you have small hands or they are slender and/or hypermobile. Use your knuckles or fist for preference and use your forearm or elbow whenever you can.

Deep tissue work involves slow, sliding pressure, generally applied without oil. Don't tense up and just use muscle power for these strokes, which is hard work and is likely to provoke an instinctive reaction in the client against this 'attack'. Instead, use your bodyweight to deliver the pressure and to keep it consistent. This saves your energy, and makes it easier to monitor the client's responses. It also enables you to be comfortable and keep the pressure consistent as you *wait* patiently for the client's tissues to accommodate to the pressure and to 'melt'. This enables you to move through them like a hot knife gradually cutting through frozen butter, rather than trying to force your way through.

As you maintain the pressure, take care that:

- The tools that you use are able to take this sustained pressure, especially your fingers;
- You use your other hand, whenever possible, to guide your working hand/forearm, to add pressure to the stroke, and to help keep it moving evenly, and;
- That you can position and lean your body to comfortably deliver and maintain the power for these strokes.

Conserving Your Fingers

When you are using your fingers, there are a number of things that you can do to reduce the pressure on them.

Avoid Hyperextending Your Fingers

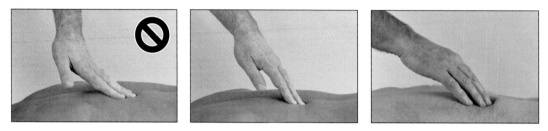

Figure 35.1: The angle of the fingers; a) hyperextended fingers, b) straight fingers, c) slightly curled fingers.

Avoid having your fingers hyperextended. Instead, have them straight or very slightly curled, which is the strongest position for pressing through them (see figure 12.7) because of the way that it engages your strong finger flexor muscles.

Use As Many Fingers As You Can

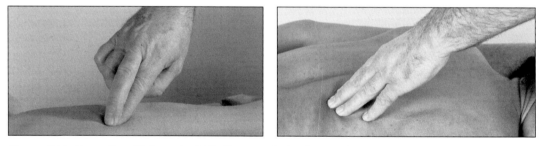

Figure 35.2: Cross-fibre friction; a) middle finger on index finger, b) group of fingers.

Because the intention in cross-fibre stroking is to focus on a small, specific area, practitioners sometimes do it with just one finger. This puts quite a pressure on that finger, so a better option is to use your middle finger on your index finger. This is still hard work on that finger and so it should be used sparingly. If you have small or slender fingers, you should probably avoid using it altogether. Instead, use a group of fingers bunched together, if you can, and support them with your other hand, or switch to using your knuckles.

Although circular friction is sometimes done with two fingers, using three or all four together will reduce the pressure on each one.

Keep Your Fingers Together

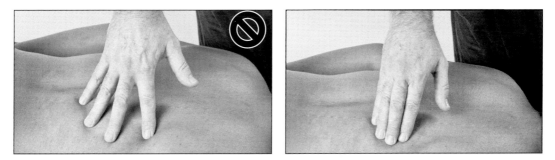

Figure 35.3: The spread of the fingers; a) widespread fingers, b) fingers together.

The wider that you spread your fingers, the more pressure that this puts on each individual finger, so keep them together to spread the workload and support each other.

Support Your Fingers With Your Other Hand

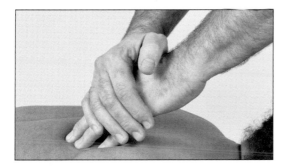

Figure 35.4: Supporting the fingers with the other hand.

When you use one hand alone, you have to tighten your arm and shoulder muscles to control the stroke. This, in turn, is likely to lead to unnecessary tension in your fingers. So, whenever you can, place your other hand over your fingers to reduce this effort and simultaneously increase the pressure that you can deliver.

Relax the Non-working Parts of Your Hand

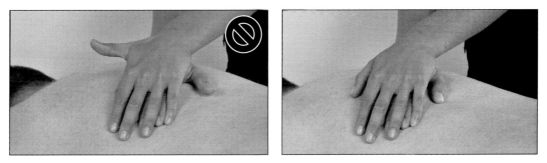

Figure 35.5: Relaxing the rest of your hand; a) stiff thumb, b) relaxed thumb.

Looking After Your Thumbs

Be Careful When Using Your Thumbs to Apply Pressure

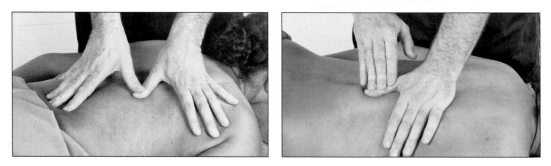

Figure 35.6: Pressing with the thumb; a) thumb-on-thumb pressure, b) fingers on the thumb pressure.

Unless you have large, strong thumbs, friction and pressure point strokes put considerable pressure on them, especially when you are working on large, well-used muscles. Even using thumb-on-thumb pressure or pressing with your fingers on your thumb puts quite a pressure through your thumb if it is small or slender.

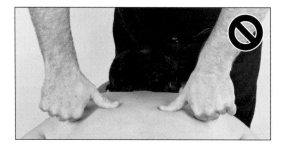

Figure 35.7: Hyperextending the thumb when applying pressure.

And of course, regularly hyperextending your thumb when you are pressing with the tip can lead to strain over time.

Conserve Your Thumb

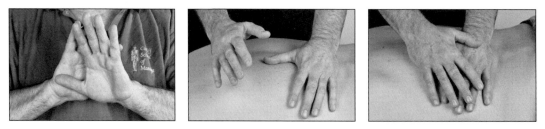

Figure 35.8: Using the reinforced thumb.

Whenever possible, use the reinforced thumb technique – using the heel of your hand to deliver power to the other thumb which rests flat and relaxed on the client's body (see figure 13.15).

Don't Try to Press On Both Sides of the Spine at Once

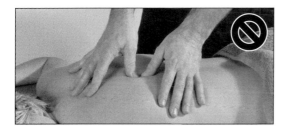

Figure 35.9: Circular friction with the thumbs on both sides of the spine from the side of the table.

Some people try to do circular friction strokes with their thumbs along both sides of the spine simultaneously, while standing alongside the massage table. This doesn't work well. You have to tense your arm and shoulder muscles to control each hand, and it puts unnecessary pressure on each hand and therefore on each thumb. In any case, it's impossible to comfortably apply equal pressure on both sides of the client's spine. Instead, use the 'reinforced thumb' technique on the close side, and then cross to the other side of the table to mirror this along the other side of the spine.

Using Your Knuckles

Support Your Index Knuckle

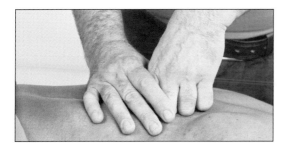

Figure 35.10: Using the index knuckle for friction strokes – holding it between the thumb and fingers.

Using your index knuckle to dig into tissue will conserve your thumb and fingers. Using it alone is hard work, so hold and guide it with your other hand. This will also enable you to work with more force and greater precision, for example when you're working close to bones such as the vertebrae.

Use a Group of Knuckles if Possible

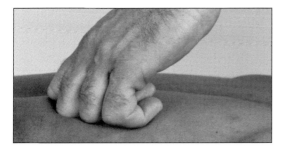

Figure 35.11: Using the knuckles together.

Whenever possible, using more than one knuckle will reduce the workload on your solo knuckle. Whether you find two or three knuckles more comfortable to use will depend on their relative lengths.

Looking After Your Hands

Move Your Whole Hand to Save Your Digits

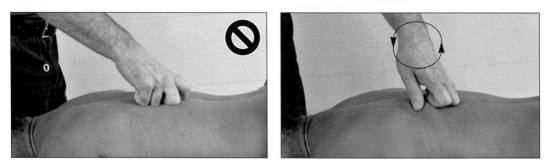

Figure 35.12: Using the knuckles; a) moving the knuckles separately, b) moving the hand as a unit.

There is a temptation in friction strokes to keep your hands still and just move your fingers, thumbs or knuckles, which would soon tire them. Try to move your hand and arm as a unit instead, to save your digits.

Keep Your Hand Relaxed

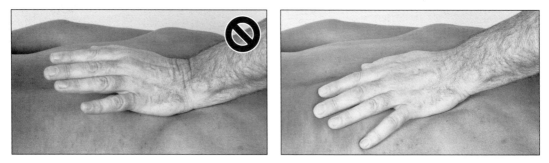

Figure 35.13: Using the palm for pressure strokes; a) with stiff fingers, b) fingers relaxed.

When using your palm for applying general pressure, keep your fingers relaxed to avoid stiffening your hand.

When Using Your Fist, Keep it Relaxed

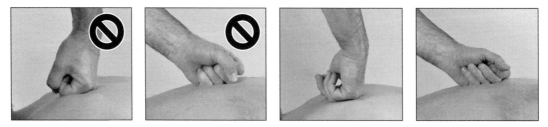

Figure 35.14: Sliding pressure with the wrist; a), b) clenched fist, c), d) relaxed fist.

Whether you are using the front of your fist (the metacarpo-phalangeal joints of your fingers, see figure 16.2), or the side of your fist (see figure 16.2), have your fist loosely curled and not clenched to avoid unnecessary and counterproductive effort.

Don't Let Your Wrist Bend Too Far

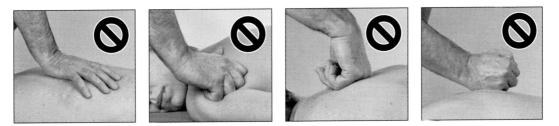

*Figure 35.15: Bent wrist; a) using the palm, b) using the knuckles,
c) using the front of the fist, d) using the side of the fist.*

Take care not to let your wrist bend or buckle when you are applying pressure, which could strain it over time if it happens regularly.

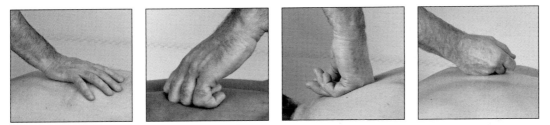

*Figure 35.16: Relatively straight wrist; a) using the palm, b) using the knuckles,
c) using the front of the fist, d) using the side of the fist.*

Keep it straight (but not rigid) to avoid straining it, so that power is transmitted relatively undiminished to your hand.

Support Your Working Hand With Your Other Hand

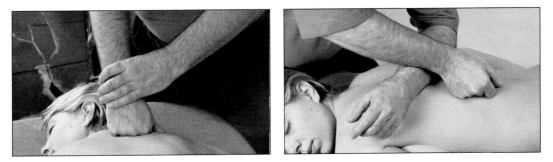

*Figure 35.17: Supporting the working hand; a) holding the wrist,
b) resting the fist over the other forearm.*

Whenever possible, use your other hand to support your working hand to increase the power and control, while reducing the pressure on your wrist. For example, when you're using your knuckles or fist, you can hold your wrist or rest it over your other hand or forearm.

Use Both Hands Together

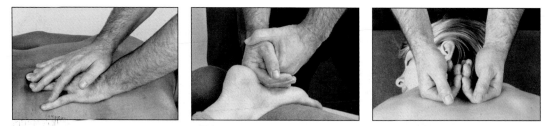

Figure 35.18: Using the hands together; a) hand-on-hand pressure,
b) one fist inside the other, c) contact between the hands.

Or you can use both hands together, to reduce the workload on each one.

Involving Your Body to Support Your Hands

Because you can't move your body at the rate of your hands in friction strokes, there is a temptation to stand still and just rely on muscle power for the strokes. This is often accompanied by tensing the shoulders and holding the breath. This puts extra pressure on your hands and makes the strokes harder work. Standing still for compression and other pressure strokes also leads to working too hard with the upper body, but delivering less effective power.

Bear in mind too that if you are straining your digits or other areas of your hands, you are likely to tense your shoulders, which would feed back into a vicious cycle of tensing your hands more. So it is important to use your body to generate the pressure, as long as this is not too much for your digits.

Lean for the Pressure

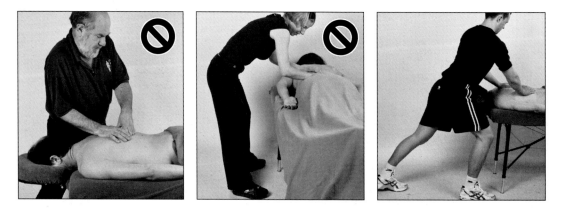

Figure 35.19: Delivering pressure; a) standing still and tensing the shoulders,
b) hunching over, c) bending the knees to lean forward.

Relax your shoulders, and lean forward to add pressure to your strokes. If necessary, sway a little every now and then to remind yourself not to tense up when you are doing friction strokes. Lean forward by bending your knees rather than hunching over which would put pressure on your lower back.

Avoid Trying to Reach Too Far

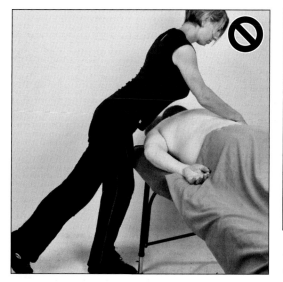

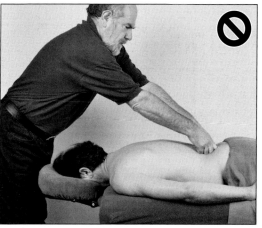

Figure 35.20: Trying to reach too far;
a) across the table, b) along the table.

Take care of your lower back by not leaning too far over the table to do friction strokes on the far side of the client's body. Instead, cross to the other side of the table to do the strokes there.

Take care not to reach further than is easily comfortable along the table as well. Either limit the stroke, or step forward to continue it.

Sway Your Body for Sliding Pressure Strokes

Figure 35.21: Moving forward; a) stiff front knee impedes the smooth movement,
b) bending the front knee to sway forward.

Sway forward for sliding strokes that move forward. Bend your knees for this, particularly your front knee so that your hips glide smoothly forward, staying on the same level.

Keep Your Arms Straight or Wedge Your Elbow Inside Your Hip

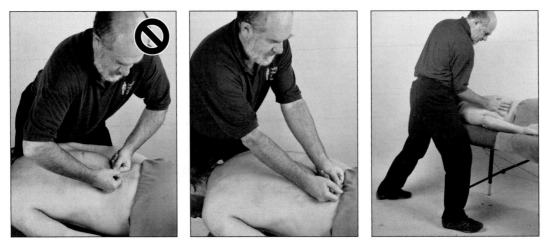

Figure 35.22: Delivering power to your fist; a) arm bent, b) arm relatively straight, c) wedging the elbow inside the hip.

As you sway forward, keep your working tools at a fairly constant distance in front of your hips for firm sliding strokes. Do this by keeping your arm fairly straight (but not rigid) to deliver the power relatively undiminished to your hand or fist. When you are using your palm or the side of your fist, you can wedge your elbow just inside your hip for the most direct transfer of power.

Bend Your Knees for Strokes in Which You Slide Your Fist Towards Yourself

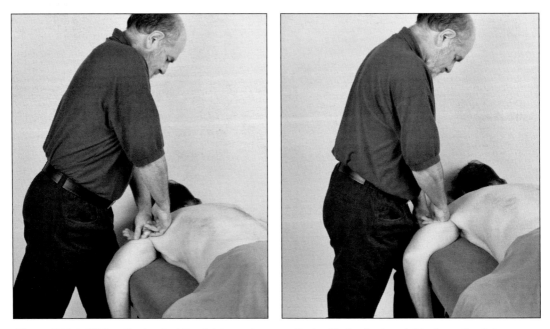

Figure 35.23: Sliding the front of the fist towards oneself; a) with the bodyweight above the fist, b) sliding it downwards.

When you are sliding the front of your fist towards yourself, start with your body above your fist. Gradually sink down by bending your knees, to slide your fist downwards.

Using the Forearm or Elbow

The forearm (see Chapter 18) is ideal for applying pressure with less effort while saving your hand and your wrist entirely.

Have Your Hand Palm Down to Use the 'Soft' Forearm for Widespread Pressure

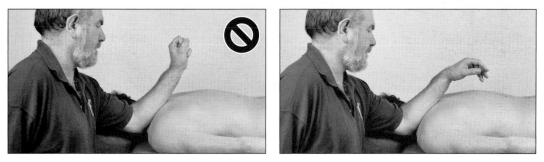

Figure 35.24: Using the 'soft' forearm, palm down, a) clenched hand, b) relaxed hand.

The 'soft' forearm (the bellies of the flexor muscles, see figure 18.3) will provide widespread general pressure. Have your palm turned down towards the client, and keep your hand relaxed, rather than clenched.

Have Your Hand Palm Up to Use the 'Hard' Forearm to Deliver More Specific Pressure

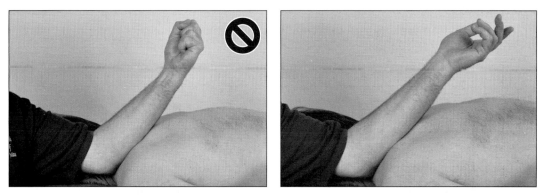

Figure 35.25: Using the 'hard' forearm, palm up; a) clenched hand, b) relaxed hand.

Turning your hand up will give you a harder working surface for sliding pressure strokes.

Guide Your Forearm With Your Other Hand

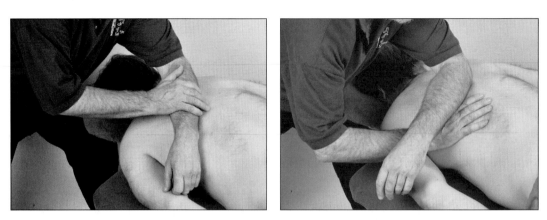

Figure 35.26: Guiding the forearm; a) pressing on the forearm, b) guiding it from underneath.

Whenever possible, guide your working forearm with your other hand (or forearm). Place it on top of your working forearm to increase the pressure, or have it underneath for guiding the forearm with more precision.

Use the Point or Back of Your Elbow for More Focused Pressure

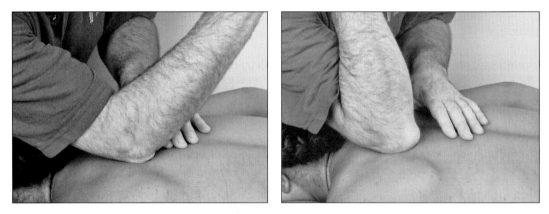

Figure 35.27: Using the elbow; a) the point of the elbow, b) the back of the elbow.

To focus pressure on a small area, use the point of your elbow, which should be used sparingly because it is such a sharp tool, or the back of your elbow, which also concentrates pressure on a small area, but is a blunter tool.

Control the Depth of Elbow Work by How Much You Bend Your Arm
Control how deep and sharp your working elbow is by the amount that you bend it.

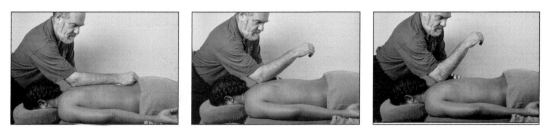

Figure 35.28: Bending the elbow for a deeper 'cut'.

Drop into a Low 'Chimp' Stance to Save Your Back

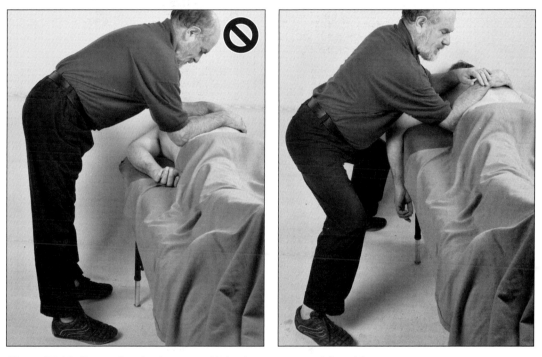

Figure 35.29: Supporting the forearm with body movement; a) hunching over,
b) wider stance to get lower.

Don't hunch over to get closer to the table. Instead, save your back by widening your stance and bending your knees to get lower (the 'chimp' stance, see figure 18.24).

Review

Be careful of your hands when doing pressure strokes, particularly if you have small hands, slender fingers and thumbs, and/or hypermobile digits.

Friction and pressure point techniques probably won't cause you problems if you have large, strong hands, unless you use them too often, too forcefully, or with your digits hyperextended.

However, if you have small, slender, or hypermobile fingers and thumbs, use these strokes carefully and sparingly.

If you feel discomfort developing in your digits, reduce how much you use these strokes or avoid using them altogether.

Whenever possible, switch to larger appropriate tools, such as your palm, your fist, or your forearm.

To reduce the pressure on your fingers and thumbs, avoid:

- Having your digits or wrist hyperextended;
- Only using one or two fingers when you can use them all together;
- Just moving your fingers or thumb when you could move your whole hand;
- Consistently applying more pressure than is comfortable for them;
- Using your fingers or thumbs when you could use your knuckles or fist.

As you maintain the pressure in compression and deep pressure strokes, take care that:

- The tools that you use are able to take this sustained pressure;
- You use your other hand, whenever possible, to guide your working hand/forearm, to add pressure to the stroke, and to help keep it moving evenly, and;
- You can position and lean your body to comfortably deliver and maintain the power for these strokes.

To conserve you fingers:

- Avoid hyperextending them;
- Use as many fingers as you can at a time, rather than using them solo;
- Keep your fingers together rather than having them spread;
- Support your fingers with your other hand, and;
- Relax the non-working parts of your hand.

When using your thumbs for applying pressure:

- Don't let them hyperextend;
- Use the reinforced thumb techniques to conserve them, and;
- Don't try to press on both sides of the spine at once from the side of the table.

When using your knuckles:

- Support your index knuckle if you need to use it alone;
- Use a group of knuckles whenever possible, instead of one on its own.

Look after your hands by:

- Moving your whole hand rather than just moving each digit separately;
- Keeping your hand appropriately relaxed;
- Not letting your wrist bend;
- Supporting your working hand with your other hand, and;
- Using both hands together whenever possible.

Support your hands by:

- Leaning forward for pressure, rather than standing still and overusing the upper body;
- Not trying to reach too far;
- Swaying your body for sliding strokes;
- Keeping your arms relatively straight to deliver pressure from your body to your hands, or wedging your elbow inside your hip;
- Bend your knees to gradually drop down in strokes in which you slide your fists towards yourself.

When using your forearm:

- Have your hand palm down and relaxed to use the 'soft' forearm for widespread pressure strokes;
- Have your hand palm up (and relaxed) to use the 'hard' forearm to deliver more specific pressure, and;
- Widen your stance and bend your knees to drop into a chimp stance in order to save your back.

Use the point or the back of the elbow for more focused pressure, controlling the depth of your elbow by how much you bend your arm.

CHAPTER 36

Massage Without Oil

For various reasons it may not be possible or desirable to use oil for a massage, for example in situations in which it wouldn't be appropriate for the client to disrobe, or the client prefers not to have oil on his/her skin. It extends the practitioner's versatility to be able to work without oil on either clothed or unclothed clients on the massage table. It is also the way that much seated massage is done (see Chapter 41).

Many massage strokes can be used in much the same way as for oil massage. These include percussion (see Chapter 37), vibration (see Chapter 38), passive stretches and lifts (see Chapter 39), body rocking and limb rolling (see Chapter 40), and the sliding pressure strokes of deep tissue massage which are applied without oil on the skin (see Chapter 35).

The main differences from oil massage are that:

- You can't do sliding strokes in the same way while maintaining pressure, which primarily affects effleurage and compression strokes, and;
- You have to modify petrissage strokes.

As well as affecting your choice of techniques, working without oil also makes it a little harder to feel muscles and identify tensions (and it takes even more practise to learn to palpate through clothing). Therefore practitioners can find non-oil massage at first daunting and difficult, and treat it like a poor relation of the 'real thing'. It is different, but can be quite effective in its own way once you have developed a feeling for this way of working.

Working on Bare Skin Without Oil Vs Working Through Clothing

Many techniques can be done in much the same way for both of these situations. However some techniques are more restricted and/or harder work when you are working through clothing. Small kneading strokes, for example, are not worth doing on clothed clients as they are very hard work on your thumbs for little effect.

There are some advantages to having the client clothed. It enables you to do massage in public situations, whether you are taking a massage chair to offices (see Chapter 41), or working without any special equipment in other situations such as a sports locker room. And, when you are using a massage table, having the client clothed makes it easier to do extensive stretches (see Chapter 39) and body rocking (see Chapter 40) without fear of embarrassing the client through putting them in compromising or exposing positions.

Bear in mind that it is harder work to massage through clothing, especially if it's made of a stiff material such as denim. Therefore, to make life easy for yourself, encourage your clients to disrobe if they feel comfortable doing so. Or, if it's possible to give people advance notice, encourage them to wear the sort of loose clothing that they would wear to an exercise class – a T-shirt and track suit bottoms get in your way the least. If this is not an option, for example in public situations such as doing massage in an office, get clients to take off jackets and sweaters and to loosen collars.

General Principles

Looking After Your Hands
Working without oil is more demanding on your hands than oil massage. Take care not to overuse your thumbs and fingers, especially for kneading and applying pressure. Be particularly careful if your hands are small or you have long, slender or hypermobile digits.

Whenever you can, save your digits by switching to larger tools, such as your knuckles, fist, forearm or elbow. If you are going to do extended non-oil work, it is crucial to learn to use your forearm and elbow skilfully (see Chapters 18–19) in order to save your hands.

Involving Your Body
Because you are using your hands more, there is a great temptation to stand still, tense your shoulders and rely on arm muscle power. This puts even more pressure on your hands, especially in petrissage strokes. Instead, take up a dynamic posture, with your back long but not rigid (see figure 26.14) and your knees soft enough that you can sway (see figure 28.5). Relax your shoulders and breathe easily. Change position regularly to keep your bodyweight behind your hands. Sway for effleurage strokes, and lean forward to deliver power in compression strokes. Take care to not put pressure on your lower back by leaning too far across the table.

Rhythm
Involving your whole body not only takes pressure off your upper body, it is also essential for providing an even rhythm to your strokes. Because you are not sliding (as you would with oil), it is harder to create a feeling of fluidity in the massage session. The way to create this is by establishing an even rhythm to your strokes and by moving from one area to another in a way that fits the rhythm of the strokes. This needs more attention than in oil massage, and generally takes more practise to master.

In petrissage strokes, for example, pick up and release the tissues rhythmically, rather than doing it jerkily or suddenly. Similarly, in compression strokes, slowly lean forward to increase the pressure, sustain it for a time, and slowly release it. Then pause for a few moments, so that the timing of applying pressure again doesn't cut across the pacing that you've established for the strokes. (This applies whether you are pressing on the same area again or you are moving to another area).

Proportioning Strokes
Because of the demands on your thumbs and fingers, try to reduce the amount of kneading that you do, especially if you have small hands or slender or hypermobile digits. Instead, use large areas of your hands to stretch the tissues, such as the 'squeeze and lift' technique or 'double-handed wringing' (see figure 34.19). If it is appropriate to work firmly, move quickly into pressure techniques such as compression techniques or deep tissue massage techniques.

However, all of these strokes can be demanding on your hands, so learn to use your forearm and elbow whenever possible. And make more use of other strokes which are less demanding on your hands, such as stretches (including 'anchor and stretch' techniques, see figure 36.12), moving the client rhythmically (body rocking and limb rolling, see Chapter 40) and percussion (see Chapter 37).

In relaxation massage, it is quite useful to do more joining strokes than in oil massage in order to give the client a clear sense of interconnectedness throughout his/her body.

Effleurage

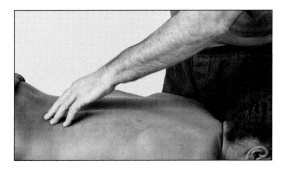

Figure 36.1: Light effleurage.

Effleurage can't be done with the same pressure as with oil. Sliding strokes need to be light enough that you can slide over the skin/clothing without dragging or getting stuck.

It takes practise to get accustomed to reducing the pressure enough for this. Some people are used to using these light, sliding strokes over the drapes to 'join up' areas of the client's body after more detailed work on the area. However, if it is unfamiliar, this will be quite a challenge as firm sliding strokes are such a feature of oil massage. One way to develop this is to begin by just using your fingertips. Sway with your hands' movements to give fluidity and evenness to the strokes. Then when you feel comfortable with this, try using more of the front of your fingers and finally incorporate the whole front surface of your hand. It is generally easier to do light stroking towards yourself, so begin with this. It takes more practise to get the right pressure and keep the movement even when you are pushing away from yourself.

Petrissage

There is a great temptation to use petrissage strokes (kneading, wringing, and squeezing) more than in oil massage to make up for other strokes that you can't do. However, because you can't glide without oil, this is harder work on your hands, so be careful about how you use them. If you have small hands or long, slender or hypermobile digits, use these strokes sparingly, especially if most of your work is non-oil massage, for example if you regularly work in offices or hospitals.

If you are using both hands together, for example for squeezing or double-handed kneading, rhythmically pick up and release the tissue. If you are using your hands alternately, establish a rhythm of smoothly releasing the tissues with one hand as you take hold of them with the other.

Taking Care of Your Thumbs

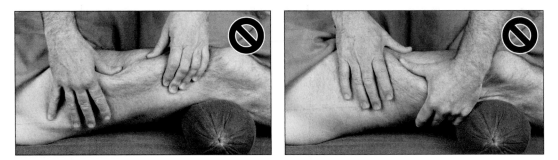

Figure 36.2: Conserving the thumbs; a) kneading with hyperextended thumbs, b) wringing with hyperextended thumbs.

As with oil strokes, take special care of your thumbs. Don't work with them hyperextended, which is a great temptation in clothed massage.

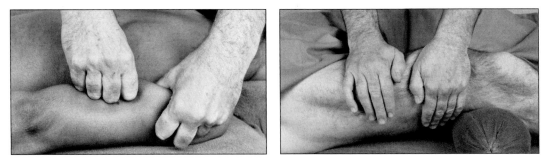

Figure 36.3: Conserving the thumbs; a) knuckle kneading, b) thumbs with the fingers in wringing.

And conserve your thumbs. Use your knuckles instead for kneading and keep them with your fingers for wringing strokes.

Use Your Hands Together to Reduce the Workload On Each

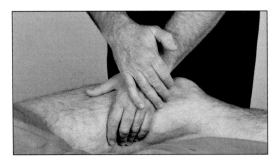

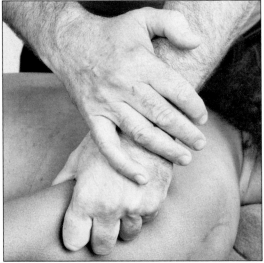

Figure 36.4: Using the hands together; a) supported kneading, b) supported knuckle kneading.

Use Double-handed Strokes to Save Your Digits

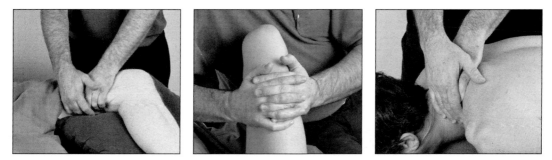

Figure 36.5: Double-handed strokes; a) circular kneading, b) double-handed squeezing, c) double-handed wringing.

Wherever possible, use your hands together to take the pressure off your digits.

Look After Your Hands in Pressure Strokes

Pressure strokes demand a lot of your hands, so it's important to constantly monitor them, especially your fingers and thumbs. Be especially careful of them if you have small, slender or hypermobile digits. This is crucial in deep tissue massage, in which you are not only applying great pressure, but also sustaining it.

Take Care of Your Fingers and Thumbs

There is a great temptation to rely on your fingers and thumbs for non-oil pressure strokes, and consequently to strain them by:

•   Using them too often (when you could use other larger tools),
•   Consistently putting too much pressure through them, and/or;
•   Hyperextending them when applying pressure.

Avoid Hyperextending Your Fingers and Thumbs

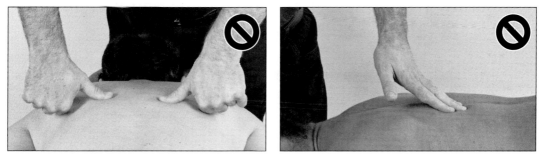

Figure 36.6: Pressing with the digits; a) hyperextended thumbs, b) hyperextended fingers.

If you are using your thumbs or fingers, don't let them hyperextend as you apply pressure. And support them with your other hand if possible.

Use the Reinforced Thumb for Applying Thumb Pressure

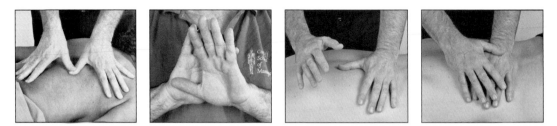

Figure 36.7: Pressing with the thumbs; a) thumb-on-thumb pressure – use cautiously; b), c), d) the reinforced thumb.

Be wary about using thumb-on-thumb pressure. Instead, if possible, use the 'reinforced thumb' technique (see figure 13.15) to focus pressure on a single point.

Use Larger Tools to Save Your Digits

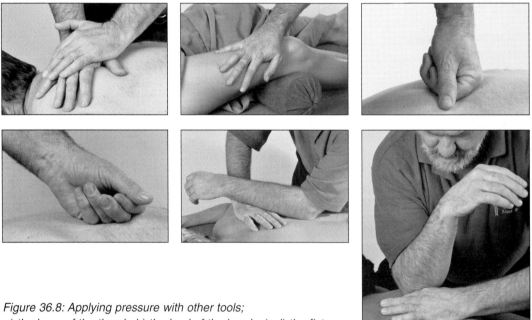

Figure 36.8: Applying pressure with other tools; a) the base of the thumb, b) the heel of the hand, c), d) the fist, e) the forearm, f) the elbow.

Whenever you can, conserve your thumbs and fingers by switching to larger tools such as the base of your thumb or the heel of your hand (see Chapter 14), your fist (see Chapter 16), your forearm (see Chapter 18) or your elbow (see Chapter 19).

Look After Your Wrist

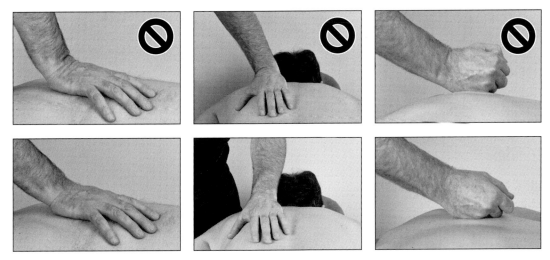

Figure 36.9: Looking after the wrist; a), b), c) bent wrist, d), e), f) straighter wrist.

Whichever part of your hand that you are using, take care not to hyperextend your wrist as you apply the pressure.

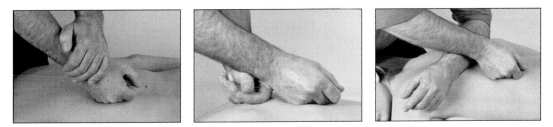

Figure 36.10: Supporting the wrist.

Whenever possible, support your wrist by holding it with your other hand, or by resting it over your other hand or forearm.

Using Your Body for Pressure Strokes

Stationary pressure can be applied in much the same way as in oil massage by leaning your body for the power. However, you can't do sliding pressure techniques in the same way when you are working without oil, so this requires quite a shift in technique. Three ways of getting moving pressure over muscles are:

1. The 'press and stretch' technique in which you maintain the pressure while sliding the skin and/or clothing over the muscles;
2. The 'anchor and stretch' technique in which you press on a muscle while moving a distal part of the body to move the muscle under your pressure, and;
3. The slow, focused sliding pressure of deep tissue massage techniques, which is generally done without oil anyway.

The first two can be done with the client clothed or unclothed; the third is done on bare skin.

Take care to use your bodyweight by positioning, leaning and swaying your body, to avoid standing still and relying on upper body muscle power (and take care of your working tools, particularly your fingers and thumbs, because of the extra pressure that you are putting through them).

Lean Your Body Forward to Apply Stationary Pressure

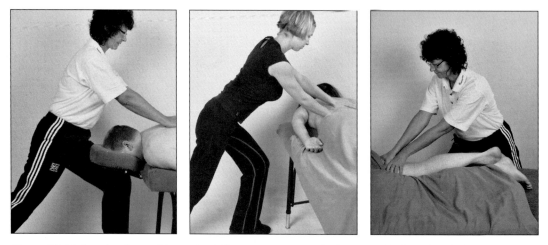

Figure 36.11: Leaning forward to apply stationary pressure – the 'press and release' technique.

A way of applying stationary pressure, which is a major feature of shiatsu and acupressure massage, is the 'press and release' technique. Don't try to just press with your arm power. Put your hand or forearm into position and then slowly lean forward to apply the pressure, stay in position to sustain the pressure for a short time and then slowly sway back to release it.

Sway Your Body While Maintaining the Pressure for the 'Press and Stretch' Technique
In the 'press and stretch' technique, you apply pressure in the same way as for stationary pressure. Sustain the pressure (by continuing to lean forward) as you sway your body to stretch the skin and/or clothing as far as it will comfortably go. Sway back to let it return and then release the pressure.

Lean Your Body to Sustain the Pressure in the 'Anchor and Stretch' Techniques

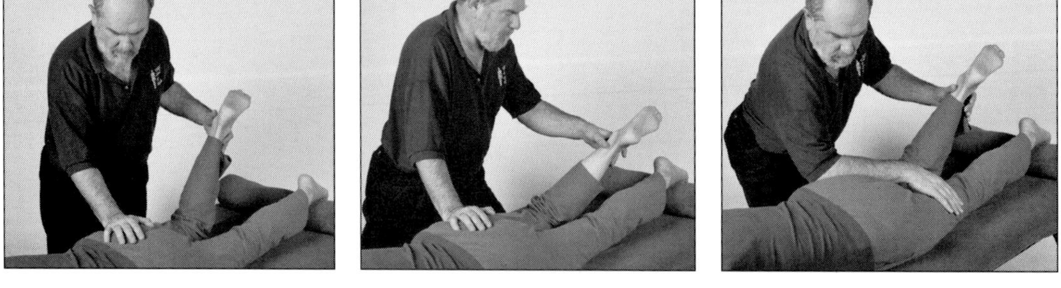

Figure 36.12: 'Anchor and stretch' – leaning to sustain the pressure while moving the leg.

The 'anchor and stretch' technique is done by putting pressure on muscles and then moving a distal part of the body to move the muscles under your pressing hand or forearm. This is commonly used on the buttocks, for example by moving the client's leg whilst maintaining pressure on the gluteals. Face towards where you are applying pressure so that you can lean your bodyweight forward onto that area for the pressure. This makes it easy to maintain the pressure with one hand/forearm as you use the other hand to move the limb.

Sway Your Body Forward for the Power of Deep Tissue Massage

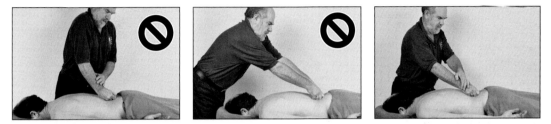

Figure 36.13: Swaying forward for deep tissue massage; a) standing stiffly and overusing the shoulders, b) trying to reach too far from one position, c) swaying forward.

Don't stand in one position and rely on upper body power, or try to reach too far when doing deep tissue strokes. Instead, get into a position that you can comfortably sustain for a time as you wait for the tissues to 'melt' and let you through. And make sure that this position also enables you to sway forward easily when you are able to move forward along the muscle.

When you can't reach further on long muscles, slowly release the pressure, step forward and then pick up the pressure again in this new position (ideally overlapping with the previous one).

Review

Many massage strokes can be used in much the same way as for oil massage, including percussion, vibration, passive stretches, body rocking and limb rolling, and deep tissue massage strokes.

Because you can't do sliding strokes while maintaining pressure, you'll need to modify effleurage, petrissage and pressure strokes.

Practise palpating the tissues when you are working without oil, including through clothing.

Massaging through clothing is hard work, especially if it's made of a stiff material, so encourage client's to wear soft, loose clothing if possible.

Having the client clothed enables you to do massage in public situations, and on the massage table, makes it easier to do extensive stretches and body rocking.

Working without oil is more demanding on your hands than oil massage.

Don't overuse your thumbs and fingers. Be particularly careful if your hands are small or you have long, slender or hypermobile digits.

Whenever possible, use larger tools, such as your knuckles, fist, forearm or elbow for firm pressure techniques.

Don't stand still, tense your shoulders and rely on arm muscle power.

Do strokes rhythmically to give an even rhythm to the massage.

Effleurage strokes need to be light enough to slide without jerkiness.

Small kneading strokes are not worth doing on clothed clients as they are very hard work on your thumbs for little effect.

Take care of your thumbs in petrissage strokes by:

- Using thumb kneading sparingly;
- Not hyperextending your thumbs;
- Conserving them by using your knuckles for kneading, and;
- Not using them in wringing strokes.

Reduce the workload on your hands in petrissage strokes by supporting your working hand with your other hand, or using them together for double-handed strokes.

In pressure strokes:

- Use your thumbs and fingers carefully and sparingly;
- Avoid hyperextending your digits;
- Use the reinforced thumb for applying thumb pressure;
- Save your digits by using larger tools, such as the base of your thumb, the heel of your hand, your fist, your forearm or your elbow;
- Avoid hyperextending your wrist, and;
- Support your wrist by holding it with your hand, or resting it across your other hand or forearm.

Don't stand still and rely on upper body strength for pressure strokes but position, lean and sway your body to use your bodyweight.

CHAPTER 37

Percussion Techniques

This chapter looks at general bodyuse practices that are effective when you are using percussion techniques (*tapotement*), and ways of taking care of your hands in specific percussion strokes. Common problems to watch out for are:

- Not aligning your body behind your working hands;
- Standing stiffly, tensing your shoulders and/or hunching over;
- Trying to reach too far across the table, which can strain your back;
- Just using your hands and not involving your forearms;
- Tensing your hands, and using them in a stiff, awkward or heavy-handed way, and;
- Trying to work faster than is easy or comfortable (so that you are likely to tense up and become heavy-handed).

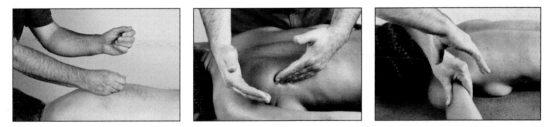

Figure 37.1: Types of percussion strokes; a) 'hitting'/'striking', b) flicking, c) plucking.

Percussion strokes can range from very light strokes used for their sedating effect to the heaviest pounding strokes on the client's back to vibrate the lung tissue. For convenience of description, I have grouped them according to the way that they are applied:

- *'Hitting'/'striking'* strokes, the most commonly used, which range from light tapping to the heaviest pounding;
- *Flicking'* strokes, ranging from light brushing to 'scooping' up muscles, and;
- *Plucking* strokes, ranging from small, light 'pinching' to full-hand 'grabbing'.

Rhythm, Pacing and Continuity

Before covering effective hand and bodyuse for specific types of percussion strokes, it is useful to look at some general aspects of delivering percussion that will influence how you use your body.

Work at a Pace That Is Comfortable for Your Non-dominant Hand

Percussion strokes can be done with a range of speeds and pressures – it is *vibrating* the muscles and not just applying force that encourages them to soften. So, even if you are working slowly, you can be effective with percussion strokes as long as you are not being heavy-handed.

However, there is an unfortunate misconception that percussion is only effective when it is done fast and firmly. This belief can lead practitioners to tense up as they try to work faster and heavier than is comfortable for them, becoming stiff and awkward with their hands and losing their rhythm. This is potentially jarring for the client and also for the practitioner's hands.

It is important to work at a pace that is *comfortable for your non-dominant hand*. This can be frustrating for your faster hand, but it will enable you to avoid tensing up. It can be useful for beginners to start doing percussion slowly and lightly, and only for short bursts. With practice, you will build up your stamina for maintaining percussion strokes for longer and be able to increase the speed and pressure without tensing up.

Keep the Rhythm Even

Working at a comfortable rate will enable you to keep an even rhythm. This is important, as a disjointed rhythm is jarring to the client. If you don't find it easy to keep an even rhythm, practice working with music that has a steady beat and is slow enough for you to relax into it and maintain the rhythm for some time. With practise, you will be able to gradually increase your speed without tensing up or losing your rhythm. If you are getting tired, slow it back down to a pace that you can maintain.

Avoid Being Heavy-handed

Percussion that aims to 'pummel the client into submission' is counterproductive – clients flinch from it, tensing their muscles against these 'blows', which could lead to bruising. This heavy-handedness can also jar your own hands. Bear in mind that the vibrational aspect of percussion is as important as the force that you are applying. Keeping your wrist loose and avoiding tensing your hands will help you to do this.

Monitor the Effects of Percussion Strokes

Because the contact with the client is intermittent in percussion strokes, it's harder to palpate the client's structure and monitor their responses than with other strokes. However, by this stage of the massage, you will generally have covered the area with other strokes and therefore have a good sense of it. If not, do some more sliding strokes. Then, in percussion, use the moments of contact to feel for the familiar structural 'landmarks' and the elasticity, pliability and resilience of the tissues, and to monitor the client's responses. This is like making sense of a broadcast on a crackling radio or of a scene viewed under a strobe light. Return to sliding strokes if you need to palpate in a more familiar way again. With practise, your palpation skills during percussion will develop, and you will learn to sense with whichever part of your hand that you are using.

Some Practicalities of Percussion Strokes

Involve Your Forearms

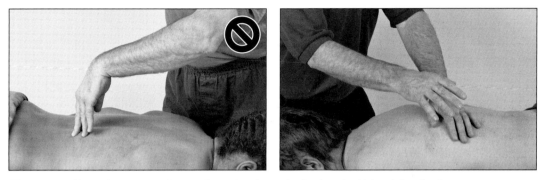

Figure 37.2: Powering percussion strokes; a) using only the hands, b) involving the forearms.

In each type of percussion stroke, your forearm provides an essential part of the effect. In the 'striking' strokes, for example, initiating the movement from your forearm will help you to rebound easily and fluidly. Flicking strokes require a movement like a cat or a bear scooping a fish out of a stream. In plucking percussion, you stretch the tissues by lifting your forearm as you 'grab' them momentarily with your fingers.

Why Involve Your Forearm in Percussion Strokes

There is a temptation to hold your forearms still and just use your hands for percussion strokes. This would be much harder work, especially for your wrists, than involving your forearms. If you try holding your forearms still while doing a percussion stroke, you will feel how this requires extra effort in your hands and puts more pressure on your wrists (and you probably still won't be as effective). You would be quite likely to also tense your shoulders, and quite possibly hold your breath, which would lead into a vicious cycle of further stiffening your arms and hands.

Soften your hands and initiate the percussion by lifting each forearm in turn and letting them 'flop' down in turn, to feel how much easier this is. It enables you to keep your wrists softer and your hands relatively relaxed, and makes it much easier to keep the rhythm and the pressure even. This will also help you to avoid being heavy-handed and thus jarring the client. Even in strokes in which you tighten your wrist, such as pounding, it is important to move your forearm as part of the stroke.

Alternating Your Hands

Some people find it difficult to alternate their hands, and begin by using both hands at the same time for percussion. However, there are good reasons for using your hands alternately. You only have to go at half the speed to achieve the effect. This enables you to stay more relaxed and makes it much easier to maintain an even rhythm. You're more likely to be tensing up and becoming stiff and heavy-handed if you're trying to 'hit' down with both hands at the same time (unless your hands are in contact, as in double-handed hacking, (see figure 37.5), and you focus on not being too heavy).

Practising Alternating Your Hands in Percussion Strokes

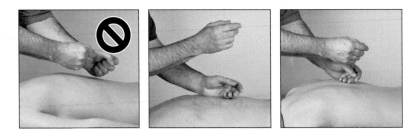

*Figure 37.3: Percussion stroke; a) with both hands at the same time,
b) practising large alternating hand movements,
c) smaller alternating hand movements.*

It's worth taking time to get used to alternating your hands if this is unfamiliar or you find it difficult. It's easiest to practise initially with strokes in which your hands are relaxed, such as 'pounding' lightly with the side of a soft fist (see figure 37.28). Start slowly with big, floppy movements of your forearms, allowing one hand to drop as you raise the other. As this becomes more familiar, gradually make the movements smaller and speed them up, but only at a rate that enables you to keep your arms and hands relatively relaxed. You will probably find that you need to focus more on your non-dominant hand in order to achieve an even balance between your hands.

When you feel comfortable with alternating your hands with these percussion strokes, practise those in which you need to tighten your hands such as cupping, and those which use your fingers more actively, such as plucking.

'Hitting'/'Striking' Vs 'Bouncing'

The group of strokes which 'hit' down onto muscles can energise them if they are done briskly or can press deeply into the muscles if they are done more firmly. Although these are generally referred to as 'hitting' or 'striking' strokes, students often find it more helpful to think of them as *bouncing* strokes. This image helps steer them away from beating heavy-handedly down onto the client with clenched hands and tense wrists. Instead, they learn to treat the client's body like a trampoline that they *drop* their hand onto, which *rebounds* them up for the next stroke. A feeling of bouncing is easiest to incorporate into light percussion strokes, but it's also essential for firm percussion in order to avoid heavy-handed 'striking' which can bruise the client and your own hands.

Comparing 'Hitting' and 'Bouncing' in Percussion Strokes

Try this with a partner who can give you clear feedback, and then get them to do it on you to feel the effect. Use the side of your soft fist so that you don't have to tense your hand. Begin by focusing on hitting down into the tissue, as if you were trying to push through it. Both you and your partner will probably find this jarring, so just do it once or twice to clarify the effect, and to avoid bruising them or your own hand.

To help you focus on the feeling of 'bouncing', it can be useful to focus initially on one hand at a time. Firstly, lift your forearm and then let it drop lightly towards your partner. Don't push your hand down, but just let it fall with gravity. People often find it helpful to let their breath go as they let the forearm drop in order to avoid using any effort. Let your hand bounce off and drop back again a few times, like a tennis ball gradually bouncing less and less before finally coming to rest.

Next, start in the same way, but, after the initial drop, use a little extra effort to keep your hand and forearm rebounding in a small way at a steady, even rate. Find out how little effort is required to maintain this – how relaxed you can be when doing percussion. When you feel comfortable with this, experiment with increasing the speed or the force *without tensing up*.

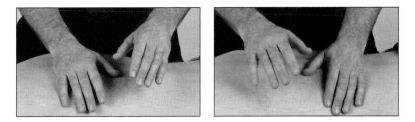

Figure 37.4: One hand 'bouncing' up as the other drops.

When you have done this with each arm separately, use both together. (This builds on the alternating hand exercise – above). Lift both forearms, and let one drop. As it rebounds, let the other drop. Keep them alternately rebounding in this way, focusing on staying relaxed in your shoulders, arms and hands and not holding your breath. Get your partner to give you feedback on the rhythm and evenness from the receiving side. (Get your partner to do this on you as well, so that you can appreciate how effective slow, rhythmical percussion can be, as long as it's not done in a heavy-handed way).

When this feels comfortable, develop the speed and power at a rate that enables you to stay relaxed as you do it.

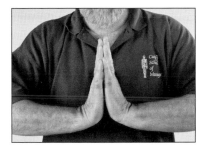

Figure 37.5: Holding the hands for double-handed hacking.

The most common stroke in which the hands are used together is double-handed hacking. Place your hands together as in the photo to 'hit' gently down with them together. Spend time practising how to use it in this relaxed, 'bouncing' way to avoid losing the rhythm or becoming heavy-handed with it.

Smooth Transitions into Percussion Strokes

If a practitioner launches suddenly into heavy percussion in a massage, s/he is quite likely to tense up. (This can also be jarring for the client and cause them to tense against you). Similarly, practitioners often tense up if they change abruptly from one type of percussion to another. So it is useful to practise making smooth transitions between other strokes and percussion so that you maintain the same body ease (and also between different percussion strokes, below). Transitions into percussion can easily be reversed to exit from percussion.

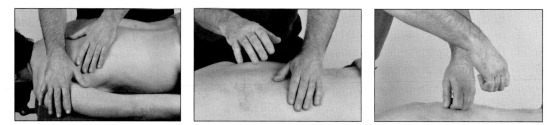

Figure 37.6: A transition from effleurage to percussion; a) 'thousand hands' stroking, b) 'patting' with the hands, c) 'knuckle brushing'.

It is a very easy step from short hand-over-hand stroking ('thousand hands' stroking) to 'brushing' with the fingers, as if you were brushing dust off your clothes. This leads easily into 'patting' with the hands. It can also be a bridge into knuckle percussion such as 'knuckle brushing'.

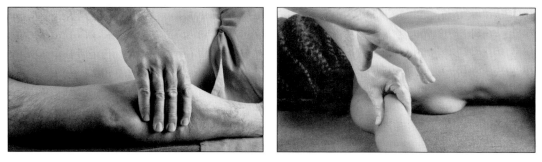

Figure 37.7: A transition from kneading to percussion; a) kneading, b) plucking.

Another easy transition is between kneading and 'plucking' percussion.

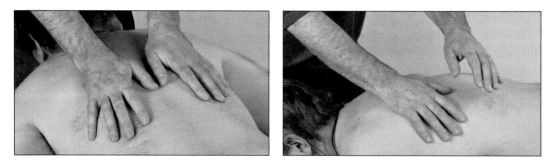

Figure 37.8: Transitions between vibration and percussion; a) muscle vibration, b) 'patting'.

It is also useful to practice moving smoothly between vibration and percussion strokes, which are often mixed together. From muscle vibration (see Chapter 38), the easiest percussion stroke to move to and from, is 'patting'.

Transitions Between Different Percussion Strokes
It is easiest to link different percussion strokes smoothly by just changing one aspect at a time.

For example, it is very easy to change from tapping softly with your fingertips to 'patting', or to the 'big bird peck' ('emu peck'), in which you cluster your fingers together to focus pressure on a single point.

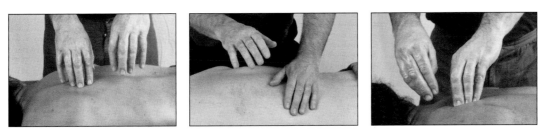

Figure 37.9: Percussion transition 1; a) tapping, b) patting, c) 'big bird peck'.

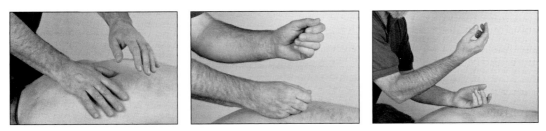

Figure 37.10: Percussion transition 2; a) 'clapping', b) soft hand 'pounding',
c) back of the hand percussion.

Another easy sequence is to turn your hand so that you use different parts, whilst maintaining the same force. For example, you could gradually change from clapping to light 'pounding' with the side of a soft fist and then to using the back of your hand.

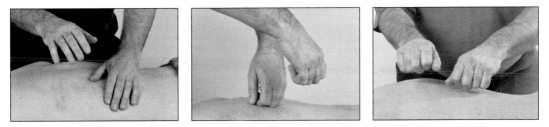

Figure 37.11: Percussion transition 3; a) brushing with the fingers, b) 'knuckle brushing',
c) rapping with the knuckles.

You can also easily link light brushing with the fingers, to 'knuckle brushing' to rapping with the knuckles.

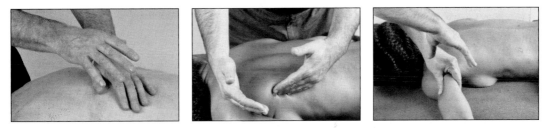

Figure 37.12: Percussion transition 4; a) 'patting', b) flicking, c) plucking.

Or you could move from 'patting' to flicking the muscles and on to plucking them.

Looking After Your Hands

The Practitioner's Build
Of course your build will affect how you are able to do percussion. If you have long, slender fingers don't overuse them or use them too forcefully, especially in hacking. Instead, do firm percussion strokes with the larger areas of your hands, such as the side of your fist or the back of your hand.

And, if you have small hands, don't strain them by trying to be too forceful in percussion strokes, or overuse them for plucking.

Vary Your Hand Use
Some practitioners limit themselves to tapping (with the fingertips), hacking (with the side of the hand) and cupping (with a cupped hand). However, varying the strokes by using different parts of your hands for a range of effects will spread the workload throughout your hands, save you from overusing particular areas, and give you more versatility.

Use the Largest, Strongest Parts of Your Hands
This is a related point. Use the largest and strongest parts of your hands that are appropriate. For example, only use your fingertips for light percussion such as tapping or light brushing and on areas that are too small for larger parts of your hand. Switch to your knuckles or your fist for firmer strokes, especially when you are working on clients with large, well-used muscles.

However, although your knuckles (the IP/interphalangeal joints, see figure 15.1) can be effective on large, firm areas of muscle, they are more vulnerable than your fist so don't overuse them either. (Practitioners with prominent knuckles obviously need to be more careful about how they use them).

Keep Your Hands Relaxed
It is important to keep your hands relaxed to avoid jarring yourself or the client.

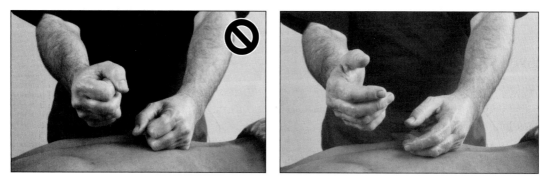

Figure 37.13: 'Pounding'; a) with a stiff, clenched fist, b) with relaxed hands.

This is particularly important when using your fist. Although the names of the heaviest strokes, such as 'pounding' or 'beating', suggest a fierce attack, they should not be done as heavy-handedly as this might imply. So, even for these very firm strokes, don't clench your fist tightly, which uses unnecessary energy and could jar your hands and the client. Have your fist a little relaxed so that it can 'bounce' easily.

Keep Your Wrist Relaxed
Having your wrist stiff would also reduce the 'bounce' and is potentially jarring.

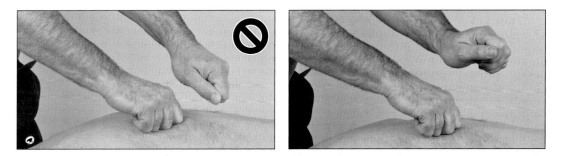

Figure 37.14: 'Rapping' with the knuckles; a) with a stiff wrist, b) with a loose wrist.

Keep your wrist relaxed so that your hands are 'floppy' and able to bounce easily in light strokes, such as rapping. Even with firm strokes such as pounding, don't have your wrist rigid which is likely to jar your hand (and the client). And don't stiffen it when you are using your fingers for plucking strokes.

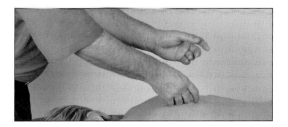

Figure 37.15: Soft 'hacking'.

Similarly, using a soft hand with your fingers slightly curled for hacking enables you to do this stroke without the 'attack' that the name implies, and which is often delivered with the hand and fingers held stiffly.

Involving Your Body to Support Percussion Strokes

There's quite a temptation to stand stiffly and tense your shoulders and/or hunch over when doing percussion strokes, which would lead to working stiffly. Instead, take up a dynamic posture, with your back long but not rigid (see figure 26.14) and soft knees (see figure 29.5) so that you can easily sway to move your hands over an area of the client's body. Lean forward with your whole trunk, rather than hunching over. Keep your shoulders relaxed by working at a comfortable pace.

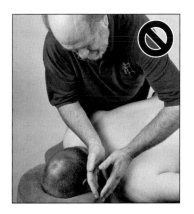

Move your body to stay aligned behind your working hands, and don't try to reach too far.

Figure 37.16: Leaning over further than is comfortable for the practitioner's back.

Review

Percussion strokes can range from very light strokes used for their sedating effect to the heaviest pounding strokes on the client's back to vibrate the lung tissue, and from 'hitting' to 'flicking' to 'plucking' strokes.

When doing percussion strokes:

- Involve your forearms, rather than just moving your hands;
- Work at a pace that is comfortable for your non-dominant hand, and that enables you to keep an even rhythm and avoid being heavy-handed;
- Monitor and adapt to your client's responses;
- Working with the feeling of bouncing easily off the client's tissues rather than hitting down into them in the 'hitting' strokes;
- Find ways of making smooth transitions from other strokes into percussion strokes, and between different percussion strokes.

Look after your hands by:

- Varying how you use them;
- Use the largest parts of your hands whenever possible, and;
- Keeping your hands and your wrist relaxed.

Look after your body by:

- Taking up a dynamic posture that enables you to easily sway;
- Move to keep your body aligned behind your hands;
- Lean forward with your whole trunk, rather than hunching over, and;
- Keep your shoulders relaxed by working at a comfortable pace.

CHAPTER 38

Vibration Techniques

In the classic Swedish massage sequence, percussion and vibration techniques are often used together, one leading into or out of the other. In percussion (see Chapter 37), the hand contact with the client's body is intermittent, whereas in vibration there is continuous contact to vibrate the soft tissues. As with percussion, an even rhythm is essential to making them work, whereas a disjointed application would be unpleasant to receive and much less effective.

There are two vibrating techniques commonly used in massage.

1. *Tremoring'/'wobbling'* the muscles can be done lightly to merely soften the muscles, or with more pressure to encourage deeper release (in a similar way to the 'shuddering' effect of many vibrating massage machines). It is generally done by 'gluing' your fingers or palm onto the skin and 'wobbling' the soft tissues around.

2. *'Rolling'* muscles from side to side to soften and stretch them, like rolling out a stiff lump of pastry into a long bread roll, is done with the fingers or palms. In classic muscle 'rolling', the hands are moved backwards and forwards together; in 'shearing' the muscle (a variation of muscle 'rolling') they are moved in opposite directions.

(Body rocking and limb rolling, which are sometimes considered types of vibration techniques, are looked at in Chapter 40).

Looking After Your Hands

Avoid Hyperextending Your Fingers

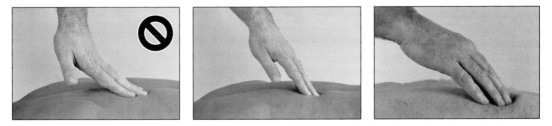

Figure 38.1: 'Tremoring' soft tissue with the fingers; a) hyperextended fingers,
b) straight fingers, c) slightly flexed fingers.

The fingertips are used for the lightest 'tremoring' strokes and sometimes for rolling muscles. In these strokes, you can also slide your fingers so that they gradually snake along an area. Take care not to hyperextend your fingers as you do this. Even holding them straight is harder work than having them slightly flexed, which is simultaneously the strongest and least effortful position to maintain (see figure 12.7).

When Using Your Fingers, Have Them Together

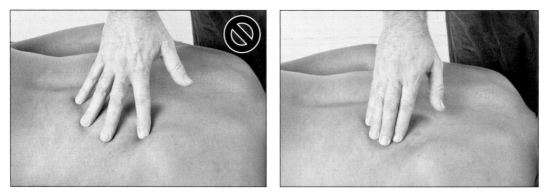

Figure 38.2: Using your fingers; a) spread; b) together.

Keep your fingers together. Having your fingers spread increases the workload on each individual finger, so keep them together to support one another.

Use Your Other Hand to Increase the Pressure

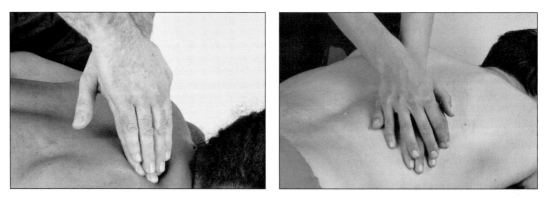

Figure 38.3: Use the other hand to increase the pressure; a) on the fingers, b) on the whole hand.

Use your other hand on top of your fingers if you want to increase the pressure whilst still directing it onto a small area.

Use Your Palm to Save Your Fingers
Whenever possible, switch to using your palm to spread the effect over a wider area and to work more firmly and vigourously. Whenever you are working on limb muscles, relax your hand enough so that it moulds to the client's body, rather than holding it stiff.

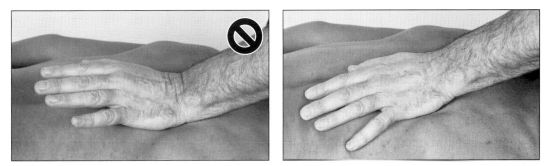

Figure 38.4: Using the palm to save the fingers; a) with tense fingers, b) with relaxed fingers.

Avoid Stiffening Your Fingers or Hyperextending Your Wrist

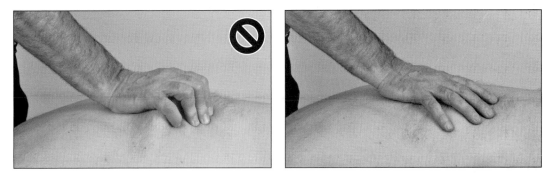

Figure 38.5: Vibrating muscles with the whole hand; a) tensing the fingers and bending the wrist,
b) working with a more relaxed hand and straighter wrist.

Avoid the temptation to stiffen your fingers or bend your wrist back too much. Relax your fingers so that your hand is not stiff and find a comfortable angle for your wrist. Drop down lower, if necessary, to save your wrist.

This is particularly important in 'shearing' because of the extra challenge of simultaneously moving your arms in opposite directions to soften the muscles. Obviously these movements are done with your arms and not just your hands. Remember to keep your shoulders relaxed and your body moving as you work over an area of muscle. Keep your hands firm enough to deliver the push and pull without rigidifying them.

Do the Movement With Your Whole Arm

Do the movement with your arm, and not just by moving your hand, which would quickly become tiring and put unnecessary pressure on your wrist and could strain if you persevered. Although you need to keep your hand and wrist firm to translate the movement from your forearm to your fingers, make sure that they are not rigid.

Establish an Even, Relaxed Rhythm

If you find that you are uneven or disjointed in the 'tremoring' and 'shearing' techniques, take time to practise the movements. As with percussion strokes, start at a pace that suits your slower hand, and focus on increasing the ease and evenness of the movement of that arm. Do this for short periods at first, focusing on getting the rhythm even between your hands. Then practise building up your speed and stamina whilst keeping your shoulders and hands relaxed and not holding your breath.

And practise making smooth transitions to and from other techniques, such as percussion strokes (see figure 37.8) and kneading (see Chapter 34).

Stay Relaxed When Rolling Muscles

Avoid the temptation to tense up when you are rolling the muscles, especially in 'shearing'. To see these movements done in a relaxed but efficient and rhythmical way, treat yourself to a meal at a pizza restaurant. Watch how the chef rolls out the balls of dough, starting with his hands together to soften it and then moving them oppositely to stretch it out.

Incidentally, the chef will probably also do some kneading – called 'impastimento' ('breadmaking') in Italian – which points out the affinity between kneading and 'shearing' strokes, and therefore how easy it is to make smooth transitions between them. (This is probably enough to copy from this source – don't try rolling your client back into a ball and slamming him on the bench, or spinning him around in the air!).

Involving Your Body

Keep Your Shoulders Relaxed

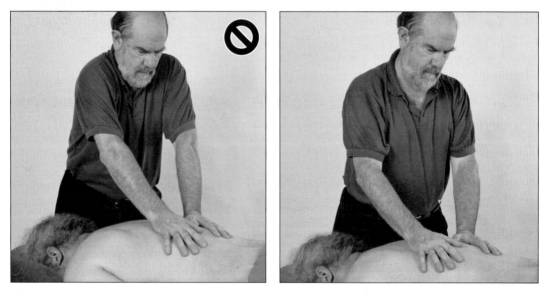

Figure 38.6: Monitoring the shoulders; a) tensing the shoulders, b) relaxing the shoulders.

These techniques demand considerable use of your arms. So there is quite a temptation to stand stock still, tense your shoulders and to work harder than necessary with your arms and hands. This leads to working stiffly, which quickly becomes tiring and creates disjointed, jarring rhythms. So monitor that you are keeping your shoulders relaxed.

Keep Your Hands in Front of Your Hips

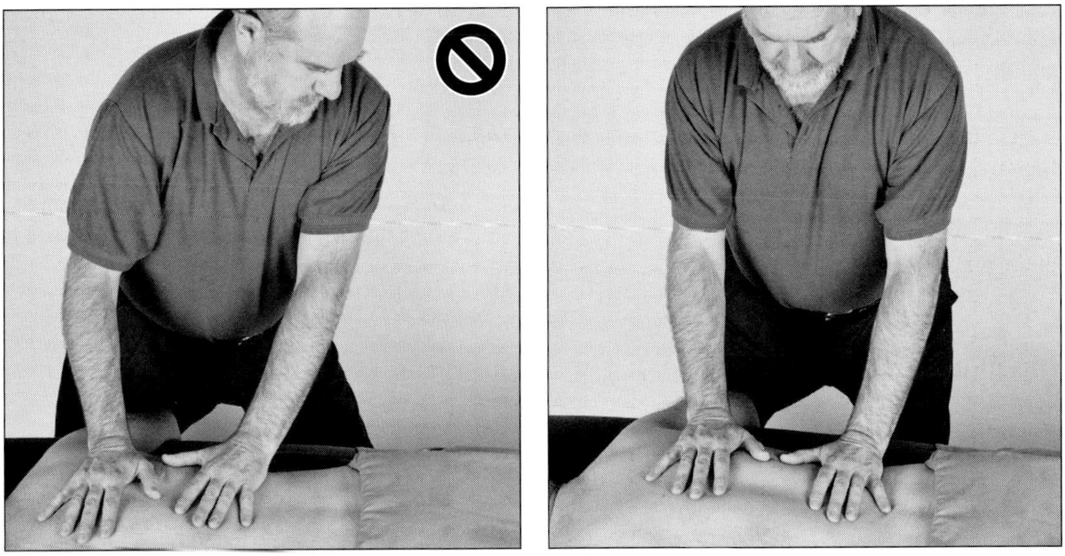

Figure 38.7: Keeping the hands in front of the hips; a) hands and hips not aligned,
b) aligning the body behind the hands.

As you work your way along the length of a muscle, sway or step sideways to keep your body behind your hands and to avoid working with your trunk twisted. When necessary, reposition yourself to keep your hands in front of your hips.

Don't Try to Reach Too Far Across the Client's Body

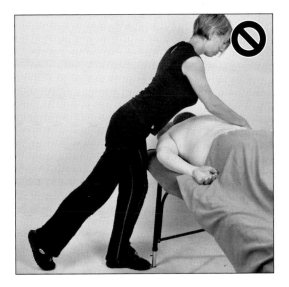

Figure 38.8: Straining to reach across
the client's back.

Review

When you're doing vibration strokes on muscles:

- Avoid hyperextending your fingers in light 'tremoring' strokes;
- Use your fingers together rather than separated;
- Use your other hand to increase the pressure that you are applying with your fingers or palm;
- Use your palm to save your fingers;
- Avoid stiffening your fingers or hyperextending your wrist;
- Do the movement with your whole arm not just by moving your hand;
- Establish an even, relaxed rhythm, and;
- Keep your hands relaxed.

Look after your body by:

- Keeping your shoulders relaxed;
- Moving your body to keep your hips behind your hands, and;
- Not trying to reach too far across the client's body.

CHAPTER 39

Lifting and Stretching Techniques

This chapter focuses on good handling practices for lifting and stretching techniques which are used to mobilise joints and to encourage muscle release. Many of the principles of good lifting also apply when you add a stretch by pulling and some in pushing stretches also. (Many of the ways of handling the client and using your body are also relevant when you're doing rhythmical body movements, see Chapter 40).

At the end of the chapter, there is a brief look at using your body for some of the other stretches in common use:

•   'Anchor and stretch' techniques, in which you apply pressure to a muscle while moving a limb to stretch the muscle, and;
•   Assisted / resisted stretches, which involve the active participation of the client.

Creating Trust Vs Forcing

It is important for the client to feel that they can trust you, especially when you are moving them into unfamiliar or vulnerable positions. Working awkwardly or straining your hands or body as you apply stretches would be conveyed to the client through your hands. This would tend to evoke an unconscious wariness in clients, making it harder for them to relax. However, using your body and your hands in a relaxed (but effective) way will help you to establish trust, and therefore encourage them to 'go with' the stretches. It will also make it easier for you to monitor and adapt to your client's responses.

So, when you are applying stretches, it is important that you:

•   Make the stretches *slow* and *easy* to avoid the client tensing against sudden, vigorous movements;
•   Coach the client to extend his/her range but *don't* attempt to *force* stretches beyond the client's obvious limits;
•   *Don't strain yourself* as you apply stretches, for example by working in an awkward position or trying to pull or push further than *you* can comfortably manage.

A Note About the Client's Clothing

This chapter focuses on using stretches when the client is wearing loose clothing that won't restrict his/her range of movement. In oil massage sessions, take care that the stretches don't leave the client feeling exposed or vulnerable. Use drapes to cover the client's body and, when necessary, tuck them in well. You can also use the drapes to provide you with a non-slip gripping surface.

Accommodating Lifting, Pulling and Pushing to Your Build

Whilst this chapter covers general principles of good bodyuse for lifting parts of the client's body and applying stretches, it is important to make sure that you can accommodate them to your own build.

Don't Lift a Limb That's Too Heavy For You
Don't try to lift a limb that is too heavy for you, which could strain your back. Obviously, practitioners with small builds need to monitor this very carefully. In some stretches, you could save your body by asking the client to move into the stretched position themselves.

Tall Practitioners – Look After Your Back When Reaching
If you are a tall person with long arms, you will often find it easier to do pulling stretches, as long as you look after your back by not trying to reach too far over the client. Save your back in this situation by dropping down to reach across. Be careful when doing pushing stretches that you don't get into cramped, awkward positions.

Short Practitioners – Focus On Pushing Stretches
Conversely, if you are short, and especially if you have short arms, you are likely to find it much easier to execute stretches by pushing. When pulling, make sure that you're not trying to reach too far across the client's body.

Good Lifting Practices

Because you often lift a part of the client's body to lead into a stretch, there's no clear-cut distinction between lifting and stretching. So this section of the chapter overlaps with the next sections on pulling and pushing stretches.

Whenever you are lifting any part of the client's body, incorporate good lifting practices in order to save your back – holding the weight close to your body, using your knees to lift and moving in the direction of the lift.

Hold the Weight Close to Your Body

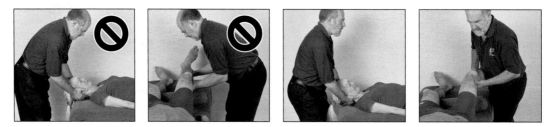

Figure 39.1: Lifting position; a), b) standing too far away, c), d) standing closer.

Don't stand too far away which would put strain on your lower back. Move in close, so that you are lifting the weight as close to your body as you can.

Don't Lean Over to Lift the Client's Legs From the Foot of the Table

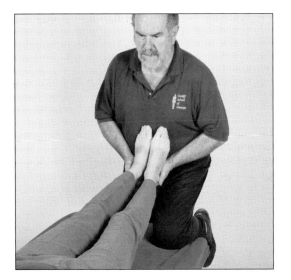

Figure 39.2: Kneeling one knee on the table to get closer when lifting the client's legs.

Try not to lift the client's legs from the foot of the table, unless you are swaying back into a stretch. If you do lift them from this position, take care not to hunch over or lean too far forward. If necessary, kneel one knee on the table to get in close enough under the weight of the leg to avoid straining your back.

Lift With Your Knees to Save Your Back

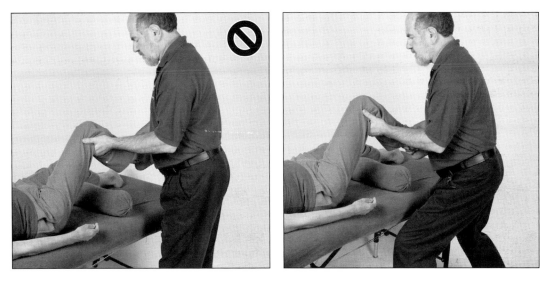

Figure 39.3: Lifting; a) just lifting with the arms, b) using your knees.

Don't stand still and just use your arms to lift, which overuses your upper body and puts strain on your back. This might also cause you to hunch over as you lift. Instead, bend your knees so that you can rise up under the client's head or limb to lift it.

Face in the Direction That You Are Moving as You Lift

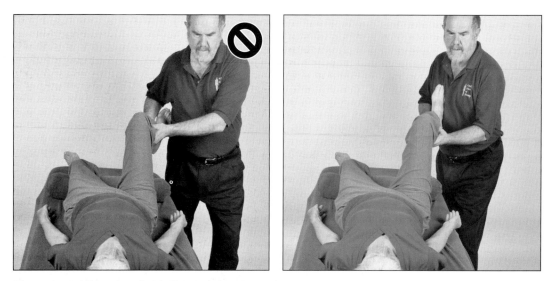

Figure 39.4: Lifting the client's leg over the chest; a) turned away from the direction of the movement, b) facing the direction of the movement.

If you intend moving a limb as you lift it, face your intended direction of movement, so that you can easily sway forward as you lift. If you were turned away from this direction, your body would be twisted which would make the movement awkward. And you would have to carry the full weight of the client's limb with your arms. These factors would put pressure on your back, especially when you're lifting a heavy leg.

Change Direction by Turning Your Feet, Not Just Twisting Your Body

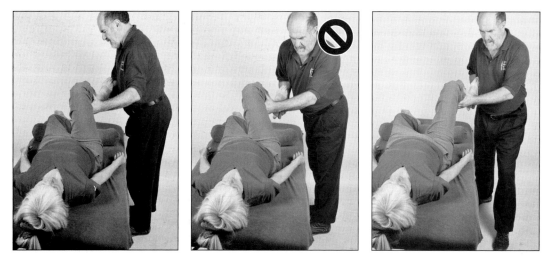

Figure 39.5: Turning in mid-movement; a) starting the movement, b) turning the upper body without changing feet positions, c) turning the feet.

If you need to change direction during the movement, turn smoothly by turning your feet. If you don't turn your feet, your body will be twisted with the potential for straining your back. And you would lose the impulse from your lower body and would therefore have to work much harder than necessary with your upper body.

Avoid Lifting the Full Weight of the Client's Leg Unless it is Essential

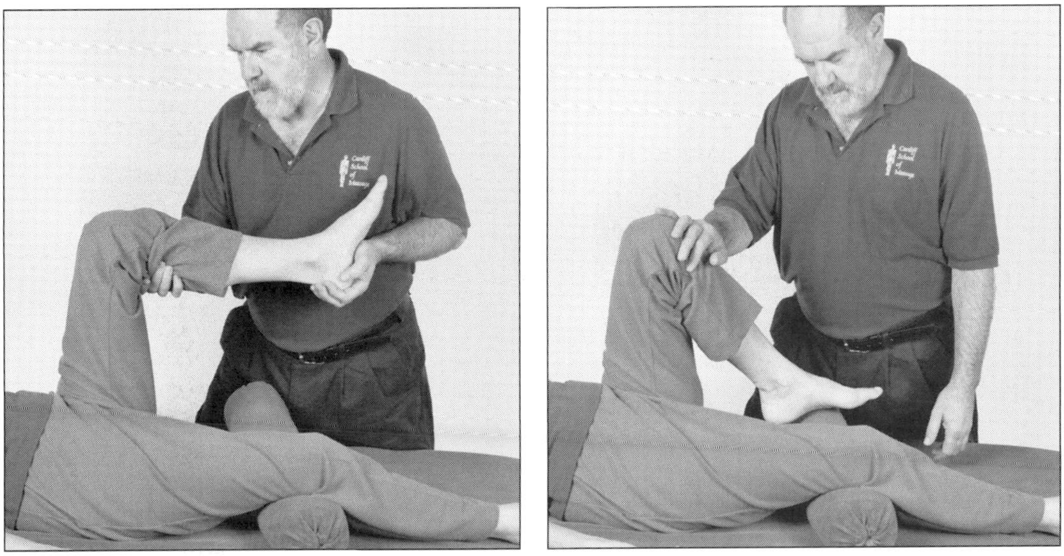

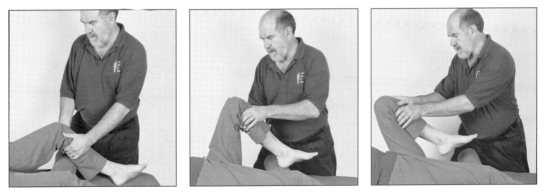

Figure 39.6: Lifting the client's leg; a) lifting the full weight of the client's leg – do cautiously,
b) lifting it with the foot dangling.

When the client is supine and you are just lifting one leg, you will have most control of the movement if you hold under the client's knee. Unless you have a definite reason for lifting her lower leg up, let it hang down so that her foot dangles near the table. This considerably reduces the effort needed to move the leg. You might even let her foot slide along the table to make the movement easier. In fact, if you are a small-framed practitioner working on a large client, this may be the only way that it's possible for you to comfortably move the client's leg over her chest.

Lift the Client's Leg at the Knee if You Can

Figure 39.7: Using the hands; a), b) hands under the knee to lift it,
c) hands on the shin to push the knee over the chest.

Begin lifting the leg by swaying forward to push up with your hands under the back of the knee. Once the back of the client's knee begins to fold onto your hand(s), reposition them at the front of the tibia just below the knee, and continue to sway forward in order to push the knee over the chest.

Don't Lift Both of the Client's Legs at Once if They're Too Heavy
Only lift both of the supine client's legs at once if they're not too heavy for you.

Hold the Client's Ankles Together to Lift Their Legs

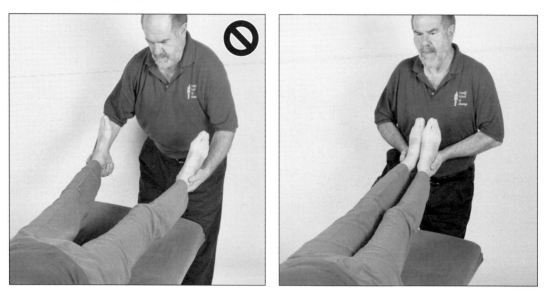

Figure 39.8: Lifting the client's legs together; a) holding the legs apart, b) holding the ankles together.

Take care not to hunch over as you lift. To lift their legs together in preparation for stretching them, hold their ankles next to one another to reduce the workload on your separate arms.

If the Client's Arm is Heavy, Support it on Your Hip When She is Supine

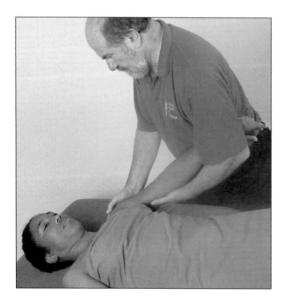

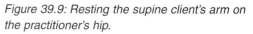

Figure 39.9: Resting the supine client's arm on the practitioner's hip.

There is less potential problems in lifting the client's arm as long as you use good lifting practices – holding the weight close to your body (see figure 39.1), using your knees to save your back (see figure 39.3), and facing and moving in the direction of your lift (see figures 39.4 & 39.5). When the client is supine you can guide the movement by holding under her elbow. Placing your other hand under her shoulder will provide more support and precision. If the client's arm is quite heavy, you might rest it on your hip to support the weight and then guide it with both of your hands. (In an oil massage, use a small towel to protect your clothing from the oil).

Avoid Gripping Too Tightly

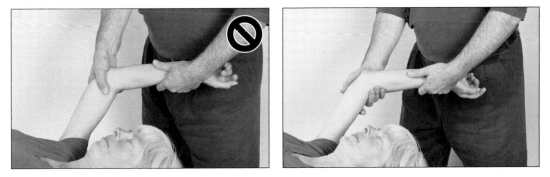

Figure 39.10: The 'grip'; a) tense grip, b) loose 'grip'.

How you use your hands is important. Don't grip tightly, which uses unnecessary energy, and is likely to produce wariness and 'resistance' in the client and to obscure your ability to feel the client's subtle responses.

Support the Limb From Underneath

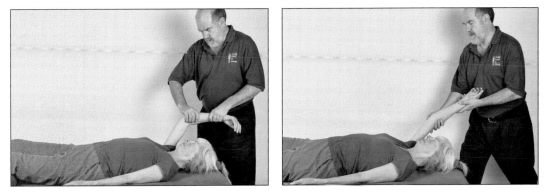

Figure 39.11: Hand support underneath; a) hold from above – use sparingly,
b) supporting from underneath.

Although you might take hold of the client's arm, leg or head from above, it's hard work to keep holding it up. So, whenever possible, try to support the client's head or limb from underneath. This takes less effort and enables you to keep your hands more relaxed, so that you are more able to feel the client's responses. It is also easier for the client to trust this support.

Stretch the Prone Client's Arm at the Elbow or Wrist

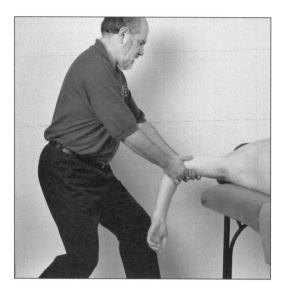

Figure 39.12: Stretching the prone client's arm.

You can stretch and move her arm by holding (but not grabbing) around the elbow, when the client is prone.

Whenever Possible, Let Your Arms Straighten for Lifting

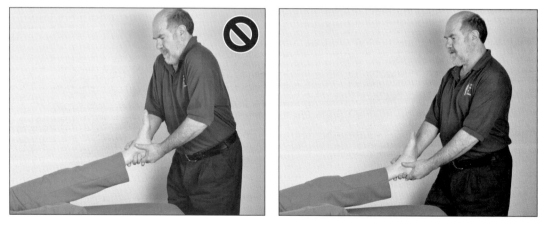

Figure 39.13: Using the arms in stretches; a) bent arms, b) letting the arms straighten.

Try to avoid bending your arms when you are pulling, as this makes an unnecessary demand on your upper arm muscles. Instead, as you pull back by swaying your hips backwards, let your arms straighten so that the power for pulling comes more directly from your body while your arms remain relatively relaxed.

Use Your Hands Like a 'Sling' Rather Than Grabbing

One way to make this easier is to put your hands together, one cradled inside the other, and 'sling' them under the body part that you are lifting.

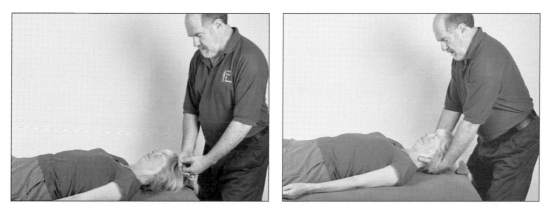

Figure 29.14: Using the hands like a 'sling'.

Pulling Stretches

Many of the good lifting principles are also relevant for pulling stretches. These stretches are not only effective for clients, they are also very useful for the practitioner. They give you an opportunity to relax your hands, and open out the joints of your own arms and shoulders as a break from applying pressure through your upper body. This is particularly useful in non-oil massage sessions (see Chapter 36), which demand more use of your hands than oil massage.

(Stretches can also be done by pushing, for example by moving the client's knee over her chest to stretch her gluteals, see figures 39.25 & 39.31).

Align Your Body With Your Hands for Pulling

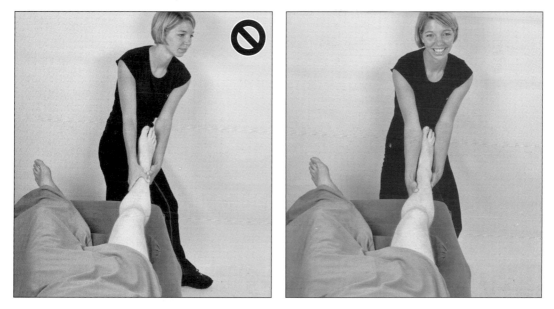

Figure 39.15: The practitioner's position for a stretch; a) turned away, b) aligned.

Position yourself for pulling with your hips facing your hands and the back of your hips facing your intended direction of movement.

Pull by Swaying Backwards

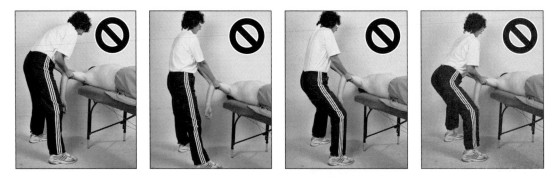

Figure 39.16: Pulling awkwardly; a) hunching over, b) stiff legs, c) tense shoulders, d) stiff, sway back.

Even when practitioners know how to use their bodies well for sliding, petrissage and pressure strokes, unconscious postural habits can come to the fore in applying stretches.

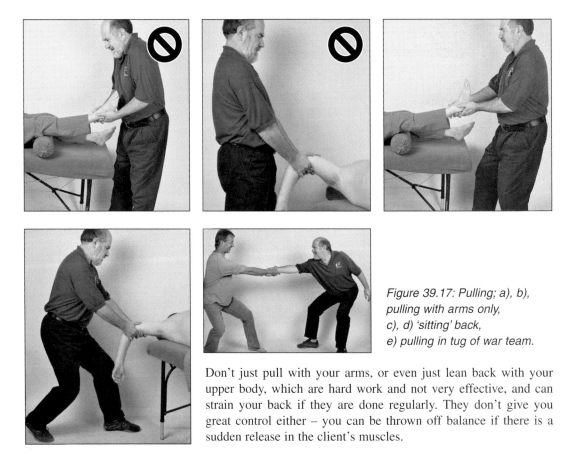

Figure 39.17: Pulling; a), b), pulling with arms only, c), d) 'sitting' back, e) pulling in tug of war team.

Don't just pull with your arms, or even just lean back with your upper body, which are hard work and not very effective, and can strain your back if they are done regularly. They don't give you great control either – you can be thrown off balance if there is a sudden release in the client's muscles.

Instead, sway back *with your whole body* to give power and evenness to the stretch. It can be useful to imagine that you are 'sitting' back (towards an imaginary chair) to help get a sense of pulling with your bodyweight rather than just your upper body. Another image which some people find helpful are to imagine that you are pulling in a tug of war team.

'Reach' Back With Your Back Leg to Pull More Strongly

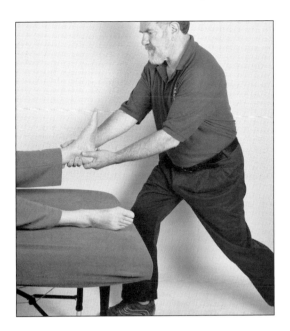

Figure 39.18: Increasing the pull – reaching back with one leg.

Rather than pulling back suddenly, which the client is likely to react against, gradually sway back to slowly increase the pull. If this begins to feel like hard work, increase the momentum by 'sitting' back more and/or by reaching back with one leg. (Of course, as you do this, you will need to keep the stretch within comfortable limits for the client).

Sway Your Body for Moving a Sustained Stretch

You can also add movement to a sustained stretch by swaying your body.

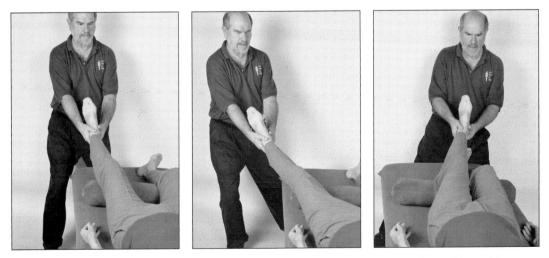

Figure 39.19: Swaying whilst sustaining a stretch; a) the stretch, b), c) swaying from side to side.

For example, you can move the client's leg sideways. Hold around the ankle to stretch the leg lengthwise, and then sway your body sideways as you maintain the traction of the stretch. You can use this to encourage release in the hip joint when the client is either supine or prone. It is also the easiest way of moving the client's leg away from her other leg, so that you have space to massage her inner thigh.

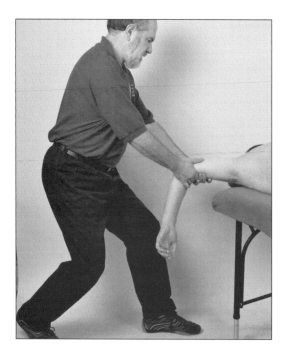

Figure 39.20: Stretching the arm.

When the client is prone, you can stretch her arm out to the side by swaying backwards, and then sway from side to side while maintaining the stretch in a similar way.

Save Your Hands by Using Your Forearm to Pull

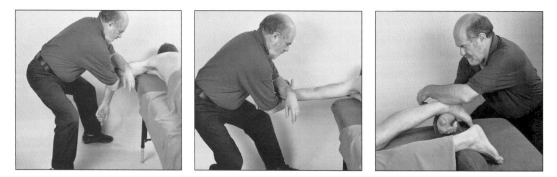

Figure 39.21: Doing stretches with the forearms.

Whenever you can, conserve your hands by 'hooking' your forearm around a client's limb to stretch it, for example inside the client's bent elbow or knee. Don't tense your arm more than necessary to maintain the effective 'crook' of your elbow. Using both forearms together, whenever it is possible, will enable you to keep your upper arm and shoulder muscles relatively relaxed. Be careful to use the inner 'soft' forearm (the flexor muscle bellies, see figure 18.3), especially if you have thin arms, to avoid cutting into the client with your 'bony' forearm (the proximal ulna, see figure 18.7).

When Using Your Forearm, Drop into the 'Chimp' Position to Save Your Back

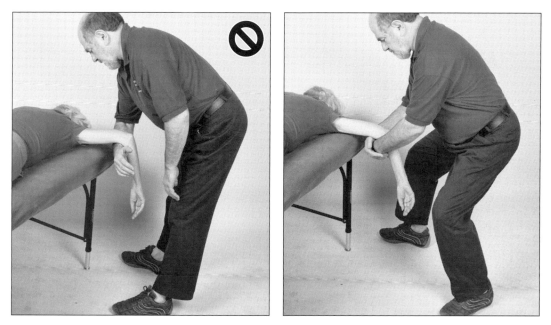

Figure 39.22: Using the body; a) standing stiff-legged, b) bending the knees.

When using your forearm, save your back by widening your stance and bending your knees to get low enough (into the 'chimp' position, see figure 18.24). Once you are in position, apply the stretch by swaying back rather than just pulling with your arm and shoulder muscles.

Avoid Hunching Over to Pull When You Are Sitting on the Table

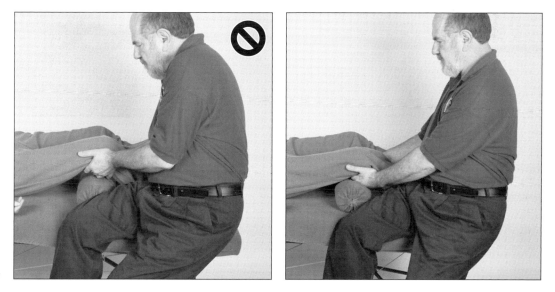

Figure 39.23: Sitting on the table to stretch the supine client's leg from the knee; a) crumpling to pull, b) swaying the whole trunk.

If you are sitting on the table, for example to stretch the supine client's leg at the knee, lean back with your whole trunk rather than just crumpling your back.

Pushing Stretches

Some stretches, including some of those described above, can be done by pushing. In fact, if you are short, you may find this easier as it will save you from straining to reach across the client's body. And pushing is most effective for certain stretches, for example pushing the client's leg over their chest for a gluteal stretch (see below). The main elements to focus on in pushing stretches are using your body rather than relying on muscle power, looking after your hands as you push (especially your wrists), and the angle of the push.

Look after your hands by:

- Using larger areas of your hand such as your palm rather than just using your fingertips, especially if you have small or slender fingers;
- Avoid hyperextending your wrist as you apply pressure (see figure 17.7);
- Conserve your hands whenever you can by using your forearm (see Chapter 18);
- Swaying forward to push.

Use Your Forearm for Pushing to Save Your Hand/s

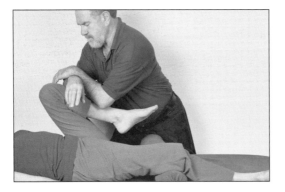

Figure 39.24: Using the forearm for a push.

Learn to use your forearm so you can reduce the workload of your hands.

Face the Direction of Your Push – Orientate Yourself to Push at Different Angles
Align your hips with your hands for the push and then move in that direction to apply the stretch.

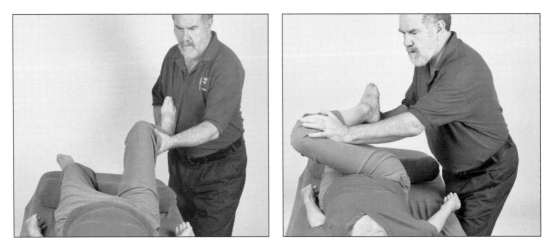

Figure 39.25: Directing the direction of the push; a) towards the same-side shoulder,
b) diagonally across the trunk.

As you move forward, you can fine-control the direction of your movement by the angle that you aim towards. For example, you could go straight forward to take the supine client's knee further over the chest, or aim more diagonally (towards the client's opposite shoulder) to move the knee across the client's body.

Drop Down to be Able to Push Upwards

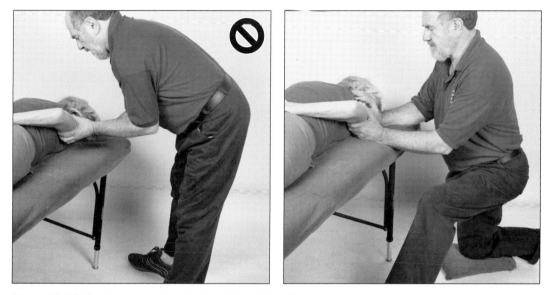

Figure 39.26: Pushing up under the shoulder; a) hunching over, b) dropping down to be able to push forward and upwards.

When pushing up under the prone client's shoulder, don't hunch over. If necessary drop one knee down to the floor, so that as you push, you are able to rise up as you sway forward for the push.

Pushing and Pulling at the Same Time

When you are pushing and pulling at the same time, the temptation is to stand still and rely on arm muscle power. This is hard work.

Turn Your Hips to Power Each Hand
Instead, position yourself so that you can turn your body a little to power each hand. Twist your hips so that one moves forward to push its respective hand forward, and your other hip simultaneously moves backwards to initiate the pull of your other hand.

Anchor and Stretch

In the 'anchor and stretch' technique (also called 'pin and stretch'), you press on a muscle while moving a distal part of the client's body to stretch the muscle under your pressure. For example, you can bend the prone client's leg and tilt it from side to side to encourage release in the gluteus maximus as you press on it.

Lean Your Body to Sustain the Pressure in 'Anchor and Stretch' Techniques

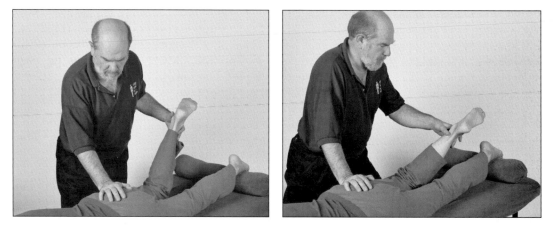

Figure 39.27: 'Anchor and stretch' – leaning to sustain the pressure while moving the leg.

Face towards where you are applying pressure so that you can lean your bodyweight forward onto that area for the pressure. This makes it easy to maintain the pressure with one hand/forearm as you use the other hand to move the limb.

Avoid hyperextending your wrist as you apply the pressure with your hand.

Although you'll need to turn a little towards the client's leg as you tilt it from side to side, make sure that you don't turn so far that you feel twisted in your trunk or lose the pressure (in which case, you would be trying to maintain the pressure by muscle power alone).

Use Your Forearm to Save Your Hand

If you are using your forearm to apply the pressure, widen your stance to lower your body (into the 'chimp' stance, see figure 18.24) in order to avoid hunching over. Have your palm turned down so that you are using the 'soft' forearm (the area of the flexor muscle bellies, see figure 18.3) and keep your hand relaxed so that you are not unnecessarily tensing your flexor muscles (see figure 18.4).

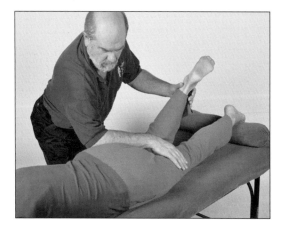

Figure 39.28: Using the forearm.

Assisted / Resisted Stretches

Assisted stretches (also called 'facilitated stretches' or 'resisted stretches') are used by many practitioners, particularly in the sports massage field, to help clients extend their movement range. They are known by many technical names, such as *Proprioceptive Neuromuscular Facilitation* (PNF), *Neuromuscular Technique* (NMT) or *Muscle Energy Technique* (MET). They involve the client stretching or being stretched by the practitioner to a point of challenge (the 'end-range'), pushing forward or pulling back at this place against a resistance (provided by the practitioner), relaxing for a few seconds and then moving into the extra range that has been opened up.

In doing these techniques, the challenge is to avoid tiring or straining yourself:

*   While you are guiding the client into the initial stretch position, or;
*   When you are bracing yourself to provide the resistance.

Obviously you need to pay particular care when you are working with large-framed and/or fit clients, especially in leg and trunk stretches. And you need to conserve your body and your energy when these techniques make up a large part of your work, particularly if your clientele is largely sportspeople.

Save Your Back by Standing Closer to Lift Parts of the Client's Body into Position

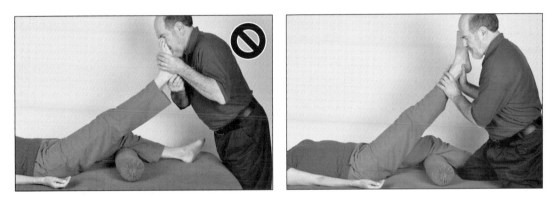

Figure 39.29: Lifting the supine client to position the leg; a) leaning from the end of the table, b) kneeling one knee on the table.

When moving the client's limb or trunk into position, position yourself so that you can use your body for this rather than standing still and just lifting with your arms. For example, when lifting the supine client's leg in preparation for a hamstring stretch, get your weight under the leg and move forward to lift it.

Use Your Body to Provide the Resistance
The temptation in these stretches is to provide resistance for the client just by *tensing your upper body*. This is hard work, especially if you're doing a lot of these stretches in a session. So lean and sway forward with your bodyweight. When you are providing resistance, keep your back relatively straight (but not stiff) and use your knees to push instead of standing still and just using your arms. If necessary, step back to make it easier to lean your body forward to brace the movement. Make it easy on yourself in these stretches by:

*   Having the client move into position herself for the stretch, perhaps guiding her with your hands;
*   Align your hips and hands and use the lunge stance to provide resistance;
*   Push forward or pull back *with your body* to provide the resistance.

Support the Client's Leg on Your Shoulder

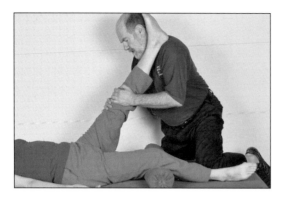

Figure 39.30: Supporting the client's leg.

When holding the client's leg, putting it on your shoulder will reduce your hard work while enabling you to use both hands for the resistance, if necessary.

Move Your Body to Provide the Resistance
Sway forward if you intend to provide resistance by pushing. When you need to provide the resistance by pulling, there is a temptation to tense your shoulders and just pull with your arms. Instead, 'sit' back in order to pull with your whole bodyweight. Of course, even when you are using your bodyweight like this, you are still directing the pull through your arms. If this feels too much, move to a position in which you can *push* with your bodyweight which is an easier and stronger action.

Minimise the Pressure on Your Body
The following guidelines will also help you to minimise the pressure on your body:

* Guide your client to begin the stretch slowly so that you're not taken by surprise or pushed off balance.
* These stretches are *isometric*, so tell the client to only stretch enough to engage muscles, not to pull or push enough to move you.
* Look after yourself by providing resistance only up to the level *that is comfortable for yourself*, and then ask your client to hold at that level of effort.
* If either of you feels pain, stop the stretch, talk it through and make adjustments.
* If the client is recruiting other muscles to do the work, only stabilise them if it's easy and comfortable for you.
* Alternatively, direct them to do the work of self-stabilising, using verbal instruction and guiding them with your hands. As well as saving your body, this is useful learning for the client.

Review
Lifting and stretching techniques are used to mobilise joints and to encourage muscle release.

It is important for the client to feel that they can trust you, especially when you are moving them Using your body and your hands in a relaxed (but effective) way will help you to establish trust, and therefore encourage clients to 'go with' the stretches.

Apply stretches in a *slow* and *easy* manner to avoid the client tensing against them.

Coach the client to extend his/her range but *don't* attempt to *force* stretches beyond his/her obvious limits.

Don't strain yourself by working in an awkward position or trying to pull or push further than *you* can comfortably manage.

In oil massage sessions, use drapes to ensure that the stretches don't leave the client feeling exposed or vulnerable.

Tall practitioners often find it easiest to do pulling stretches, as long as they don't try to reach too far over the client, whilst short practitioners often find pushing stretches easier.

When lifting parts of the client's body:

- Don't lift a limb that's too heavy for you;
- Hold the weight close to your body to save your back;
- Lift with your knees to save your back;
- Don't lean over when lifting the client's legs from the foot of the table;
- Face in the direction that you are moving as you lift;
- Change direction by turning your feet, not just twisting your body;
- Try to avoid lifting the full weight of the client's leg;
- Lift the client's leg at the knee if you can;
- Don't lift both of the client's legs at once if they're too heavy;
- Hold their ankles together to ease the workload if you do lift them, and;
- Support the clients arm on your hip if it is heavy.

In addition:

- Avoid griping tightly by 'slinging' your hands underneath the limb to support it;
- Whenever possible, let your arms straighten as you lift or apply a stretch.

In pulling stretches:

- Align your body with your hands and pull by swaying backwards;
- Increase the stretch by 'reaching' back with your back leg;
- Sway your body for moving a sustained stretch;
- Save your hands by widening your stance and bending you knees to drop into a 'chimp' stance in order to use your forearm to pull, and;
- Avoid hunching over to pull when you are sitting on the table.

In pulling stretches, look after your hands by:

- Using larger areas of your hand such as your palm rather than just using your fingertips;
- Avoid hyperextending your wrist as you apply pressure;
- Conserve your hands whenever you can by using your forearm;
- Face and sway your whole body in the direction of your push;
- Drop lower to be able to push upwards.

When pushing and pulling at the same time, twist your hips so that each hip delivers power to the respective hand.

In the 'anchor and stretch' technique:

- Face towards your pressing hand;
- Lean your body to sustain the pressure;
- Avoid hyperextending your wrist as you apply the pressure with your hand, and;
- Use your forearm for pressing to save your hand.

In assisted stretches, avoid tiring or staining yourself while you are guiding the client into the initial stretch position, or when you are bracing yourself to provide the resistance, by:

- Standing close to lift any parts of the client's body;
- Getting the client to move his own leg into position;
- Providing resistance by moving your body, not just using your arms;
- Supporting the client's leg on your shoulder, and;
- Guiding the client to do the stretch in ways that don't stress your body.

CHAPTER 40

Rhythmical Body Movements – Body Rocking and Limb Rolling

This chapter looks at good bodyuse practices for establishing rhythmical to-and-fro movements of the client's body for two of the most commonly used rhythmical movements:

- *Body rocking*, in which you push the client's hips to move the body from side to side;
- *Limb rolling*, which is done either by facing across the limb to push or pull it with both hands together, or facing the axis of the limb and rolling it from side to side between your hands.

These techniques can be done lightly to encourage relaxation throughout the client's body or more vigourously for energising.

The general principles covered in this chapter also apply to other rhythmical ways of moving the client's body, such as adding a rhythmical element to stretches. (It's beyond the scope of this book to cover the extensive repertoire of rhythmical/vibratory techniques of Hawaiian kahuna massage, Tragering®, Pulsing and RhythmMobility®).

An Important Caution

Rhythmical movements are designed to give the client a sense of mobility and suppleness which, for many people, is an antidote to gradually stiffening up in a sedentary lifestyle. However, sometimes rhythmical movements are *totally inappropriate* because of injuries or weak or inflamed areas. Spinal problems, for example, can preclude rocking the body or longitudinal push-pull movements.

Even when rolling a limb to give the client a sense of movement, you may need to restrict the amplitude of the movement. This will be the case, for example, when you are feeling your way with a client who has shoulder or hip joint problems. Use your hands to contain the movement and carefully monitor the client's responses, so that you give them a feeling of safety, and that you're not going to push them beyond their comfort zone into pain.

Some General Principles

Monitoring the Effects

Tracking how the rhythm spreads through the client's body, especially in body rocking, will tell you about the areas of suppleness in the client's body (which move easily) and the areas where tightness restricts the movement.

With practice, you will learn to distinguish how the distant parts of the body affect the central movement that you're initiating – for example, following the central movement easily or dragging behind it so that you have to slow it down, or forcing you to push harder because the whole limb/body moves as one stiff unit. This is like learning to make accommodations in the rhythm, momentum or direction of the movement when you're pushing a child on a swing who is kicking out with her legs or spinning around as she swings.

Many people find that watching rhythmical movement can interfere with their ability to feel it. So shutting your eyes, defocusing or at least looking away (see figure 24.2) is often helpful in feeling the rhythm through your hands more easily.

Finding the Client's Rhythms
It is crucial to search out the 'natural' rhythms of the client's body by pushing and waiting for the body's natural return, instead of trying to impose a rhythm that doesn't fit. This would be like trying to push a child on a swing at an arbitrary speed, rather than following the pace that they naturally settle into because of their weight and the length of the ropes/chains.

It takes time to gain a feel for this, as there is no single rhythm that fits everyone. Each body has its own rhythm ('every-body got rhythm'), and so does each body part or area, due to the individual's build and the distribution of their weight. You will only discover this through experiment, feeling for the rhythm that is easiest for you to maintain because it's the client's natural rhythm.

You will notice that the lighter the body part, the faster the cycle of oscillation will be. And when you are rocking the whole body, clients with short, stocky builds will generally oscillate faster with the whole body moving more as a unit, whilst tall clients with long limbs will tend to go slower as the movement ripples out through the length of their limbs.

Finding this basic rhythm is also crucial for developing this way of working further. For example, movements can be amplified, or you can set up related overriding rhythms or complementary counter-rhythms in other body parts, as long as they remain *in relation* to the basic rhythm.

Looking After Your Hands

The main thing to think about in delivering rhythmical body movement is that you are applying a potentially strong force at regular intervals, and therefore it's important to consider how to minimise the potentially jarring impact on your hands. So the main focus of this chapter is on ways of reducing and containing the impact, and how to position and use your body to help you to do this.

Start the Movement Slowly to Minimise the Jarring to Both Client and Practitioner
There are many aspects of initiating rhythmical movements, especially body rocking, that are akin to pushing a child on a swing. Pushing firmly and abruptly to begin the movement would be disturbing to the client (as it would be for a child) as well as being hard work for your hands. So initiate the movement slowly, pushing firmly and relatively continuously, to get movement started. As it builds up, you can make your touch briefer and lighter, as you would do to maintain a child's swinging once the motion is fairly well established.

Use Larger Parts of Your Hands for Larger Areas of the Client's Body and to Get the Movement Started
Therefore it makes sense to use the large areas such as your whole palm to initially get the movement happening, especially if you are rocking the whole body, even if you switch to using your fingers to maintain the movement once it's established. This can be done by having your hands on either side of the client's hips or on the back of the sacrum.

Have Your Hand Relaxed

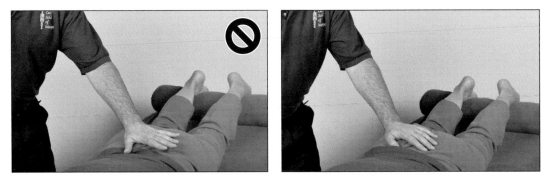

Figure 40.1: Using the whole hand; a) stiff hand, b) relaxed hand.

When you are initiating the movement from the sacrum with your palm, there's quite a temptation to stiffen your hand in impatience to get the movement happening. Relax your hand and trust that you can build the movement slowly.

Use Two Hands for More Control

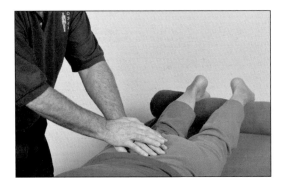

Figure 40.2: Using two hands – hand on hand.

There are two ways of using both of your hands to have more control and therefore to build the movement faster. One is to use hand on hand pressure, which makes it easier to involve your own body.

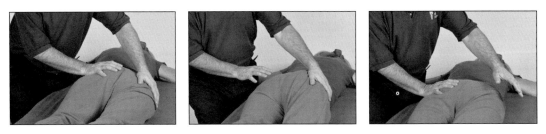

Figure 40.3: Hands on either side of the hips; a) continuous contact, b), c) non-continuous contact.

The other way is to start with one hand on each side of the client's hips, either with continuous or non-continuous contact. For most people, this is an easier way of initiating the movement, especially when you're first learning to get these movements happening.

Don't Let Your Fingers Hyperextend When You Push

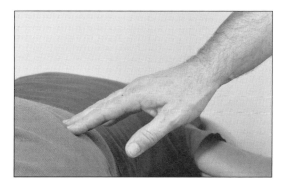

Figure 40.4: Keeping the fingers straight when pushing.

When the movement is established, you can use your fingers for the pushing. However take care that they're not consistently bending as you push, particularly when you're pushing with the tips.

Pull as Well as Push to Vary Your Hand Use
Switch to pulling at times to give your fingers a rest from the impact of pushing.

When Rolling the Limbs, Don't Grab the Muscles or Stiffen Your Fingers

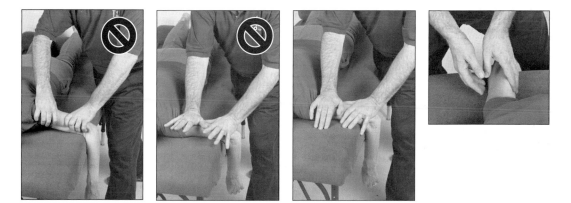

Figure 40.5: Using your hands to push; a) gripping too tightly, b) tense fingers, c), d) relaxed but alert hands.

When you are rolling a limb, try not to grip the muscles too tightly or stiffen your hand unnecessarily. These both use unnecessary energy, and are less comfortable for the client. Find the 'middle way' of having your hands relaxed but 'alert'.

Avoid Hyperextending Your Wrist When Pushing With Your Palm

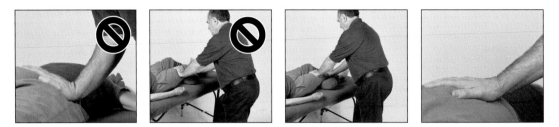

*Figure 40.6: The angle of the wrist; a) pushing with the wrist hyperextended,
b) positioning oneself with the wrist hyperextended, c), d) moving the hands to a higher position.*

Lower your body, or make contact at a higher point on the client's body, to make sure that your wrist is not bent back too much as you push.

Involve Your Arms in the Movement, Not Just Your Hands
Don't just do these movements with your hands which would make it much harder work, and your movements would be stilted. Move your arms so that your hands can stay freer to combine the qualities of relaxation and liveliness.

Conserve Your Hands by Using Your Forearm for Pushing

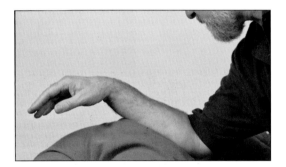

Figure 40.7: Using the forearm.

If you can use your forearm skilfully for pushing, you can conserve your hands.

Involving Your Body to Support Your Hands

Face Your Hands
Don't stand stiffly in one place but keep your body moving so that you can keep facing your working hands (so that they stay within the area of the 'hip spotlight', see figure 28.11). This will avoid twisting and potentially straining your body which would also lead to overusing your upper body. In body rocking, face across the client's body. In limb rolling you can face across the limb to roll it like a rolling pin, or face the central axis of the limb and roll it by 'flipping' it from side to side between your hands.

Don't Stand Still and Just Use Your Arms

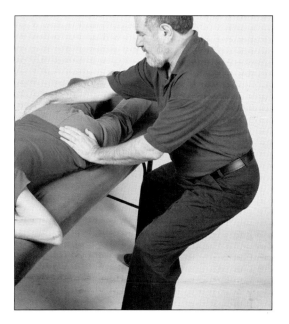

Figure 40.8: Involving the body in rocking movements.

Although rhythmical work is mainly done by your hands (and arms to support them), try not to stand still and just rely on upper body muscle power alone.

Lean Forward for Pushing Movements

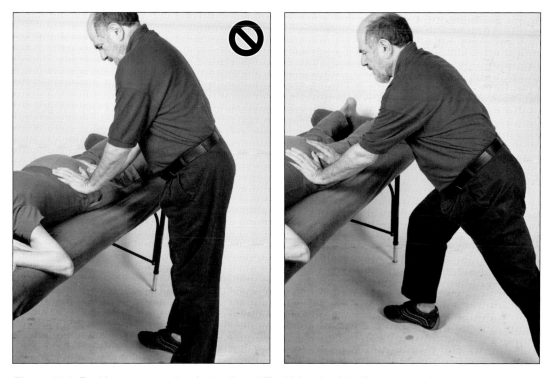

Figure 40.9: Pushing movements; a) standing stiffly, b) leaning into the movements.

Lean forward to add power when you are focusing on the pushing aspect of the movement.

Lean Back for Pulling Movements

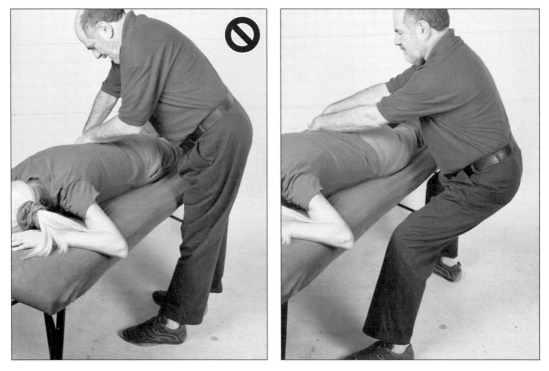

Figure 40.10: Pulling movements; a) standing stiffly, b) leaning back for the movements.

Lean back to add power to pulling.

Don't Reach Too Far Across the Table

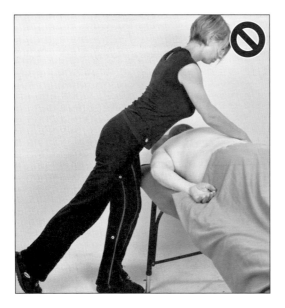

Figure 40.11: Trying to reach too far.

Take care that you are not putting strain on your back by trying to reach further than is comfortable across the table. If you have short arms, you might consider focusing on pushing strokes on the close side of the client's body and not try to pull on the far side.

Sway From Side to Side for Rolling a Limb Between Your Hands

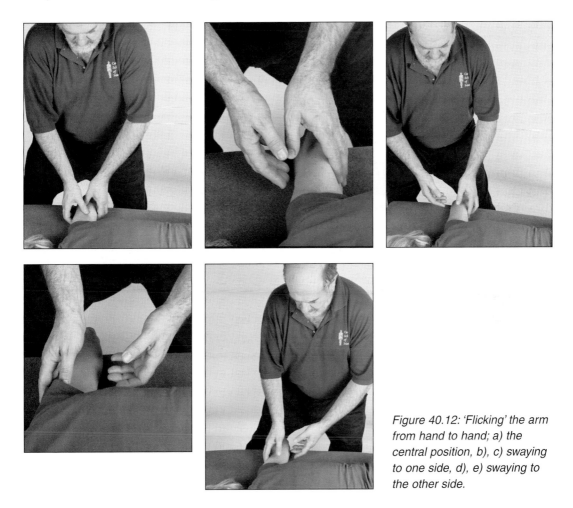

Figure 40.12: 'Flicking' the arm from hand to hand; a) the central position, b), c) swaying to one side, d), e) swaying to the other side.

When you are facing across a limb or the whole body in order to roll it from the side, swaying from side to side will enable you to gradually move your hands along the length of it. When you are facing the axis of a limb to roll it between your hands, you can sway forward and back to move your hands up and down along the sides of the limb.

Review

Rhythmical movements may be inappropriate for some clients because of injuries or weak or inflamed areas, and spinal problems.

Search out the 'natural' rhythms of the client's body by pushing and waiting for the body's natural return, instead of trying to impose a rhythm that doesn't fit.

Look after your hands by:

- Starting the movements slowly to minimise jarring yourself or your client;
- Using larger parts of your hands for large areas of the client's body and to get the movement started;
- Keeping your hand/s relaxed;
- Using two hands for more control;
- Not letting your fingers hyperextend when you push;
- Pulling as well as pushing to vary your hand use;
- Not grabbing the muscles or stiffening your fingers when you're rolling the limbs;
- Not hyperextending your wrist when pushing with your palm;
- Involving your arms in the movement, not just your hands, and;
- Conserving your hands by using your forearm for pushing.

Involve your body by:

- Facing your hands;
- Not standing still and relying on your arms only;
- Leaning forward to emphasise the pushing part of rhythmical movement and leaning back to emphasise the pulling aspect of the movement;
- Not trying to reach too far across the table, and;
- Swaying from side to side when you're rolling a limb between your hands.

Varied Working Situations

While most of this book focuses on doing massage with the client on a massage table, this is not the only working situation. So this section of the book looks at applying good bodyuse principles to look after your body and hands in the two other situations that are most commonly used in Western massage.

People have always done a quick shoulder massage with the client seated, and the development of portable massage chairs has hugely increased the use of seated massage.

Floor massage (with the client on a mat or futon) is very natural in cultures where people live more happily on the floor than most Westerners do. Although many of the Asian massage traditions tend to work without oil (with the client clothed), Swedish massage can be adapted for working on the floor when there isn't a table handy. However, it is harder work on the floor, and so needs more care to look after your body.

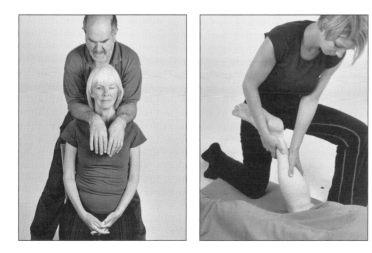

CHAPTER 41

Working With a Seated Client

Having a client seated enables you to work on his/her upper body, and, in a portable massage chair, to work down his/her back as well. This is generally done without oil. While much seated massage training is based on pressure point work derived from shiatsu / acupressure, this chapter (in line with the rest of the book) mainly focuses on techniques adapted from Swedish massage to release muscle tension and to mobilise joints.

The first part of the chapter looks at the particular challenges of working with clients when they are seated in an ordinary chair, or a portable massage chair, or leaning forward onto a chair back, a table or a desktop unit. The rest of the chapter focuses on good working practices when the client is seated, for looking after your hands and, using your forearm and elbow for applying pressure and doing passive stretches. This summarises information in other chapters and refers you back to the relevant parts of the book.

Having the Client Sitting Upright

You can have the client sitting upright in an ordinary upright chair. This position enables you to work on the client's shoulders (the most common area of tension), including applying pressure. You can also mobilise the client's shoulders, work on the neck and do a head massage.

Support the Client's Back
The backs of many chairs tilt back, so you will often need to put cushions behind the client's back to get her sitting comfortably upright. This will enable you to press down on her shoulders without causing her to just crumple down in the chair.

Don't Stand Too Close
It is crucial to move around the chair to reposition yourself effectively for each stroke. This includes stepping in close to the chair for some strokes and stepping further away for others.

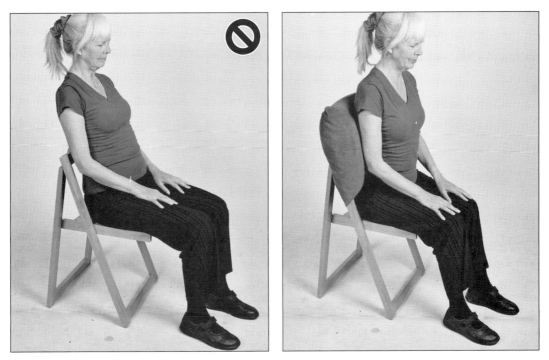

Figure 41.1: The chair back; a) tilting the client back, b) cushions to support her back.

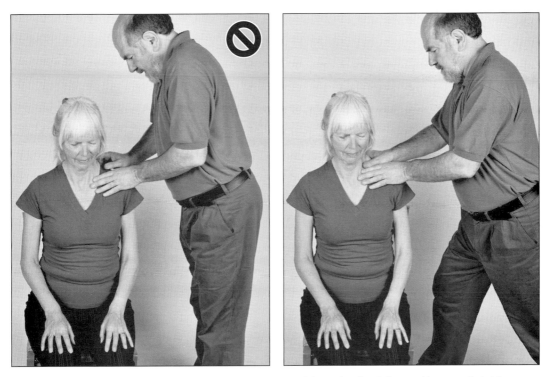

Figure 41.2: Distance from the chair; a) being too close, b) moving back for working comfortably.

Having Enough Space Around the Chair

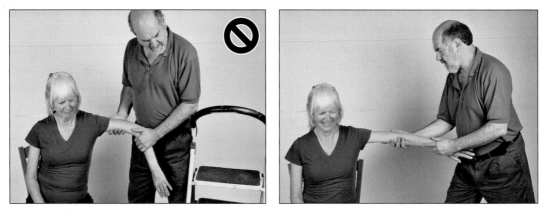

Figure 41.3: Having space; a) hemmed in by furniture, b) space for a stretch.

If you feel cramped or restricted as you move around the chair, you are likely to stiffen up and work awkwardly. So, in order to move freely, you need to have as much uncluttered space around the chair as possible.

If your working space precludes doing certain strokes easily, you will either need to modify those strokes or to leave them out of your massages entirely. If you have less space on one side of the chair, take extra care of your body on the restricted side.

Bracing the Client's Shoulder
At times, you will want to brace the client's shoulder as you work on them.

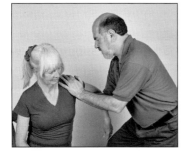
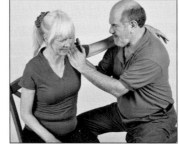
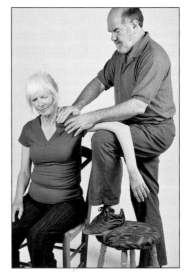

*Figure 41.4: Supporting the client's arm; a) by hand,
b) across the practitioner's shoulder, c) across the thigh.*

You can do this by hand. However, this is tiring for your hands if you want to do extensive work around her shoulder while holding her arm up. To save your hands, you could rest her arm over your own shoulder by sitting alongside her on another chair. This will stabilise her shoulder and enable you to use both hands simultaneously to massage around the shoulder and to mobilise it.

Another option is to place your foot on the side of the client's seat, or onto another chair, so that you can rest her arm across your thigh. This also enables you to use both hands at once. By getting above her shoulder in this way, you can press down on it, as well as mobilising it by rolling it forward and back on your thigh. When you need to, move your standing foot to alter your position for different strokes.

Use Your Forearm

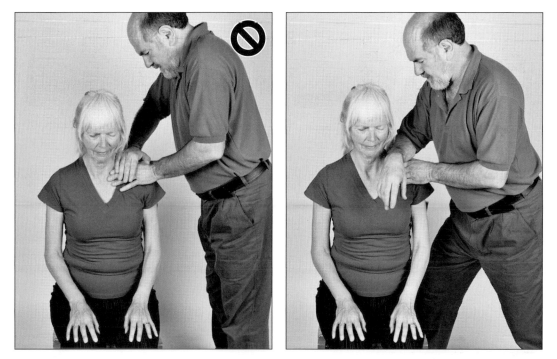

Figure 41.5: Applying pressure; a) not able to get far enough above, b) using the forearm.

When you can't easily get your bodyweight above your hands, for example when you're working on the client's shoulder, switch to using your forearm (see figure 41.36).

When the Client is in a Wheelchair
Much of this applies when the client is sitting in a wheelchair. It is also important to monitor that you are not leaning over too far to reach over the chair frame. Sit for as much of the treatment as you can to take pressure off your back, especially when you are doing small work, such as extensive nurturing movements or small coaching movements on holding patterns that have followed an accident or stroke.

Having the Client Leaning Forward

This section of the chapter looks at how to position and move your body when the client is leaning forward in a supported position. Having the client leaning forward and supported enables you to apply pressure all the way down her back and to use percussion over her whole back. You can apply pressure on the shoulders and mobilise them without having to support her. You can work on her arms and mobilise the wrist by resting them on the desktop, table or the arm rest of a portable chair. Although you can only work on the client's neck and scalp in this position, you can get them to sit upright for a head massage and trunk stretches.

You can have the client leaning forward:

*   Leaning over a cushion on the back of a chair;
*   Onto a table with cushions for support;
*   Onto a desktop unit on a table, or;
*   Seated in a portable massage chair.

Avoid Getting Too Close, Standing Stiffly and Tensing Your Shoulders

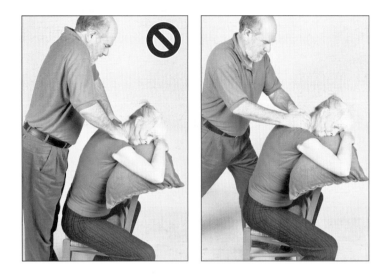

Figure 41.6:
Working with the client leaning over a chair back;
a) standing stiffly and too close,
b) moving away and leaning.

If you stand stiffly or stand too close to the client, you are likely to tense your shoulders as you massage. Instead, stand a little further away in a lunge stance. This will enable you to lean and sway in order to use your bodyweight and keep your shoulders relaxed.

Don't Stiffen Up to Work Over the Chair Back

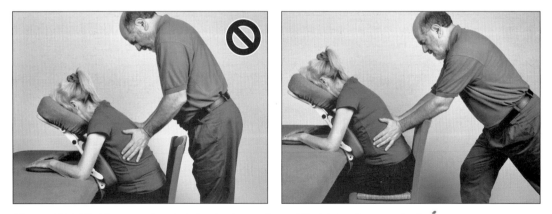

Figure 41.7: Working over the chair back; a) standing stiffly, b) leaning your body.

When the client leans forward onto cushions or a desktop unit on a table, take care not to stiffen your back to work over the chair back. Step back into the lunge stance and work around the chair back as best you can.

Step to the Side to Avoid Trying to Reach Too Far From Behind the Chair

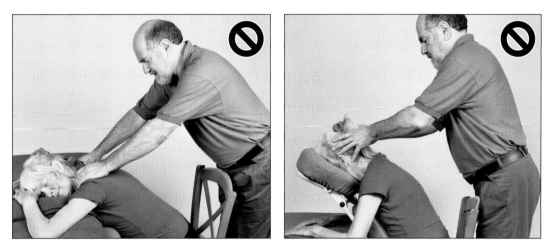

Figure 41.8: Working over the chair back; a) straining to reach the client's shoulders, b) straining to reach the client's head.

And don't try to reach too far when you are standing behind the chair, which could lead to back strain.

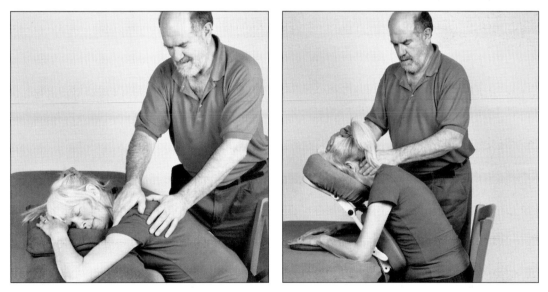

Figure 41.8 (cont.): c), d) moving to the side to work comfortably.

Instead, move to the side of the client to comfortably reach her shoulders and neck.

Find a Comfortable Position for Massaging the Client's Arms

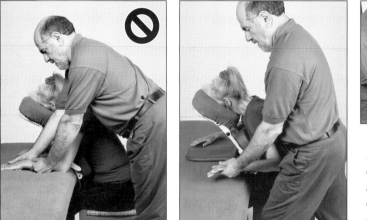

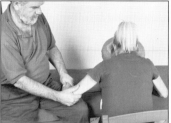

Figure 41.9: Massaging the client's arms; a) leaning over, b) having the client's arms close to the edge of the table, c) sitting on the desk.

Similarly, avoid leaning over when you are working on the client's arms. Get the client to move her arm towards you, or, if you can, sit on the table.

Having the Client in a Portable Massage Chair

As well as paying attention to how you are using your body when you are working, take care of your back when you are carrying the chair around and take care getting it in and out of cars (as for getting massage tables into cars, see figure 7.9).

Adjust the Client's Level to Suit Yourself

Of course, when you set up the chair, you will need to make adjustments to the seat and the face cradle to get *the client comfortable*. However, it is also important to take *your own* height and ease of working into account in raising or lowering the client's level.

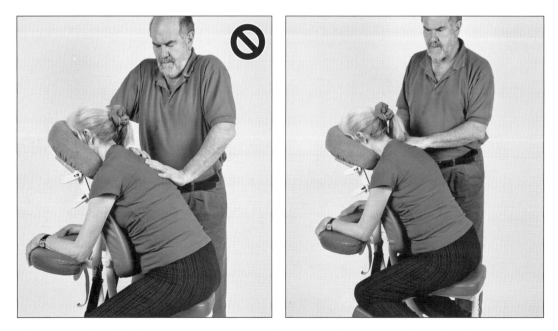

Figure 41.10: The client's level; a) too high for comfortable working, b) a comfortable height.

If the client is too high, you will be straining and probably tensing your own shoulders to work on her upper back and shoulders. A good height is to have the client's shoulders just below the level of the practitioner's elbow.

Therefore a short practitioner will need to lower the seat before the client sits on the chair. Conversely, a tall practitioner will need to raise the seat. If you are tall and the client is not high enough, take up a wide stance and bend your knees to avoid straining your back by hunching over.

Avoid Standing Stiffly or Leaning Over Too Far From Behind

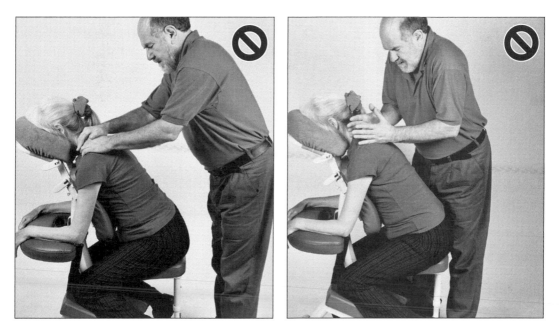

Figure 41.11: Leaning over too far to work on the client's shoulders;
a) doing petrissage strokes, b) doing percussion.

Take care of your back by not standing with stiff knees or leaning too far over from behind your client, for example to work on her shoulders. Be particularly careful about this if you have short arms.

Change Position to Keep Your Hands in Front of Your Hips

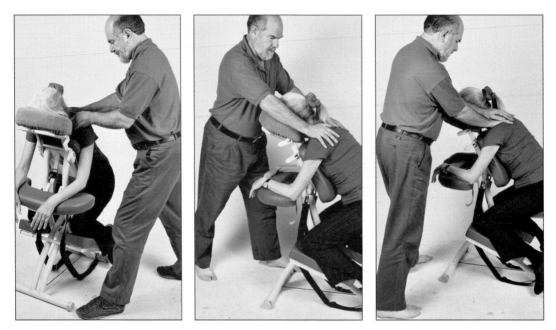

Figure 41.12: Working on the client's shoulders from different angles.

Instead, move around the chair to work on the shoulders from different angles. Use the lunge stance so that you can lean in and sway in order to use your bodyweight for power. Remember to keep your hands within the 'hip spotlight' area (i.e. in front of your hips, see figure 28.11).

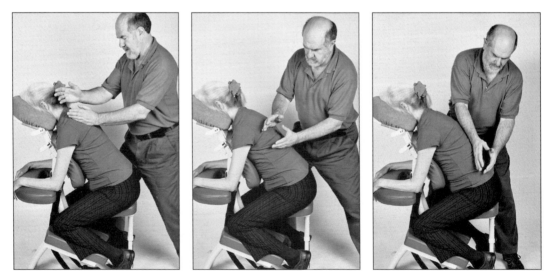

Figure 41.13: Applying percussion.

Change your direction also to work on different areas of the client's back, for example with percussion. Kneel down, if you need to, in order to get at the client's lower back and buttocks.

Let Your Height Determine How Far You Try to Reach

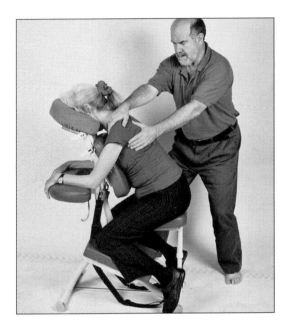

Figure 41.14: Working comfortably on the opposite shoulder.

When you are standing at the side of your client, only reach across to massage the opposite shoulder if your arms are long enough for you to comfortably reach without straining your back. If your arms are short, just work on the close shoulder.

Have Your Arms Straight to Deliver Pressure

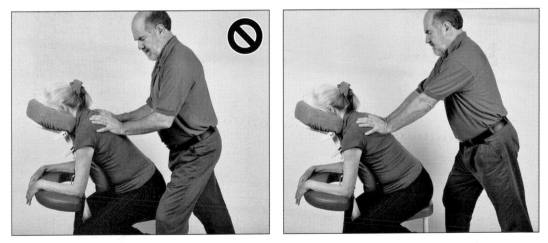

Figure 41.15: Applying pressure on the client's back; a) bent arms, b) arms straight.

When you are leaning forward to apply pressure on the client's back, keep your arms straight (but not stiff) in order to transmit the power relatively undiminished from your trunk to your hands. If you were to bend your arms significantly, you would be scattering this power (and therefore reducing how much is transmitted to the client), as well as having to tighten your upper arm muscles unnecessarily to direct the force to your hands.

Don't Let Your Wrist Hyperextend

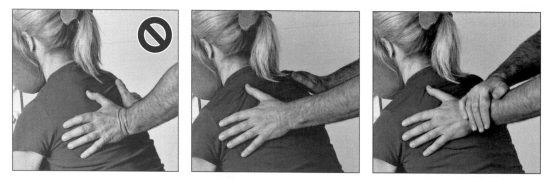

Figure 41.16: Looking after the wrist; a) hyperextended wrist, b) relatively straight wrist, c) supporting the wrist.

Having the client lean forward in a supported position enables you to apply pressure all the way down her back. When you are doing this, particularly when you are working on both sides of her back at once, take care that your wrists don't get hyperextended, which is not good for them (see Chapter 17). Keep your wrist relatively straight if necessary by changing position, and support it with your other hand whenever you can.

Step Back or Kneel Down to Avoid Getting Cramped as You Work Down the Client's Back

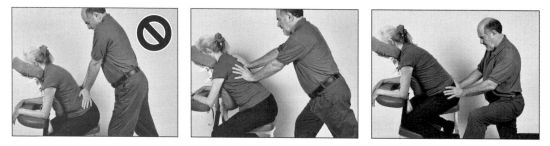

Figure 41.17: Applying pressure on the client's back; a) getting cramped, b) stepping back, c) kneeling.

Don't let yourself get cramped in as you work further down the client's back. Step back if you can so that it is easier to lean forward behind your hands, or even to kneel down to work on the client's lower back and/or buttocks.

Sit or Kneel to Work on the Client's Forearm

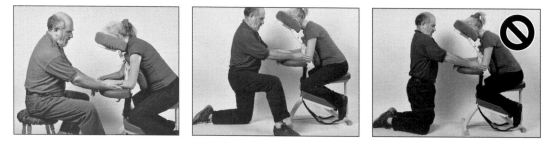

Figure 41.18: Massaging the client's forearm; a) sitting, b) kneeling in the proposal position, c) kneeling up on both knees.

When you are working on the client's forearm, place it on the arm rest of the chair. Sit or kneel down to avoid hunching over, and to enable you to work with more precision. Use the proposal position for kneeling so that you can move, rather than kneeling up on both knees, which restricts your ability to move and can strain your back over time.

Move Your Body to Apply Stretches

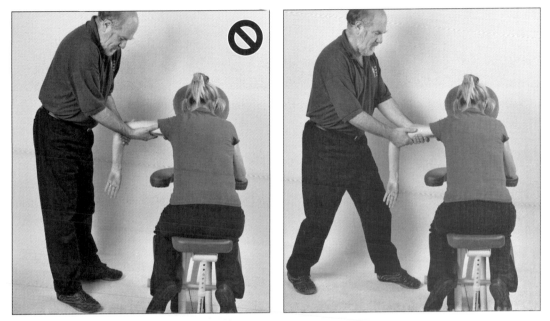

Figure 41.19: Stretching the client's arm; a) standing still, b) swaying back.

Don't stand still and just use your arm for stretches. Sway backwards to stretch the client's arm.

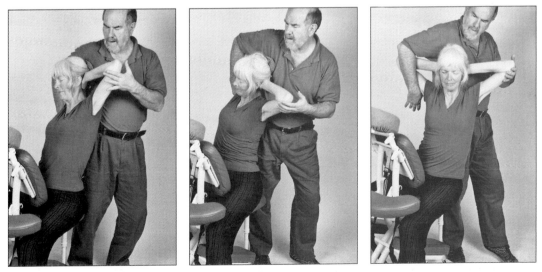

Figure 41.20: Stretching and rotating the seated client's trunk.

When the client is sitting upright with her feet on the floor for stability, put your hip against her back and sway and twist your body to stretch and rotate her trunk.

Good Hand Use Practices

Non-oil massage (see Chapter 36) is intrinsically harder work on your hands than oil massage, so you need to monitor them carefully. And, if you are working in an office or public situation, you will probably be doing many short sessions (sometimes 3 or 4 people per hour) in which you are likely to constantly repeat a limited repertoire of strokes.

(In fact, some on-site massage employers expect you to do the same 'house-style' routine on every client. In my opinion, having no leeway for adapting the massage to suit your build or abilities or to vary it for each client puts you at risk of strain).

Be particularly careful if your hands are small or you have long, slender or hypermobile digits. Don't overuse your thumbs or fingers. Reduce the pressure on them by using the largest appropriate parts of your hands whenever you can (particularly your knuckles and fist). Whenever possible, conserve your hands by using your forearm and elbows, if you're trained to do this skilfully.

Adapt strokes to suit your own build and strength. Develop a range of techniques so that you can vary the treatment according to the client's build, tensions, needs, and responses. And give yourself a break from constantly applying pressure by using stretches (see Chapter 39) to mobilise the client's joints.

Applying Pressure in Non-oil Massage

Applying sliding pressure is relatively easy when you are using oil. However, a major challenge of working without oil is to find a comfortable way of applying pressure and moving it across muscles, particularly when you are working through clothing.

There are two simple ways of applying pressure with your palm, fist, forearm or elbow when you don't have oil (see Chapter 36):

1. '*Press and release*' technique – slowly applying stationary pressure by leaning your bodyweight forward, maintaining it for a short time and then slowly swaying back to release it, or;
2. '*Press and stretch*' technique – applying the pressure, and then doing a short stretch of the skin and clothing over the underlying muscles whilst maintaining the pressure by swaying forward.

Keep Your Fingers Relaxed When Using Your Palm

You can use your palm for applying widespread pressure. Take care not to hyperextend your wrist. And conserve your hand, whenever you can, by using your forearm instead.

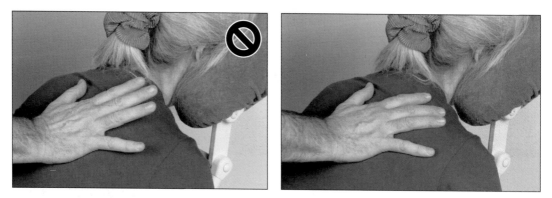

Figure 41.21: Using your palm; a) with stiff fingers, b) with relaxed fingers.

Don't tense your fingers when using your palm, which would use extra energy and reduce your effectiveness by stiffening your hand.

Use Hand-on-hand Pressure Whenever You Can

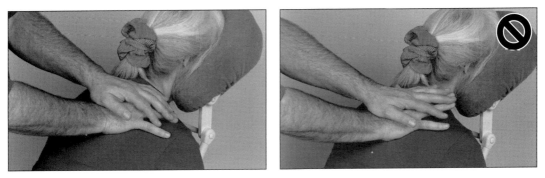

Figure 41.22: Hand-on-hand pressure; a) relaxing the fingers, b) stiffening the fingers.

Whenever possible, use your other hand on top to reduce the workload on your lone hand. This will make it easier to transfer the power of swaying your body forward for both the pressure and the stretch. As with using one hand, keep your fingers relaxed.

Use 'Double-handed Wringing' to Save Your Hands

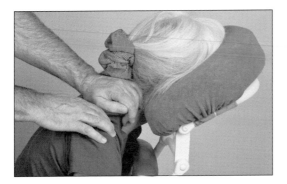

Figure 41.23: Classic wringing.

When the client is sitting in an upright chair, you will need to use classic wringing – one hand pushing forward as the other pulls back in order to stabilise her in the chair as you work on her shoulders.

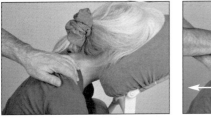
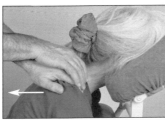
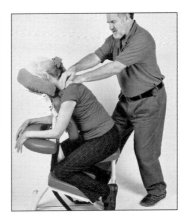

Figure 41.24: 'Double-handed wringing'– pulling;
a) the shape of the under-hand, b) the other hand on top,
c) swaying back.

However, when the client is leaning forward in a supported position, such as in a portable chair, you can use 'double-handed wringing'. Have one hand on the other. Use your upper hand to power and control the movement. Sway back to pull your hands back, dragging a little with your fingers as you do so.

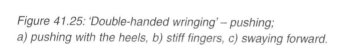
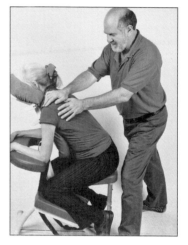

Figure 41.25: 'Double-handed wringing' – pushing;
a) pushing with the heels, b) stiff fingers, c) swaying forward.

When you are pushing forward with the heels of your hands by swaying forward, keep your fingers relaxed.

Look After Your Thumbs

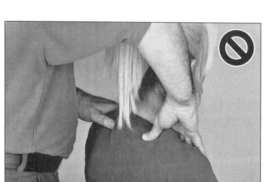

Figure 41.26: Looking after the thumbs;
applying pressure with hyperextended thumbs.

Your thumbs (and wrists) are the parts of your hands most at risk in massage. You need to take particular care of your thumbs when you are working without oil, as there is a great temptation to overuse them for kneading or applying pressure, particularly on the client's shoulders. Unless you have large, strong hands, it is very easy to tire your thumbs in this way, without achieving much effect. You are particularly at risk of straining them if you regularly work with them hyperextended (see figure 13.3–13.6).

Reduce Thumb Kneading

Thumb kneading is often used on the client's shoulders (on the upper trapezius) in two ways in seated massage – to move and stretch the muscles, and to dig into them. This is quite hard work, especially if you are doing a series of seated massages, and not particularly effective. Reduce the workload on your thumbs by using substitutes:

1. Stretching the muscles by wringing them, including 'double-handed' wringing (see figure 41.25), and;
2. Applying pressure with the 'reinforced thumb' (next), or the knuckles, fist, or elbow (below).

Using the Reinforced Thumb for Precise Pressure

When you feel the need to use your thumb for applying precise, firm pressure, use the 'reinforced thumb' technique (see figure 13.15).

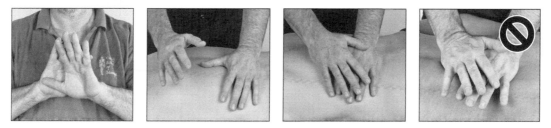

Figure 41.27: The 'reinforced thumb'; a) how the thumb fits the heel of the top hand, b), c) pressure applied through the thumb, d) having stiff fingers.

Keep your thumb relaxed and press the heel of your other hand onto the phalanges of your thumb. Have the interphalangeal joint of your thumb in the groove between the thenar and hypothenar eminences so that you don't press directly onto it. Keep the fingers of your top hand relaxed to avoid tensing it unnecessarily.

Apply pressure by leaning your bodyweight to transmit it through your top hand. This enables you to palpate the effect through your sensitive thumb while it remains relatively relaxed. Stay within the range of pressure that is comfortable for your thumb.

Substitutes for the Thumb for Pressure Work

However that still puts pressure on your thumbs. Save them entirely by using your palm for widespread pressure. For more focused pressure, switch to using your knuckles, your fist or your elbow.

Take Care of Your Fingers

It is also important to be careful of your fingers, as it is easy to use them too often or to put too much pressure through them when you're working without oil. Conserve them whenever possible, by using other parts of your hands to apply pressure, such as your knuckles or fist, or switch to using your forearm or elbow.

Don't Hyperextend Your Fingers

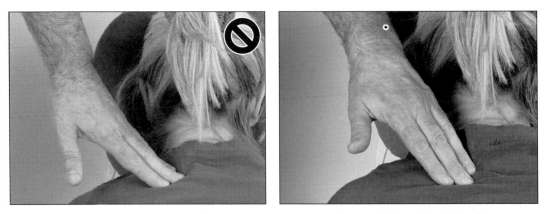

Figure 41.28: Applying pressure with the fingers; a) hyperextending the fingers, b) straight fingers.

If you use your fingers for applying pressure, don't let them hyperextend which puts considerable pressure on them and would strain them if you did it regularly. Instead have them straight or slightly flexed (see figure 12.7).

Keep Your Fingers Together

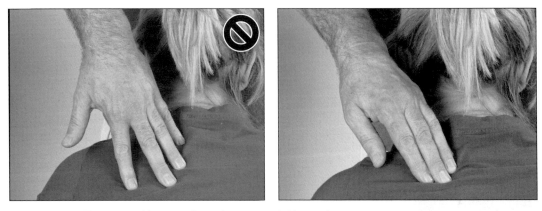

Figure 41.29: Fingers working together; a) separated, b) together.

Pressing with your fingers spread apart would put extra pressure on each one.

Support Your Fingers

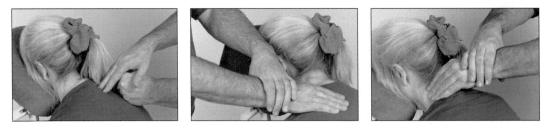

Figure 41.30: Supporting the fingers; a) resting over the other hand, b) holding the hand, c) supported squeeze.

Whenever you can, reduce the workload on your fingers by using the other hand to support your working hand. You can rest your working hand over your other hand or fist to help you to control the movement. Another option is to hold your hand or wrist, in order to add pressure to your stroke while stabilising your wrist. It is also good to support your working hand when you are squeezing muscles, for example when you are working on the client's neck.

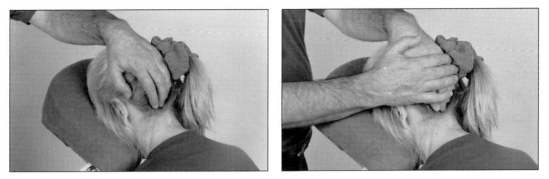

Figure 41.31: Supporting a stretch; a) the under hand, b) supported stretch.

You can also support your fingers for a stretch. When the client is in a portable chair, you can stretch her neck by 'hooking' the fingers of one hand under the occiput and using the other hand to pull.

Using Your Knuckles

You can use your knuckles to save your thumb and fingers for kneading or applying pressure. This is harder work than the equivalent oil massage strokes, so use your knuckles sparingly. Because of the pressure that this can put on your knuckles, conserve them, by switching to your fist, forearm or elbow, whenever possible.

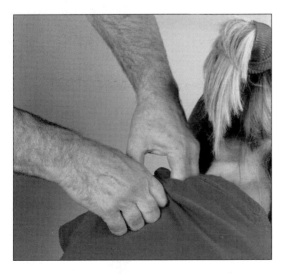

Figure 41.32: Knuckle kneading to stretch the tissue.

Whenever you can get your hands around the muscles, you can stretch and move the tissue by kneading it with your knuckles (see figure 15.4). This works well, for example, on the client's arms or the shoulders of a small to medium built client. You can also press to dig into the tissues more. Move your whole hand as a single unit (see figure 15.7), rather than moving the individual knuckles separately, which would be harder work and would quickly tire them.

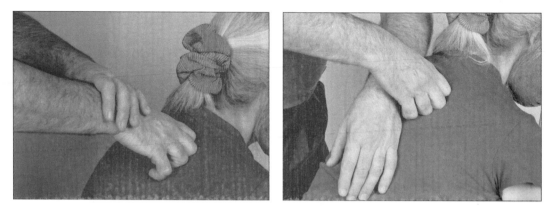

Figure 41.33: Supporting your working knuckles; a) holding the wrist, b) resting over the other forearm.

Use your other hand to reduce the pressure on your working hand, either by resting your working hand over your arm or by supporting your wrist. Both of these methods will also reduce the pressure on your wrist.

Don't Let Your Wrist Bend When You Are Using Your Fist

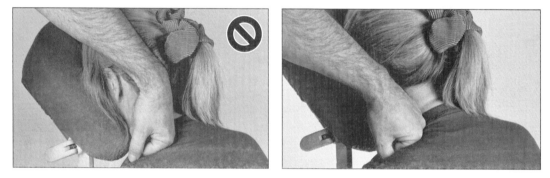

Figure 41.34: Using the fist; a) with a bent wrist, b) with a straight wrist.

When using your fist for pressure strokes in order to save your knuckles, take care not to let your wrist bend too much.

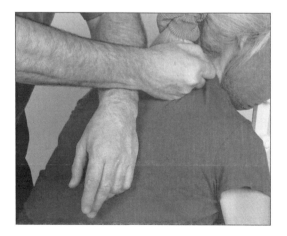

Figure 41.35: Supporting your wrist – resting it over your other forearm.

Look after it in the same way as for your knuckles – resting it over your other forearm or hand, or hold your wrist to support it directly.

Using Your Forearm

Whenever you can, conserve your hands by using your forearm or elbow for pressure strokes. The forearm provides a wide pressure area, while the elbow is effective for focusing pressure on a small area. This section of the chapter covers some basic pointers for using these tools, which are covered in Chapters 18 and 19 in more detail. If using these tools is new for you, get individual coaching or training from an experienced colleague/teacher, to avoid straining yourself or brutalising clients.

Work in the Wide 'Chimp' Stance to Save Your Back

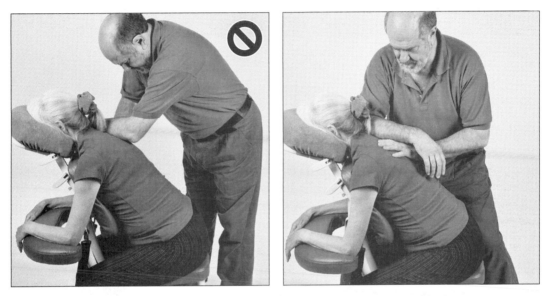

Figure 41.36: Saving the back; a) hunching over,
b) the 'chimp' stance – widening the feet and bending the knees.

When using either tool, you need to allow for having 'shortened' your working arm. Work in the 'chimp' stance – widen your stance and bend your knees – to avoid hunching over with consequent strain to your back.

Have the Hand of Your Working Forearm Relaxed

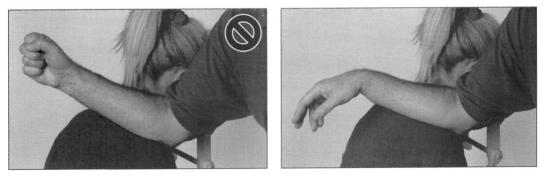

Figure 41.37: The hand of your working forearm; a) clenched, b) relaxed.

To avoid tightening the muscles of the working area of your forearm, let your hand relax (see figure 18.4).

Have Your Hand Turned Down to Use the 'Soft Forearm'

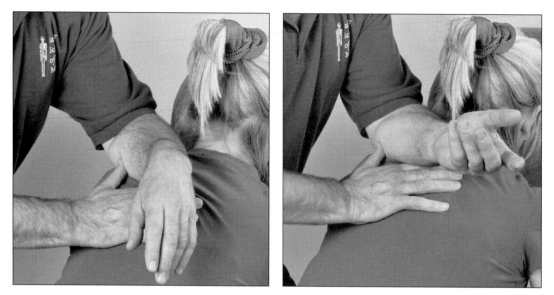

*Figure 41.38: Using the forearm; a) palm down for the soft forearm,
b) palm up for the hard edge of the ulna.*

Turn your palm down to use the soft, 'fleshy' forearm (the bellies of the flexor muscles, see figure 18.3) as a substitute for the palm/heel of your hand for applying general pressure over a wide area, unless you specifically want to use the harder area of the edge of the ulna by turning your hand up (see figure 18.7).

Use the Area Close to Your Elbow for Applying Pressure

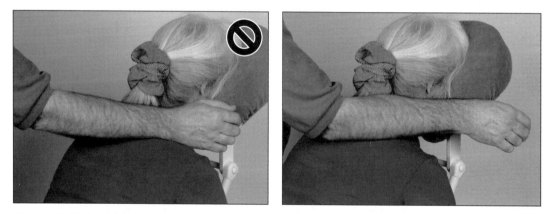

Figure 41.39: Applying pressure; a) close to the wrist, b) close to the elbow.

Bear in mind that it is most effective to apply pressure towards your elbow rather than close to your wrist (see figure 18.5).

Use Your Other Hand/Forearm to Guide Your Working Forearm

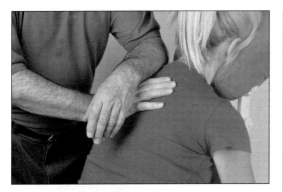

*Figure 41.40: Guiding the forearm
with the other hand below.*

Use your other hand underneath your forearm to guide it with precision.

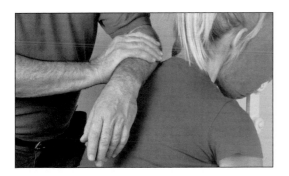

Figure 41.40 (cont.): with the other hand on top.

Using your other hand on top of your forearm enables you to increase the pressure.

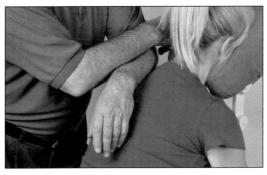

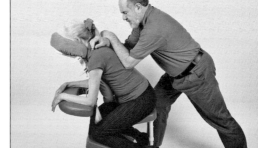

Figure 41.40 (cont.): with the other forearm.

With practise, you will be able to use your other forearm for this.

Involve Your Body to Apply Pressure

You can use your forearm, as you did with your hands, to apply pressure by:

- Leaning forward for stationary pressure ('press and release');
- Swaying forward whilst maintaining the pressure to stretch the skin and clothing over the underlying muscles ('press and stretch').

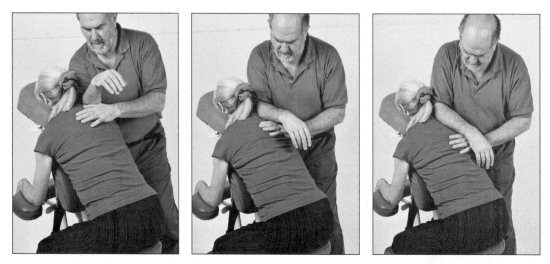

Figure 41.41: The 'rocking chair'; tilting the forearm over the client's shoulder.

Another technique that works well on the seated client's shoulder is the 'rocking chair'. This involves moving your body forward and back to maintain the pressure as you tilt your forearm over the client's shoulder muscles (upper trapezius) without sliding it.

Using Your Elbow

For more concentrated pressure, use your elbow, *as long as you can do so skilfully*. It can be a brutal tool if it's used indiscriminately, which, unfortunately, it too often is. This section summarises the main principles covered in Chapter 19. Use your elbow for applying stationary pressure or for 'press and stretch' techniques.

Control the Depth and Intensity of Your Techniques by How Much You Bend Your Elbow

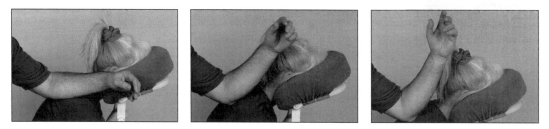

Figure 41.42: Bending the elbow for the depth of elbow 'cut'; a) small bend for shallow pressure, b) more bent elbow for firmer, deeper pressure, c) bent more for deepest pressure.

When using the point of your elbow (the olecranon), bending and straightening your arm will enable you to control the depth of working for different areas. Begin by having your arm relatively straight. Only bend it to make more of a penetrating 'dagger' when it feels appropriate to dig more deeply into well-developed, tight muscles.

Lean Your Body to Deliver Pressure

In order to avoid tensing your shoulders, control the pressure by how much (or little) you lean forward. Remember to take up the low 'chimp' stance (see figure 41.36) to save your back and to work effectively. Bear in mind that the olecranon is a very strong tool when your bodyweight is positioned behind it. So monitor the client's responses carefully, as it's easy to apply more pressure than you realise.

Guide Your Elbow With Your Other Hand

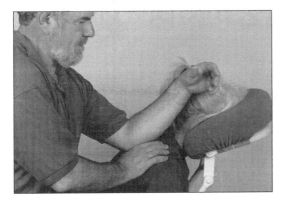

Figure 41.43: Guiding your elbow with your other hand.

Guide your elbow with your other hand for ease and precision in your pressure techniques.

Relax the Hand of Your Working Elbow

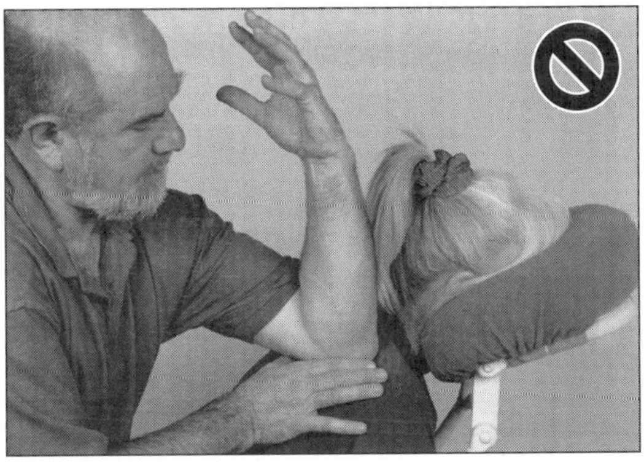

Figure 41.44: Having a stiff hand.

As with using your forearm, keep the hand of your working elbow relaxed (above), to avoid the unnecessary effort and tension of holding it tightly.

Use the Other Hand as a Guide When Using the Back of the Elbow

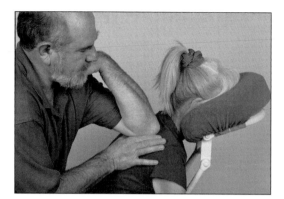

Figure 41.45: Guiding the back of the elbow with the other hand.

Because it is a wider, 'blunter' area, the back of the elbow will enable you to deliver hard pressure over a slightly wider area, which 'stabs' in less (see figure 19.16). When you are using it, use your other hand to guide it so that you can work with precision.

Rest Your Hand on Your Shoulder, Neck or Face When Using the Back of the Elbow

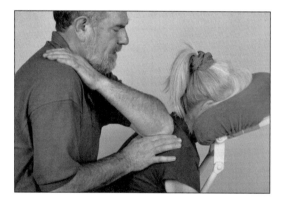

Figure 41.46: Rest your hand on your shoulder.

Resting the hand of your working elbow on some part of your upper body (such as your shoulder, your neck or your face, see figure 19.13) will enable you to 'steer' your elbow from two places. When you try this, you will feel how this enables you to use it with precision, whilst keeping your shoulder muscles relatively relaxed.

Review

Having a client seated enables you to work on his/her shoulders, neck and head, and, in a portable massage chair, to work down his/her back as well.

When the client is in an upright chair:

- Support her back to have her sitting comfortably upright;
- Have enough space around the chair to be able to move comfortably around it;
- Don't cramp your work by standing too close to the chair, and;
- Brace her shoulder when necessary.

If your client is in a wheelchair:

- Take care not to lean over too far to reach over the chair frame, and;
- Sit when you're doing small, focused work.

You can have a client leaning forward:

- Leaning over a cushion on the back of a chair;
- Onto a table with cushions for support;
- Onto a desktop unit on a table, or;
- Seated in a portable massage chair.

When the client is leaning forward:

- Avoid getting too close, standing stiffly and tensing your shoulders;
- Don't tense up when you have to work over the chair back;
- Step to the side to avoid trying to reach too far from behind the chair, and;
- Find a comfortable position for massaging the client's arms.

When the client is sitting in a portable massage chair:

- Adjust the client's level to suit yourself;
- Avoid standing stiffly or leaning over too far from behind;
- Regularly change position in order to keep your hands / working forearm in front of your hips;
- Don't try working beyond your comfortable reach;
- Have your arms straight to deliver pressure;
- Don't let your wrist hyperextend when you're applying pressure;
- Step back and/or kneel down to avoid getting cramped in or hunching over as you work low down the client's back;
- Sit or kneel to work on the client's forearm, and;
- Move your body to apply stretches, rather than standing still and just using muscle power.

Look after your hands by:

- Being very careful about how you use them if they are small, long and slender;
- Adapt strokes to suit your own build and comfort;
- Use the largest appropriate areas of your hands that you can;
- Switch to using your forearm and elbow, whenever you can, to save your hands;
- Vary the techniques that you use;
- Incorporate mobilising stretches into treatment sessions to give yourself a break from constantly applying pressure;
- Use stationary pressure techniques and the 'press and stretch' technique to deliver pressure;
- Keep your fingers relaxed when using your palm;
- Use hand-on-hand pressure whenever you can, and;
- Use 'double-handed wringing' to save your digits.

Look after your thumbs by:

- Using them as little as possible for applying pressure and for kneading;
- Not letting them hyperextend when you do so;
- Use the reinforced thumb technique if you feel the need to use them for precise pressure, and;
- Save them by using substitutes such as your knuckles, fist or elbow.

Take care of your fingers by:

- Not letting them hyperextend when you're applying pressure;
- Using them together to reduce the pressure on each one, and;
- Supporting them with your other hand.

When you are using your knuckles or fist:

- Don't overuse your knuckles when you could use your fist, forearm or elbow;
- Support your working hand with your other hand, and;
- Don't let your wrist bend when you're applying pressure.

When you are using your forearm:

- Work in the wide 'chimp' stance to save your back;
- Have the hand of your working forearm turned palm down in order to use the 'soft' forearm (the bellies of the flexor muscles) and keep this hand relaxed;
- Use the area close to your elbow for applying pressure;
- Use your other hand / forearm to guide your working forearm, and;
- Lean your body to provide the pressure.

When you are using your elbow:

- Control the depth and intensity of your techniques by how much you bend your elbow;
- Relax the hand of your working elbow, and guide your elbow with your other hand;
- Rest your hand on your shoulder, neck or face when you're using the back of the elbow to help guide it, and;
- Lean your body to deliver pressure.

CHAPTER 42

Floor Massage

This chapter focuses on how to use your body safely and effectively when massaging a client 'on the floor' (i.e. lying on a camping / yoga mat or futon). It firstly looks at the commonly used sitting and kneeling positions. Then it covers general principles for looking after your back and your hands, which are crucial areas to monitor in floor massage.

Although Swedish massage was developed for a massage table, it can be done on the floor when there isn't a table handy. In fact, oil massage is often done on the floor in many parts of North Africa and the Middle East. However, it is harder work and more difficult to maintain the fluidity and continuity of the massage. And some strokes which work well on a table don't work on the floor (and vice-versa).

Floor massage traditions that don't use oil, such as Thai yoga massage and shiatsu, generally focus on applying stationary pressure and doing stretches. It is easier to involve your body for these techniques than swaying forward and back to establish the rhythm of an oil massage. So working with oil needs extra care to look after your body. It is particularly important to pay attention to your back – taking care not to hunch over, twist, or try reaching too far forward or too far under the client, or to lift them when you are leaning over. You also need to look after your hands, making sure that you're not hyperextending your wrists when you are applying pressure or putting too much pressure through your thumbs.

Floor massage can be challenging for Westerners who are unaccustomed to sitting and working on the floor. In many Asian floor massage traditions, training includes yoga or a martial art training which helps students to develop their strength and flexibility in sitting, kneeling and squatting positions. Training often also includes instruction on working from the hara, the physical and energy centre of the body (see figure 27.15). If you want to do floor massage but find the positions awkward, it's worth doing some yoga or similar training to help make it easier.

> **Note:** *Much of the information in this chapter also applies when you are sitting on the floor to massage a baby. There is a great temptation to hunch over the baby. As well as incorporating the suggestions for looking after your back, place the baby higher, for example on cushions, in a bouncer or on a low coffee table, to make life easier for yourself.*

Looking After Your Hands

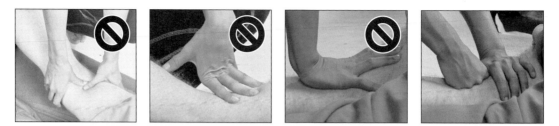

*Figure 42.1: Monitoring the hands; a) pressure through hyperextended thumbs,
b) hyperextended fingers, c) hyperextended wrist, d) using the fist.*

There is a great temptation to make extensive use of your thumbs in this position for applying pressure. Use them carefully and sparingly, make sure that you are not hyperextending them, use the reinforced thumb (see figure 13.15) and switch to using your knuckles and fist whenever you can.

Look after your fingers too (see Chapter 12). Use them sparingly for applying pressure and make sure that they are not hyperextended as you do this.

And take care of your wrist too (see Chapter 17). Because you are mostly positioned above the client in floor massage, it is all too easy to hyperextend your wrist when pressing with your hand. If you find yourself doing this, move back a little so that you can lower your wrist to a less bent angle (see figure 17.8).

You can use your knees and feet for applying pressure in order to save your hands at times. And interspersing stretches throughout the massage will also enable you to give your hands a rest from pressing (and an opportunity to open out the joints of your arms and shoulders).

Saving Your Back

One of the great dangers in floor massage is straining your back. To look after your back:

- Avoid hunching over and twisting which can put strain on the lower back;
- Avoid leaning too far over the client;
- Avoid awkward lifting;
- Sway your body with your hand movements, rather than sitting or kneeling still, relying on upper body strength only, and overreaching.

Have Space Around the Client

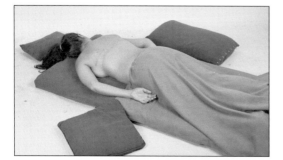

*Figure 42.2: Space around the client, and
cushions available for the practitioner.*

Being able to move around is dependent on having enough free space around your client. If you are hemmed in, monitor your body carefully and don't do strokes that are consequently awkward.

Sitting on the Floor

Watch Your Back When Sitting on the Floor

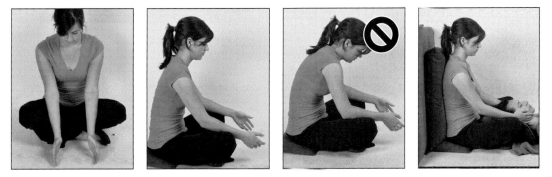

Figure 42.3: Sitting cross-legged on the floor; a) the sitting position, b) sitting on a cushion, c) hunching over, d) supports behind the back.

Some people are comfortable sitting cross-legged on the floor, perhaps sitting on a cushion. If you sit in this position, take care of your back. Don't let yourself fall into hunching over. If necessary, lean up against a wall with a large cushion behind your back.

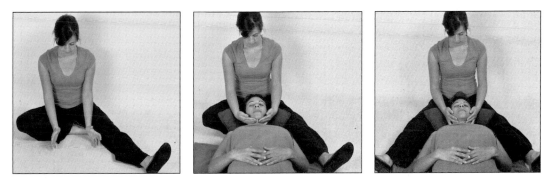

Figure 42.4: Other sitting positions; a), b) with one leg bent in front, c) with both legs straight.

In each of these positions too, you need to be careful of your back because of the way that they limit movement in your hips.

Sitting on Your Heels

Cushion Your Ankles and Knees if Necessary for Your Comfort

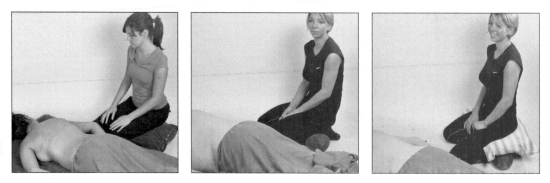

Figure 42.5: Sitting on the heels; a) sitting on a cushion, b) cushion/bolster under the ankles, c) cushion between heels and ankles.

Many of us have prominent bones in our feet and ankles that are not comfortable on the floor. If you find it comfortable, sitting on your heels enables you to get your weight more easily behind your hands. You may need to place a small cushion / bolster under your ankles to make this comfortable. If you can't comfortably sit directly onto your heels, placing a thick cushion on your heels may make this possible. And you may want a cushion for your knees as well as for your feet.

Don't Twist Your Trunk

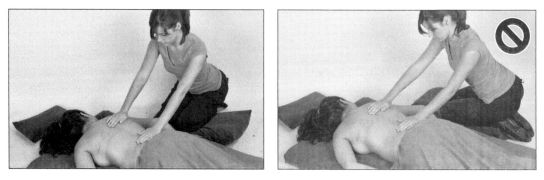

Figure 42.6: The angle of sitting; a) facing the working area, b) working twisted.

Take care to sit facing the area that you are working on. If you were to sit at an angle, for example sitting alongside the client when working across her back, watch out that you don't twist your trunk too much for any length of time, as this would put pressure on your back.

Look After Your Back When You Lean Forward
Avoid putting pressure on your back as you lean forward to deliver pressure, by not:

- Hunching over;
- Having your knees together;
- 'Standing up' on both knees;
- Lifting your feet off the floor.

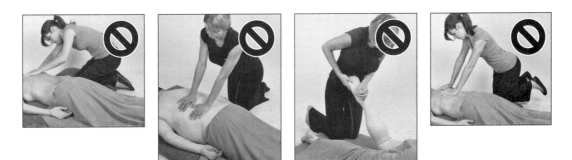

Figure 42.7: Looking after your back; a) hunching over, b) having the knees close together, c) 'standing up' on the knees, d) lifting the feet off the floor.

Having your knees right next to one another restricts your movement when you are sitting up and also puts pressure on your lower back. So does lifting your feet from the floor as you lean forward.

'Standing up' on your knees in order to reach further puts considerable strain on your lower back. It also limits your ability to move with massage strokes compared to sitting on one heel (next), or working in the 'proposal position'.

Instead, have your knees comfortably spread to provide a stable base, lean with your whole trunk, even for small movements of your hands.

Sitting on One Heel

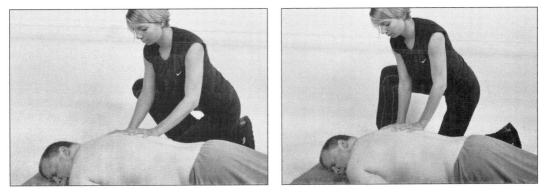

Figure 42.8: Sitting on one heel; a) leaning forward, b) rising up and moving forward.

If it is comfortable for you, sitting on one heel is a more dynamic position which makes it easier to sway and lean your trunk. When leaning forward, you can step forward with your foot to be able to reach further without strain. It's also easy to rise up into the 'proposal position' (below), or to sit back down, rest a moment and then rise up again when appropriate.

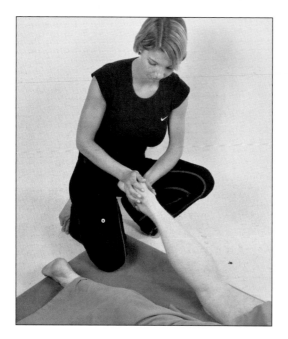

Figure 42.9: Rising up and leaning forward with the whole trunk.

The 'Proposal' Position

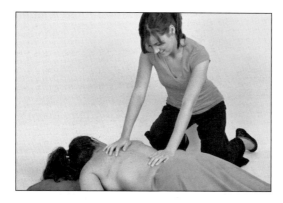

Figure 42.10: The 'proposal' position.

The 'proposal' position (being on one knee and one foot) is used extensively in the Asian floor massage styles because it is such a dynamic position. It enables you to cover the greatest area without losing balance or power, and you are able to use your legs for the power and the movement of your massage strokes, rather than relying on your back.

Have Cushioning Under Your Knee

Kneel on the mat / futon or put a cushion under your knee if you need to protect it from a hard floor. (It is useful to have a number of cushions scattered around so that there's always one close by without a scrabble).

Don't Have Your Hips Turned Away From Your Hands

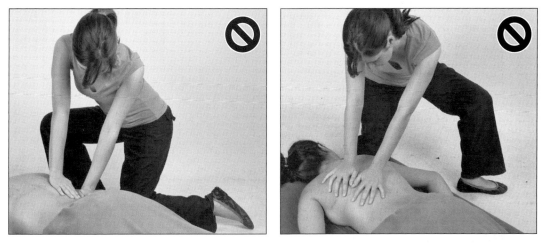

Figure 42.11: Working twisted.

Don't work in positions in which your lower body is turned away from your hands and your trunk is twisted.

Changing Direction When Necessary to Keep Facing Your Hands

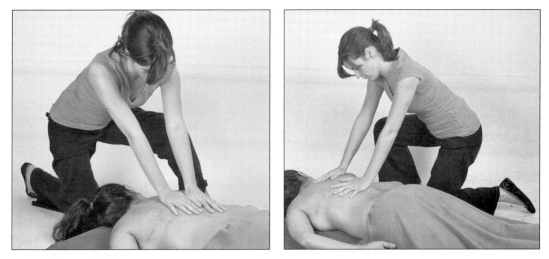

Figure 42.12: Changes of direction.

Regularly change position to avoid twisting your trunk. Move your foot and change the angle of your back leg to change direction slightly for each shift of focus. This keeps your hips behind your hands.

When necessary, change the foot that you are standing on and the knee that you are kneeling on to change the direction that you are facing.

Position and Use Your Feet to Support Your Body Movements

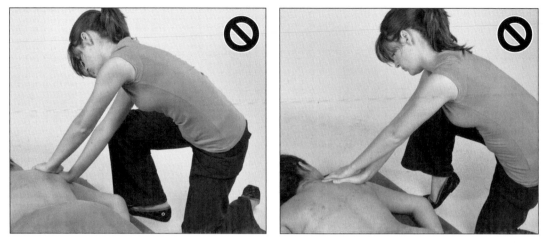

Figure 42.13: Poor leg use; a) having the back leg turned away from the direction of movement, b) having the front heel off the floor.

Note that having your back lower leg turned away from the direction of your hips and hands will restrict your ability to move easily forward and back with your massage strokes. And that having your front heel off the floor for extended periods is not nearly as stable as having your whole foot on the floor.

Move With Your Strokes

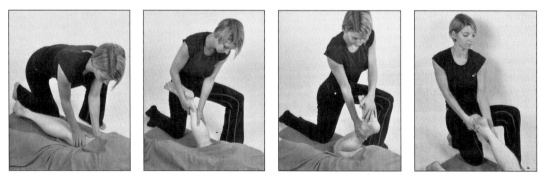

Figure 42.14: Moving to give power to massage strokes; a) leaning over – do cautiously, b) swaying forward for pressure, c) swaying forward for a stretch, d) swaying back to apply a stretch.

Don't try and reach too far which will put pressure on your back in the proposal position. Instead take advantage of the way that this position enables you to sway forward and back quite easily to initiate the power and movement of your massage strokes. This gives fluidity and evenness to sliding strokes in oil massage. It also enables you to use your bodyweight effectively for applying stationary pressure, leaning slowly forward to increase the pressure and swaying back to release it, and to sway back for stretches.

Step Forward if Necessary to Reach Further Forward
Even though the 'proposal' position will extend your reach, don't try to take it too far. Step forward to move forward with the stroke when you need to. If you then need to move further forward, slide your knee forward as well.

To Enable You to Work With Both Hands, Rest Parts of the Client's Body Across Your Thigh

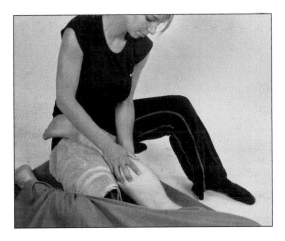

Figure 42.15: Supporting the client's limb across the thigh.

You can sometimes rest the client's limbs over your thigh to save reaching over so much or having to hold it up.

Sitting back onto your heel and resting the client's bent ankle on your thigh, will enable you to use your thigh as a 'third hand' – swaying to move his bent leg while you are using both of your hands for the massage.

Incorporating Stretches
Incorporating stretches into massage treatments has great merit for both the client and yourself. After you have loosened the client's muscles through direct massage and pressure, it is very useful to stretch and mobilise that area of the body. And it gives you a rest from delivering pressure, which compresses all of the joints of your upper limb. This is particularly important when you're working on the floor.

Don't just pull with your arms for stretches, but sway back with your body (see Chapter 39). This will help you to make the stretches more powerful and smooth with less effort. Take advantage of this to give your own body a good stretch in the process, to balance the tendency to sit or kneel in one position for long periods. For small stretches, you may be able to just sit back on one knee. Larger stretches are easiest in the proposal position.

Standing in Floor Massage

The main thing when standing is to make sure that you don't hunch over. Take hold of the client's body and use you legs to initiate stretches. If you enjoy this aspect of floor massage, it is well worth receiving treatments and studying some Thai yoga massage, which has developed these stretches into quite an art form.

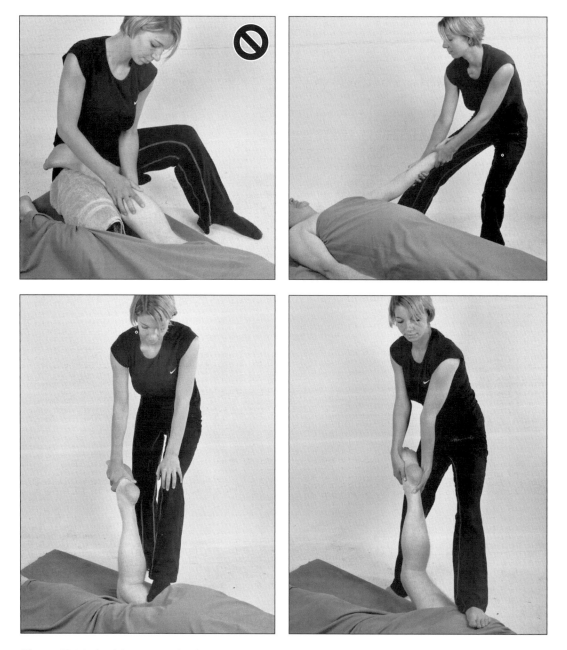

Figure 42.16: Applying a stretch; a) hunching over, b), c), d) Thai massage style stretches.

Review

When doing floor massage, look after your hands by:

- Using your fingers and thumbs carefully and sparingly;
- Make sure that you are not hyperextending them;
- Use the reinforced thumb;
- Switch to using your knuckles and fist to save your digits;
- Avoid hyperextending your wrist; and do stretches as well as applying pressure.

Look after your back by:

- Not hunching over or working with your trunk twisted;
- Not leaning too far over the client;
- Avoiding awkward lifting;
- Swaying your body with your hand movements, and;
- Having enough space around the client in which to move freely.

When you are sitting on the floor, look after your back by:

- Sitting on a cushion;
- Leaning you whole trunk to lean forward rather than hunching over;
- Supporting your back with a cushion against a wall.

When sitting on your heels:

- Have cushions under your ankles and knees, if necessary, for comfort;
- Have a cushion on your heels to sit on;
- Position yourself so that you're not working with your trunk twisted;
- Have your knees apart so that you don't strain your back when you lean forward and;
- Don't 'stand up' on both knees.

In the proposal position:

- Have cushioning under your knee if necessary;
- Have your hips facing towards your hands, and regularly change position to continue facing towards your hands;
- Don't bend your back leg away from your direction in which you are facing;
- Move your body with your strokes, and step forward if necessary to avoid trying to reach too far forward;
- Rest the parts of the client's body, such as the lower leg, across your thigh, and;
- Include stretches in your sessions.

If you stand up at times in floor massage, take care not to hunch over.

SECTION 9
Self-maintenance for the Practitioner

This section of the book covers ways of looking after yourself around massage.

The first chapter covers ways of managing your working environment and your workload in order to avoid 'burn-out'. It also looks at other aspects of your life that will impact on your body and your energy and covers ways of balancing up the demands of doing massage. Chapter 44 outlines activities that can help you to stay strong, supple and energised. Chapter 45 looks at ways of addressing problems that have already been created through massage.

Chapter 46 covers the potential problems that can arise in each part of the body through doing massage. It lists the massage practices that can cause these strains and also identifies other common activities that can contribute to these problems. It refers you to the relevant parts of the book that address the particular problem.

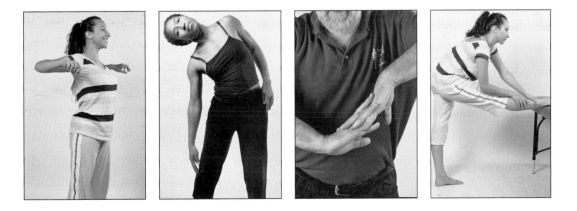

CHAPTER 43

Looking After Yourself Around Massage

The main focus of this book is on looking after your body while you are delivering massage treatments (and warming-up to prepare for this and winding-down to relax at the end of the day, see Chapter 10). However many other factors can also affect your ability to maintain your energy and stamina for massage, and influence how you are able to work. This chapter looks at:

- Your working environment and your workload;
- How you structure treatment sessions;
- Having realistic expectations;
- Not pushing yourself to the limits;
- Ways of keeping yourself physically, mentally, and emotionally nourished;
- The role of supervision to sort through problems that arise with clients;
- Factors in the rest of your life that can impact on your body and your energy.

What affects you will, of course, vary from person to person, and can also vary at different times for the same person.

The Working Situation

There are a number of things that you can do to make your working situation pleasant and easier.

The Physical Working Environment

Keep your working environment pleasant and uncluttered, and organise the space and your equipment so that it functions best for you.

Try to get some natural light into your room. If you can't get any and/or you can't get fresh air because of the heating/air conditioning, try to spend some time in light, airy rooms or out of doors during your working day.

Because you always need to keep the working space warm enough for the client, be sure to drink enough fluid to avoid getting dehydrated. And consider having a dish of water on or near the heaters to keep the air from dehydrating.

If you are going into work places to do on-site massage, make sure that you have the maximum uncluttered space around your massage chair, even if this involves shifting some furniture.

Your Workload

Set a realistic number of working hours per day, and give yourself enough preparation time each day, and 'wind-down' time afterwards. When you know you've got busy times coming up, organise non-pressured time for rest and replenishment, including regular treats and holidays for yourself.

Bear in mind that if you are regularly exceeding what you can easily do by consistently working beyond your comfortable physical capabilities – regularly doing too many massages in a day, not taking enough breaks during your working day, or doing techniques that are strainful for you – you will begin to wear yourself out. And if you consistently work in this way, you are likely to damage your health.

Take account of the fact that events in the rest of your life can affect your capacity for work. If you are able, organise your workload to reflect this. For example, you may need to cut down your workload at times of significant life changes or stressful family events. When my mum died (suddenly), I took a month off work as I knew I had no energy to give to clients. Many colleagues have had to monitor and ration their energy carefully when looking after their ageing parents or ill partners or children.

Structuring Your Working Day

Massage is a demanding physical activity, which also requires mental focus. It can also be emotionally challenging as well when clients are distressed by pain, loneliness or illness. So it is important to build elements into your working day that start you off well, give you breathing space which enables you to re-centre yourself and replenish your energy during the day, and help you to switch off at the end of your day. Much of this is covered in Chapter 10: *Warming-up and winding-down.*

Make sure that you structure breaks into your working day so that you are not on the go for the whole time, and that you are not exhausting yourself by working too many hours.

Pacing Yourself

It is worth taking stock of your energy at the beginning of each working day (see Chapter 5). Some days you will have boundless energy and on other days you will need to pace yourself carefully. Pacing yourself is particularly important when your energy is fluctuating, for example when you are undergoing a stressful time, affected by hormonal cycles, or recovering from a cold or illness.

And, if you have regular low energy times during the day, you will need to pace yourself carefully to get through these. For example, you may find it hard to get going in the morning, or you may be a morning person who starts to flag toward the end of the working day, or you may regularly hit a low spot after lunch. If it's in your control, you could consider not booking clients for the low energy parts of your day.

Review Your Techniques

Take stock of your body and your energy at the end of the day (see Chapter 5), and take note of any aches or pains that you've developed. Think about the techniques or ways of working that may have contributed to these, and how you might change them. Reduce how much you use them, adapt them or find easier substitutes to reduce the strain on your body.

Structuring Individual Treatment Sessions

Try to reduce the potential for misunderstandings between you and your clients by being clear about what you can offer, giving them information about reasonable expectations for the session and getting feedback during the session.

Being Clear About What You Can Offer

If you are self-employed, state the nature of your services clearly on your publicity. If necessary, remind your clients of the range of skills that you can offer, and give them information on reasonable expectations of outcomes for the session and the likely time/number of sessions necessary to achieve these.

If you are employed in a spa/health centre, tell clients of your particular skills, which may be different from those of other people at the spa from whom they've received treatments.

Involving the Client

When you're meeting new clients, find out their needs and desires and let them know the skills that you have to offer. Offer them a plan of treatment that fits their needs, being realistic about what you offer (for example, "I can't guarantee to cure your condition, but I can pretty certainly ease it" or, "My speciality is sports / relaxation massage, so you'll need to go to a physiotherapist / osteopath / chiropractor for more specific attention to your vertebrae"). With regular clients, it's good to ask them about any relevant events that have happened since the last session, and what they want from the present session.

Get the client's agreement on the overall focus of the session so that you're not at cross-purposes between their expectations and your intentions. For example, you could ask them to choose between either having a general all-over massage or having you just focus on particular areas that need more attention. You could discuss whether they would like you only to do hands-on work, or whether they would also find it useful for you to guide them through exercises that they could take away for 'homework'. You could suggest a treatment plan for a series of sessions. Obviously the choices that you offer will depend on your particular skills.

Getting feedback from the client during the session will help *you* to work effectively, and to ensure that *they're* involved and happy with what you're doing. Feedback could be about the pressure, the time and focus of working on each area and the type of techniques that you are using.

Finishing the Massage Session

Setting Clear Limits

Set clear limits in the working situation, as far as you are able, so that you can look after yourself and not to get 'drained' by clients – either during the session or by demands that they might make afterwards.

Have a clear-cut finishing point for each treatment session, after which you (or your receptionist) deal with payment and setting up the next appointment. Make it clear that you then need to get on with other things. You are no longer available for the client, even if s/he is taking time to sit and 'recover' from the massage before leaving your premises.

Incidentally, when you are talking to a potential new client on the phone or in person, don't let them take up too much of your time. Give them a reasonable time to gain relevant information about your skills and the appropriateness of your work for their needs. If they remain uncertain about booking a session, suggest that they take time to think further about it and contact you again when they want further specific information or to make a booking.

Finishing With the Client

It is important to be able to disengage from the last client so that you can be ready and available for the next person. In addition to being good hygiene, many people use washing their hands after each session as a useful cleansing ritual to 'dissolve' the connection with that client and prepare for the next one.

Of course, you might think about clients between sessions, for example researching medical information about their conditions, thinking about homework exercises that you might offer them, or revising or learning new hands-on techniques that could be relevant, or considering professional referrals that you might offer them. However, no matter how much the client's situation has affected you, obsessively thinking about them won't help them and will drain you.

Obviously, when you first start doing massage, each individual client will have a major impact on you. However, after a time, most practitioners find that they develop an automatic 'switch' that enables them to 'let go' of the client as they walk out of the door, while remaining happy to see them again next time and remembering their story (perhaps with prompting from case notes). This may sound callous but is an essential survival mechanism for professional life.

As mentioned above, you may need winding-down time at the end of the day for thinking through your day and 'laying it to rest'. It's particularly important if you are working with people with serious injuries or illnesses that you are able to 'leave your work at work'. Ways of doing this may include having time after work with colleagues that enables you to talk things through and/or let off steam (see Chapter 10).

Left Over Feelings and Client Reactions

Dealing With 'Left Over' Feelings

If, after a massage, you are left with some uncomfortable thoughts or feelings, do something immediately to clear yourself as best you can and to reenergise yourself. You might do something physical such as stretches or more vigorous jogging on the spot, or incorporate some imagery such as shaking out your hands while visualising that you are 'shaking it off', or you could do some mental re-centering.

This process may not be enough. If the feelings are persistent or you find that you are regularly left with unresolved thoughts, feelings or client issues, make time to discuss this with colleagues or a supervisor who can help you sort though the issues involved (see *Supervision* below).

Client's Negative Reactions

Be aware that clients can sometimes feel very tired, low or sore after massage sessions through no fault of yours. Most of the time, if you get verbal feedback from clients that they're comfortably managing the pressure and pacing during a massage, they won't feel sore afterwards. However, when people have held tension in areas of their bodies for a long time, it can feel quite sore when this is brought back into their attention and released through massage (even if the massage wasn't especially deep). In a similar way, athletes usually only feel the aches and pains after the adrenaline 'high' of a sporting event is over.

Clients who constantly push themselves to their limits may 'let down' enough in a massage session to uncover the longstanding cost of this attitude to themselves. As they relax, they may get in touch with their underlying exhaustion, for example, which may need much more time and attention than is possible in a single massage session. Many of us have experienced a similar effect when going on holiday. It's not unusual to spend the first days of a holiday feeling a bit down and tired as you recover from the daily pressures of life and work (as well as the stress of preparing to go on the holiday).

Occasionally clients will have reactions to massage that are entirely unpredictable. As long as you've checked the pressure and their general comfort throughout the massage session, this is not anyone's fault. It may be due to medical conditions (diagnosed or undiagnosed), the effects of an old injury resurfacing, or to associations with forgotten experiences. Sometimes these passing feelings are not explicable in simple physical or mental terms. A once-off experience of this sort is not something to be unduly concerned about.

However, if the reaction is a strong physical one such as dizziness or specific pain, and particularly if it persists, recommend that the client seek medical advice. Physical reactions can be due to medical conditions. For example, multiple sclerosis (MS) can produce unpredictable reactions to activity or massage, and low blood pressure can give rise to dizziness if the client sits up suddenly after lying down for a long time. Mild medical conditions such as low blood pressure may be previously undiagnosed and the client may have forgotten about old injuries.

If clients have strong emotional reactions or persistent unpleasant mental images, it can be useful for them to see a counsellor / therapist to help sort this through.

Adapting to Client Responses
You may sometimes feel it necessary or appropriate to warn clients that they may feel sore or achy on the next day, either because you have a sense that they have held tension for a long time that may come back into awareness, because you've worked firmly, or because they have conditions that may get stirred up by massage. Tell them that this will usually pass within a day or two (and to talk to you if it doesn't – about reasons and possible avenues of relief).

Sometimes, even if you've monitored the client's reactions and got verbal feedback, they will have negative reactions. For example, their verbal feedback may be at odds with their body responses (they may be asking you for more pressure or stretching than their body can comfortably handle). Or, whilst the massage is manageable moment by moment, the cumulative effects that they experience after the session may be negative. Or you may not have properly 'got the measure' of the client in the first session, or your style of massage, or at least the particular way that you chose to work on them in the session, may not be what they need.

Whether the reaction is passing or persists, you need to talk it through together so that you can modify your approach at the next session (or occasionally to mutually decide that massage, or at least your style of massage, is inappropriate). Massage is a two-way process (see below), so it needs the two of you to sort it out together as much as possible. In this process, bear in mind that you have professional information and experience that the client doesn't have, and therefore can offer informed suggestions (e.g. "I could work much more lightly in this session"; or, "We could try a different approach, with more active involvement from you in doing stretches" etc.), and that, no matter how reasonable these offers, the client may decline to have another session with you.

Some General Attitudes

This section of the chapter looks at some common attitudes to massage held by both practitioners and clients, that can lead to practitioners wearing themselves out.

Not Exhausting Yourself in Each Session
There is a common attitude that the practitioner should give *everything* that they have to *every* client, no matter the cost to themselves. Women, who are more often socialised to be the caregivers, need to be especially alert to this.

Obviously, constantly working at your limit will lead to a very short career. So it is important to pace yourself so that you will get through each working day, with some energy left for the rest of your life and for tomorrow. It is also important to:

- Maintain your time boundaries (see *Setting clear limits* above);
- Mentally 'let go' of each client when you've finished with the session (see *Finishing with the client* above);

- Make sure that you have breaks during the day, and;
- Look after yourself outside of the massage situation (see *Nourishment* below).

There are limits to every person's strength, stamina and resilience. These will be determined by such things as your build and inherited constitution, your level of fitness and medical history, and the pressures that exist in the rest of your life.

This can be hard to accept. Practitioners who are used to constantly pushing themselves to the limit often feel that they are short-changing the client if they give anything less than 200% of themselves in every session. You can survive this for a time in your youth, but it cannot be sustained day in and day out, especially as you get older. At the very least, you will begin to wear yourself out if you are regularly exceeding what you can comfortably do (the number of massages that you do in a day, having enough rest between massages, working beyond your comfortable physical capabilities). You may even damage your health, and become a liability rather than an asset to your community.

Realistic Expectations
It is important to approach each massage session with realistic expectations about the possible outcomes, and to refer clients to other professionals if their needs are outside your area of professional competence or if you're not able to get satisfactory results within a few sessions. Two experiences in my early years of practice helped me put this into perspective.

One involved a client who told me on the phone that she had pain all over her body. A friend had told her that massage would be helpful. I approached the session with naive optimism about 'curing' her. However, in talking to her, I discovered that in twenty years of having this pain, she'd had treatments from nearly every type of medical practitioner and alternative therapist. Not only had their treatments been unsuccessful, but most of them had exacerbated the condition. I gave her a massage, which she seemed to enjoy for the relaxation, but it gave her no relief from the pain and she later informed me that it too had caused a flare-up.

On another occasion, a young woman who was going through a traumatic time in her personal life came for a massage, which had been recommended by a friend who had told her that massage was good for calming down. Within a few minutes of talking, it became clear that, never having had a massage before, she was very apprehensive about it. It would clearly create extra anxieties for her rather than calming her. What she really needed was a sympathetic person to listen to her talk through her situation and feelings. I didn't give her a massage, but gave her the contact details of a good counsellor.

So aim to do your best within your capabilities and your energy on any given day. Try to approach each session with enthusiasm, but don't exhaust yourself for each client. And bear in mind that it generally takes more than one treatment to deliver long-term effects.

Clients may expect you to have all the answers. Sometimes you will have the pertinent knowledge and sometimes not. And you may only be able to deal with effects of problems and not the causes such as a past injury or the effects of a sedentary job. In any case, many massages are primarily for maintenance – keeping your clients going by balancing out the rigours of a physically demanding job, such as building work, a stressful computer-based job or being a musician – rather than necessarily solving particular problems.

Massage is a Two-way Process
There are two people involved in the massage process. You can only do your best to help clients, but it also requires *their* willing cooperation. Some clients want to be involved in the process, asking questions and taking on your advice and exercises that you offer. Others expect *you* to do all the work, with no effort at all on their part. However, you can't *make* clients let go of their tensions, you can only

offer them the opportunity to do so. Similarly, you can't make clients do the 'homework' exercises that you offer them.

Bear in mind that a massage session is only one hour in a client's life, so don't be hard on yourself for not fixing all of their problems in one session. Their tensions / problems will generally have been accumulating over some time, so it will take time to reverse that process. And clients are generally only able to 'let go' a certain amount in each session. Generally clients are able to 'let down' more in a series of sessions as they get to know and trust you and your work, and get more in touch with their own bodies. But sometimes they have reached their comfortable limits in that first session and aren't able to let go any further in subsequent sessions.

And some problems will be impossible to resolve because they are so entrenched, either because of the client's medical history or because the client would need to change more of their attitudes, habits and lifestyle than they're able or prepared to.

So bear in mind that massage is a two-way process, which depends on both parties. If you have done your best within your capabilities, then it is also up to the client to come to the party. If they are unable to, whatever the reason, then you have nothing to reproach yourself about, *even if they want to blame you* for the lack of a result. (This is why it's important to get their agreement about the treatment strategy, see *Structuring Individual Treatment Sessions* above).

Remember that *you can't please everyone all of the time*. This can be hard to accept because most of us enter the profession with a strong desire to help people. However, you and a client may just not 'click'. Or they may be the type that always needs to find fault. Or your skills may not be what they most need. So refer clients to other massage practitioners or other professionals when it's appropriate – it is the professional thing to do, and it is the best thing for both you and the client.

And there's one other aspect of this, which is sometimes even harder to accept. Even if clients absolutely *love* your massage, events in their life (including their finances) may stop them coming back for more massages.

Replenishing Yourself

Massage is an easy profession in which to 'burn out' – to feel overloaded and empty by constant giving. Symptoms of 'burn out' can include:

* A loss of resilience and perspective, such as constant irritability;
* A reduced ability to cope;
* Physical symptoms such as backache, headaches, stiff shoulders, and constant tension in the hands, and;
* A general inability to relax.

So it is important to make sure that you are replenishing yourself in the rest of your life, especially if you have responsibilities there too (such as bringing up children or looking after ageing parents). Three areas need attention – general self-maintenance, doing things that nourish and replenish you, and getting support to deal with client and work issues.

General Self-maintenance
Massage is a demanding physical activity, so you need to treat your body as an athlete would. Get enough restful sleep, eat healthy nourishing food, and drink enough water. Keep yourself flexible and energised through stretches and exercise (see *Warm-ups* in Chapter 10).

Self-massage can be helpful to keep you going during your working day, even if it is just a few minutes between clients. Receiving regular massage or other bodywork treatments is important for nourishing both body and soul (as we so often tell our clients).

It can be important to have an exercise programme for looking after and building up your body (see Chapter 44). A well-rounded programme would include exercises for:

*   Developing *muscle strength* (without rigidity);
*   *Flexibility* – to keep you supple;
*   *Aerobic conditioning* to keep your heart healthy;
*   Some *relaxation* procedures so that you're not just tightening muscles.

Make sure that what you do suits your needs and abilities, so get guidance and coaching from a personal trainer, sports trainer or sports physiotherapist. And pace yourself with this. As you build up this type of programme, cut back or have a break when you need to.

Breathing exercises and meditation can help you to mentally 'switch off', and to calm and re-centre yourself. Many practitioners in the nurturing / healing area of massage also use images and rituals from meditation, yoga, martial arts or healing to energise themselves during and after massages.

Leisure and Daily Life Activities
It's important to have leisure activities that nourish you (below). However, if you find that these put pressure on your body, particularly if you are feeling strain in your body, you may need to reduce some of them or even avoid them. For example, if you are feeling strain in your wrist (see Chapter 45), you need to be careful of how much time you spend on the computer and/or to cut down on other hand-intensive activities such as craft work, DIY or playing a musical instrument.

You may also need to think about how to protect your hands in daily life, for example, by:

*   Investing in hand saving devices such as electric can-openers and dishwashing machines;
*   Getting other people to do some of your cleaning and washing to save your hands, and;
*   Not carrying heavy things – by getting travel luggage on wheels, being careful about carrying large, heavy shopping bags, and getting help to move furniture, etc.

This is covered in more detail at the end of Chapter 45.

Time Out
You may need to take time off work on occasions to deal with life problems and/or give your body a rest at times of stress or when you've been working too hard, especially if you notice strains developing in your hands or wrists (see Chapter 45). Even if you are not self-employed, you may be able to reduce your working hours, either for a time or permanently.

It is also important to have breaks from work / daily life, whether it is the occasional long lunch break, a special day out, a weekend away or a longer holiday. A 'sabbatical' can also help you to replenish yourself – an extended time out, to do some extensive research into an area of work or indulge yourself in some other activity entirely.

Nourishment
It is crucial to do things that nourish you, so that you can maintain your spirit and energy. Some practitioners find it hard to take time off to play and indulge themselves, but it is essential to avoid work (and life) just becoming a grind. ("All work and no play makes a dull person.").

What delights, nourishes and energises you varies from person to person, of course, and will also vary on different occasions for the same person, so this section of the chapter just touches on a few general ideas. The main thing is to balance up from the intense demands of massage.

Having *'time out'* from the demands of life is quite important. This can range from solo activities such as day dreaming, soaking in a warm bath/tub, reading, hobbies, or going for a walk (or formal procedures such as meditation) to activities with other people such as going to parties, spas, restaurants or attending sports or arts events or outdoor pursuits.

Social connections with friends and family are important, rather than only having our social needs met through clients. Connections with friends and family can be deeply nourishing. Playing with children can rekindle your delight in life. 'Letting off steam' is important too – a fun evening with friends can remind you of the joy of laughter and frivolity to balance up the serious business of dealing with people in discomfort and distress.

Many people maintain balance in their lives by having interests and activities in which they focus on *developing themselves*, for example:

- *Physically* through sports, martial arts, dance, playing a musical instrument or juggling, etc.;
- *Mentally* through doing puzzles and quizzes, learning languages or other studies;
- *Expressively* through the performance of music, singing, theatre, dance, etc.;
- *Spiritually* through study, meditation, chanting, religious activities, etc., or;
- Activities that *combine* some of these aspects.

These activities may feed directly or indirectly into their massage work or be quite separate.

And many people also search for *something bigger* in their lives, such as working in organisations that focus on more than just individual or professional concerns, in an enjoyment of nature or in religious or spiritual activities that connect them to the deeper threads of life.

Continuing professional development is also important to maintain your freshness and interest in your work. Receiving treatments from other practitioners was mentioned above, and peer support and supervision are covered below. Taking regular courses helps you to stay fresh and to expand your toolkit, and provides you with the opportunity to mix with colleagues. You might also consider regularly trading skills with colleagues, or forming a study group to practice what you've learnt in a course or to work your way through a book or a DVD. And it's good to stay up to date with developments in your field via professional journals, and by attending conferences and getting involved in your professional organisation.

Supervision
Massage is an isolated activity. You can get weighed down by problems with your clients or your work situation, and they can get out of proportion if you can't share them with anyone. It is good to have *safe, confidential* situations in which you can talk about issues, get support and suggestions and work out solutions.

Some people have individual colleagues with whom they have mutual arrangements for doing this, either as the need arises or on a regular basis. Other people get professional supervision or join a support / supervision group. Some groups are led by an experienced practitioner, and others consist of professionals sharing with each other. Supervision might include counselling, to help you understand and change unproductive patterns in relation to clients.

Your Massage Career

Working full time in a spa situation is primarily a young person's activity. As you get older, you may use your knowledge and experience to work differently in treatment sessions, and/or build on this experience to create a related career in administration of a clinic or health facility, teach massage or exercise classes, or sell health-related products.

Make Changes in Your Work Situation

Changing treatment sessions: If you are self-employed, it may be possible to gradually change how you work with clients, or at least the nature of treatments that you offer new clients. For example, you could incorporate more assisted stretches in your treatments (see Chapter 39) to get the client working more and reduce your own work. You could focus on myofascial release and reduce your deep tissue work. You could offer to coach clients in more self-maintenance procedures, such as relaxation or exercises routines.

Changing your clientele: You might consider changing your clientele, for example by referring on clients who want deep pressure work. You might focus on the nurturing side of massage, for example working in hospices, or doing baby massage (and teaching it to new mothers/parents).

Changing your career: However, these changes may not be enough, so you may be forced to look at changing your career. Many people view full-time general massage work in a sauna/spa/health resort as more of a younger person's activity. Many of us who are still working in the field in our 40s and 50s have developed some specialist skills in our treatments, and/or combine part-time clinical work with teaching, administrating, promoting health products or exercise coaching, etc.

Some people work part-time at massage, balancing out the physical and mental demands by doing another very different professional (or voluntary) activity. The possibilities are as wide as your interests and imagination can make them.

Review

Keep your working environment pleasant and uncluttered, and organise the space and your equipment so that it functions best for you.

If you are going into other work places, try to have uncluttered space around your massage chair.

Set a realistic number of working hours per day, and give yourself enough preparation time each day, and 'winding-down' time afterwards.

When you're busy, organise non-pressured time for rest and replenishment, including regular treats and holidays for yourself.

Don't wear yourself out by exceeding what you can comfortably do, working too many hours, not having breaks, and take account of events in the rest of your life which can affect the energy that you have to give.

If possible, start your working day with warm-ups and/or centering exercises, have breathing spaces during the day to re-centre yourself and renew your energy, and find ways of winding-down and switching off at the end of the day.

Monitor your energy and pace yourself during your working day so that you can sustain yourself.

If it's in your control, consider not booking clients for the low energy parts of your day.

At the end of the working day, take stock of your body and your energy, and think about changes that you could make in the techniques that you use and/or how you apply them.

In massage sessions:

- Be clear with clients about what you can offer, including reasonable expectations for the session;
- Negotiate a treatment approach that is agreeable to the client;
- Get feedback during the session and adapt your massage accordingly;
- Have clear limits for the session (including a clear-cut finishing time).

Even if you get consistent feedback, clients can have negative reactions to sessions (that are not your fault) due to:

- Catching up with underlying soreness of muscles, or tiredness / exhaustion;
- Physical reactions such as dizziness or pains, which need to be checked by a medical practitioner;
- Strong emotional reactions or persistent unpleasant mental images, which a counsellor / therapist could help them to sort through;
- Occasional unpredictable reactions (which need talking through before future sessions), which can be due to physical conditions such as ME or MS.

Refer clients on if:

- They need different treatments than those you can offer;
- They require a firmer treatment than you can comfortably deliver;
- Their problems are outside of your area of expertise, or;
- If you are making no headway after a few treatments.

Do your best within your capabilities and your energy. Try to approach each session with enthusiasm, but don't exhaust yourself. And bear in mind that it generally takes more than one treatment to deliver long-term effects.

Be realistic about what you can do with massage;

- Offering maintenance for people with sedentary jobs, hard physical work, or old injuries;
- Teaching people to look after their bodies better *if they are willing to be involved in this*;
- Offering clients 'homework' exercises if they're willing to do them;
- Sometimes only dealing with effects and not causes, or;
- Calling on specialised skills (such as sports massage) to sort out particular problems.

To avoid wearing yourself out through doing massage:

- Get enough restful sleep, eat healthy nourishing food and drink enough water;
- Drink enough fluid to avoid getting dehydrated when keeping your working space warm;
- Keep yourself flexible and energised through stretches and exercise;
- Use self-massage and swaps with colleagues to make sure that you receive enough massage;
- Have social activities and interests outside of work that nourish and replenish you;
- Balance out or cut down on activities that put similar pressure on your body as massage does, especially on your wrists and fingers;
- Have time out to replenish yourself;
- Take part in continuing professional development activities to regularly refresh yourself, such as training courses, conferences, reading journals, discussion and study groups, etc.;
- Get supervision with either colleagues or a supervisor.

You may need to make changes in your work situation to sustain your career, including:

- Changing how you work with clients in sessions, for example using other modalities or offering exercise coaching;
- Changing your clientele;
- Working part-time, or;
- Moving into administration, teaching, fitness coaching or teaching exercise classes, or making and/or selling health-related products.

CHAPTER 44

Helpful Approaches

This chapter briefly surveys some of the many 'exercise' disciplines and health maintenance treatments that are widely available to help you, the massage practitioner, to stay strong, fit, supple and energised. It firstly lists methods of developing and maintaining a range of qualities that are important to the massage practitioner such as strength, flexibility, coordination and relaxation. It then covers individual treatments that will help you to look after your own body. This is just a brief listing of possibilities, not an exhaustive guide – this *could* easily be another book (or two) in itself.

I am not suggesting that you should do all of these activities (although, if you have a few lifetimes to spare, it could be fun to work through the list). It is offered more as a guide to activities that you could undertake if you feel the need to develop or refine certain aspects of your physicality.

> **Caution:** You are strongly advised to have a general health check before undertaking an exercise programme. This is *absolutely crucial* if you have any physical problems or health concerns, or if you unaccustomed to physical exercise. It is also strongly recommended if you are over 40.

'Exercises'

In this section of the chapter, exercise systems are grouped together according to their effects. Obviously, many disciplines have a number of effects and will appear in more than one place in the list. Bear in mind that the considerations of this list may only be a small part of the area that each of these disciplines covers. So, if you join a class, expect to be encouraged, challenged, and stretched in ways that are beyond the focus of this book.

Most are taught as group classes, but many teachers will also give you individual coaching. Two that are listed in this section are also repeated in the section on individual treatments. The Feldenkrais Method® takes a different form in individual treatments than in group classes. Although the Alexander Technique is primarily taught via individual treatments, it focuses on many of the qualities listed here.

Bear in mind that *how* a class is taught and its focus will depend on the interests, experience and skill of the individual teacher. You may find that, although you like the method, you can't get on with a particular teacher's style.

A note about '*Dance*'. This probably encompasses the broadest range of qualities of any activity on the list below, ranging from solo to couples to groups, from gentle to strong, from graceful to wild, and from learning highly structured sequences to the open expressivity of 'free dance' forms (including doing household chores to music). Moving to music can be helpful if you feel that you're 'not rhythmical'. Couples dances, such as ballroom and salsa, can give you a feeling for the give-and-take of movement, which is readily applicable to rhythmical techniques such as body rocking and limb rolling (see Chapter 40).

Strength

Gym workouts under supervision, can help you to build up strength on the weight machines. Get individual instruction from a trainer to assess and advise you, especially if you intend undertaking specific body development programmes, such as building up your upper body, strengthening your back or developing the muscles that stabilise your wrist.

The Upper Body

Working with free weights will help you to develop upper body strength in action. Areas of focus can include the chest, shoulders and upper back, the forearm muscles, the muscles that stabilise the wrist, and hand strength.

'Core' Strength

The Pilates method addresses this directly – developing the strength of the 'core' muscles of the lower trunk, which are often neglected in our sedentary society. This is useful for back problems, and for improving posture. Yoga classes can also focus on this.

Spinal Suppleness

Yoga, the Feldenkrais Method® and the throwing martial arts such as judo and aikido develop a combination of strength and suppleness in the trunk.

Poise/Posture

The Alexander Technique, yoga, Pilates and many forms of dance address posture in action directly. It is also a by-product of many martial arts and some sports such as basketball.

The Lower Body

If you are working out in the gym, don't just build up the static strength of your legs, but also use equipment such as rowing, cycling and running machines to develop strength in action. Outside of the gym, you can develop this through running / jogging, via sports that involve running such as soccer and basketball, and through many forms of dance. Solo activities such as skiing, skating, skipping, skateboarding, surfing, snowboarding and trampolining will also strengthen the lower body in action, while also helping balance.

Lightness on the Feet

As mentioned in Chapter 28 (see figure 28.14), you may feel 'over-grounded' at the end of a day's massage – heavy and sluggish in your legs. Lighten and energise them to balance this out by activities such as running, skipping, jumping, or trampolining. Many forms of dance also promote nimbleness in the feet.

Stretching – Flexibility

Many exercise classes and sports warm-up routines include stretches for encouraging flexibility. It is a central feature of many styles of yoga. Flexibility in action is also a feature of both the group classes and the individual treatments of the Feldenkrais Method®.

Dynamic Ease in Action

Some of the activities listed above just focus on developing strength in action. Others, such as Tai Chi, judo, aikido, and skiing and skating, focus more on combining ease with power (which is the balance that this book emphasises for massage).

Energy and Aerobic Fitness
Many activities will help you to develop aerobic fitness (developing your cardiovascular and respiratory fitness) and increase your energy. This can be a useful antidote to the slower, relatively restricted movements of massage. Useful activities include swimming, running, cycling, skipping, dancing, aerobic classes and sports such as tennis, soccer, and basketball. You can also do it in the gym on the cycling, running, and rowing machines.

Stamina
Most of these activities also develop stamina.

Coordination
Activities which involve rhythmical, integrated movement such as dance, martial arts and solo sports such as running, cycling and swimming, are all useful for developing general coordination.

Manual coordination can be developed through woodworking, model making, crafts and arts activities, through learning magic tricks, playing a musical instrument, some computer games, and through practising 'circus skills' such as juggling.

Coordinating Breathing With Movement
Swimming and a number of martial arts involve very specific patterns of coordinating your breathing with movement. However, more general coordination is an essential feature of most rhythmic activities such as running, skipping, and rowing.

Relaxation
Relaxation procedures are taught in stress management and relaxation classes, and in yoga and some meditation classes. Learning to relax in action is a feature of Tai Chi, the Alexander Technique and Feldenkrais classes and treatments.

Developing Self-monitoring
The Alexander Technique, the Feldenkrais Method® and Pilates are designed to directly help you to develop self-monitoring of your body in action. However, doing any activity that encourages you to focus on how you do it will encourage this.

Developing Your Kinaesthetic Memory
As well as their particular use in keeping you fit, strong, flexible, etc., most of the activities suggested here will also have the general effect of helping you to develop your kinaesthetic memory (your memory for movement). If you have a physical background, this will be probably already familiar.

However, for those who don't, immersing yourself in physical activity (the medium of massage) will help you to develop your appreciation, understanding, and memory for movement. In addition, you may gain perceptions of movement that are useful with clients, and perhaps even specific movement ideas that you can take directly to the massage table. You might also offer exercises from these classes to clients for self-maintenance 'homework'.

Another way of developing your memory of movement is through 'people-watching' – sitting at a café and watching how passers-by walk. And, as you walk down the street, mimicking the movements of others (if you can do it discreetly) is even more helpful in developing your feeling for movement and gaining active insights into people's movements and restrictions.

When you are with clients, it can be quite useful to copy their posture for the same reason. Stating clearly that you are doing it to help you understand their postural habits so that you can work with them more effectively will make it professional and take any potential offence out of it.

Receiving Treatments

This last part of the chapter looks at some of most widely available individual treatments. As mentioned above, many of the 'exercise' classes can also be done as personalised individual coaching. However, only three are repeated here – the Alexander Technique, which is primarily taught via individual treatments, Pilates which can be taught in groups or via individual coaching, and the Feldenkrais Method®, which takes a different form in individual treatments than in group classes.

Relaxation, nurturing and replenishment are the goals of a range of (generally) lighter massage styles.

Physical release and rebalancing is more often the focus of deeper massage such as Rolfing and its offshoots.

Energy rebalancing is the focus of shiatsu, Thai yoga massage, Hawaiian kahuna massage and zero balancing treatments.

Spinal problems are the focus of osteopathy, chiropractic and physiotherapy.

Posture and body awareness are addressed in Alexander Technique sessions, in Feldenkrais treatments and in individual Pilates sessions.

Review

There are a great number of 'exercise' disciplines and health maintenance treatments that are widely available to help you, the massage practitioner, to stay strong, fit, supple and energised.

You can use them:

- To develop and/or maintain qualities that are important to the massage practitioner such as strength, flexibility, coordination, and relaxation, and;
- To look after your own body through receiving individual treatments.

CHAPTER 45

Addressing Established Problems

The central focus of this book is on a preventative approach to massage – looking after your body and hands by monitoring yourself and making adjustments in action. However, problems can still arise. This may be due to the general cumulative effects of doing massage for years, but can also arise from:

*   Strains in massage sessions, such as lifting a client's leg which is unexpectedly heavy;
*   Regularly working too hard in massage sessions – on too many large clients and those with rock-hard muscles, working too many hours, pushing yourself too much in each session;
*   The cumulative effects of other activities and the stresses of the rest of your life, or;
*   Accidents and injuries, including the continuing effect of old injuries.

Practitioners with small or slender builds and those with hypermobile joints need to be especially careful of their bodies because they are more vulnerable to strain. People who are unaccustomed to this sort of physical activity need to learn to monitor their bodies carefully too, and to learn to distinguish between extending themselves to develop strength and stamina and the overload of pushing themselves too far.

This chapter focuses on ways of dealing with the problems that most commonly arise for massage practitioners. It looks at the effects and treatment options for the four main areas where this can happen:

1. Shoulders and upper back;
2. Lower back;
3. Thumbs, and, to a lesser extent, the fingers, and;
4. Wrists.

An Important Note About Back Pain and Overuse Strains
A large percentage of the population has some back pain at some stage of their lives. This pain can come and go. The causes are not always clear (or agreed by specialists), so it is not necessarily going to be clear what part doing massage has played, and the contribution of other factors, such as your build and other life activities. There are also many factors that experts agree can contribute to overuse strain in the upper limbs (which is also called *Repetitive Strain Injury* – RSI, or work-related upper limb disorders – WRULD, see below), which can lead to wrist problems.

So the information in this chapter covers possible causes and effects in a general way. As you read through it, you may find it helpful in pinpointing causes in your massage work or other life activities. Hopefully it will help you to work out possible treatment options, helpful self-maintenance exercises, and useful adjustments to consider in your way of working.

It must be emphasised that the information in this chapter is offered as a *general guide only*. Any medical conditions need individual diagnosis and specialist treatment and exercise advice.

Terminology

The terminology of methods of treatment and the professions that carry them out is used in a variety of ways. These can be confusing and sometimes conflicting because of the areas of overlap and of professional demarcations, and the variations between countries and often from state to state. And, of course, there is also a difference in each profession between the basic professional skill and those of the specialist. Therefore, to try and take a simple path through this complex territory, I will use the following terms in this chapter to cover groups of skills and professional groups (and please bear with me on this if it's not your familiar terminology).

I will use *massage* as an umbrella term to cover general soft tissue work ranging from a spa massage to basic therapeutic massage, including the soft tissue work of manipulative therapists. I will use *deep tissue massage* to refer to working firmly and more specifically into the muscles.

I will use the term *mobilisation* of joints to refer to moving parts of the client's body to promote general mobility (which many massage therapists do). And use *manipulation* to refer to more specific joint adjustments, both the 'classic' high velocity thrusts (HVT) of osteopathy, chiropractic, and physiotherapy / physical therapy, and also the specific non-HVT joint work of these professions.

I will therefore also use broad terms for these two groups – *massage practitioners* and *manipulative therapists*.

A Few Notes About Treatments

Throughout this chapter, I make recommendations about receiving treatments or getting individual coaching to address particular problems. However, I am not suggesting that you have treatments from just *any* practitioner / coach. I think that it is important to find one who suits you, who listens sympathetically, and is *willing to adapt their treatment according to your feedback*, especially if you are already in pain.

So, for example, when you are receiving massages (of any type), make sure that the masseur / masseuse or manipulative therapist appreciates the difference between 'good pain' and 'bad pain' and is willing to adapt their pressure and techniques to suit you, particularly when you are already in pain. (If you are tensing against the massage because the pressure is too much, he/she is likely to bruise you if they try to push through your 'resistance'. And the muscle tension may be a protective body reaction, which is guarding an area of vulnerability. This is most often seen near the spine, where specific muscle tensions may be working to stabilise the vertebrae (and maybe the discs), perhaps to take over the work of stretched ligaments. So it's important that the practitioner feels his/her way, encouraging release in the areas where you are able to let go and respecting the tensions that won't let go).

There is another important thing to look for with manipulative therapists – that they do some preparatory work on the joint or soft tissue before performing a joint manipulation.

And it is also crucial that all practitioners are prepared to refer you to the appropriate medical specialist for X-rays, MRI scans, blood tests, etc. for investigations and advice which are outside of their area of expertise.

Part 1: The Shoulders and Back

The Shoulders and Upper Back

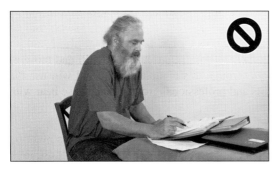

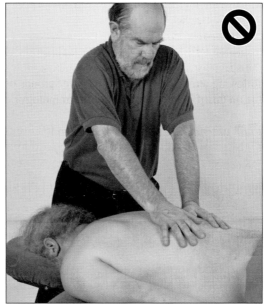

Figure 45.1: Shoulder tension;
a) tension (shoulders up 'around the ears'),
b) working hard with the shoulders.

Most massage practitioners, like most of our clients, carry the stresses of everyday life and how we deal with them (or don't cope) in our shoulders. In addition, we can get tight here:

- Through the constant physical activity of doing massages;
- From working too hard;
- From overusing the upper body and/or the hands (rather than involving the whole body), or;
- In reaction to strain in our hands, and;
- Due to poorly set up working environments.

The accumulated stress here can be painful, and can contribute to a vicious cycle of further winding us up. However, it can be released through massage and other treatments and via mobilising stretches.

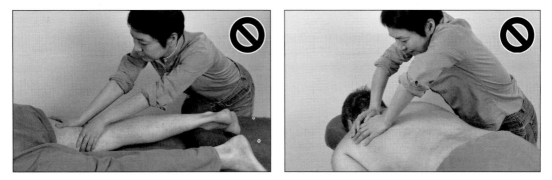

Figure 45.2: Upper back stiffness; a) consistently reaching forward, b) hunching over.

Upper back stiffness and pain is often related to shoulder tension. It generally arises from hunching over, often with the shoulders forward, both in the massage situation when we are focusing on the client on the table and in everyday life activities.

Maintenance of these areas includes getting regular massages, especially deep massage, and doing release and mobilising exercises.

Yoga and the Feldenkrais Method® offer useful exercises for the shoulders, and, along with the Alexander Technique, for the upper back. Not only will these approaches give you ways of releasing accumulated tension, with time and practice you can develop good self-monitoring and new postural habits (see previous chapter).

The Lower Back

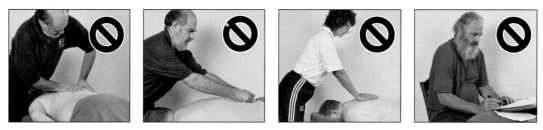

Figure 45.3: Lower back tension; a) working awkwardly, b) leaning over too far, c) only leaning with the upper body, d) hunching over a desk.

Muscle tension can arise over time from regular activities such as exercises or doing massage. Specific lower back tension can also come from:

• Hunching over or slouching;
• Standing with stiff legs and only leaning with the upper body;
• Trying to reach too far;
• Regularly working in awkward positions at the massage table;
• Working twisted (not having your hips aligned behind your hands), and;
• Regularly sitting hunched over at a desk;
• Weaknesses and/or old injuries can also contribute to these problems.

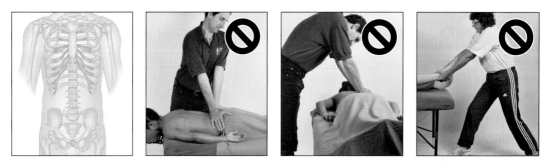

Figure 45.4: The tall, slender practitioner; a) the distance between the lowest ribs and the ilium, b) twisting, c) bending, d) hunching down.

As a broad generalisation, people with tall, slender builds are a little more vulnerable to lower back problems. The relatively long gap between the lower ribs and the top of the ilium at the back makes a bigger demand of the spinal muscles and the lumbar vertebrae in turning, bending, and reaching. Tall people also tend to hunch down more to fit into a world that's designed for shorter people (see figure 9.8).

Lower Back Stiffness
Lower back stiffness can be helped by:

- Massage;
- Mobilising treatments (from chiropractors, osteopaths, and physiotherapists), and;
- Self-help mobilising exercises (see figures 25.16–25.18).

Any exercise that involves *gentle* back mobilisation can be helpful, as long as you're not trying to force it or holding stressful positions for extended periods of time. Yoga, Feldenkrais, the Alexander Technique and Pilates all offer useful ways of learning to use your back differently through a combination of mobilising and strengthening. Experienced physiotherapists and personal trainers can also guide you in exercise programmes that will help you to develop this.

These treatments and self-maintenance exercises may provide some relief from back discomforts, making the worst conditions manageable or at least bearable for some people. For others, they may offer a way of maintaining their back if they are combined with changing postural habits at the massage table and in other activities, particularly desk work.

Back Pain

A large percentage of the population has some back pain at some stage of their lives, which can come and go for reasons that are not always clear. Most specialists would agree that the following factors can contribute to back problems:

- Poor sitting posture, especially for prolonged periods (e.g. hunching over a computer);
- Working in stooped or awkward positions;
- Poor work station ergonomics;
- Lifting awkwardly;
- Prolonged standing with stiff knees;
- Genetic factors, such as having different length legs or inherent weaknesses, or;
- Injuries.

Sometimes, there's no obvious cause for a back pain episode. Or sometimes a small movement, such as bending down to pick something up or reaching up to a high shelf, triggers a disproportionate response, for example shooting pains or even getting stuck in the position. In these instances, it seems safe to assume that an underlying weakness or accumulated problem have just been pushed that little bit further.

Some physical conditions (either cause or effect) are detectable by medical tests and some are not. Restrictions in the movements of ligaments and muscles can generally be ascertained by diagnostic tests done by relevant medical specialists. X-rays can show conditions of bones but not soft tissues. Most people over 60 would show some bone degeneration, but only a percentage will have pain. MRI scans can indicate disc problems too, although the scan may not show small disc protrusions. And here too, the direction of protrusion (whether it affects the spinal cord or nerves) will have different effects, ranging from none, to manageable effects with professional guidance, to major pain. Nerve impingement is indicated by sensations such as numbness, pins and needles and sharp aches, but this doesn't pinpoint the cause – whether it's due to:

- Damage within the spinal cord;
- Impingement as the nerve leaves the spinal cord (via a misaligned vertebra, or a bulging or prolapsed disc);
- Pressure from muscles on the nerve (e.g. tight shoulder muscles pressing on the brachial plexus, or the piriformis pressing on the sciatic nerve);
- Pressure on the blood supply to the nerve, or;
- Damage to the nerve along its length.

Muscle Strains

Back pain can arise from doing unfamiliar activities, which make unaccustomed demands on the back muscles, particularly if they involve awkward positions. This might be a single burst of activity, for example moving house, a long gardening session, or house maintenance or repairs. Increases in familiar activities, such as stepping up exercise or having a sudden increase in your massage workload, can also cause muscle tension and sometimes pain. Muscle pain due to unaccustomed activity generally goes away by itself after a time. It can often be helped along by massage and gentle exercises. Some people also find acupuncture / acupressure / shiatsu helpful in calming the tension / pain cycle.

Having treatments from manipulative therapists can also be of benefit (as long as it incorporates soft tissue work, see above). If spinal muscles tighten as a protective body reaction to pain or damage to ligaments, discs or the vertebrae (see below), massage, including deep tissue massage, *may* be able to provide regular short-term relief from the cycle of accumulating tension. Obviously it won't deal with the underlying causes.

Stretched Ligaments

Longer-term pains have less clear-cut causes and therefore treatments. There may be ligament overstretching, which can be due to poor sitting posture over a long period. Or it can be due to regularly twisting and bending into awkward positions, especially when you are lifting objects. These latter activities can leave a lasting legacy of weakness and a predisposition to problems and pain. The factory production lines that I worked on when I was young, which involved reaching and twisting to place and retrieve metal components and then stacking them behind me, did my back no favours. Nor did a stint of stacking beer barrels into restricted spaces in railway trucks. Similarly, a friend who spent his late teens and early adult years driving a tractor while constantly turned to look behind, has a permanent weakness in one side of his spine and has to always take care when turning to that side.

Sometimes there's a particular instance (or instances) of strain, such as an injury or an awkward movement, such as lifting a heavy object. These may tear ligaments as well as stretching them. If the ligaments no longer have the ability to maintain the integrity of the vertebral column so that there's a potential risk of damage to the spinal cord or the emerging spinal nerves, the body will take protective measures by tightening up spinal muscles to take over the job of the ligaments.

Many exercise systems can help you to regain back suppleness, and carefully applied massage can help the muscle tightness from becoming solidly locked-in. Pilates and similar ways of developing the 'core' muscles of the lower trunk provide the most effective method of strengthening and stabilising this area. This can reduce the regularity and severity of future problems (but not necessarily totally eliminate them).

Prolapsed Discs and Damaged Vertebrae

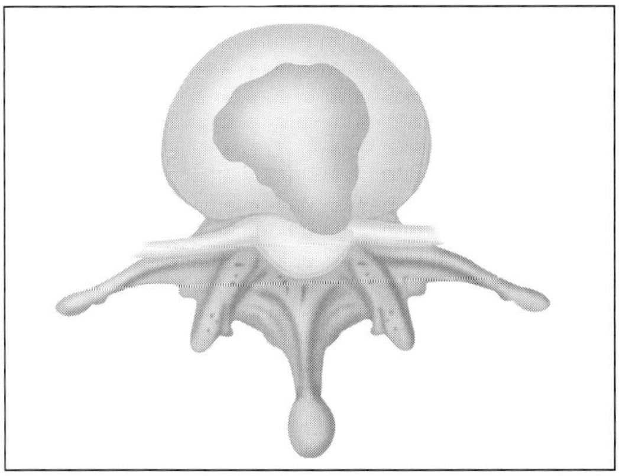

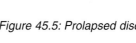

Figure 45.5: Prolapsed disc.

Strainful movements can also affect the intervertebral discs, stretching or tearing the disc wall, which, over time, may allow the central pulp (nucleus pulposus) or the outer wall of the disc to protrude. These protrusions may press on the spinal cord or the emerging nerves. This can cause anything from mild aches or discomfort to debilitating back pain, which can be intermittent or constant.

If X-rays / MRI scans reveal that vertebrae are damaged (for example, thinning or degenerating in parts), medical people usually advise you to:

*   Modify aspects of your lifestyle;
*   Avoid heavy lifting and bending activities, and;
*   Do an ergonomic evaluation of your home and working situation.

In these situations, it's good to do muscle strengthening exercises that will help stabilise your back (such as Pilates or yoga). It's also time to think seriously about:

*   Changing your treatment approach so that you don't have to work so hard;
*   Just doing nurturing massage (e.g. with babies or senior citizens);
*   Switching to teaching stretching / exercise classes, or;
*   Totally changing your career.

Part 2: Hand Problems

The Thumbs and Fingers

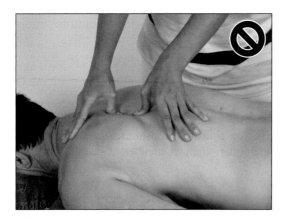

Figure 45.6: Straining the thumbs when applying pressure; the hyperextended thumb.

The thumbs are the most commonly strained part of the massage practitioner's body. The commonest cause is through having them consistently hyperextended when applying pressure (see figure 13.5). However, strain can arise just from using them too much to apply pressure. You are especially at risk of this if you have small thumbs, long, slender thumbs or if they are hypermobile.

It is important to take the pressure off them by using them less, supporting them with the other hand (for example, using the 'reinforced thumb' technique, see figure 13.15), and switching to using your knuckles, fist or elbow to save them entirely whenever you can.

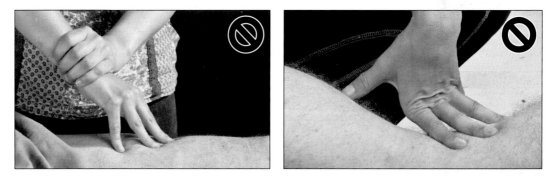

Figure 45.7: Straining the fingers when applying pressure; a) putting too much pressure through them, b) having them hyperextended.

Finger strains are a lot less common. However, putting too much pressure through them, particularly with them hyperextended, can strain them. People with slender and/or hypermobile fingers are most at risk of this.

Thumb Strain
Thumb strain generally develops as pain in the joints of the thumb (dull, aching or sharp). There can also be pain in the muscles – soreness in the thenar eminence (the muscles at the base of the thumb) and/or burning pain in the forearm (in the thumb muscles on the radial edge of the forearm). This can also lead to consequent tension in the arm and shoulders which sets up a vicious cycle of tensing up, which may lead into WRULD strain in the arm (see below).

Some of the hand mobilising exercises such as shaking out the hands (see figure 11.47) and closing and stretching the hands open (see figure 11.46), can release some of the accumulated tension. Make sure to do wrist mobilising exercises (see figure 11.50) to help stretch and release the thumb muscles in the forearm. Because thumb strain is likely to lead to a reflex tightening up in the shoulders, it is also important to do releasing exercises for them too (see figures 22.7–22.11). As with wrist strain (below), it is very useful to do self-massage of your forearm and wrist, especially if you've learnt to do it with your other forearm (see figures 11.44 & 11.45). Self-massage of your hand is also useful. Focus particularly on the thenar eminence.

It is also good to receive massages, especially from skilled deep massage practitioners. Ask the practitioner to focus on your forearms, wrists and hands, and to work thoroughly on your shoulders too. Manipulative therapy treatments can be helpful to relieve the common complications of shoulder and neck nerve impingement. Specialist therapists can give you guidance on using ice / heat / splinting procedures for the management of pain and to avoid further strain. A number of people also find acupuncture useful for relieving the tension / pain build-up cycle.

As well as looking after your thumbs in this way, it is important to deal with the causes of thumb problems. As mentioned above, conserve your thumbs when you're applying pressure by using the reinforced thumb technique. And save them, whenever you can by using your knuckles, fist, forearm or elbow.

The Wrist

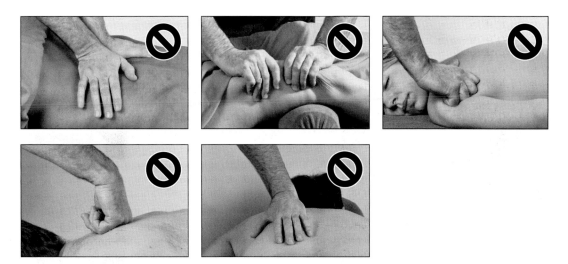

Figure 45.8: Working with the wrist bent; a) hyperextended when applying pressure,
b) squeezing muscles, c) knuckle kneading, d) fist pressure with the wrist flexed,
e) having the wrist bent to the side.

Wrist strain is probably the second most common massage strain. It is primarily the cumulative effect of applying pressure with the wrist hyperextended that causes problems in massage (see figures 17.4–17.9). Although having it flexed or bent to the side is less common, working with your wrist consistently in these positions can also cause problems (see figures 17.10 & 17.11). Having your wrist hyperextended in other activities (especially working at a computer keyboard, or activities such as driving) can also contribute or sometimes even be the main cause. If you spend time at the keyboard, be careful of ulnar deviation (having your hand bent outwards at the wrist), and, if necessary, look at ergonomic equipment (such as ergonomic keyboards and mouse and also wrist supports). You are more at risk of problems if you have a small or slender wrist.

Chapter 17 has information on keeping your wrist straight (but not rigid) in massage. And, of course, learning to use your forearm for massage takes the pressure off your wrist entirely (see Chapter 18). This can sometimes ease some of the strain through the incidental massage of your flexor muscles that this way of working offers.

Wrist Stiffness
Wrist mobilising exercises (see figure 17.2) can be useful preventative exercises, and can also release accumulated stiffness. Don't forget to do releasing exercises for the commonly related areas of tension – your hands (see figures 11.46–11.49) and your shoulders (see figures 22.7–22.11). Self-massage of your forearm, wrist, and hand (see figure 11.44) is also very useful, especially if you have learnt to do it with your other forearm. Supervised gym work and exercise routines can also be helpful in building up the strength of your wrists, especially if you have small or slender wrists.

It is good to receive massages too, especially from skilled deep massage practitioners. Get the practitioner to focus on your forearms, wrists and hands, and to work thoroughly on your shoulders too. Manipulative therapy treatments can be helpful to relieve the common complications of shoulder and neck nerve impingement. A number of people also find acupuncture useful for relieving the tension / pain build-up cycle.

Whilst massage and exercises are useful for looking after your wrists, they don't deal with the causes of wrist problems. So rest your wrists whenever you can, and look at the factors of poor wrist use and overuse in massage and in the rest of your life. Avoid working with your wrist bent in massage, and learn to use your forearm and elbow to save it. Watch out for having it bent for long periods in other activities, such as computer work (or play) and driving.

However, regular sharp wrist pain, or persistent pain when you're not working, especially at night, is an indication of more serious problems. Don't ignore these symptoms. These are common indicators on the road to developing WRULD (see below). So take heed of them. Look at the additional changes that you need to make in your work and the rest of your life to reduce the causes, and think about further treatments that may help you to deal with them.

Overuse Injuries

These are commonly called *Repetitive Strain Injury (RSI), Work-related Upper Limb Disorder (WRULD), Repetitive Stress Injury, Cumulative Trauma Disorder* or *Occupational Overuse Syndrome.* These terms are all hedged with medical contention and litigation issues, so none is universally accepted. For simplicity in this text, I will refer to this as WRULD.

These are all terms used for a range of problems affecting the muscles, tendons, joints, nerves, and vasculature (blood vessels) of the upper limbs. It generally occurs through prolonged and repetitive use of the hands in restricted and/or repetitive activities, often in awkward positions. The main contributing factor is the cumulative micro-traumas that affect tissues when they are subjected to repeated strain without sufficient recovery time.

Although, it was most associated in the past with production line workers (e.g. screwing lids on jars), the ubiquitous use of computers in recent years has brought the condition into the public eye. Therefore the focus of WRULD has mostly been on symptoms that develop in the wrist and hands, although these can have consequent effects in the other parts of the upper body, particularly the shoulder and neck, and sometimes also the arm and upper back. Massage practitioners can also strain their thumbs, which will produce a similar chain of events in these upper body areas. WRULD is also an occupational hazard for dentists, hairdressers, supermarket checkout workers, film / videotape editors, carpenters, plumbers, factory workers, and musicians.

The Symptoms
There are a range of symptoms that develop from wrist strain. If you regularly monitor your wrists, you will be able to adjust your massage techniques in response to small discomforts that you notice. (Bear in mind that strain doesn't usually develop evenly in both wrists. It generally develops much more in one wrist, although it can then develop in the second wrist if you begin to rely on that hand in order to save the strained one).

The pain and loss of function of full-blown WRULD in the wrist is quite unmistakeable. However, there is usually a long, slow build up that precedes this. DO NOT IGNORE THESE SYMPTOMS. Common signs to watch out for include:

- Soreness or pain – dull, aching, throbbing, sharp, sudden or stabbing;
- Tingling ('pins and needles'), numbness (loss of sensation), burning sensations, hands falling asleep, or tremors;
- Unusual stiffness in the hands, difficulty opening and closing the fingers or the whole hand;
- Clumsiness (in holding things, getting dressed, etc.), loss of control (dropping things), and difficulty in carrying things;
- Sudden or unfamiliar weakness, loss of endurance, heaviness in the arms;
- Cold hands (when they're usually warm), or your hands won't warm up;
- Night symptoms (waking with dull or shooting pain);
- Observable physical symptoms such as swelling in the wrists;
- Positive responses to diagnostic tests for carpal tunnel syndrome, etc. (done by a skilled sports medicine doctor or physiotherapist);
- Finding it uncomfortable to hold onto poles or straps on public transport;
- Guarding an affected area to avoid bumping it, or avoiding using it altogether.

Intermittent symptoms are an early warning. An increase in the severity or regularity of these symptoms, or the symptoms becoming persistent, indicates that the problem has developed further.

The Development of WRULD
In the first stage of problems developing, practitioners are only likely to notice discomfort in their wrists while they are actually working. Initially, these may be dull twinges or just a feeling that you are putting too much pressure through your wrist. If these small niggles are ignored, they are likely to develop into sharper pain when you are working.

If you continue to work in ways that put strain on your wrist, the next stage is aches or pain that persist when you are *not* working, initially intermittently and then more permanently. These can range from a sore or aching wrist to sharper, niggling pains or even throbbing pain. A further warning sign at this stage is sudden pain that comes on when you are relaxed, especially in the night. Waking at night on occasions with shooting pains in my wrists was the warning signal that drove me to research and develop 'hands-free' massage to save my hands and wrists – working extensively with my forearm and elbow (see Chapters 18 and 19).

After a while, if you keep working in the same way, persistent pain will often be aggravated in massage sessions, initially just by the type of massage strokes that sparked off the problems, then by other strokes that put pressure on your wrists, and later even by softer strokes. These pains will also start to flare up in other hand-intensive activities such as computer work and driving. If it gets worse, pain can even be set off by everyday activities such as cleaning one's teeth, turning keys, opening doors, cooking, washing the dishes, and, in extreme cases, dressing and feeding oneself. Ultimately, you can reach a stage where you are in pain, even when you are not using your hands. Obviously, this is quite debilitating and can be a very frightening experience.

Reaching this stage has put paid to the careers of a significant number of massage practitioners who hadn't received information about the likelihood of this happening, about how it develops, or how to monitor and avoid it. For many people this was the wake up call that spurred them into researching preventative / alternative ways of working and rehabilitation options (see, for example, the books of Laurianne Green and Gerry Pyves).

This all sounds quite alarming. *It is.* It is scary for the individual practitioner who is not only at risk of losing his/her livelihood but also of becoming debilitated in everyday life. It is also alarming for a profession whose aim is to *help others* to look after their bodies. It is an aspect of massage that needs to be highlighted much more than it currently is, because wrist problems are unfortunately prevalent in the profession, and they are largely *preventable* by using the guidelines in this book (especially in Chapter 17) and by learning the skilled use of the forearm and elbow.

Responding to Wrist Strain
Therefore, treat any discomforts or pains that you feel in your wrists as a warning sign. *Do not* continue doing strokes that strain your wrists. Work out how to vary the massage techniques that you use, so that the pressure is not constant and not always on the same part of your wrists. Include pulling, lifting, and stretching techniques, wherever possible, to lessen the compressive forces through your wrist. With many strokes, you can further reduce the pressure on your wrist by using your other hand to support and stabilise it (see figures 17.13–17.17). Get a skilled teacher or movement coach to watch you in action and give you suggestions.

Rest your hands and wrists whenever you can, for example when you're watching TV, at the cinema or sports / music events, travelling on public transport, etc.

Of course, if you are a massage practitioner and *also* doing other hand-intensive activities such as computer work (or games), gardening, DIY, craftwork or playing musical instruments, you need to be especially careful of your wrists in your massage sessions *and also* in these other activities. You may need to stop some of these activities for awhile.

As mentioned above, regular massage can help as a preventative measure. It can also provide some relief from the pain / tensing cycle if you already have problems. If you are receiving deep massage, get the practitioner to focus particularly on your shoulders, upper back, and the flexor and extensor muscles in your forearms. Regular self-massage of your forearm muscles can also be helpful (see figure 11.44).

However, it is vital that treatments and exercise are pain-free to be helpful. Once an area is sensitised to pain, it's easy to feed into the pain / tensing vicious cycle. Therefore, with any treatment (especially massage, mobilising and manipulations) and also self-massage and exercise, MONITOR DURING SESSIONS THAT THE TREATMENT IS NOT AGGRAVATING YOUR CONDITION. If it is, tell the therapist and get them to scale down the treatment or stop. This is also crucial in self-massage and exercise too.

Seek help from medical people too who can direct you to useful medical specialist and pain management help. Coordinated approaches over time with care and support from a range of avenues has helped many people to reverse the process.

If necessary, take some time off work to give your wrists recovery time, and then plan ways of changing how you work when you return to it. Don't return to the habits, techniques, and workload that you had before.

Managing Chronic WRULD

If you have persistent pain, especially if the pain persists when you're *not* working, seek specialist help. It needs clear assessment by a knowledgeable medical specialist, physiotherapist or specialist who is *experienced* in diagnosing and treating this sort of problem and is *sympathetic* to your experience.

You need to be sure that this person tests you thoroughly (or refers you to the appropriate specialist/s) to find out exactly what *your* specific problems are and therefore what *you* need to do, rather than treating you in a general way. Because this is a new (and still contentious) area of trauma, you may need to search around to find such a person.

There are no single or simple cure-alls for WRULD. Different people have different needs and different experiences of what most helps their WRULD. So the rest of this chapter covers a range of approaches, which some people have found of benefit in dealing with WRULD. You need to address *all* of the following areas:

- Taking time out for rest and recovery;
- Getting professional help;
- Making changes in your work situation;
- Reorganising other aspects of your life.

> The best book that I know of which addresses this area is *The Repetitive Strain Injury Recovery Book* by Deborah Quilter. Bear in mind that she comes from a computer background, which creates somewhat different problems than those which massage practitioners encounter. Computing, as well as putting strain on the wrists (especially if they are hyperextended) and the mouse finger, has other aspects which compound the wrist problems and which don't necessarily apply to massage practitioners – sitting still, often in a poor posture, sticking the head forward to look at the screen, holding the arms still and only moving the fingers. However, massage practitioners, while (hopefully) moving their arms and bodies more (especially if they've read this book), have the extra challenge of regularly applying pressure, which in turn puts compressive pressure through all of the joints of the hands, arms, and shoulders. Of course, if your massage problems are compounded by spending time on the computer, all of the information in Quilter's book will be particularly relevant.

Get Professional Help
This has four aspects: getting clear medical diagnosis and guidance, getting treatment to reduce pain and to stop or reverse the trauma, getting coaching to establish a self-help exercise programme, and getting support through the process.

Medical diagnosis and guidance: Find a medical person who is:

- *Experienced* in dealing with this type of problem for diagnosis of your individual problem;
- *Sympathetic* to your experience;
- Able to offer you appropriate *personalised guidance* on dealing with it, and;
- Willing to *be available* on your journey to adaptation and recovery.

Pain reduction: The second aspect is to find professionals who can offer you help to step out of the vicious cycle of tension and pain and consequent diminished functioning. Many people find acupuncture, hypnosis and/or training in relaxation procedures can help them to break out of the cycle of pain and tension. However, this doesn't deal with the causes, so it remains important to change the way that you work, and the way that you function and what you do in other parts of your life (below).

Gentle massage can be calming. A range of firmer massages, such as deep tissue massage, shiatsu, Thai massage and Hawaiian kahuna massage, can be helpful in relieving tensions, *provided that the practitioner adapts to the client's feedback*. So can manipulative therapy. Bear in mind that when there's strain in the wrists, there is always related tension in the shoulders, so these areas need thorough attention in such treatments.

Developing a self-help programme: It is important to develop a self-help programme for looking after and building up your body again. A well-rounded programme needs to includes exercises for:

- Developing *muscle strength* (without rigidity);
- *Flexibility* – to keep you supple;
- *Aerobic conditioning* to keep your heart healthy;
- Some *relaxation* procedures so that you're not just tightening muscles.

Get guidance and coaching from a personal trainer, sports trainer or physiotherapist with experience in the area. It is crucial that s/he develops a programme that fits your specific needs. Get them to adapt the programme according to your abilities and the ways that your body responds, and refuse to do things that aggravate your condition. Find another trainer if s/he won't listen to your particular concerns and needs.

Pace yourself. Don't overdo it, especially at the beginning, in your eagerness to regain control of your hands.

Getting support: Get support through the ups and downs of what can be a slow process of:

- Accepting and working with the situation;
- Changing or even relinquishing your work and perhaps other parts of your life;
- Adapting to the challenge to your self-image, and;
- Setting realistic goals whilst also maintaining optimism.

It is only recently that this problem has even begun to be acknowledged in massage circles as a potential occupational hazard. So in the past, people have often felt very isolated with WRULD problems and blamed themselves (for being careless, for not being strong enough). Even now, you may feel the need to hide your injury at work to protect your job, or because of possible taunts from co-workers, or because of the possible reactions of clients.

So it is important to find somewhere that you can express your feelings *safely*, to avoid isolation (in which the problem just magnifies), and to talk through your options and get support for your situation and how you're handling it. This could be with trusted friends or colleagues, in a supervision group, or with a professional massage teacher/supervisor or counsellor (see Chapter 42).

At the same time, you might want to call on friends, etc. to help you with the practical tasks of life, which might otherwise further strain your wrists, such as house repairs, maintenance tasks such as washing dishes or clothes, cleaning, driving, and carrying groceries.

Take Time Out for Rest and Recovery
It is important to make time for rest and recovery. This might include taking time off from work if you need a break from activities that aggravate your condition, and also reducing other hand-intensive activities. As mentioned above, get help with these tasks if you need to.

When you start doing self-maintenance / recovery exercises, pace yourself with them. Start doing them gently, and, if necessary, spread them out (perhaps initially just doing a few exercises every few days). As you build them up, cut back or have a break whenever you need to.

In the long term, also build rests into your day. Take at least a minute to switch off from your worries as much as you can and to relax your shoulders, arms, and hands.

Be careful if you are using painkillers to keep going. Because they mask pain, you may worsen problems without feeling it.

Make Changes in Your Work Situation

Look at your work situation to see the changes that you could reasonably make to reduce your present wrist problems and to reduce the development of further strain. Obviously, if you are self-employed, you have more control over your working conditions, the sort of treatments that you do and the range of clientele that you see.

Changing hand and body use: Thinking about how you use your body and hands, and how to look after them and conserve them is the focus of this book. So look back over Section 3 (see Chapters 11–17) for ideas on saving your hands by doing less kneading and squeezing, using your knuckles and fist instead of your fingers and thumbs, and learning to use your forearm and elbow more. Monitor what is comfortable and what isn't, reduce the stressful techniques and find substitutes for them.

Reorganising your work situation: Even if you are not self-employed, you may be able to reduce your working hours, either for a time or permanently. If you are able, you might break your workload up during the day, for example by having a few hours break in the middle of the day between your morning and afternoon work. When I had a severe bout of back pain (through pushing myself too hard and not doing regular back maintenance exercises), there was a month in which I had to take a half hour break between clients, so that I could lie down and do some stretches and regather my energy

Changing treatment sessions: If you are self-employed, it may be possible to gradually change how you work with clients, or at least the nature of treatments that you offer new clients. For example, you could incorporate more assisted stretches in your treatments (see Chapter 39) to get the client working more and reduce your own work. You could focus on myofascial release and reduce your deep tissue work. You could offer to coach clients in more self-maintenance procedures, such as relaxation or exercises routines.

Changing your clientele: You might consider changing your clientele, for example by referring on clients who want deep pressure work. You might focus on the nurturing side of massage, for example working in hospices, or doing baby massage (and teaching it to new mothers/parents).

Changing your career: However, these changes may not be enough, so you may be forced to look at changing your career. Many people view full-time general massage work in a sauna/spa/health resort as primarily a younger person's activity. Many of us who are still working in the field in our 40s and 50s have developed some specialist skills in our treatments, and/or combine part-time clinical work with teaching, administrating, promoting health products, exercise coaching, etc.

You might consider expanding 'sideways' into related fields, which build on your experience, as long as they don't involve long hours on the computer or hauling around equipment to the detriment of your wrists. Some possibilities might be light reception duties, promoting massage / healthy life products, or teaching non-strenuous exercises classes (for example for senior citizens). Teaching massage is a possible but trickier option – it can involve a lot of paper / computer work, students are wary of damaged role models (unless you can clearly present your problems as a productive warning), and teaching that is not consistently renewed and reshaped by regular clinical experience can become dry, idealised and ungrounded.

Some people work part-time at massage, balancing out the physical and mental demands by doing another very different professional (or voluntary) activity. The possibilities are as wide as your interests and imagination can make them.

Reorganise Other Parts of Your Life
Whichever of these changes that you make, it's good to also look at other parts of your life to see how you could support them.

Diet: Make sure you're getting a good balance of carbohydrates, fat (preferably from vegetable oils rather than meat), protein (but not too much), and drinking enough water. Although there are different views on their usefulness, many people are enthusiastic advocates of the 'joint food' capsules / powders that are now readily available. These contain the two major building blocks of cartilage – glucosamine and chrondoitin.

Sleep: Getting enough good sleep can be difficult if you are worried about your condition (or life in general). Many people find it helpful to do things that help them to wind-down before going to bed – learning relaxation processes, soaking in a hot bath, or receiving a soothing head, hand, or foot massage.

Leisure activities: In order to look after your wrists, you may need to cut down on hand-intensive leisure activities, and get help with household chores (such as shopping, cleaning, and washing) and with house maintenance and repairs. This can be frustrating, especially if you have to forego pleasurable activities that help you to relax, such as computer activities (playing games, sending e-mails, going on the internet, etc.), art or craft activities or playing musical instruments.

Exercise helps maintain circulation and energy. However, when you have weak or strained wrists, avoid those that pressure your hands – such as racquet, bat and ball sports, hitting martial arts (such as kung fu), and exercises such as push-ups.

Computer work: If you need to work on a computer, do it for short periods with breaks. One way of doing this is to have it set up so that you stand to work on it. This encourages you to step away and move around regularly.

Whether you are standing or sitting, try to have the screen and keyboard at heights that don't encourage you to slouch. If you are seated, have a seat that is horizontal or even tilts you forward slightly. When you are sitting, lean forward by rolling your hips, not by bending in your lower back (see figure 31.10).

Increase the font size that you use, so that you don't have to strain so much to see.

It can be helpful to have an expert conduct an ergonomic assessment of your computer home/work place set up. Simple changes can often make a big difference in your ease at the computer. (But bear in mind that hours of *constantly* sitting at a computer will take its toll on your body, no matter how good the setup).

Be aware that laptops are the worst culprits for computer-induced body strain. While they have the convenience of portability, their structure forces you into having either your hands or your eyes (or both) at the wrong height, and working in a cramped way. So try to reduce how much you use them, or at least how much unbroken time you spend on one. And try to get it off your lap. For example, whenever possible, lift the screen up and use a separate keyboard to minimise the effect on your posture.

Protecting your hands and shoulders in daily life: It is also worth looking at ways of protecting your hands and reducing shoulder tension in everyday life. Simple changes can include using:

- Soap dispensers;
- Headsets if you have long phone conversations;
- Travel luggage on wheels to avoid carrying it on your back;
- Shopping trolleys instead of carrying shopping by hand;
- Prepared food (good food) in easy-to-open containers to reduce cooking and washing;
- Clothing that is easy to put on and doesn't need ironing, and;
- Taking non-essentials out of your wallet / purse / waist pouch / day, pack, etc.

There are now many gadgets available that are designed to make it easier to open fliptop cans and jar lids. In fact, with the ageing population of most Western countries, there are a growing selection of aids that are designed for those with weak wrists and hands. Look at disability equipment catalogues, or, if possible, visit a store so that you can see them demonstrated to assess how specifically helpful they would be for you.

If your wrist condition is severe, you might also consider investing in labour-saving devices such as electric toothbrushes, electric can-openers, dishwashers, etc.

Review

Strains can arise over time from working too hard in massage sessions, or from the effects of other activities or of accidents or injuries.

Upper back strain can arise from;

- The stresses of everyday life and how we deal with them;
- The constant physical activity of doing massages;
- Working too hard;
- Overusing the upper body and/or the hands;
- In reaction to strain in our hands;
- Due to poorly set up working environments.

Maintenance of these areas includes:

- Getting regular massages, especially deep massage, and;
- Doing release and mobilising exercises.

Lower back tension can come from:

- Hunching over or slouching;
- Standing with stiff legs and only leaning with the upper body;
- Trying to reach too far;
- Regularly working in awkward positions at the massage table;
- Working twisted (not having your hips aligned behind your hands);
- Regularly sitting hunched over at a desk, and;
- Weaknesses and/or old injuries.

Lower back stiffness can often be helped by:

- Massage;
- Mobilising treatments and manipulations, and;
- Self-help mobilising exercises;
- Combined with changing postural habits at the massage table and in other activities.

A range of factors can contribute to general back problems, including:

- Poor sitting posture, especially for prolonged periods (e.g. hunching over a computer);
- Working in stooped or awkward positions;
- Poor work station ergonomics;
- Lifting awkwardly;
- Prolonged standing with stiff knees;
- Genetic factors, such as having different length legs or inherent weaknesses, or;
- Injuries.

Nerve impingement can be due to:

- Damage within the spinal cord;
- Impingement as the nerve leaves the spinal cord (via a misaligned vertebra, or a bulging or prolapsed disc);
- Pressure from tight muscles on nerves;
- Pressure on the blood supply to the nerve, or;
- Damage to the nerve along its length.

Muscles strains can arise from doing unfamiliar activities, or increases in familiar activities, such as a sudden increase in your massage workload.

Ligament overstretching can be due to;

- Poor sitting posture over a long period;
- Regularly twisting and bending into awkward positions, especially when you are lifting objects;
- Accidents or injuries.

Disc prolapses / protrusions can be due to:

- Regular strainful or awkward movements;
- Wear and tear on the spinal ligaments and/or the walls of the discs;
- If these protrusions press on the spinal cord or the emerging nerves they can cause nerve effects ranging from mild aches or debilitating back pain, which can be intermittent or constant.

Many exercise systems can help you to develop 'core' strength, and/or regain back suppleness; and carefully applied massage can help release muscle tightness.

You may also need to:

- Change your massage treatment approach so that you don't have to work so hard;
- Just do nurturing massage (e.g. with babies or senior citizens);
- Switch to teaching stretching / exercise classes, or;
- Totally change your career.

Thumb strain can develop as:

- Pain in the joints of the thumb (dull, aching or sharp);
- Soreness in the thenar eminence (the muscles at the base of the thumb);
- Burning pain in the forearm (in the thumb muscles on the radial edge of the forearm) – all of which may lead to arm and shoulder tension.

Take pressure off your thumbs and fingers by:

- Using them less, especially for strokes that involve pressure;
- Supporting them with your other hand;
- Using the reinforced thumb technique;
- Avoiding having them hyperextended when you are applying pressure.

Wrist pain can arise from the cumulative effects of applying pressure, especially with the wrist hyperextended, or bent forward or sideways. Look after your wrists by:

- Keeping your wrist straight and supporting it with your other hand, and;
- Learning to use your forearm and elbow;
- Doing wrist mobilising exercises, and wrist strengthening exercises (under supervision);
- Doing self-massage and receiving massages, manipulative treatments, and acupuncture.

Overuse syndromes can affect the upper body, especially the wrists. Common symptoms include:

- Soreness or pain – dull, aching, throbbing, sharp, sudden or stabbing;
- Tingling, numbness, burning sensations, hands falling asleep, or tremors;
- Unusual stiffness in the hands, difficulty opening and closing the fingers or the whole hand;
- Clumsiness, loss of control, and difficulty in carrying things;
- Sudden or unfamiliar weakness, loss of endurance, heaviness in the arms;
- Cold hands (when they're usually warm), or your hands won't warm up;
- Night symptoms (waking with dull or shooting pain);
- Observable physical symptoms such as swelling in the wrists;
- Finding it uncomfortable to hold onto poles or straps on public transport;
- Guarding an affected area to avoid bumping it, or avoiding using it altogether.

Intermittent symptoms are an early warning. An increase in the severity or regularity of these symptoms, or the symptoms becoming persistent, indicates that the problem has developed further.

Overuse strains develop through a series of stages, getting progressively worse if you continue to work in the same way:

- Beginning with dull twinges and niggles in the wrists only when the practitioner is working;
- Developing into sharper pain when you are working, and;
- Then aches or pain that persist when you are *not* working, initially intermittently and then more permanently;
- Then a sudden pain that comes on when you are relaxed, especially in the night, and;
- Then persistent pains that are aggravated in massage sessions (initially by the type of techniques that started the problem, and later by any strokes that put pressure on your wrists, and later even by soft strokes), and;
- Later as pain that flares up in other hand-intensive activities, and;
- If it gets worse, pain can be set off by everyday activities.

Therefore, if you feel wrist strains developing:

- Don't continue doing strokes that strain your wrists;
- Vary the massage techniques that you use;
- Increase the pulling and stretching techniques that you use;
- Use your other hand to support and stabilise your wrist;
- Learn to use your forearm and elbow;
- Rest your hands and wrists whenever you can;
- Have regular massages and manipulative treatments, (but don't have a treatment or level of pressure that aggravates your condition);
- Do self-massage of your hands and forearms and do exercises (as long as these don't aggravate the condition);
- Consult a doctor for referral to medical specialists.

You may also need to:

- Take time off work to give your wrists recovery time;
- Get professional help to get a clear diagnosis, help with pain reduction, develop a self-help programme, and get support;
- Make changes in your work situation, such as changing your hand and bodyuse, reorganising your working hours, changing the type of treatments that you do, and changing your clientele;
- Consider moving into other areas of massage such as teaching or administration, or;
- Doing other related activities that build on your experience such as teaching exercise classes, doing personal coaching or health promotion, or;
- Consider changing your career entirely, and;
- Also consider reorganising other parts of your life, such as reducing the amount of other hand-intensive activities that you do;
- Protect your hands in everyday activities, and;
- Get help with any chores, DIY, etc. that puts pressure on your wrists.

CHAPTER 46

Trouble Shooting

While massage practitioners can strain themselves through sudden, taxing efforts, such as picking up a client's leg which is unexpectedly heavy, the focus of this chapter (and the book) is on the gradual *accumulation* of strain over time that develops from poor working habits. It summarises the information contained in the previous sections of the book about the common causes of strain in each area of the body, and directs you to the relevant parts of the book for more detailed information.

Using This Chapter as a Reference
This chapter provides a reference for when you encounter problems. You might, for example, notice strains or soreness during and/or after doing a massage in areas of your body that weren't previously sore. You may notice particular aches after a busy massage day or soreness developing in certain areas over time, or that old injuries are flaring up. Or that aches or discomforts that you experience in other activities are being aggravated. You may find yourself waking at night with sudden shooting pains, for example in your wrist. Or you might just feel that you're tensing up and sense that aspects of your way of working could be building up towards future problems.

This chapter highlights the aspects of the practitioner's bodyuse that are *common* causes of particular problems and covers ways of addressing them. (While focusing on these specific elements, bear in mind that the overall ideal is to involve your whole body and attention in the massage 'dance' in an integrated way). While the book cannot deliver a *specific* prescription for any individual, this chapter points to possible causes of strain on each area to watch out for – both direct causes such as straining your wrists by having them bent when applying pressure, and also how the way that you use the rest of your body may contribute, such as tensing your shoulders which puts strain on your wrists.

This chapter also points out possible contributing factors to be aware of in the rest of your life, such as using your hands extensively for other activities. There is also a list of *some* exercises, which are useful in stopping the accumulation of tension and may reverse it. They will also help you to make adjustments in your postural and movement habits. Of course, this is just a few of the possible exercises to provide some examples – most sporting, fitness, aerobic, etc. systems have useful exercises to contribute. You can use them as part of regular warm-ups, exercises between clients or during winding-down at the end of the day (see Chapter 10), or when you need to focus on particular developing tensions or strains.

Look at the previous two chapters for ideas on exercise systems and individual treatment modalities that will help you develop and maintain strength, stamina, and suppleness in each area (see Chapter 44) and to help deal with problems (see Chapter 45).

Note: that the references in the tables are to the figure numbers (not the page).

Get Help From an Experienced Teacher / Colleague

As has been noted throughout this book, if you are unsure of what's being suggested or you run into difficulties, *enlist the help of an experienced teacher or colleague* who can provide you with coaching that is *tailored to your individual needs*. And consider finding a mentor/ supervisor or joining a supervision / support group to talk through problems and get support and helpful ideas

The Hands

Symptoms	Commonest causes	Other bodyuse factors that can contribute	Possible contributing life factors	Massage solutions	Helpful exercises
Tired, sore, aching hands.	Overusing the hands. Too much kneading or squeezing. Not supporting hand when applying pressure.	Tense shoulders and arms (22.6). Standing still and overusing upper body (2.10).	Too much desk work, e.g. computers, etc. Other hand intensive activities, e.g. DIY, hobbies, driving, etc. Small or slender hands.	Support your working hand & work double-handed (11.10–11.15). Involve your body = move with hands. Use forearm & elbow (chaps. 18 &19).	Shake out hands & arms (11.47). Wrist stretches (11.50). Guided gym work to build strength (incl. arms). Massage & self-massage.

The Fingers

Symptoms	Commonest causes	Other bodyuse factors that can contribute	Possible contributing life factors	Massage solutions	Helpful exercises
Stiff, sore, painful fingers.	Overuse. Too much pressure. Working unsupported. Working with stiff fingers (12.5). Having fingers hyperextended (12.6).	Tense shoulders and arms (22.6). Standing still and overusing upper body (2.10).	Digital machines. Computers.	Work with fingers straight / slightly flexed (12.7). Have fingers together, not spread for pressure (12.8). Support your fingers (12.9–12.15). Use larger parts of hands or forearm.	Squeeze and open fingers (11.46). Stretch fingers (11.48). Shake out hands (11.47). Fine-tuning finger movements (11.51–11.52).

The Thumbs

Symptoms	Possible causes	Other body/use factors that can contribute	Possible contributing life factors	Massage solutions	Helpful exercises
Sore, aching thumbs. Sharp pain at base of thumb.	Overusing the thumbs. Applying too much pressure through them. Having thumbs hyperextended (esp. applying pressure) (13.3–13.5). Using them unsupported.	Tense shoulders (22.6). Standing still and overusing upper body (2.10).	Digital technology. Texting. Musical instruments.	Support thumb with curled fingers & other hand (13.12–13.13). 'Reinforced thumb' (13.15). Switch to knuckles, fist or elbow.	Stretches, shake out hands (11.46–11.47). Massage & self-massage.

The 'Knuckles'

Symptoms	Possible causes	Other body/use factors that can contribute	Possible contributing life factors	Massage solutions	Helpful exercises
Sore, aching knuckles	Overusing them. Too much pressure. Proximal phalanges hyperextended. Using them clenched or unsupported.	Stiff shoulders (22.6). Wrist unsupported.	Arthritis.	Keep wrist straight (15.8 & 16.5). Use fist to save IP knuckles (ch.16). Switch to elbow.	Curl & uncurl fingers (11.46). Shake out hands (11.47).

The Wrists

Symptoms	Possible causes	Other bodyuse factors that can contribute	Possible contributing life factors	Massage solutions	Helpful exercises
Painful wrist, incl. when not working. Sharp shooting pain or pins & needles or numbness. Episodes of loss of control of hand (see Overuse Injuries in Chapter 45).	Working with it consistently hyperextended (17.4). Having it unsupported. Putting too much pressure through it.	Reaction to strain in fingers & thumb. Using hands stiffly. Body not behind hands.	Bent wrists at computer. Overusing hands in other activities, e.g. leisure, driving, DIY – esp. with wrists bent.	Only work with wrist at safe angle (17.8). Hold your wrist (17.13–17.14) or support from underneath (17.15–17.16). Wear wrist support (8.5). Learn to use elbow and forearm (chaps. 18 & 19).	Wrist stretches (11.50). Shake out hands & arms (11.47). Guided gym work to build wrist muscles.

The Arms

Symptoms	Possible causes	Other bodyuse factors that can contribute	Possible contributing life factors	Massage solutions	Helpful exercises
Aching, sore (feeling overused).	Trying too hard. Tense shoulders (22.6). Elbows bent wide when applying pressure (23.8). Body not behind arms (25.4 & 25.5). Using forearm too close to wrist (18.5).	Tense / trying too hard. Little / no previous exercise using arms. Standing too close to couch (2.11).	Building clientele quickly. Lots of driving.	Relax, esp. shoulders (22.7–22.11). Learn to use forearm well (ch. 18).	Guided gym work to build muscles.

The Shoulders

Symptoms	Possible causes	Other bodyuse factors that can contribute	Possible contributing life factors	Massage solutions	Helpful exercises
Stiff, sore, painful. Tense = up 'around ears'. Rounded shoulders.	Table too high (22.3). Standing still to massage (2.10). Unconscious postural habits of shoulders 'around ears' (22.2). Hunching over (22.4). Standing too close to couch (22.5). Body not behind hands (25.4–25.5). Not leaning trunk for power (25.12). Push/pull with shoulders not whole body (22.14–22.15). Breath held or inhale as press (26.3). Reaction to putting too much pressure through fingers or thumbs. Reaction to strain in hands or wrist. Over reliance on hands instead of using forearm and elbow.	Stress of workload. Demands of clients. Not bending your knees (28.4). Working too hard with hands.	Habitual tense shoulders (22.2). Hunching over writing table (22.2). Straining hands, wrist in other activities. Life stresses.	Lower table (22.3). Breathe out as press (26.3). Focus on relaxing shoulders (22.13). Involve body for pressure and movement, incl. bend & sway knees (28.5). Use forearm & elbow to save hands.	Shoulder circles; stretch arms back (22.7–22.12). Practise push/pull table with relaxed shoulders (22.14–22.15).

The Neck and Head

Symptoms	Possible causes	Other bodyuse factors that can contribute	Possible contributing life factors	Massage solutions	Helpful exercises
Stiff, sore neck.	Jaw tension (24.11). Hold head – neck tension. Standing too upright (22.4). Standing too close to couch (22.5). Look by dropping head only, not lean body (24.1).	Not moving body enough.	Eyes on computer; stress in life.	Regularly shut/defocus eyes (24.2). Bend with whole trunk to look (24.1). Relax jaw (24.12 & 24.13). Keep body moving.	Neck movements (24.8). Jaw release exercises (24.12). Self-massage (24.13).

Breathing

Symptoms	Possible causes	Other bodyuse factors that can contribute	Possible contributing life factors	Massage solutions	Helpful exercises
Held in breath.	Breathe in or hold breath when press (26.3). Unconscious habit of holding breath.	General tension. Trying too hard. Working too hard with rest of body.	General tension. Habit of trying too hard / pushing self.	Monitor breathing (ch. 26). Find breathing patterns with strokes (26.2). Breathe out when pushing / pressing (26.3). Bend knees to sway (28.5)	Breathing exercises, yoga, etc. Breathing exercises (26.6–26.10). Practice breathing in rhythm with movements (26.2).

The Upper Back

Symptoms	Possible causes	Other bodyuse factors that can contribute	Possible contributing life factors	Massage solutions	Helpful exercises
Stiff, sore midback.	Tense shoulder (22.6). Hunching over (22.4). Standing stiffly upright (25.1). Standing too close to couch (25.1). Holding breath (ch. 26). Stance too narrow (28.7). Stiff legs (28.4). Looking by just tilting head down (24.1). Not in 'chimp' stance for forearm & elbow work (18.24).	Standing too long in one position. Standing stiffly instead of swaying (28.4). Table too low (7.1).	Hunching over a desk = much of everyday life (esp. computers). Habitual posture. Stress in life, e.g. feeling weighed down, overloaded. Life stresses. Tall person fitting into a short world.	Bend knees to lean and sway forward (28.5). Lean with whole trunk (25.9). Reposition self to keep body behind hands (25.5–25.7). Widen stance & bend knees for forearm / elbow work (18.24). Eyes closed or defocused (24.2).	Trunk movements (esp. hyperextension & side-bend, (25.16–25.19)). Practice push / pull table without hunching over (22.14 & 22.15). Stretch arms up & back to open chest (22.7 & 22.8). Breathing exercises (26.6–26.10).

The Lower Back

Symptoms	Possible causes	Other bodyuse factors that can contribute	Possible contributing life factors	Massage solutions	Helpful exercises
Stiffness. Pain. Lumbar 'niggles'.	Trying too hard. Overusing arms = not involving legs. Crumple back = bend from lower back, not knees (28.4). Working twisted = hips not aligned with upper body (27.9–27.14). Standing with stiff legs (28.4). Too narrow or too wide a stance (28.7). Slouch when working seated (31.10). Kneel up on both knees instead of 'proposal' position (32.2). Trying to reach too far, esp. when applying pressure (25.3–25.4).	Table too low (7.1). Table too high (work on tiptoes too much) (28.13). Knee problems.	Hunching over a desk = much of everyday life (esp computers). Habitual posture (esp. slouch when seated). Tall person – fitting into a short world.	Involve legs = bend knees (28.5). Sway & lean forward to push/press, & sway back to pull (28.12). Lean with whole trunk = not hunching (25.14). Get table at right height for self (7.1). Move to avoid overreaching (25.2–25.3). Kneel in 'proposal' position (32.3).	Trunk suppleness (25.16–25.18). Postural development (Alexander Technique, Feldenkrais, yoga, etc.). Strengthen 'core' muscles (Pilates).

The Hips

Symptoms	Possible causes	Other bodyuse factors that can contribute	Possible contributing life factors	Massage solutions	Helpful exercises
Sacroiliac pain. Stiffness. Pain (sharp or aching) in hip joints / butts. Referred lumbar 'niggles'.	Standing with stiff legs = not swaying body with hands (28.4). Working twisted = hips not aligned with upper body or hands (27.9). Back foot turned away in lunge stance (28.20). Feet splayed out (28.21). Bent knee not above foot (28.26 & 28.27).	Bending in lower back instead of leaning whole trunk (25.12). Trying to reach too far (30.5–30.7).	History of S-I (sacroiliac) problems. Knee problems. Too much desk sitting = not used to using knees.	Sway forward and back with hands (29.17–29.19). Push and pull from legs (28.10–28.12). Reposition self to keep hips behind hands (27.9–27.11). Keep feet turned towards hips (28.23).	Mobilise hips (27.5). Strengthen core muscles (Pilates).

The Knees

Symptoms	Possible causes	Other bodyuse factors that can contribute	Possible contributing life factors	Massage solutions	Helpful exercises
Stiffness. Sharp, aching pain.	Working twisted (27.9–27.10). Stiff legs instead of swaying (28.4). Bent knees not over feet (28.26 & 28.27). Knees sagging inwards (28.40). Back foot turned away in lunge position (28.20–28.21). Too narrow a stance (28.7).	Stiff hips. Stiff ankles / feet.	Sedentary – not used to using legs. Previous knee problems / injuries.	Keep hips, knees & feet aligned with hands (28.3). Sway body (28.5). Wide enough stance (28.7). Keep bent knees over feet (28.6–28.7).	Hip & knee circles to mobilise (28.42–28.45). Strengthen legs (gym, sports, dance).

The Ankles

Symptoms	Possible causes	Other bodyuse factors that can contribute	Possible contributing life factors	Massage solutions	Helpful exercises
Stiff, sore ankle. Sore arch.	Stiff legs instead of swaying (28.4). Bent knees not over feet (28.26–28.27). Knees sagging inwards (28.40). Back foot turned away in lunge position (28.20–28.21). Too narrow a stance (28.7).	Flat (collapsed) arch. Stiff ankles. Stiff hips.	Sedentary – not used to using legs.	Sway body (28.5). Keep hips, knees & feet aligned (28.3). Keep knees over feet when bend (28.26–28.27). Stretch your calves as you work (by lowering heel to floor, 28.41).	Mobilise knees (28.44). Stretch calf muscles (28.41). Mobilise ankles (ankle circles, 28.45).

Bibliography

Alexander, F. M.: 1985. *The Use of the Self.* Victor Gollancz Ltd., London

Alon, R.: 1996. *Mindful Spontaneity: Lessons in the Feldenkrais Method.* North Atlantic Books, Berkeley, California

Anderson, B.: 1980. *Stretching.* Pelham Books, London

Andrade, C.-K., and Clifford, P.: 2001. *Outcome-based Massage.* Lippincott, Williams and Wilkins, Philadelphia

Bertherat, Thérèse and Bernstein, C.: 1976. (English translation, 1977) *The Body Has Its Reasons: Anti-exercises and Self-awareness.* Avon Books (1979), New York

Butler, S. J., 1996. *Conquering Carpal Tunnel Syndrome.* New Harbinger Publications, Oakland, California

Cash, M.: 1996. *Sport and Remedial Massage Therapy.* Ebury Press, London

Cassar, M.-P.: 1999. *Handbook of Massage Therapy.* Butterworth-Heinemann, Oxford

Clay, J. H., and Pounds, D. M.: 2003. *Basic Clinical Massage Therapy: Integrating Anatomy and Treatment.* Lippincott, Williams and Wilkins, Philadelphia

Downing, G.: 1974. *Massage and Meditation.* Random House Inc., New York

Fagg, A. and Pritchard, D.: 1999. *Dynamic Body Use in Massage.* (40), *Positive Health Magazine*, Bristol

Feldenkrais, M.: 1952. *Higher Judo: Ground Work.* F. Warne & Co. Ltd., London

Feldenkrais, M.: 1972. *Awareness Through Movement: Health Exercises for Personal Growth.* Harper & Row, New York

Fox, S. and Pritchard, D.: 2001. *Anatomy, Physiology and Pathology for the Massage Therapist.* Corpus Publishing, Lydney

Frye, B.: 2000. *Body Mechanics for the Manual Therapist.* Fryetag Publishing, Standwood, WA

Gerzabek, U.: 1999. *The Power of Breathing.* Marshall Publishing, London

Greene, L.: 1995. *Save Your Hands!* Infinity Press, Seattle, WA

Harris, J., and Kenyon, F.: 2002. *Fix Pain: Bodywork Protocols for Myofascial Pain Syndromes.* Press4Health Press, Santa Barbara, CA

Hessel, S.: 1978. *The Articulate Body.* St. Martin's Press, New York

Huang, Al Chung-liang: 1973. *Embrace Tiger, Return to Mountain: the Essence of Tai Chi.* Real People Press, Moab, Utah

Juhan, D.: 1998. *Job's Body: a Handbook for Bodywork.* Station Hill Press, Barrytown, NY

Kauz, H.: 1974. *Tai Chi Handbook: Exercise, Meditation and Self-defence.* Doubleday & Co., New York

Kravette, S.: 1979. *Complete Relaxation.* Para Research, Rockport, Massachusetts

Lidell, L.: 1984. *The Book of Massage.* Gaia Books, London

Lidell, L. (ed.): 1987. *The Sensual Body.* Gaia Books, London

Lordi, J. M.: 1998. *Tai Chi Massage.* June Lordi Publications, Maine

McAtee, R. E., and Charland, J.: 1999. *Facilitated Stretching.* Human Kinetics, Champaign, Ilinois

Napier, J.: 1980. *Hands.* George Allen and Unwin Ltd., London

Olsen, A.: 1991. *Body Stories: a Guide to Experiential Anatomy.* Station Hill Press, Barrytown, New York

Osborne-Sheets, C.: 1990. *Deep Tissue Sculpting.* Body Therapy Associates, Poway, California

Petrasz, Vèronique: 1973. *New Outlook on Yoga.* Sharp-Petrasz Ltd., Halifax

Pyves, G.: 2000. *The Principles and Practice of No-hands Massage.* Shi'Zen Publications, Huddersfield

Pritchard, D.: 2001. *RhythmMobility®.* (63) *Positive Health Magazine*, Bristol

Pritchard, D.: 2002/2003, 2006/2008. *Dynamic Bodyuse for Massage* (series). *Massage World Magazine*, London

Pritchard, D.: 2003/2004. *Dynamic Bodyuse for Massage* (series). *Massage Australia Magazine*, Sydney

Qilter, D.: 1998. *The Repetitive Strain Injury Recovery Book.* Walker Publishing Company, New York

Salvo, S.: 1999. *Massage Therapy: Principles and Practice.* W.B. Saunders Co., Philadelphia

Sharma, Pandit Shiv: 1971. *Yoga Against Spinal Pain.* George G. Harrap & Co. Ltd., London

Stephens, R. R.: 2006. *Therapeutic Chair Massage.* Lippincott, Williams and Wilkins, Philadelphia

Tappan, F. M.: 1980. *Healing Massage Techniques – a Study of Eastern and Western Techniques.* Reston Publishing Company, Reston, Virginia

Trew, M., and Everett, T. (eds.): 1997. *Human Movement: an Introductory Text, third edition.* Churchill Livingstone, New York

Walker, B.: 2007. *The Anatomy of Stretching.* Lotus Publishing/North Atlantic Books, Chichester/Berkeley

Williams, P. L. (ed.): 1995. *Gray's Anatomy, thirty-eighth edition.* Churchill Livingston, Edinburgh

Wilson, F. R.: 1998. *The Hand: How Its Use Shapes the Brain, Language and Human Culture.* Pantheon Books, New York

Biography

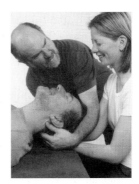

Darien Pritchard has been a bodyworker for three decades, including twenty-five years delivering professional massage training. Having back problems in his teens was Darien's initial motivation for entering the field of bodywork and studying physically based disciplines that aim at personal development. He has taught regular classes in the Feldenkrais Method® of movement awareness since qualifying (California, 1987) and holds a Certificate in Education (University of Wales College Newport, UK, 1998).

Darien is a co-director of the Massage Training Institute (MTI), a UK-wide organisation of holistic massage schools, and served on the inaugural committee of the General Council for Massage Therapy (UK), to which MTI is affiliated. He established and ran the Massage Study Centre in South Australia (1981–89) and the Cardiff School of Massage in South Wales, UK (1991–2002). He teaches bodywork modules in a degree course in Complementary Therapies at the University of Wales Institute, Cardiff, and is a guest teacher on training programmes for blind and visually impaired massage practitioners in Britain and Scandinavia.

For two decades Darien has run training programmes for massage teachers, and professional development courses for massage practitioners. These include *Working Easier – Working Stronger* (Dynamic Bodyuse for Massage), *'Hands-free' Massage* (using the forearm and elbow to save the practitioner's hands), *RhythmMobility*® (rhythmical rocking and vibratory techniques for release and energising), *Subtle Stretch* (gentle release and mobilising techniques), *The Art of Touching* (using touch skilfully in massage), *Creativity in Massage* (getting out of a rut), *Seated Massage* (western massage for the seated client), *The SuppleSpine Programme* for back care, and a series on *Releasing the Neck, Freeing the Shoulders,* and *Releasing the Lower Back and Hips.*

In addition to writing articles on massage for alternative health publications and a series on *Dynamic Bodyuse for Massage Practitioners* for *Massage World* magazine (UK) and *Massage Australia* magazine, Darien has written massage training manuals, contributed to handbooks for massage tutors and been involved in syllabus development. With Su Fox, he co-authored *Anatomy, Physiology and Pathology for Massage* (Corpus Publications, UK, 2001) which is designed for students and practitioners in the early years of practice. He is currently planning training DVDs and teaching aids on the material covered in this book and other aspects of massage and anatomy.

Alongside his professional life, Darien has nurtured his interest in movement, rhythm and release through dancing and playing music. He has worked with dancers on greater ease and flexibility in performance, run courses on *'Dancing for the Joy of It'* (helping people to discover the 'dancer within'), and designed a programme for actors on the physical embodiment of character (*'I Feel a Character Coming On'*). For two decades he has also taught the body release sections of the training courses run by the singer Frankie Armstrong for people wishing to learn the Natural Voice / Voice Liberation approach that she pioneered in Europe and Australia.

Index

11/2